Acta Neurochirurgica Supplement 131

Series Editor
Hans-Jakob Steiger
Department of Neurosurgery
Heinrich Heine University
Düsseldorf, Germany

ACTA NEUROCHIRURGICA's Supplement Volumes provide a unique opportunity to publish the content of special meetings in the form of a Proceedings Volume. Proceedings of international meetings concerning a special topic of interest to a large group of the neuroscience community are suitable for publication in ACTA NEUROCHIRURGICA. Links to ACTA NEUROCHIRURGICA's distribution network guarantee wide dissemination at a comparably low cost. The individual volumes should comprise between 120 and max. 250 printed pages, corresponding to 20-50 papers. It is recommended that you get in contact with us as early as possible during the preparatory stage of a meeting. Please supply a preliminary program for the planned meeting. The papers of the volumes represent original publications. They pass a peer review process and are listed in PubMed and other scientific databases. Publication can be effected within 6 months. Hans-Jakob Steiger is the Editor of ACTA NEUROCHIRURGICA's Supplement Volumes. Springer Verlag International is responsible for the technical aspects and calculation of the costs. If you decide to publish your proceedings in the Supplements of ACTA NEUROCHIRURGICA, you can expect the following: • An editing process with editors both from the neurosurgical community and professional language editing. After your book is accepted, you will be assigned a developmental editor who will work with you as well as with the entire editing group to bring your book to the highest quality possible. • Effective text and illustration layout for your book. • Worldwide distribution through Springer-Verlag International's distribution channels.

More information about this series at http://www.springer.com/series/4

Bart Depreitere • Geert Meyfroidt
Fabian Güiza
Editors

Intracranial Pressure and Neuromonitoring XVII

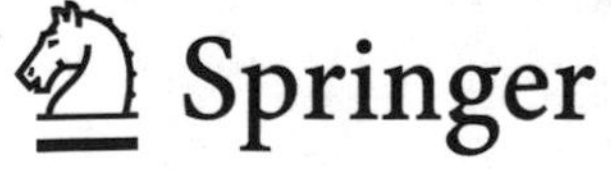

Editors
Bart Depreitere
Department of Neurosurgery
University Hospitals Leuven
Leuven
Belgium

Geert Meyfroidt
Department of Intensive Care Medicine
University Hospitals Leuven
Leuven
Belgium

Fabian Güiza
Department of Intensive Care Medicine
University Hospitals Leuven
Leuven
Belgium

ISSN 0065-1419 ISSN 2197-8395 (electronic)
Acta Neurochirurgica Supplement
ISBN 978-3-030-59438-1 ISBN 978-3-030-59436-7 (eBook)
https://doi.org/10.1007/978-3-030-59436-7

This Springer imprint is published by the registered company Springer Nature Switzerland AG
The registered company address is: Gewerbestrasse 11, 6330 Cham, Switzerland

Preface (17th International Conference on Intracranial Pressure and Neuromonitoring)

Since its first edition in 1972, the International Symposium on Intracranial Pressure and Neuromonitoring (also called the ICP Conference) has been an excellent high level and multidisciplinary forum for the exchange of ideas and results on clinical management and research associated with the monitoring of intracranial pressure, cerebrovascular autoregulation, and additional physiological and metabolic signals of the brain relevant to conditions as traumatic brain injury, subarachnoid hemorrhage, stroke, spinal cord injury, hydrocephalus, and cerebrovascular fluid disorders. What initially started with the investigation of the information concealed within the ICP signal and the association with clinical variables, has expanded over the past decades to include advanced imaging methods, metabolic monitoring, and sophisticated mathematical modeling. One of the great strengths of the ICP Conference has always been that it brings together all the disciplines involved and facilitates direct communication between neuroscientists, engineers, computer scientists, mathematicians, and clinicians from a variety of backgrounds. In all of the fascinating developments that were subjects of the ICP Conferences, the dedication to those who suffer devastating acute brain and spinal cord injuries and cerebrospinal fluid disorders has always remained central.

The 17th ICP Conference was held in Leuven, Belgium from September 8 through 11 2019 and we were proud to host it. The Conference welcomed 360 delegates from all over the world. It featured 202 contributed presentations and attained a high level of interaction and discussion. In addition, it hosted four satellite events, amongst which a data challenge, ICM+ users group meeting, annual meeting of the Brain-IT group and the 9th annual meeting of CARNet. A cross-section of the research presented in Leuven is included in this Proceedings volume. The 70 papers that were selected for this volume give an accurate insight into current thought and direction in the research on brain monitoring. We are happy to present them and are confident that these contributions will inspire future work and ideas. Therefore, we are already looking forward to the 18th edition of the ICP Conference, that will take place in Cape Town, South Africa in 2022, at which the 50th anniversary of the ICP Conference will be celebrated.

The editors wish to thank the ICP2019 Scientific Committee, the International Advisory Committee and Mrs. Marie-Laure Bettens and Ann Moerenhout for their enormous administrative support.

Leuven, Belgium

Bart Depreitere
Geert Meyfroidt
Fabian Güiza

Contents

Part I

Neuromonitoring and Management in Adult Traumatic Brain Injury

Microcirculatory Biomarkers of Secondary Cerebral Ischemia in Traumatic Brain Injury

Alex Trofimov, Antony Dubrovin, Dmitry Martynov, Darya Agarkova, Ksenia Trofimova, Ann Zorkova, and Denis E. Bragin

Introduction

Secondary cerebral ischemia (SCI) is still one of the leading causes of mortality and disability in patients who have experienced a traumatic brain injury (TBI) [1]; however, changes in microcirculation parameters that occur with posttraumatic SCI still remain underinvestigated [2]. The purpose of this work was to study changes in cerebral microcirculation parameters in the development of SCI.

Materials and Methods

This retrospective, observational, nonrandomized, single-center study was conducted as an analysis of a prospectively maintained database cohort (2013–2018) and included patients with a head injury and unilateral foci of posttraumatic ischemia. The protocol of the study was reviewed and approved by the institutional ethics committee, and conformed to the standards of the Declaration of Helsinki. Neuromonitoring parameters were measured as part of standard patient care, and the data were archived in a physiological monitoring database. Age, sex, injury severity, and clinical condition data were recorded in this database at the time of monitoring. The study inclusion criteria were as follows: moderate or severe TBI within 6 h after head injury, with a Glasgow Coma Scale (GCS) score $\leq$ 12, and unilateral foci of posttraumatic ischemia on perfusion computed tomography (PCT). We excluded patients who were younger than 16 years or had an Injury Severity Score (ISS) greater than 60. All patients were subjected to multiphase PCT using a 64-slice Philips Ingenuity CT tomograph (Philips Medical Systems, Cleveland, OH, USA). PCT was performed 1–4 days after TBI (mean 3.3 ± 0.5 days). The perfusion examination report included initial contrast-free CT of the brain. Further extended scanning with a contrast agent was performed within 60 s, focusing on 16 areas of interest, 160 mm in thickness. The scanning parameters were 160 kVp, 160 mA, 70 mAs, 512 × 512. The contrast agent Ultravist 370 (Schering, Berlin, Germany) was administered, using a syringe injector (Medrad Stellant, Bayer HealthCare, Whippany, NJ, USA), into a peripheral vein through a standard 20 G catheter at a rate of 4–5 mL/s in a dose of 30–50 mL per examination. After the scanning, the data were transferred to a KIR picture-archiving and communication system (PACS) (JSC, Kazan, Russia) and a Philips Extended Brilliance Workspace workstation (Philips HealthCare, Amsterdam, the Netherlands) with MATLAB 2013b (The MathWorks, Natick, MA, USA). Artery and vein marks were automatically recorded, followed by manual control of indices in the time–concentration diagram. The region of interest was established on the basis of subcortical areas of the middle cerebral artery (MCA). Errors introduced by delay and dispersion of the contrast bolus before arrival in the cerebral circulation were corrected by use of a block-circulant deconvolution algorithm. Quantitative perfusion indices, including cerebral blood flow (CBF), were calculated on a voxel-wise basis and were used to generate color-coded maps. Voxels with CBF >100 mL/100 g/min or cerebral blood volume (CBV) >8 mL/100 g were assumed to contain vessels and removed from the perfusion map [3]. Core infarction on PCT was defined as CBV <2.0 mL/100 g or a relative decrease in CBF >38% in comparison with the contralateral hemisphere [4]. Immediately after PCT, Doppler ultrasound of the MCA was recorded bilaterally with 2 MHz probes (Sonomed 300 M, Spektromed, Moscow, Russia). A Centaurus 2.0 neuromonitor (Privolzhsky State Medical University, Nizhny Novgorod, Russia) was used to monitor the cerebral complex during the

A. Trofimov (✉) · A. Dubrovin · D. Martynov · D. Agarkova
K. Trofimova · A. Zorkova
Department of Neurosurgery, Privolzhsky Research Medical University, Nizhniy Novgorod, Russia

D. E. Bragin
Lovelace Biomedical Research Institute, Albuquerque, NM, USA

Department of Neurosurgery, University of New Mexico School of Medicine, Albuquerque, NM, USA

B. Depreitere et al. (eds.), *Intracranial Pressure and Neuromonitoring XVII*, Acta Neurochirurgica Supplement 131,
https://doi.org/10.1007/978-3-030-59436-7_1, © Springer Nature Switzerland AG 2021

study. Arterial blood pressure and its amplitude (MAP_{amp}) were measured noninvasively using a Cardex MAP-03 monitor (Cardex, Nizhny Novgorod, Russia). The cerebrovascular resistance (CVR), cerebral arterial compliance (CAC), cerebrovascular time constant (CTC), and critical closing pressure (CCP) were measured using a complex neuromonitoring, as described previously [5, 6].

Statistical Analysis

To determine whether the data were normally distributed, a Shapiro–Wilk test was used. The data were expressed as mean ± standard deviation. A statistical analysis of all results was performed using a paired Student's *t* test. To specify the structure of the relationship of the variables, factor analysis was performed. We used a two-factor model with a raw varimax rotation. *P* values <0.05 were considered statistically significant.

Results

The patients' sex distribution had a male predominance (15 women, 187 men). The mean age was 54.7 ± 15.6 (range 17–87) years. The mean level of wakefulness, according to the GCS score, was 9.1 ± 0.5 (range 5–12). The distribution of TBI patients according to the Marshall Classification is shown in Table 1. Analysis of the studied parameters (Table 2) showed that in all patients with TBI, the mean CVR values were significantly higher than normal reference values ($P < 0.05$) and there was a significant difference in the CVR between the SCI zone and the opposite locus of the contralateral hemisphere (4.06 ± 2.16 vs. 2.7 ± 1.1 mmHg × 100 g × min/mL, $p = 0.0009$). In all patients with TBI, the mean CAC values were significantly lower than normal reference values ($P < 0.05$) and the CAC was significantly lower in the hemisphere with SCI than in the opposite hemisphere without SCI (0.026 ± 0.017 vs. 0.049 ± 0.035 mL/mmHg, $p = 0.017$). The mean CTC, as a product of the CAC and CVR in both hemispheres in patients with SCI, appeared to be significantly shorter than the mean normal value ($p < 0.05$). We also saw a small but significant decrease in the CTC between the hemispheres with and without SCI (0.10 ± 0.07 vs. 0.08 ± 0.08 s, $p = 0.015$). Analysis of the studied parameters showed that the mean CCP values appeared to be significantly higher than the mean normal value ($p < 0.01$). There was a significant difference in the CCP between the hemisphere with SCI development and the hemisphere without SCI (46.88 ± 14.05 vs. 45.44 ± 10.73 mmHg, $p = 0.65$). In factor analysis of potential risk factors for SCI development, the CVR and CCP were significant risk factors for SCI ($P < 0.05$).

Table 1 Distribution of patients with traumatic brain injury according to the Marshall Classification

Classification			
Class	Definition	Number	Percentage
I	No visible intracranial pathology	0	0
II	Midline shift of 0–5 mm, basal cisterns remain visible, no high- or mixed-density lesions >25 cm^3	24	11.9
III	Swelling	28	12.7
IV	Shift	37	16.8
V	Evacuated mass lesion	113	51.4
VI	Nonevacuated mass lesion	0	0

Discussion

Microcirculatory disturbances remain the cornerstone of development of cerebral hypoperfusion and SCI in patients with TBI [7]. Evaluation of the pial bed status is necessary since it can serve as a predictor of SCI development. This study showed that with development of SCI in the acute period (on days 2–3) after craniocerebral injury, the CAC and CTC significantly decrease while the CCP and CVR significantly increase in comparison with normal reference values. In our opinion, there may be a few reasons for these CAC and CTC reductions and CCP and CVR augmentations, but all of them seem to be associated with brain edema. First, development of combined (vasogenic and cytotoxic) edema due to blood–brain barrier disruption and SCI development may lead to compression of the pial vessels [8]. CT signs of brain edema found in all 202 patients in our study indirectly confirmed this assumption. The second reason may be

Table 2 Acquired and analyzed data

	CVR (mmHg × 100 g × min/mL)	CAC (cm^3/mmHg)	CTC (s)	CCP (mmHg)
Hemisphere with SCI[a]	4.06 ± 2.16	0.026 ± 0.017	0.10 ± 0.07	46.88 ± 14.05
Hemisphere without SCI[a]	2.7 ± 1.1	0.049 ± 0.035	0.08 ± 0.08	45.44 ± 10.73
P value (for comparison between hemispheres)	0.0009[*]	0.017[*]	0.015[*]	0.65

CAC cerebral arterial compliance, *CCP* critical closing pressure, *CTC* cerebrovascular time constant, *CVR* cerebrovascular resistance, *SCI* secondary cerebral ischemia

[a]The data are expressed as mean ± standard deviation

[*]*P* values <0.05 are statistically significant

regional microvascular vasospasm due to increases in the concentrations of blood degradation products trapped in the subarachnoid spaces. This effect results from auto-oxidation of oxyhemoglobin to methemoglobin with the release of ferric" [i.e., Fe(III)]. Furthermore, it is supposed that superoxides change the NO concentration [9], which leads to development of microvascular vasospasm [10]. In our study, Doppler ultrasound revealed no signs of MCA vasospasm in patients suffering from TBI. However, this ultrasound method does not provide the possibility to evaluate microvascular spasm. The third cause of pial bed compression may be swelling of astrocyte endfeet directly adjacent to the capillary wall [11]. Such swelling evolving in the first hours after TBI may persist for a week thereafter [12]. Finally, compression of pial vessels both in brain injury and in vasospasm is associated with dysfunction of pericytes located in the basal pericapillary membrane. It has been shown that narrowing of arterioles and capillaries occurs because of disturbance in the expression of endothelin-1 and pericytial receptor types A and B, as well as migration of over 40% of pericytes from the basal membrane [13].

Our study had the following limitations. First, it was impossible to carry out dynamic assessment of microcirculatory parameters without repeated PCT. Second, we have to admit that we failed to completely eliminate a mathematical error associated with measurement of the "area of interest" space. Third, the obtained data incorporated therapeutic and surgical influences, which could not be removed. Fourth, the data artifacts were removed manually by two experts (AT and DM), and we could not exclude the possibility that some artifacts went unnoticed. Lastly, no corrections for multiple testing were performed.

Clearly, this new approach to the concept of microcirculatory biomarkers in TBI still needs to undergo more thorough scrutiny. Further studies need to be performed to confirm these findings and provide better insight into how to interpret data derived from patients with TBI [14].

Conclusion

In this study, changes in cerebral microcirculation parameters (the CVR, CAC, CTC, and CCP indices) in patients with traumatic intracranial hemorrhage were associated with progression of secondary ischemia ($P < 0.05$), suggesting they have promising potential for use as early biological markers of SCI development. Further studies are needed to confirm these findings.

Acknowledgments Alex Trofimov was supported by a grant-in-aid for exploratory research from the Privolzhsky Research Medical University. Denis Bragin was supported by National Institutes of Health grant number R01NS112808-01.

Conflict of Interest: **The authors declare that they have no conflict of interest.**

References

1. Walder B, Haller G, Rebetez M (2013) Severe traumatic brain injury in a high-income country: an epidemiological study. J Neurotrauma 30:1934–1942
2. Spaite D, Hu C, Bobrow B, Chikani V (2017) Association of out-of-hospital hypotension depth and duration with traumatic brain injury mortality. Ann Emerg Med 70:522–530
3. Miles K, Eastwood JD, Konig M (eds) (2007) Multidetector computed tomography in cerebrovascular disease: CT perfusion imaging. Informa, Abingdon
4. Donahue J, Wintermark M (2015) Perfusion CT and acute stroke imaging: foundations, applications, and literature review. J Neuroradiol 42(1):21–29
5. Sheludyakov A, Martynov D, Yuryev M (2020) The cerebrovascular time constant in patients with head injury and posttraumatic cerebral vasospasm. Acta Neurochir Suppl 127:191–194
6. Trofimov A, Kalentyev G, Voennov O (2018) The cerebrovascular resistance in combined traumatic brain injury with intracranial hematomas. Acta Neurochir Suppl 126:25–28
7. Rhodes JK, Chandrasekaran S, Andrews PJ (2016) Early changes in brain oxygen tension may predict outcome following severe traumatic brain injury. Acta Neurochir Suppl 122:9–16. https://doi.org/10.1007/978-3-319-22533-3_2
8. Marmarou A (2007) A review of progress in understanding the pathophysiology and treatment of brain edema. Neurosurg Focus 22(5):E1
9. Rey FE (2002) Perivascular superoxide anion contributes to impairment of endothelium-dependent relaxation: role of gp91(phox). Circulation 106(19):2497–2502
10. Ehlert A, Schmidt C, Wölfer J (2016) Molsidomine for the prevention of vasospasm-related delayed ischemic neurological deficits and delayed brain infarction and the improvement of clinical outcome after subarachnoid hemorrhage: a single-center clinical observational study. J Neurosurg 124(1):51–58. https://doi.org/10.3171/2014.12.JNS13846
11. Bullock R (1991) Glial swelling following human cerebral contusion: an ultrastructural study. J Neurol Neurosurg Psychiatry 54(5):427–434
12. Jha RM, Elmer J, Zusman BE (2018) Intracranial pressure trajectories: a novel approach to informing severe traumatic brain injury phenotypes. Crit Care Med 46(11):1792–1802. https://doi.org/10.1097/CCM.0000000000003361
13. Bhowmick S, D'Mello V, Caruso D et al (2019) Impairment of pericyte–endothelium cross-talk leads to blood–brain barrier dysfunction following traumatic brain injury. Exp Neurol 317:260–270. https://doi.org/10.1016/j.expneurol.2019.03.014
14. Carpenter K, Czosnyka M, Jalloh I (2015) Systemic, local, and imaging biomarkers of brain injury: more needed, and better use of those already established? Front Neurol 6:26

Visualization of Intracranial Pressure Insults After Severe Traumatic Brain Injury: Influence of Individualized Limits of Reactivity

Joseph Donnelly, Frederick A. Zeiler, Fabian Güiza, Erta Beqiri, Simon J. Mitchell, Marcel J. Aries, Marek Czosnyka, and Peter Smielewski

Introduction

Raised intracranial pressure (ICP) is an important secondary brain injury after traumatic brain injury (TBI), as it leads to hypoperfusion and, in some cases, brain herniation [1, 2]. Therefore, preventing elevated ICP is an important facet of modern neurocritical care. However, knowing what constitutes a prognostically important ICP insult is largely based on clinician experience. A method has recently been elucidated that allows for assessment of how the duration and magnitude of ICP insults relate to patient outcomes [3].

Individualized cerebral perfusion pressure (CPP) targets have been offered as an alternative to a 'one size fits all' approach [4]. In this method, the individualized lower limit of reactivity (LLR) can be calculated continuously to give an indication of whether a patient's CPP is above or below their LLR. Having a CPP below the LLR has been shown to relate to unfavourable outcomes and mortality even after adjustment for other important prognostic factors [5].

In this study we aimed to illustrate how having a CPP below the LLR affects how ICP insults relate to patient outcomes. We hypothesized that with a CPP below the LLR, even relatively mild ICP insults would be related to poor patient outcomes.

Materials and Methods

This study was conducted as a retrospective analysis of a prospectively maintained database cohort (treated between 1997 and 2017), in which high-frequency physiological monitoring data were archived. Monitoring of brain modalities was conducted as a part of standard patient care and archived in an anonymized database of physiological monitoring. Data on each patient's age, injury severity and clinical status were recorded at the time of monitoring of this database, and no attempt was made to re-access clinical records for additional information. Since all data were extracted from hospital records and fully anonymized, no data on patient identifiers were available; therefore, formal patient or proxy consent and institutional ethics approval were not required.

Participants

TBI patients with a clinical need for ICP monitoring and computerized signal recordings were included in the analysis. A total of 729 head-injured patients admitted to the Addenbrooke's Hospital Neurocritical Care Unit between 1997 and 2017 were included. The inclusion criteria were TBI, computerized invasive monitoring of ICP and arterial blood pressure (ABP) for

J. Donnelly (✉)
Academic Neurosurgery, University of Cambridge, Cambridge, UK

Department of Anaesthesiology, University of Auckland, Auckland, New Zealand
e-mail: joseph.donnelly@cantab.net

F. A. Zeiler
Section of Neurosurgery, Department of Surgery, Rady Faculty of Health Sciences, University of Manitoba, Winnipeg, MB, Canada

Division of Anaesthesia, University of Cambridge, Cambridge, UK

F. Güiza
Intensive Care Medicine, KU Leuven, Leuven, Belgium

E. Beqiri · M. Czosnyka · P. Smielewski
Academic Neurosurgery, University of Cambridge, Cambridge, UK

S. J. Mitchell
Department of Anaesthesiology, University of Auckland, Auckland, New Zealand

M. J. Aries
Department of Intensive Care, University of Maastricht, Maastricht, The Netherlands

B. Depreitere et al. (eds.), *Intracranial Pressure and Neuromonitoring XVII*, Acta Neurochirurgica Supplement 131,
https://doi.org/10.1007/978-3-030-59436-7_2,

at least 12 h, available admission Glasgow Coma Scale (GCS) and available 6-month mortality data. Patients were managed according to contemporaneous TBI guidelines.

All patients were sedated, intubated and ventilated. The stepwise ICP management included appropriate positioning and head elevation, prevention of hypotension and hypoxia, maintenance of end-tidal partial pressure of carbon dioxide (pCO_2) levels, sedation, muscle paralysis, ventriculostomy, osmotic agents, induced hypothermia, barbiturate coma and decompressive craniectomy. CPP was maintained at target levels using intravenous fluids, vasopressors and inotropes. Tight glucose management was achieved with an insulin sliding scale, with target blood glucose levels of 6–8 mmol/L (108–144 mg/dL). Seizure management was achieved using phenytoin and levetiracetam as appropriate. Each patient's initial GCS score was obtained prior to sedation. Patients without a point breakdown of their GCS were included in the analysis, as data on patients treated prior to the introduction of electronic medical records frequently included only the total GCS score. The Glasgow Outcome Scale (GOS) score was assessed at 6 months post-injury.

Data Acquisition

ICP was monitored with an intraparenchymal Codman ICP MicroSensor (Codman & Shurtleff, Raynham, MA, USA) inserted into the frontal cortex, and ABP was monitored in the radial or femoral artery using a standard pressure transducer (Baxter Healthcare, Deerfield, IL, USA) with a zero calibration at the level of the right atrium (in patients treated between 1997 and 2015) or at the foramen of Monro (in patients treated between 2015 and 2017). Between 1997 and 2002, data trends (1-min time averages) were collected with nonproprietary intensive care monitoring (ICM) software developed in-house and 1-min trends were stored. From 2002 to 2017, data were collected using ICM + ® software (Cambridge Enterprise, Cambridge, UK; http://www.neurosurg.cam.ac.uk/icmplus). The moving Pearson correlation coefficient (PRx) was calculated as the Pearson correlation of 30 consecutive 10-s average values of ABP and ICP. CPP was calculated as ABP minus ICP. A 10-s average was used to reduce the influence of respiratory and pulse waveforms. A 300-s moving window was used to generate continuous PRx values.

Lower Limit of Reactivity Calculation

CPP–PRx curve fitting was calculated as described previously [6]. Briefly, 5-min periods of the mean CPP values (updated every minute) were collected alongside 1-min mean values of PRx. These PRx values were then binned into 5-mmHg-wide CPP intervals. These data were plotted as an error bar chart with CPP on the x-axis and PRx on the y-axis. A second-order polynomial curve was fitted after 4 h of data collection with predefined heuristics. A moving window with 1-min updates was used to generate a trend in the CPP LLR. Instead of a single-calculation window (of 4 h) being used to produce the CPP LLR, multiple calculation windows were applied during a period of 2–8 h (in 10-min increments) to yield up to 36 estimations. The means of these estimates were calculated and updated every minute [7].

The defined CPP–PRx curve was extrapolated to both sides to include the full range of plausible CPP values (from 40 to 120 mmHg) to obtain the CPP values at which the curve crossed the threshold PRx value for impaired pressure reactivity (PRx = +0.30). The lower value of CPP at these two points of intersection was denoted as the CPP LLR.

ICP Visualization

Episodes of increased ICP were extracted from each patient's recording, as described previously [3]. For each episode, the average difference between the CPP and CPP LLR was also calculated. ICP hypertensive episodes were defined as being above a given intensity threshold I, for at least a given duration D. For each pair of intensity and duration thresholds $<I,D>$, the total number of corresponding episodes per patient was calculated separately in each 6-month GOS score group [2]. Thereafter, the Pearson correlation between the average number of ICP episodes and the GOS was calculated for each $<I,D>$ and colour coded according to a predefined colour map. The point of zero correlation was termed the transition curve and denoted in black. Colour maps were produced for ICP hypertensive episodes where the CPP was above or equal to the CPP LLR and for episodes where the CPP was below the CPP LLR.

Results

Demographic information regarding this cohort is available in a previous publication [5]. When the CPP was above or equal to the LLR, we found a curvilinear relationship whereby even prolonged durations of low-intensity ICP insults were not associated with poor outcomes but short durations of high-intensity insults were (Fig. 1, *left panel*). However, when only ICP insults with a CPP below the CPP LLR were considered, even much lower-intensity and shorter ICP insults were associated with poor patient outcomes (Fig. 1, *right panel*).

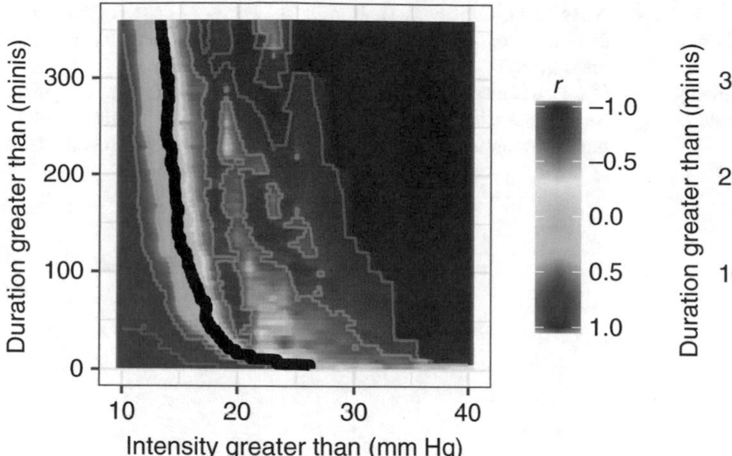

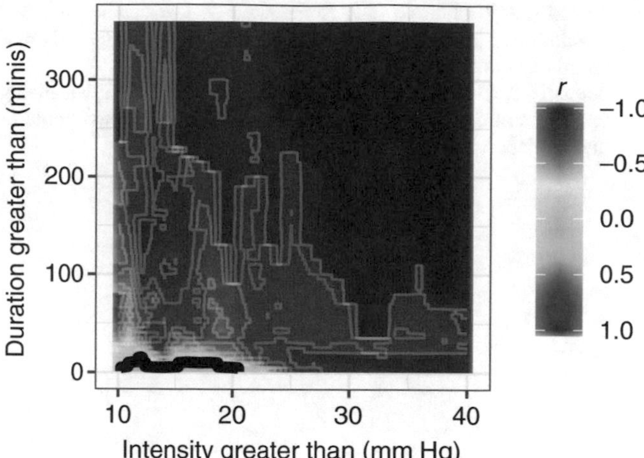

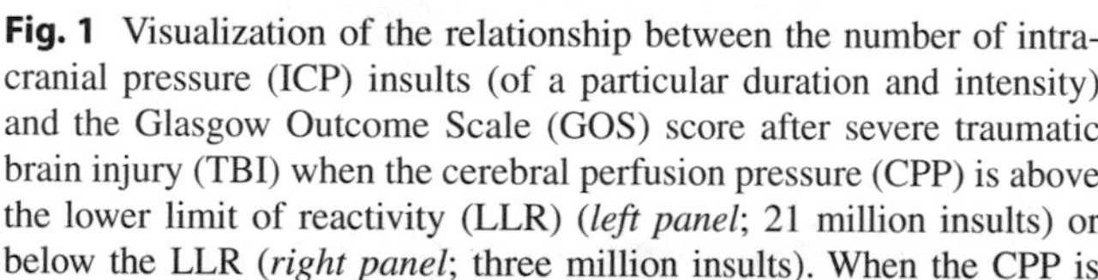

Fig. 1 Visualization of the relationship between the number of intracranial pressure (ICP) insults (of a particular duration and intensity) and the Glasgow Outcome Scale (GOS) score after severe traumatic brain injury (TBI) when the cerebral perfusion pressure (CPP) is above the lower limit of reactivity (LLR) (*left panel*; 21 million insults) or below the LLR (*right panel*; three million insults). When the CPP is above the LLR, a curvilinear transition zone is seen (shown in black in the *left panel*) whereby the longer the episode of raised ICP lasts, the lower the level of raised ICP that is associated with poor outcomes. In contrast, when the CPP is below the LLR during an insult, even low-intensity ICP insults are associated with a worse GOS score, denoted by the predominance of red in the *right panel*

Discussion

In this study we combined the concept of individualized CPP targets with an ICP insult visualization technique to show that when the CPP is below the LLR, the brain is vulnerable to even minor ICP insults. This is logical, given that both a low CPP and disturbed cerebral autoregulation have been shown in a separate data set to be associated with increased vulnerability to elevated ICP [3].

The ICP visualization technique highlights the fact that both the duration and the magnitude of ICP insults probably need to be considered during an assessment as to whether a patient's ICP warrants any treatment. For example, if a patient's ICP is 18 mmHg for 30 min and the CPP is above the LLR, aggressive ICP-lowering therapy may not be necessary, as this insult is associated with favourable outcomes (shown to the left of the black transition curve). However, if the episode lasts for 200 min, then perhaps more aggressive management could be warranted, as such an insult is associated with poor outcomes. This information could prove useful in the design of trials that assess the efficacy of ICP-lowering therapies.

Implementation of such colour-coded plots at the bedside is a possibility to assist in ICP interpretation. In this scenario, the characteristics (duration and magnitude) of a patient's current elevated ICP episode could be overlaid on the coloured contour map. Furthermore, with increasing size of the relevant data sets, detailed subgroup analyses may become possible, such as ICP insults amongst sex categories, age groups or imaging phenotypes.

This visualization technique could also be applied to other monitored signals that relate to secondary injury, such as the lactate-to-pyruvate ratio, brain tissue oxygenation or brain temperature. It is likely that the transition curves for other variables will be distinct from that of ICP, reflecting the different timescales of different forms of secondary injury. It is important to note that therapy for raised ICP is not always benign and therefore can contribute to poor patient outcomes in addition to the effects of ICP per se. In this way, harmful ICP-lowering therapies such as barbiturate coma or decompressive craniectomy could be contributing to the overall red colour profile that appears to the right of the transition zone on coloured contour maps. Unfortunately, data on patient therapies were not available in this cohort.

Conflict of Interest: **ICM+® software is licensed by Cambridge Enterprise Ltd. (Cambridge, UK) (https://icmplus.neurosurg.cam.ac.uk). Marek Czosnyka and Peter Smielewski have a financial interest in a fraction of the licensing fee.**

References

1. Donnelly J, Czosnyka M, Harland S, Varsos GV, Cardim D, Robba C, Liu X, Ainslie PN, Smielewski P (2017) Cerebral haemodynamics during experimental intracranial hypertension. J Cereb Blood Flow Metab 37(2):694–705
2. Donnelly J, Smielewski P, Adams H, Zeiler FA, Cardim D, Liu X, Fedriga M, Hutchinson P, Menon DK, Czosnyka M (2019) Observations on the cerebral effects of refractory intracranial hypertension after severe traumatic brain injury. Neurocrit Care 32:437–447. https://doi.org/10.1007/s12028-019-00748-x
3. Güiza F, Depreitere B, Piper I et al (2015) Visualizing the pressure and time burden of intracranial hypertension in adult and paediatric traumatic brain injury. Intensive Care Med 41(6):1067–1076. https://doi.org/10.1007/s00134-015-3806-1

4. Donnelly J, Budohoski KP, Smielewski P, Czosnyka M (2016) Regulation of the cerebral circulation: bedside assessment and clinical implications. Crit Care 20(1):129
5. Donnelly J, Czosnyka M, Adams H et al (2017) Individualising thresholds of cerebral perfusion pressure using estimated limits of autoregulation. Crit Care Med 45(9):1464
6. Aries MJH, Czosnyka M, Budohoski KP et al (2012) Continuous determination of optimal cerebral perfusion pressure in traumatic brain injury. Crit Care Med 40(8):2456–2463
7. Liu X, Maurits NM, Aries MJH et al (2017) Monitoring of optimal cerebral perfusion pressure in traumatic brain injured patients using a multi-window weighting algorithm. J Neurotrauma 34(22):3081–3088

Impacts of a Pressure Challenge on Cerebral Critical Closing Pressure and Effective Cerebral Perfusion Pressure in Patients with Traumatic Brain Injury

Leandro Moraes, Bernardo Yelicich, Mayda Noble, Alberto Biestro, and Corina Puppo

Introduction

Cerebral critical closing pressure (CrCP) is the arterial blood pressure (ABP) at which small cerebral vessels close and circulation stops [1–3]. It comprises intracranial pressure (ICP) and arteriolar wall tension (WT). It has been suggested that the "closing margin" [4, 5], or the "effective" cerebral perfusion pressure (CPPeff; calculated as ABP − CrCP) [12, 21], would estimate the real driving pressure gradient for cerebral perfusion and provide a more appropriate value of the real perfusion pressure than the "conventional" cerebral perfusion pressure (CPP; calculated as ABP − ICP). A schematic diagram showing the differences between the CPP and CPPeff concepts is shown in Fig. 1.

In this study, we wanted to investigate how an arterial blood increase would change CrCP and CPPeff in a cohort of patients with a traumatic brain injury (TBI), taking into account that it would probably elicit an autoregulatory response that would increase WT, decrease cerebral blood volume simultaneously, and therefore probably decrease ICP.

Patients and Methods

We retrospectively analyzed recordings of ABP, ICP, and cerebral blood flow velocity (FV), measured by transcranial Doppler ultrasound, from 11 patients (two women and nine men; median age 29 (interquartile range (IQR) 14) years) with a severe TBI and a median Glasgow Coma Scale (GCS) score of 6 (IQR 1) at admission, in whom a 20-mmHg increase in ABP was generated during a 30-min period after a 30-min basal recording as an initial part of a clinical trial studying changes in cerebral autoregulation after an infusion of tromethamine (a drug with buffer effects, which decreases intracranial hypertension). Data from the first part of this trial (obtained in the basal and hypertensive situations, without tromethamine) are presented in this chapter.

This single-center clinical trial was approved by the institutional ethics committee, and written informed consent was obtained from all participants' next of kin.

The 11 patients were admitted to our 15-bed adult general intensive care unit (ICU) at a tertiary university hospital between March 2005 and May 2007. Patients were included in the study if they were between 16 and 70 years old and had suffered a closed severe TBI with (1) a postresuscitation GCS score <9 at admission; or (2) a deterioration in the GCS score of two or more points, requiring mechanical ventilation; or (3) a requirement for neurosurgery before or after ICU admission.

The study exclusion criteria were clinical signs of cardiac failure, known renal or hepatic dysfunction, and pregnancy.

Patient Management

Management was implemented according to our ICP and CPP protocol based on (1) surgical evacuation of significant intracranial mass lesions or (2) medical treatment, including maintenance of ICP below 20 mmHg (with ventricular drainage, moderate hyperventilation, and mannitol or hypertonic saline) and CPP of 65–70 mmHg (after hydrostatic correction). Volume replacement was followed by norepinephrine if it was not sufficient to reach the required CPP. All patients were intubated and received mechanical ventilation. They were maintained in a normothermic state, sedated, and paralyzed in order to avoid CO_2 oscillations.

L. Moraes · B. Yelicich · M. Noble · A. Biestro · C. Puppo (✉)
Intensive Care Unit, Hospital de Clinicas, Universidad de la Republica, Montevideo, Uruguay

B. Depreitere et al. (eds.), *Intracranial Pressure and Neuromonitoring XVII*, Acta Neurochirurgica Supplement 131,
https://doi.org/10.1007/978-3-030-59436-7_3, © Springer Nature Switzerland AG 2021

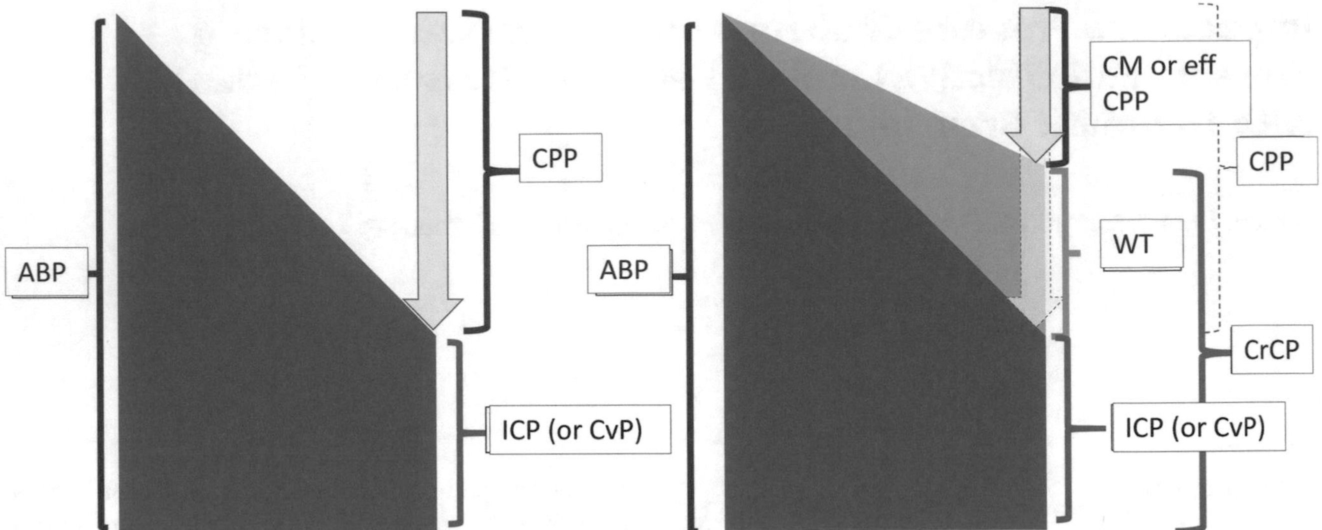

Fig. 1 Conceptual difference between (*left*) "conventional" cerebral perfusion pressure (CPP) and (*right*) "effective" cerebral perfusion pressure (CPPeff). *ABP* arterial blood pressure, *CrCP* critical closing pressure, *CvP* cerebral venous pressure, *CM or eff CPP* closing margin or "effective" cerebral perfusion pressure, *ICP* intracranial pressure, *WT* arteriolar wall tension

Pressure Challenge

After a 30-min basal recording, a norepinephrine infusion was started if it had not been necessary beforehand. A 50-mL normal saline solution containing 16 mg of norepinephrine (320 μg/mL) was started at a rate of 0.07 μg/kg/min. If the patient was already receiving norepinephrine, the basal dose was increased. The infusion rate was slowly increased to obtain a 20-mmHg slow increase in ABP. Figure 2 shows the raw and mean values of the acquired signals in the basal and hypertensive situations in one patient as an example of the study protocol.

Data Acquisition, Processing, and Analysis

The data used in this work were obtained from 11 patients with severe TBI, admitted to the ICU of the Hospital de Clinicas (Montevideo, Uruguay) between September 2005 and May 2007. The median age of the patients was 29 (IQR 14) years. An electrocardiogram, ABP, cerebral FV, and ICP were monitored continuously. Data acquisition and processing were performed with our in-house-designed CONTINE integrated neuromonitoring system including the ProcMx software system [6].

Data Acquisition

FV was measured in centimeters per second in the medial cerebral artery, using an EME TC2-64B transcranial Doppler system with a 2-MHz probe. FV was measured in the M1 segment of the middle cerebral artery through the temporal window, in accordance with the method described by Aaslid et al. [7]. The 2-MHz pulsed Doppler monitoring probe was fixed in its position and angle in order to keep the angle of insonation unchanged, using a headband. ABP (measured in millimeters of mercury) was recorded simultaneously with a Cardiocap II. ICP monitoring was performed using an intraparenchymal sensor (Codman MicroSensor) or a ventricular catheter. Both ABP and ICP transducers were zeroed at the level of the foramen of Monro in order to eliminate their hydrostatic differences. All signals were digitized with a NI-DAQ Card-6024E analogue/digital converter (A/D), at a frequency of 50 Hz, and stored on a laptop computer. The signals obtained after A/D conversion had a good signal-to-noise ratio resulting from the equipment filtering system; therefore, no new digital filtering step was needed.

Data Processing and Analysis

Each patient's signals were examined, and a short period from each phase (the normotensive and hypertensive phases) was chosen for calculation. CONTINE software incorporates an automatic CrCP calculation with four methods [8, 9]. In this chapter, we use the multiparametric method introduced by Varsos et al. [10]:

$$\text{CrCP} = \text{ABP} - \frac{\text{CPP}}{\sqrt{(\text{Ra}\cdot\text{Ca}\cdot\text{HR}\cdot 2\pi)^2+1}}\,(\text{mmHg})$$

where Ra is the cerebrovascular resistance (calculated as eCVR = CPP/FV), Ca is the pulsatile compliance of the cerebral arterial bed, and HR is the heart rate. A detailed description of the model can be found elsewhere [10].

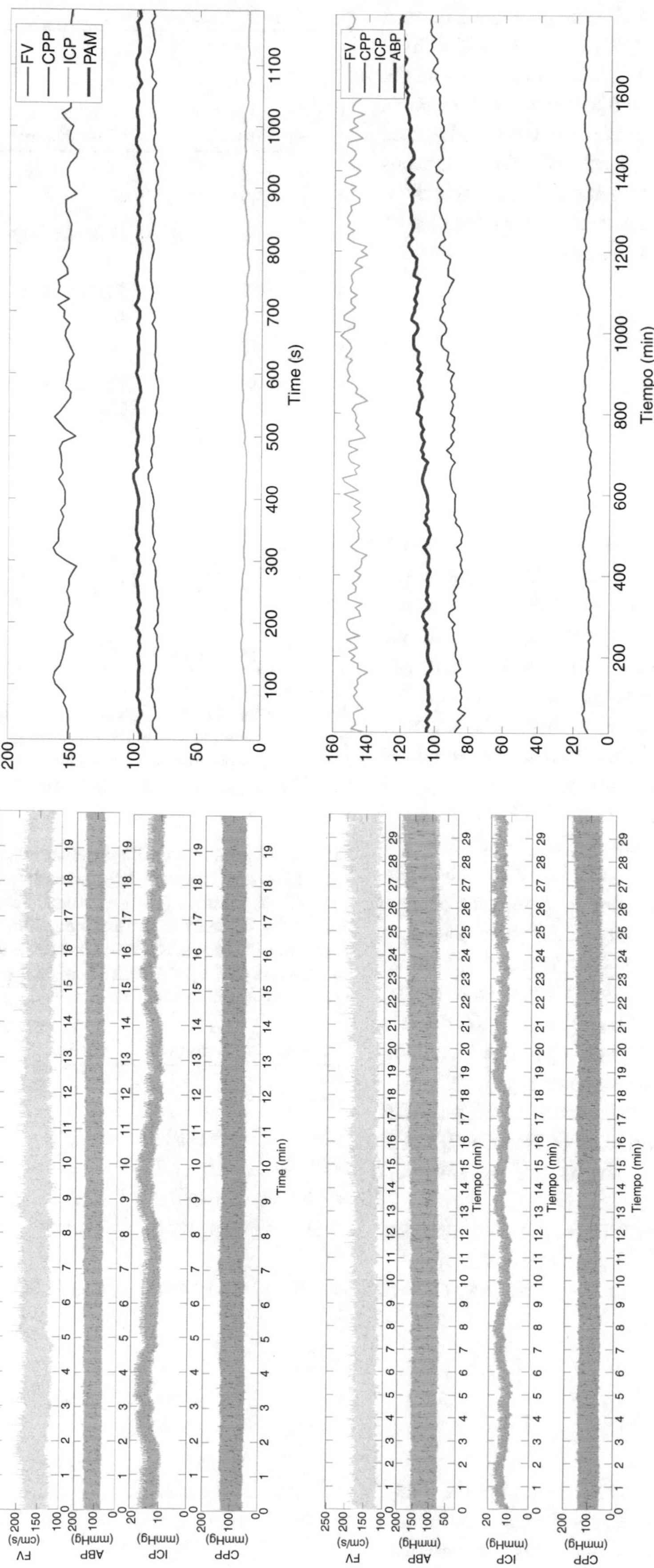

Fig. 2 Data acquired from a single patient. The *left panel* shows the raw signals in the basal situation (*top*) and during the hypertensive challenge (*bottom*). The *right panel* shows the mean signals in the same situations. The four signals shown in each panel are (*from top to bottom*) cerebral blood flow velocity (FV), arterial blood pressure (ABP), intracranial pressure (ICP), and "conventional" cerebral perfusion pressure (CPP)

Once CrCP was calculated, WT was estimated in each patient as the difference between CrCP and ICP (WT = CrCP − ICP). CPPeff (the closing margin) was calculated as the difference between ABP and CrCP (CPPeff = ABP − CrCP). The data distribution was considered nonparametric because the number of patients was small; therefore, all comparisons between numerical variables were made using the Wilcoxon signed-rank test. Statistical analyses were performed with IBM SPSS Statistics version 19 software.

Results

All values are expressed as median (IQR).

The patients described in this chapter were studied between September 2005 and May 2007. Eleven patients aged 29 (14) years were studied; nine of them were male. The time interval between admission and study was 64 (18) hours. The prehospital GCS score was 7 (7) and the admission GCS score was 7 (2). The admission GCS Motor Response score was 4 (4). The Marshall Classification was class V in five patients, diffuse injury III in two patients, and diffuse injury II in four patients. One patient died in the ICU. Table 1 shows the characteristics of each patient, the time interval from the moment of trauma until the hypertensive challenge, and the status at ICU discharge.

The increase in ABP was 20 (16) mmHg ($P < 0.005$).

ICP and WT—both parameters being included in the CrCP formula—showed different behaviors after the hypertensive challenge: ICP did not show a significant change, whereas WT increased significantly. CrCP also increased significantly by 25% (IQR 25%). CPP increased from 73 (17) to 102 (26) mmHg ($P < 0.05$), and CPPeff increased by a lesser amount from 66 (14) to 80 (20) mmHg ($P < 0.05$). The percentage change in WT showed a positive linear correlation ($P < 0.003$) with the percentage change in eCVR.

Table 2 shows the values of the recorded variables (ABP, ICP, and FV) and calculated variables (CPP, eCVR, CrCP, CPPeff, and WT), their overall changes, and the statistical significance of the changes.

Figure 3 shows boxplots of the different studied variables, each in the basal situation and the hypertensive situation.

Table 3 shows the percentage changes in CPP, CPPeff, WT, and CrCP.

Table 1 Patient characteristics

Patient number	Age (y)	Sex	Marshall Classification[a]	Time from trauma to study (h)	Condition at ICU discharge
1	16	Male	V	61	Alive
2	39	Male	V	24	Alive
3	22	Male	Diffuse injury III	81	Dead
4	17	Male	Diffuse injury II	84	Alive
5	31	Male	V	64	Alive
6	48	Male	Diffuse injury III	82	Alive
7	19	Female	Diffuse injury II	59	Alive
8	29	Male	V	72	Alive
9	32	Male	Diffuse injury II	108	Alive
10	32	Male	Diffuse injury II	46	Alive
11	18	Female	V	29	Alive

ICU intensive care unit

[a]Marshall Classification: diffuse injury II signifies cisterns intact, midline shift ≤5 mm, no high/mixed lesion ≥25 cm^3; diffuse injury III signifies cisterns compressed or absent, midline shift ≤5 mm, no high/mixed lesion ≥25 cm^3; V signifies an evacuated mass lesion

Table 2 Distribution of the different variables: changes generated in arterial blood pressure (ABP), three other directly recorded variables (intracranial pressure (ICP), cerebral blood flow velocity (FV), and "conventional" cerebral perfusion pressure (CPP)), and four calculated parameters (estimated cerebrovascular resistance (eCVR), critical closing pressure (CrCP), "effective" cerebral perfusion pressure (CPPeff), and arteriolar wall tension (WT))

Variable	Basal condition[a]	Hypertensive condition[a]	Overall change	*P* value
ABP (mmHg)	91 (17)	115 (22)	↑	0.003
ICP (mmHg)	16 (9)	17 (11)	NS	0.44
FV (cm/s)	78 (40)	87 (62)	NS	0.40
CPP (mmHg)	73 (17)	102 (26)	↑	0.006
eCVR (AU)	0.95 (0.38)	1.12 (0.58)	↑	0.003
CrCP (mmHg)	23 (11)	27 (10)	↑	0.003
CPPeff (mmHg)	66 (14)	80 (20)	↑	0.008
WT (mmHg)	7 (5)	11 (7)	↑	0.004

AU arbitrary perfusion unit, *NS* not significant

[a]The values are expressed as median (interquartile range)

Discussion

The cerebral critical closing pressure is the arterial blood pressure at which small cerebral vessels close and circulation stops [1–3]. It comprises intracranial pressure and wall

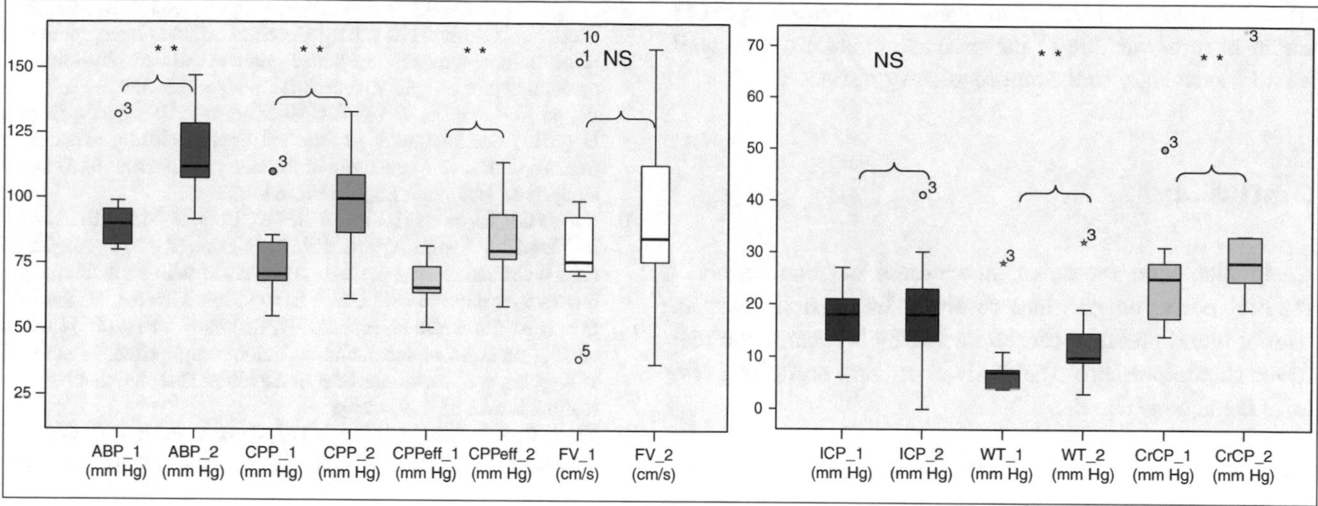

Fig. 3 Boxplots showing the median and interquartile range of each different variable studied in (*1*) the basal situation and (*2*) the hypertensive situation. *From left to right*: arterial blood pressure (ABP), "conventional" cerebral perfusion pressure (CPP), "effective" cerebral perfusion pressure (CPPeff), and cerebral blood flow velocity (FV). *In the right panel*, at a different scale, the following variables are shown, *from left to right*: intracranial pressure (ICP), arteriolar wall tension (WT), and critical closing pressure (CrCP). Two asterisks are shown when the significance reaches the level of 0.001. *NS* not significant

Table 3 Changes in "conventional" cerebral perfusion pressure (CPP), "effective" cerebral perfusion pressure (CPPeff), arteriolar wall tension (WT), and estimated cerebrovascular resistance (eCVR)

Change in variable	Percentage[a]	*P* value[b]
Change in CPP	25 (34)	0.01
Change in CPPeff	25 (25)	
Change in WT	71 (109)	0.03
Change in eCVR	25 (24)	

[a]The values are expressed as median (interquartile range)
[b]Wilcoxon signed-rank test

tension, and has been studied in different experimental and clinical settings. In patients with subarachnoid hemorrhage, it has been shown that during vasospasm, CrCP decreases both temporarily and spatially, mainly because of a decrease in wall tension due to distal vasodilatation (an autoregulatory response to vasospasm) [11, 14].

In patients with severe TBI, hypocapnia causes an increase in CrCP, which is due to an increase in cerebrovascular resistance [12]. During spontaneous ICP increases (plateau waves) [4] or controlled ICP increases (during infusion tests) [15, 16], ICH causes an increase in CrCP and, simultaneously, decreases the closing margin [17]. These changes are due mainly to the ICP increase because WT decreases. CrCP decreases in sepsis, maintaining longer adequate CPPeff, constituting a protective mechanism against ischemia [13]. To our knowledge, the changes in CrCP and CPPeff during an increase in ABP have not been specifically studied so far.

Calculation of the CrCP has been performed with different models, but some of them yield negative values, making a physiological explanation impossible [9, 18]. The model we used in this paper, introduced by Varsos et al. [10], shows a good correlation with the first harmonic method of CrCP calculation and has the added advantage that it does not yield negative values [8]. In its calculation, this multiparameter model includes the time constant (Tau) of the cerebral circulation. The tau concept, a product of cerebrovascular compliance and resistance ("CVR × Ca" in the CrCP Varsos model equation displayed above), is derived from the electrical circuits. It estimates how fast the blood entering the brain fills the arterial vascular sector. Its thorough calculation is shown elsewhere [19, 20].

In this study, we found that ICP did not change significantly. WT (calculated as CrCP − ICP) increased. Why did ICP not change if the arteriolar vessel tone did increase, probably causing a decrease in cerebral blood volume? We hypothesize that this was because the basal ICP was not high in most of the patients; therefore, their compliance (flow–volume) curves were probably working in their horizontal segment, where decreases in cerebral blood volume do not elicit significant decreases in ICP.

We also found that the CPPeff change was smaller than the CPP change. This was in accordance with our hypothesis. It has been suggested that the "closing margin" [4, 5], or CPPeff [12, 21] (calculated as ABP − CrCP), would estimate the real driving pressure gradient for cerebral perfusion and provide a more appropriate value of the real perfusion pressure than CPP (ABP − ICP). In our patients, during the basal situation, as could be predicted, CPP was higher than CPPeff. The hypertensive challenge increased both CPP and CPPeff, but the increase in CPPeff was significantly smaller. This effect was due principally to the significant increase in CrCP, which in turn was due to the increase in small-vessel wall tension, secondary to the autoregulatory response.

Conclusion

A clinician who measures an increase in "conventional" cerebral perfusion pressure resulting from an increase in arterial blood pressure can be misled by it because the real "downstream pressure" ("effective" cerebral perfusion pressure) is not considered.

Conflict of Interest **This trial (the data acquisition phase) was funded through research initiation funding to one of the authors (Leandro Moraes) by the Universidad de la Republica Comision Sectorial de Investigación Científica (CSIC) (University Scientific Research Sectorial Commission). The other authors do not have any conflict of interest to declare.**

References

1. Aaslid R, Lash SR, Bardy GH, Gild WH, Newell DW (2003) Dynamic pressure—flow velocity relationships in the human cerebral circulation. Stroke 34:1645–1649
2. Czosnyka M, Smielewski P, Piechnik S, Al-Rawi PG, Kirkpatrick PJ, Matta BF, Pickard JD (1999) Critical closing pressure in cerebrovascular circulation. J Neurol Neurosurg Psychiatry 66:606–611
3. Panerai RB (2003) The critical closing pressure of the cerebral circulation. Med Eng Phys 25:621–632
4. Varsos GV, de Riva N, Smielewski P, Pickard JD, Brady KM, Reinhard M, Avolio A, Czosnyka M (2013) Critical closing pressure during intracranial pressure plateau waves. Neurocrit Care 18:341–348
5. Varsos GV, Richards HK, Kasprowicz M, Reinhard M, Smielewski P, Brady KM, Pickard JD, Czosnyka M (2014) Cessation of diastolic cerebral blood flow velocity: the role of critical closing pressure. Neurocrit Care 20:40–48
6. Gomez H, Camacho J, Yelicich B, Moraes L, Biestro A, Puppo C (2010) Development of a multimodal monitoring platform for medical research. Presented at the 2010 Annual International Conference of the IEEE Engineering in Medicine and Biology, Buenos Aires, 31 Aug to 4 Sep 2010. https://doi.org/10.1109/IEMBS.2010.5627936
7. Aaslid R, Markwalder TM, Nornes H (1982) Noninvasive transcranial Doppler ultrasound recording of flow velocity in basal cerebral arteries. J Neurosurg 57:769–774
8. Puppo C, Camacho J, Varsos GV, Yelicich B, Gómez H, Moraes L, Biestro A, Czosnyka M (2016) Cerebral critical closing pressure: is the multiparameter model better suited to estimate physiology of cerebral hemodynamics? Neurocrit Care 25:446–454
9. Puppo C, Camacho J, Yelicich B, Moraes L, Biestro A, Gomez H (2012) Bedside study of cerebral critical closing pressure in patients with severe traumatic brain injury: a transcranial Doppler study. Acta Neurochir Suppl 114:283–288
10. Varsos GV, Richards H, Kasprowicz M, Budohoski KP, Brady KM, Reinhard M, Avolio A, Smielewski P, Pickard JD, Czosnyka M (2013) Critical closing pressure determined with a model of cerebrovascular impedance. J Cereb Blood Flow Metab 33:235–243
11. Soehle M, Czosnyka M, Pickard JD, Kirkpatrick PJ (2004) Critical closing pressure in subarachnoid hemorrhage: effect of cerebral vasospasm and limitations of a transcranial Doppler-derived estimation. Stroke 35:1393–1398
12. Thees C, Scholz M, Schaller MDC, Gass A, Pavlidis C, Weyland A, Hoeft A (2002) Relationship between intracranial pressure and critical closing pressure in patients with neurotrauma. Anesthesiology 96:595–599
13. van den Brule JMD, Stolk R, Vinke EJ, van Loon LM, Pickkers P, van der Hoeven JG, Kox M, Hoedemaekers CWE (2018) Vasopressors do not influence cerebral critical closing pressure during systemic inflammation evoked by experimental endotoxemia and sepsis in humans. Shock 49:529–535
14. Varsos GV, Budohoski KP, Czosnyka M, Kolias AG, Nasr N, Donnelly J, Liu X, Kim DJ, Hutchinson PJ, Kirkpatrick PJ, Varsos VG, Smielewski P (2015) Cerebral vasospasm affects arterial critical closing pressure. J Cereb Blood Flow Metab 35:285–291
15. Kaczmarska K, Kasprowicz M, Uryga A, Calviello L, Varsos G, Czosnyka Z, Czosnyka M (2018) Critical closing pressure during controlled increase in intracranial pressure—comparison of three methods. IEEE Trans Biomed Eng 65:619–624
16. Varsos GV, Czosnyka M, Smielewski P, Garnett MR, Liu X, Adams H, Pickard JD, Czosnyka Z (2016) Cerebral critical closing pressure during infusion tests. Acta Neurochir Suppl 122:215–220
17. Smielewski P, Steiner L, Puppo C, Budohoski K, Varsos GV, Czosnyka M (2018) Effect of mild hypocapnia on critical closing pressure and other mechanoelastic parameters of the cerebrospinal system. Acta Neurochir Suppl 126:139–142
18. Gazzoli P, Frigerio M, De Peri E, Rasulo F, Gasparotti R, Lavinio A, Latronico N (2006) A case of negative critical closing pressure. Abstracts of the 8th International Conference on Xenon CT and Related Cerebral Blood Flow Techniques: cerebral blood flow and brain metabolic imaging in clinical practice. Br J Neurosurg 20:348
19. Kasprowicz M, Diedler J, Reinhard M, Carrera E, Smielewski P, Budohoski KP, Sorrentino E, Haubrich C, Kirkpatrick PJ, Pickard JD, Czosnyka M (2012) Time constant of the cerebral arterial bed. Acta Neurochir Suppl 114:17–21
20. Puppo C, Kasprowicz M, Steiner LA, Yelicich B, Lalou DA, Smielewski P, Czosnyka M (2020) Hypocapnia after traumatic brain injury: how does it affect the time constant of the cerebral circulation? J Clin Monit Comput 34:461–468
21. Jägersberg M, Schaller C, Boström J, Schatlo B, Kotowski M, Thees C (2010) Simultaneous bedside assessment of global cerebral blood flow and effective cerebral perfusion pressure in patients with intracranial hypertension. Neurocrit Care 12:225–233

Semi-automated Computed Tomography Volumetry as a Proxy for Intracranial Pressure in Patients with Severe Traumatic Brain Injury: Clinical Feasibility Study

Ilse H. van de Wijgert, Jacobus F. A. Jansen, Jeanette Tas, Fred A. Zeiler, Paulien H. M. Voorter, Vera H. J. van Hal, and Marcel J. Aries

Introduction

Severe traumatic brain injury (TBI) is a leading cause of death and disability globally. Severe TBI is defined as a Glasgow Coma Scale (GCS) score ≤ 8 after resuscitation and abnormalities on computed tomography (CT) scanning of the brain. Admission to an intensive care unit (ICU) is necessary because the patient is in a deep coma and needs ventilation and oxygenation support. During the admission, further swelling can cause secondary damage to recovering or healthy brain tissue because of a low cerebral perfusion state and subsequent ischaemia. To monitor the intracranial volume (ICV), international guidelines recommend continuous invasive monitoring of intracranial pressure (ICP) [1]. Intracranial hypertension indicates that the total ICV is increasing. The skull volume consists of brain tissue, cerebrospinal fluid (CSF), venous blood and arterial blood. In healthy brains, the total volume and flow are kept constant by (limited) compensatory mechanisms such as CSF and venous blood displacements, and by active cerebral autoregulation. This is known as the Monro–Kellie doctrine and is based on the fact that the rigid skull prevents an unlimited rise in the ICV [2]. In severe TBI with brain swelling, compensatory mechanisms are easily exhausted, which leads to a further rise in ICV and a detrimental cascade of a decrease in arterial blood, leading to tissue hypoxia and, finally, neuronal cell death. Clinical protocols are commonly used to control ICP and to guarantee adequate cerebral perfusion pressure (CPP; defined as mean arterial pressure (MAP) minus ICP) [3]. To date, no robust alternatives to reliable and continuous ICV measurements, other than invasive ICP monitoring, are available. Trauma protocols recommend that patients with severe TBI receive CT scanning of the brain at the time of hospital admission. This is a quick and accessible way to provide an impression of the brain condition and the need for neurosurgical intervention. It can show cerebral oedema, a midline shift, haematomas, contusions and skull fractures. Radiologists are often asked whether (indirect) signs of increased brain swelling are present that might warrant intensification of ICP treatment, especially in combination with rising trends in absolute ICP levels. Detailed cerebral CT segmentations could potentially monitor the dynamics of the contused brain more closely. The ratio between the CSF volume and the ICV has previously been introduced to allow inter-individual comparisons [4]. However, manual segmentation is very time consuming. Therefore, we explored calculation of this ratio using automated CT segmentation with very limited manual input.

I. H. van de Wijgert · J. Tas
Department of Intensive Care, Maastricht University Medical Centre, Maastricht, The Netherlands

J. F. A. Jansen
Department of Radiology and Nuclear Medicine, Maastricht University Medical Centre, Maastricht, The Netherlands

Department of Neurosurgery, Maastricht University Medical Centre, Maastricht, The Netherlands

School for Mental Health and Neuroscience (MHeNs), Maastricht University, Maastricht, The Netherlands

Department of Electrical Engineering, Eindhoven University of Technology, Eindhoven, The Netherlands

F. A. Zeiler
Section of Neurosurgery, Department of Surgery, Rady Faculty of Health Sciences, University of Manitoba, Winnipeg, MB, Canada

Division of Anaesthesia, Department of Medicine, Addenbrooke's Hospital, University of Cambridge, Cambridge, UK

P. H. M. Voorter · V. H. J. van Hal
Department of Radiology and Nuclear Medicine, Maastricht University Medical Centre, Maastricht, The Netherlands

M. J. Aries (✉)
Department of Intensive Care, Maastricht University Medical Centre, Maastricht, The Netherlands

School for Mental Health and Neuroscience (MHeNs), Maastricht University, Maastricht, The Netherlands
e-mail: marcel.aries@mumc.nl

B. Depreitere et al. (eds.), *Intracranial Pressure and Neuromonitoring XVII*, Acta Neurochirurgica Supplement 131,
https://doi.org/10.1007/978-3-030-59436-7_4, © Springer Nature Switzerland AG 2021

In this pilot study, the clinical feasibility of using a semi-automated CT segmentation algorithm was investigated in patients with severe TBI and related to the current golden standard in skull volume measurements: invasively measured ICP. We hypothesized that volumetric CT measures are associated with ICP.

Materials and Methods

Patients and Data Acquisition

This study was conducted in a single academic hospital during the period between April 2017 and May 2019. Brain monitoring metrics and clinical and diagnostic data were collected from adult patients with severe TBI. The study was approved by the local medical ethics committee, and informed consent was obtained by proxy. All patients were sedated, intubated and mechanically ventilated. An intraparenchymal ICP sensor (Codman or Raumedic) was placed, and the patients were connected to a research laptop with Intensive Care Monitoring (ICM+®) software, which collected high-frequency (>100-Hz) data (e.g., ICP, blood pressure and temperature) from Philips bedside monitors. The moment of ICP sensor placement was not standardized and was thus dependent on clinical or operative indications. All physiological data were extracted from the ICM+® software, down-sampled to 1-min values and, for the purpose of this study, averaged over 24-h periods from the start of ICM+® monitoring. The first subsequent 24 h of monitoring were considered to be day 1 values. These values were compared with the values calculated from the admission CT scan (CT_1). The average time between CT_1 and the start of ICM + ® data collection was 16 (range 3–62) h. Values in patients monitored for <24 h were averaged over the available hours ($n = 3$, minimum time 12 h).

CT Volumetry

CT_1 values were used for the analysis. The CT acquisitions were obtained in DICOM file format. CT acquisitions with a slice thickness of 5 mm were used for optimal signal-to-noise properties. Brain volumes were segmented using a semi-automated algorithm (Fig. 1), based on the fast marching method of region growing in the Matlab programming language

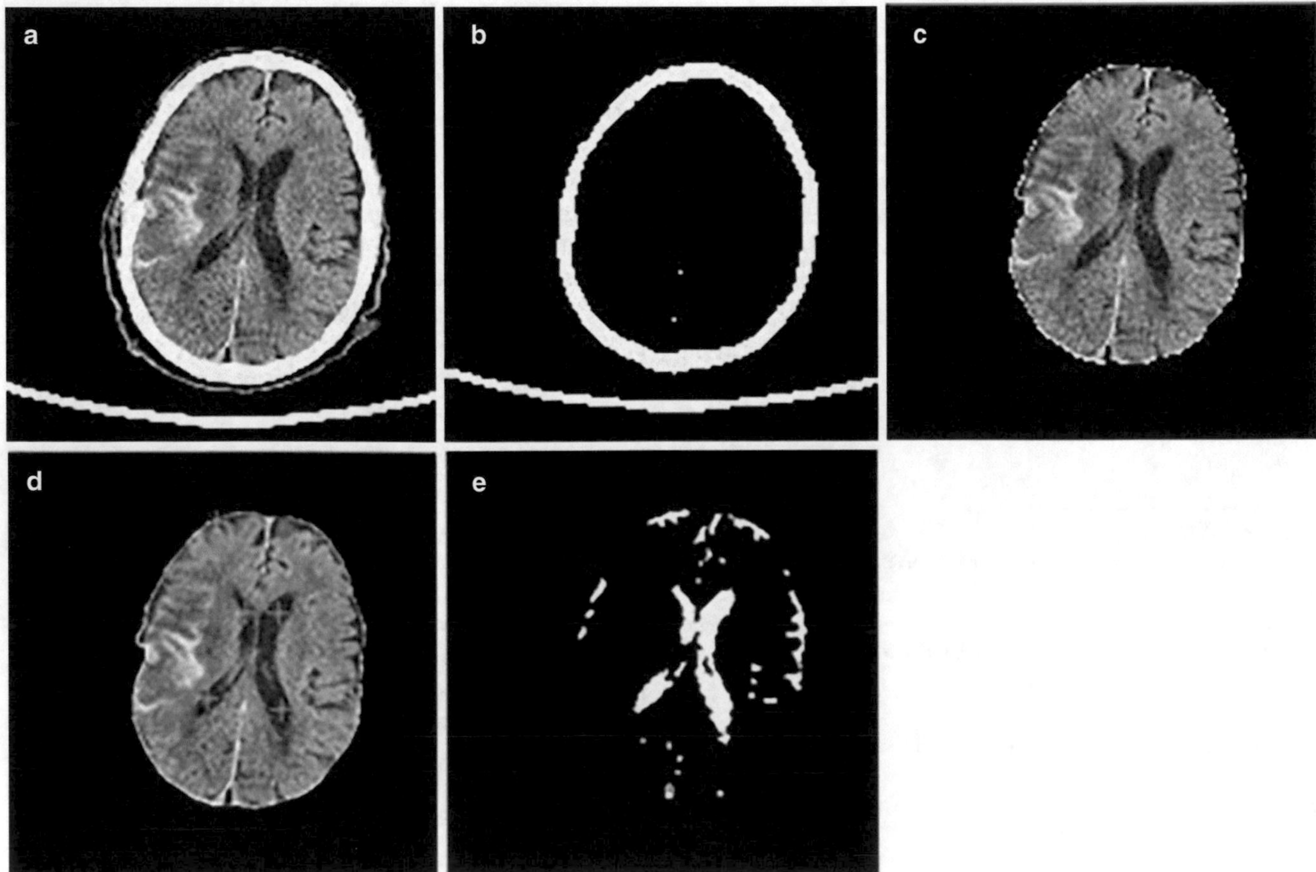

Fig. 1 Semi-automated procedure for tissue segmentation of computed tomography (CT) images. (**a**) Original transverse CT slice. (**b**) Identification of the skull on the basis of signal thresholding. (**c**) The resulting segmentation of intracranial volume after region growing. (**d**) Manual input (crosshairs) identifying the cerebrospinal fluid (CSF). (**e**) The resulting segmentation of CSF

(MathWorks, Natick, MA, USA), through which the volume of the CSF and the ICV are estimated slice by slice [5]. Manual input (by IHvdW) was needed to identify the most caudal and the most rostral slices (to establish the spatial range) and a slice at the lateral ventricle level, in which CSF was identified through selection of 5–50 voxels. Segmentation of the tissue was based on distinct Hounsfield unit values in the parenchyma, CSF and bone. In the case of skull defects (e.g., craniectomy), manual input was required to close the skull. In a final manual quality-control step, slices with artefacts were excluded. The total ICV volume and CSF volume were retrieved using the algorithm through addition of volumes per slice and calculation of the CSF/ICV ratio (expressed as a percentage) by division of the total CSF volume by the total ICV volume × 100 (Fig. 1). To limit intra-observer variability, a single rater (IHvdW) performed the CSF/ICV ratio determination three times per CT scan in all patients. The intraclass correlation coefficient (ICC) was 0.98 (95% confidence interval 0.97–.99), indicative of excellent intra-rater agreement. The validity of the method has previously been demonstrated by showing that semi-automated segmentation yields CSF/ICV ratios very similar to those obtained through manual segmentation by two independent raters (percentage point difference in CSF/ICV calculation ≤5%) [6].

Data Analysis

The relationship between the CSF/ICV ratio and ICP was assessed using nonparametric Spearman's correlation. Calculations were performed with independent data, i.e., one data point per patient for CT_1 and the mean ICP on day 1 of the data collection. Furthermore, in an explanatory assessment, the relationship between ICP and CSF/ICV was evaluated using a mono-exponential function derived from an animal experimental study in which the intracranial volume–pressure relationship was obtained with volume infusions in animals with ICP monitors [7]:

$$\mathrm{ICP} = \mathrm{ICP}_{\mathrm{cq}} \times \mathrm{e}^{\mathrm{E1}\times(1-\mathrm{CSF/ICV})} + C \qquad (1)$$

where $\mathrm{ICP}_{\mathrm{cq}}$ is a constant equal to the ICP at the equilibrium point (that is, the normal physiological steady state ICP), E1 is the elastance coefficient (a constant defining the slope of the volume–pressure curve) and C is a constant defining the intercept. In this formula, CSF/ICV is the estimate of the intracranial volume and ICP equals the measured invasive ICP. For evaluation of the different models, the squared norm of the residual (resnorm) was compared. No calculation of the required effect size or power analysis was performed in this exploratory study. The data were analysed using IBM SPSS Statistics version 25 and Matlab software.

Results

Patient characteristics are shown in Table 1. Thirty-three patient data sets were available. The median brain monitoring time per patient was 53 (range 12–293) h. An overview of the population-averaged physiological parameters and CSF/ICV ratios is shown in Table 2.

Relationship Between the CSF/ICV Ratio and Invasive ICP on the Admission CT Scan

A significant correlation between the CSF/ICV ratio and ICP was found ($r = -0.44$, $p = 0.01$) (Fig. 2). The mono-exponential function provided a better fit of the relationship between ICP and the CSF/ICV ratio than the linear model

Table 1 Patient characteristics ($N = 33$)

Variable	Value
Female/male ratio [*n*/*n*]	8/25
Median age [years (range)]	43.4 (18–91)
Mechanism of injury [*n* (%)]	
Traffic accident	17 (51.5)
Fall	15 (45.5)
Other	1 (3.0)
Median GCS score at admission (range)	7 (3–14)
Mortality [*n* (%)]	10 (30.3)
GOS score at 6 months [*n* (%)][a]	
1	10 (30.3)
2	0 (0.0)
3	3 (9.1)
4	4 (12.1)
5	7 (21.2)
Pupil reactivity [*n* (%)]	
Unreactive	3 (9.1)
Unilaterally reactive	3 (9.1)
Bilaterally reactive	27 (81.8)
Marshall Classification [*n* (%)]	
I	2 (6.1)
II	22 (66.7)
III	3 (9.1)
IV	1 (3.0)
V: Evacuated mass lesion	5 (15.2)

CT computed tomography, *GCS* Glasgow Coma Scale, *GOS* Glasgow Outcome Scale

[a]Values from 9 patients re-admitted to intensive care within the relevant 6-month period are omitted

Table 2 Mean physiological parameters and the cerebrospinal fluid/intracranial volume (CSF/ICV) ratio on day 1 of data collection from 33 patients

Parameter	Mean value (standard deviation)
CSF/ICV ratio [%]	6.3 (4.3)
Intracranial pressure [mmHg]	11.0 (6.6)
24-h TIL score	7.7 (2.5)
Arterial blood pressure [mmHg]	80.9 (8.6)
Heart rate [beats/min]	74.0 (18.3)

TIL score Therapy Intensity Level score (see Zuercher et al. [8])

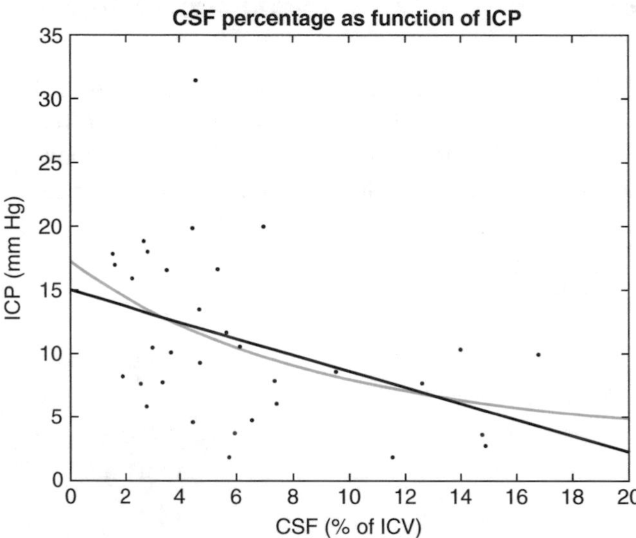

Fig. 2 Scatter plot of the mean intracranial pressure (ICP) (measured in mmHg) and the cerebrospinal fluid/intracranial volume (CSF/ICV) ratio (expressed as a percentage) on day 1. Individual data points indicate individual patients. Least-squares lines for linear regression (*black line*) and the mono-exponential formula, based on previous work by Avezaat et al. [7] (*grey line*), have been added for visualization, revealing that ICP increases with a decreasing CSF/ICV ratio

(resnorm 1156 vs. 1173), with the following estimates: ICP_{cq} = 12.2 mmHg, E1 = 0.113 and C = 3.5.

Discussion

The aim of this pilot study was to test the feasibility of using a semi-automated CT segmentation algorithm for volume estimation in severe TBI. ICP is significantly associated with the CSF/ICV ratio and best described by a mono-exponential function published previously by Avezaat et al. [7]. In comparison with controlled experimental settings, our patients with TBI were treated in accordance with a protocol recommending that ICP be kept at <20 mmHg, limiting our analysis to a small span of ICP values (Fig. 2). Our method provides a clear advantage over the classical manual segmentation methods and reduces the manual labour from hours to a few minutes per patient.

The literature on brain CT volumetric segmentation is very limited. In a study by Pappu et al. [4], 45 brain CT scans from 20 patients with severe TBI were selected. A similar negative correlation between the CSF/ICV ratio and ICP was found [4]. However, those values were not obtained independently (more scans per patient were used in the analysis). The authors discussed a cut-off value of 3.5% for the CSF/ICV ratio. Ratios higher than this cut-off were considered to have 'normal' ICP values, whereas no definite conclusion regarding ICP could be made with ratios lower than 3.5%. In our study, we were not able to define a cut-off point, probably because we had only a relatively small variety of ICP values available. Jain et al. [9] proposed automated image analysis to quantify the extent of intracranial abnormalities. Their method focused on detecting the volumes of intracranial lesions and the presence of basal cisterns and a midline shift [9], but relationships with ICP measurements and CSF/ICV ratios were not reported. Prior patient and animal experimental studies have studied the well-cited cerebral volume–pressure curve, which is best described by a mono-exponential function [7, 10, 11]. In our study, the mono-exponential function provided a better fit of the relationship between ICP and the CSF/ICV ratio than a linear model.

Our study had the limitations of being a retrospective study in a clinical setting. The variations in the timing between the admission CT scan and the start of the neuromonitoring data collection must have had an effect on the data that were collected. We tried to limit this influence by averaging the ICP values over a longer time period. Furthermore, individual patient variability has not yet been considered, although it is already known that age (i.e., brain atrophy) and clinical outcome influence the CSF/ICV ratio. Despite that, use of the presented algorithm as a clinical tool is feasible. It needs further testing in larger and more diverse patient data sets. Furthermore, segmentation features that include more tissue types (e.g., bleeding or contusions) and a further reduction in the manual input that the algorithm requires could be great improvements. Potentially, machine learning methods could be implemented in the future. Lastly, patients who subsequently develop traumatic hydrocephalus are currently assigned a higher (and more favourable) CSF/ICV ratio but have corresponding intracranial hypertension, manifested by ICP. Although hydrocephalus is found in approximately 20% of patients with severe TBI [12], only two patients in our population developed hydrocephalus at a later stage of their admission; therefore, those events did not affect the data presented here. In future studies, however, such events could cause a discrepancy in data interpretation; thus, it must be considered in order to exclude patients with different kinds of hydrocephalus from CT volumetry methods.

Semi-automated CT volumetry can be used in future studies to develop more objective criteria to guide indications for continuous invasive ICP monitoring in neuro-intensive care patients, especially when volumetry indexes are tracked over time. In addition, it could be an (objective) indicator of brain swelling in situations where contra-indications for placing an ICP monitor exist, such as a high risk of (intracranial) bleeding, hepatic encephalopathy or meningo-encephalitis. It could also be used to objectively quantify the effects of intracranial hypertension therapies.

Conclusion

Semi-automated CT volumetric measures correlate with ICP in patients with severe TBI. This proof-of-principle study demonstrates the feasibility of this approach in a clinical setting, but validation in larger and different data sets is needed. This non-invasive method could be used in the future to monitor patients who are not candidates for invasive monitoring or to evaluate therapy effects objectively.

Acknowledgments *Compliance with Ethical Standards*

Conflict of Interest: **The authors declare that they have no conflict of interest**

Ethics Approval: **All procedures performed in studies involving human participants were in accordance with the ethical standards of the institutional research committee, approval number 16-4-243, Maastricht University Medical Centre, Maastricht, the Netherlands.**

References

1. Carney N, Totten AM, O'Reilly C, Ullman JS, Hawryluk GW, Bell MJ, Bratton SL, Chesnut R, Harris OA, Kissoon N, Rubiano AM, Shutter L, Tasker RC, Vavilala MS, Wilberger J, Wright DW, Ghajar J (2017) Guidelines for the management of severe traumatic brain injury, fourth edition. Neurosurgery 80:6–15. https://doi.org/10.1227/NEU.0000000000001432
2. Mokri B (2001) The Monro–Kellie hypothesis: applications in CSF volume depletion. Neurology 56:1746–1748
3. Stocchetti N, Maas AI (2014) Traumatic intracranial hypertension. N Engl J Med 371:972. https://doi.org/10.1056/NEJMc1407775
4. Pappu S, Lerma J, Khraishi T (2016) Brain CT to assess intracranial pressure in patients with traumatic brain injury. J Neuroimaging 26:37–40. https://doi.org/10.1111/jon.12289
5. Voorter PHM (2019) Non-invasive determination of the intracranial pressure using CT images in patients with traumatic brain injury. University of Technology Eindhoven, Eindhoven
6. Berendsen AJ (2017) Volume segmentation of brain CTs for non-invasive ICP monitoring in TBI patients. University of Technology Eindhoven, Eindhoven
7. Avezaat CJ, van Eijndhoven JH, Wyper DJ (1979) Cerebrospinal fluid pulse pressure and intracranial volume–pressure relationships. J Neurol Neurosurg Psychiatry 42:687–700. https://doi.org/10.1136/jnnp.42.8.687
8. Zuercher P, Groen JL, Aries MJ, Steyerberg EW, Maas AI, Ercole A, Menon DK (2016) Reliability and validity of the Therapy Intensity Level Scale: analysis of clinimetric properties of a novel approach to assess management of intracranial pressure in traumatic brain injury. J Neurotrauma 33:1768–1774. https://doi.org/10.1089/neu.2015.4266
9. Jain S, Vyvere TV, Terzopoulos V, Sima DM, Roura E, Maas A, Wilms G, Verheyden J (2019) Automatic quantification of computed tomography features in acute traumatic brain injury. J Neurotrauma 36:1794–1803. https://doi.org/10.1089/neu.2018.6183
10. Lai HY, Lee CY, Hsu HH, Lee ST (2012) The intracranial volume pressure response in increased intracranial pressure patients: part 1. Calculation of the volume pressure indicator. Acta Neurochir 154:2271–2275. https://doi.org/10.1007/s00701-010-0765-8
11. Miller JD, Leech PJ (1974) Surgical Research Society [proceedings]. The intracranial volume–pressure response during experimental brain compression in primates. Br J Surg 61:318
12. Jiao QF, Liu Z, Li S, Zhou LX, Li SZ, Tian W, You C (2007) Influencing factors for posttraumatic hydrocephalus in patients suffering from severe traumatic brain injuries. Chin J Traumatol 10:159–162

Errors and Consequences of Inaccurate Estimation of Mean Blood Flow Velocity in Cerebral Arteries

Andras Czigler, Marta Fedriga, Erta Beqiri, Afroditi D. Lalou, Leanne A. Calviello, Manuel Cabeleira, Peter Toth, Peter Smielewski, and Marek Czosnyka

Introduction

The mean flow velocity (FVm) in the cerebral arteries is a key parameter in transcranial Doppler (TCD) ultrasonography. Many TCD devices calculate FVm using the systolic flow velocity (FVs) and diastolic flow velocity (FVd) with the traditional formula $FVm_{calc} = (FVs + 2 \times FVd)/3$ [1]. This assumes a specific linear relationship between all components. FVm can be calculated more accurately as the time integral of the current flow velocities divided by the integration period (FVm_{real}) [2, 3].

Materials and Methods

We retrospectively reviewed flow velocity (FV) and intracranial pressure (ICP) signals collected with TCD ultrasonography and intraparenchymal ICP monitors. The data were gathered from 14 patients with a traumatic brain injury (TBI) over the duration of their admission to the Neurosciences Critical Care Unit (NCCU) at Addenbrooke's Hospital (Cambridge, UK). We performed all analyses using ICM+ (Cambridge Enterprise, Cambridge, UK; http://www.neurosurg.cam.ac.uk/icmplus) and R software. All recordings contained plateau waves (transient intracranial hypertension), which resulted in a significant difference in ICP (mean ± standard deviation (SD) 25.3 ± 5.9 mmHg) between the baseline and plateau phases. Differences in the FVm_{calc} and FVm_{real} indices and the derivative pulsatility index (PI) were also assessed.

A. Czigler (✉)
Brain Physics Laboratory, Division of Neurosurgery, Department of Clinical Neurosciences, University of Cambridge, Cambridge, UK

Department of Neurosurgery and Szentagothai Research Center, University of Pécs, Medical School, Pécs, Hungary

Institute for Translational Medicine, University of Pécs, Medical School, Pécs, Hungary

M. Fedriga
Brain Physics Laboratory, Division of Neurosurgery, Department of Clinical Neurosciences, University of Cambridge, Cambridge, UK

Department of Anesthesia, Critical Care and Emergency, Spedali Civili University Hospital, Brescia, Italy

E. Beqiri
Brain Physics Laboratory, Division of Neurosurgery, Department of Clinical Neurosciences, University of Cambridge, Cambridge, UK

Department of Physiology and Transplantation, Milan University, Milan, Italy

A. D. Lalou · L. A. Calviello · M. Cabeleira · P. Smielewski
M. Czosnyka
Brain Physics Laboratory, Division of Neurosurgery, Department of Clinical Neurosciences, University of Cambridge, Cambridge, UK

P. Toth
Department of Neurosurgery and Szentagothai Research Center, University of Pécs, Medical School, Pécs, Hungary

Institute for Translational Medicine, University of Pécs, Medical School, Pécs, Hungary

Reynolds Oklahoma Center on Aging, Donald W. Reynolds Department of Geriatric Medicine, University of Oklahoma Health Sciences Center, Oklahoma City, OK, USA

B. Depreitere et al. (eds.), *Intracranial Pressure and Neuromonitoring XVII*, Acta Neurochirurgica Supplement 131, https://doi.org/10.1007/978-3-030-59436-7_5,

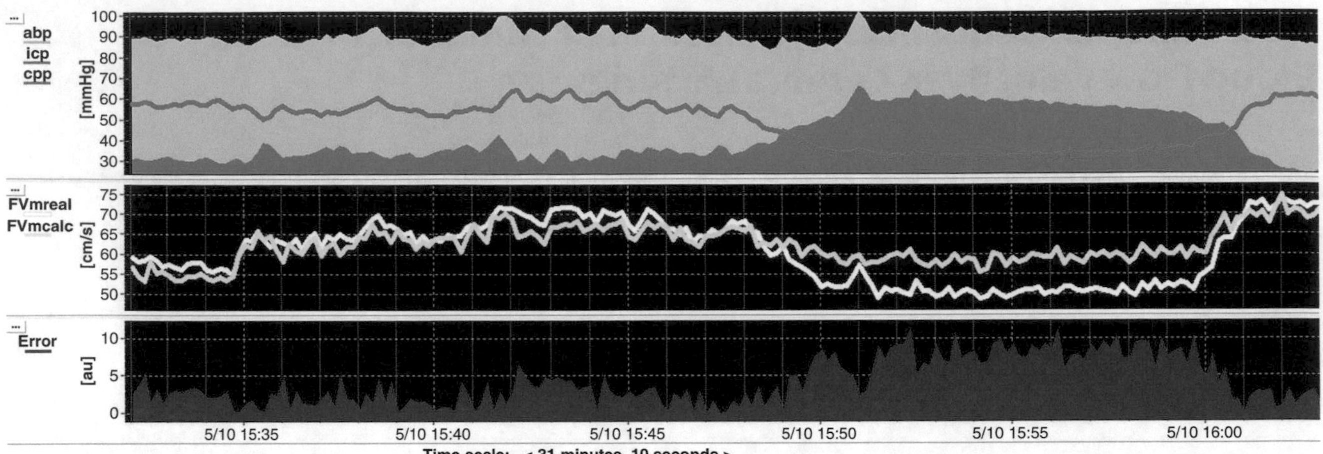

Fig. 1 Transcranial Doppler (TCD) arterial blood pressure (ABP) and intracranial pressure (ICP) monitoring using ICM+ software. *Top:* A drastic 15-min-long rise in ICP (plateau wave) is visible together with constant ABP and a consequent drop in cerebral perfusion pressure (CPP). *Middle:* The mean flow velocity in the middle cerebral arteries is calculated using both the traditional formula (FVmcalc) and the more accurate formula calculating it as the time integral of the current flow velocities divided by the integration period (FVmreal). *Bottom:* The difference between the two parameters is visible. An increase in the error coincides with the plateau wave

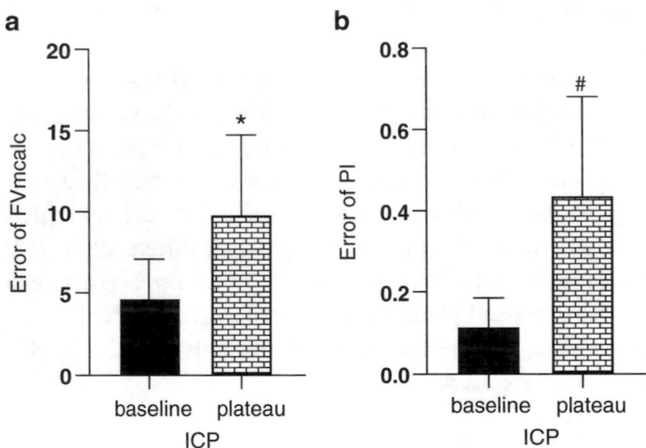

Fig. 2 Errors in both the traditional formula for calculation of the (**a**) mean flow velocity (FVmcalc) and its derivative (**b**) pulsatility index (PI) significantly increase from the baseline to the plateau. The data are expressed as mean ± standard deviation ($n = 12$ in each group). $^{*}P < 0.05$ vs. baseline, $^{\#}P < 0.005$ vs. baseline (paired Student's *t* test)

Results

During measurements, the averages of FVm_{calc} and FVm_{real} differed significantly ($P < 0.05$), and the mean ± SD of the absolute value of this difference was 6.1 ± 2.7 cm/s (Fig. 1). During plateau waves, when ICP rose, the error significantly increased from the baseline to the plateau (from 4.6 ± 2.4 to 9.8 ± 4.9 cm/s, $P < 0.05$) (Fig. 2a). Similarly, the error in PI calculated with FVm_{calc} also increased during plateau waves (from 0.11 ± 0.07 to 0.44 ± 0.24, $P < 0.005$) (Fig. 2b). In many cases, there appeared to be a strong correlation between ICP and the errors (Fig. 3).

Discussion

During plateau waves, with increasing ICP, errors in the estimated FVm and its derivatives also increase. This observation most likely occurs because the pulse waveform changes, thereby altering the FVs–FVd–FVm relationship [4, 5]. An example of such as changing relationship is when the heart rate changes and the generalization that the heart spends twice as much time in diastole as it does in systole becomes invalid; therefore, the error in the formula will increase [6]. However, in this study, we focused on elevation of ICP while the heart rate was relatively constant. This leads to the conclusion that other physiological or pathophysiological changes must happen in the brain that alter the storage of blood in the intracranial space, the compliance of the brain, the vasoreactivity of the arteries, or some other mechanism that leads to a new waveform and consequently a new link between FVs, FVd, and FVm. More research is needed to identify the driver behind this transformation; until then, if a change in the mean ICP is expected, then use of the FVm_{real} formula is recommended.

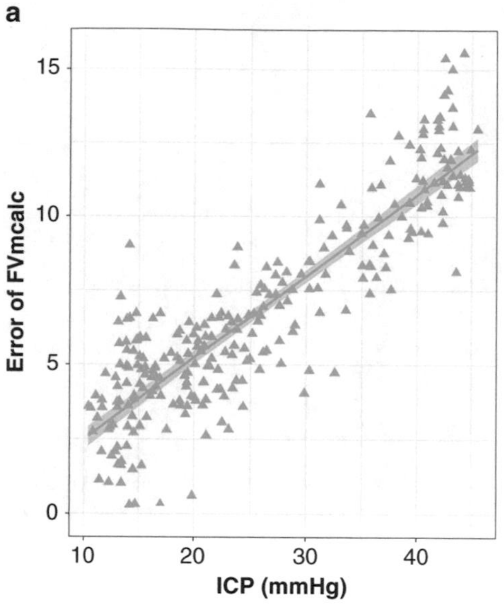

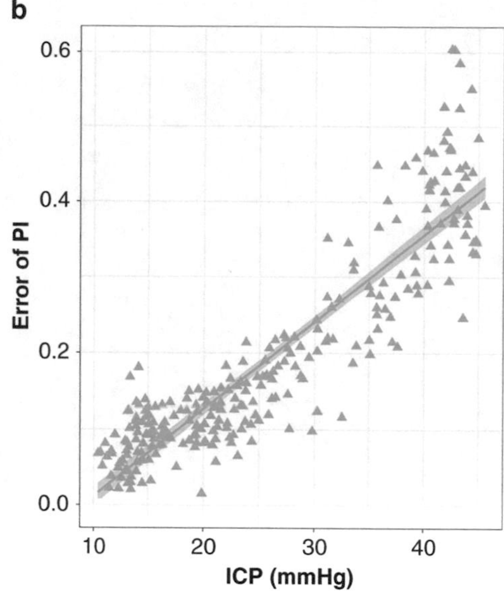

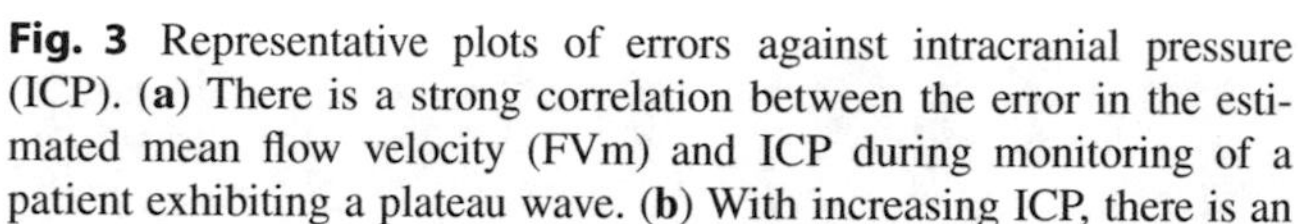

Fig. 3 Representative plots of errors against intracranial pressure (ICP). (**a**) There is a strong correlation between the error in the estimated mean flow velocity (FVm) and ICP during monitoring of a patient exhibiting a plateau wave. (**b**) With increasing ICP, there is an increasing error in the pulsatility index calculated using the traditional formula for FVm calculation (FVmcalc) instead of the more accurate formula calculating it as the time integral of the current flow velocities divided by the integration period (FVmreal)

Acknowledgments Marek Czosnyka is supported by the National Institute for Health Research, Cambridge Biomedical Research Centre (Cambridge, UK).

Conflict of Interest: **ICM+ software is licensed by Cambridge Enterprise Ltd. (Cambridge, UK) (https://icmplus.neurosurg.cam.ac.uk). Peter Smielewski and Marek Czosnyka have a financial interest in a fraction of the licensing fee.**

References

1. Bathala L, Mehndiratta MM, Sharma VK (2013) Transcranial Doppler: technique and common findings (part 1). Ann Indian Acad Neurol 16(2):174–179
2. Bryant R, Sanni O, Moore E, Bundy M, Johnson A (2014) An uncertainty analysis of mean flow velocity measurements used to quantify emissions from stationary sources. J Air Waste Manage Assoc 64(6):679–689
3. Zeiler FA, Donnelly J, Calviello L, Lee JK, Smielewski P, Brady K, Kim D-J, Czosnyka M (2018) Validation of pressure reactivity and pulse amplitude indices against the lower limit of autoregulation, part I: experimental intracranial hypertension. J Neurotrauma 35(23):2803–2811
4. Carrera E, Kim D-J, Castellani G, Zweifel C, Czosnyka Z, Kasparowicz M, Smielewski P, Pickard JD, Czosnyka M (2010) What shapes pulse amplitude of intracranial pressure? J Neurotrauma 27(2):317–324
5. Leliefeld PH, Gooskens RHJM, Peters RJM, Tulleken CAF, Kappelle LJ, Sen Han K, Regli L, Hanlo PW (2009) New transcranial Doppler index in infants with hydrocephalus: transsystolic time in clinical practice. Ultrasound Med Biol 35(10):1601–1606
6. Moran D, Epstein Y, Keren G, Laor A, Sherez J, Shapiro Y (1995) Calculation of mean arterial pressure during exercise as a function of heart rate. Appl Hum Sci 14(6):293–295

Analysis of the Association Between Lung Function and Brain Tissue Oxygen Tension in Severe Traumatic Brain Injury

Shadnaz Asgari, Chiara Robba, Erta Beqiri, Joseph Donnelly, Amit Gupta, Rafael Badenes, Mypinder Sekhon, Peter J. Hutchinson, Paolo Pelosi, and Arun Gupta

Introduction

Several researchers have attempted to find parameters that allow the clinician to assess the risk and outcome of the patient after traumatic brain injury (TBI) [1]. A major contributor to unfavourable outcomes is secondary brain damage, which progresses hours and days after TBI [2, 3]. It is widely accepted that causes of secondary injury include impaired cerebral metabolism, hypoxia and ischaemia [4]. Pulmonary complications are common in severe TBI, but few studies have investigated the association between lung function in terms of brain tissue oxygen tension ($PbtO_2$) and the ratio between the partial arterial oxygenation pressure (PaO_2) and the fraction of inspired oxygen (FiO_2) (PF ratio) [5–7]. The aim of this study was to investigate the association between lung function and brain tissue oxygenation in patients with TBI.

Materials and Methods

This was a single-centre, retrospective cohort study of 70 patients (20 females and 50 males aged 43 ± 20 years) who were admitted to the Neurocritical Care Unit at Addenbrooke's Hospital between October 2014 and December 2017. The study was approved by the relevant research ethics committee (approval number 30REC97/291) for anonymized data recording. The patients included in this study were at least 18 years old, had severe TBI with an admission Glasgow Coma Scale (GCS) score of <9 and underwent advanced neuromonitoring with invasive intracranial pressure (ICP) and $PbtO_2$ data captured using ICM+® brain monitoring software (Cambridge Enterprise Ltd., Cambridge, UK). A total of 303 simultaneous measurements of the following were considered in this work: the partial pressure of carbon dioxide in arterial blood (PCO_2), PaO_2, FiO_2, haemoglobin level

S. Asgari (✉)
Biomedical Engineering Department, California State University, Long Beach, CA, USA
e-mail: Shadnaz.Asgari@csulb.edu

C. Robba
Anesthesia and Intensive Care, San Martino Policlinico Hospital, Scientific Institutes of Hospitalization and Care (IRCCS) for Oncology and Neurosciences, Genoa, Italy

E. Beqiri
Brain Physics Laboratory, Department of Clinical Neurosciences, University of Cambridge, Cambridge, UK

Department of Physiology and Transplantation, Milan University, Milan, Italy

J. Donnelly
Brain Physics Laboratory, Department of Clinical Neurosciences, University of Cambridge, Cambridge, UK

A. Gupta · A. Gupta
Neurosciences Critical Care, University of Cambridge, Cambridge, UK

R. Badenes
Department of Anesthesiology, Hospital Clìnico Universitario, Valencia, Spain

M. Sekhon
Division of Critical Care Medicine, University of British Columbia, Vancouver, BC, Canada

P. J. Hutchinson
Department of Neurosurgery, University of Cambridge, Cambridge, UK

P. Pelosi
Department of Surgical Sciences and Integrated Diagnostics (DISC), University of Genoa, Genoa, Italy

B. Depreitere et al. (eds.), *Intracranial Pressure and Neuromonitoring XVII*, Acta Neurochirurgica Supplement 131,
https://doi.org/10.1007/978-3-030-59436-7_6, © Springer Nature Switzerland AG 2021

(Hb), pH level, base excess level (BE), temperature (Temp), sodium level, ICP, arterial blood pressure (ABP), cerebral perfusion pressure (CPP), autoregulation index (PRx), $PbtO_2$ and PF ratio.

To study the relationship between the different variables, a Pearson correlation analysis was conducted. We employed Kruskal–Wallis analysis of variance (ANOVA) for each variable within two groups of measurements: hypoxia ($PbtO_2 < 20$ mmHg) and normoxia ($PbtO_2 \geq 20$ mmHg) to indicate those variables with significant differences between hypoxia and normoxia. A multivariable forward step regression model was applied to study the independent correlation between $PbtO_2$, the PF ratio and PaO_2. For this purpose, $PbtO_2$ was considered as the response variable, while the PF ratio and PaO_2 were employed as predictor variables. We also adjusted for the following confounding factors: PCO_2, CPP, Temp and Hb.

Finally, we employed generalized estimating equations with dichotomized $PbtO_2$ (above or below 20 mmHg: PbtO2 ≥ 20 mmHg or PbtO2 < 20 mmHg) as a response variable and a dichotomized PF ratio (greater or smaller than 330: PF>330 or PF≤330) as a predictor variable to investigate whether a PF ratio of <330 is an independent risk factor for brain hypoxia, while adjusting for confounding factors such as ICP, age, sex and the GCS score.

Results

Figure 1 presents the results of correlation analysis between all variables, using a colour bar where correlations with significant p values (≤0.05) are indicated with letters on the plot, as follows:

- *W* means a significant weak correlation (correlation value <0.4).
- *M* means a significant moderate correlation (0.4 ≤ correlation value <0.7).
- *S* means a significant strong correlation (0.7 ≤ correlation value).

We observed that several variables had significant correlations with each other. For example, $PbtO_2$ had significant but weak correlations with PCO_2, FiO_2, pH, ICP and the PF ratio.

Figure 2 displays box plots from ANOVA for those variables that showed significant differences between hypoxia ($PbtO_2 < 20$ mmHg) and normoxia ($PbtO_2 \geq 20$ mmHg). The p value for the ANOVA test is accordingly indicated at the top of each plot.

We observed that among all variables we considered, only PCO_2, FiO_2, ICP, CPP and the PF ratio showed sig-

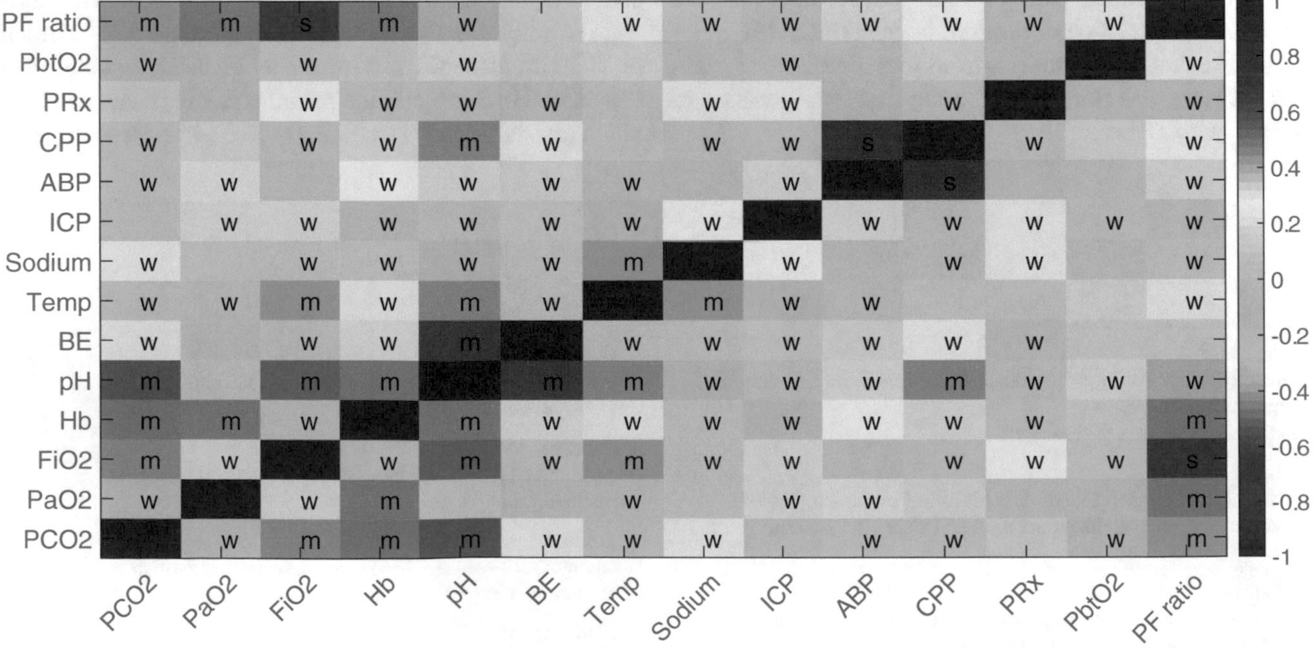

Fig. 1 Results of correlation analysis of all variables. Correlations are identified by the following letters: *W* means a significant weak correlation (correlation value <0.4), *M* means a significant moderate correlation (0.4 ≤ correlation value <0.7) and *S* means a significant strong correlation (0.7 ≤ correlation value). *ABP* arterial blood pressure, *BE* base excess level, *CPP* cerebral perfusion pressure, *FiO_2* fraction of inspired oxygen, *Hb* haemoglobin level, *ICP* intracranial pressure, *PaO_2* partial arterial oxygenation pressure, *$PbtO_2$* brain tissue oxygen tension, *PCO_2* partial pressure of carbon dioxide in arterial blood, *PF ratio* the ratio between the partial arterial oxygenation pressure and the fraction of inspired oxygen, pH level, *PRx* autoregulation index, *Temp* temperature

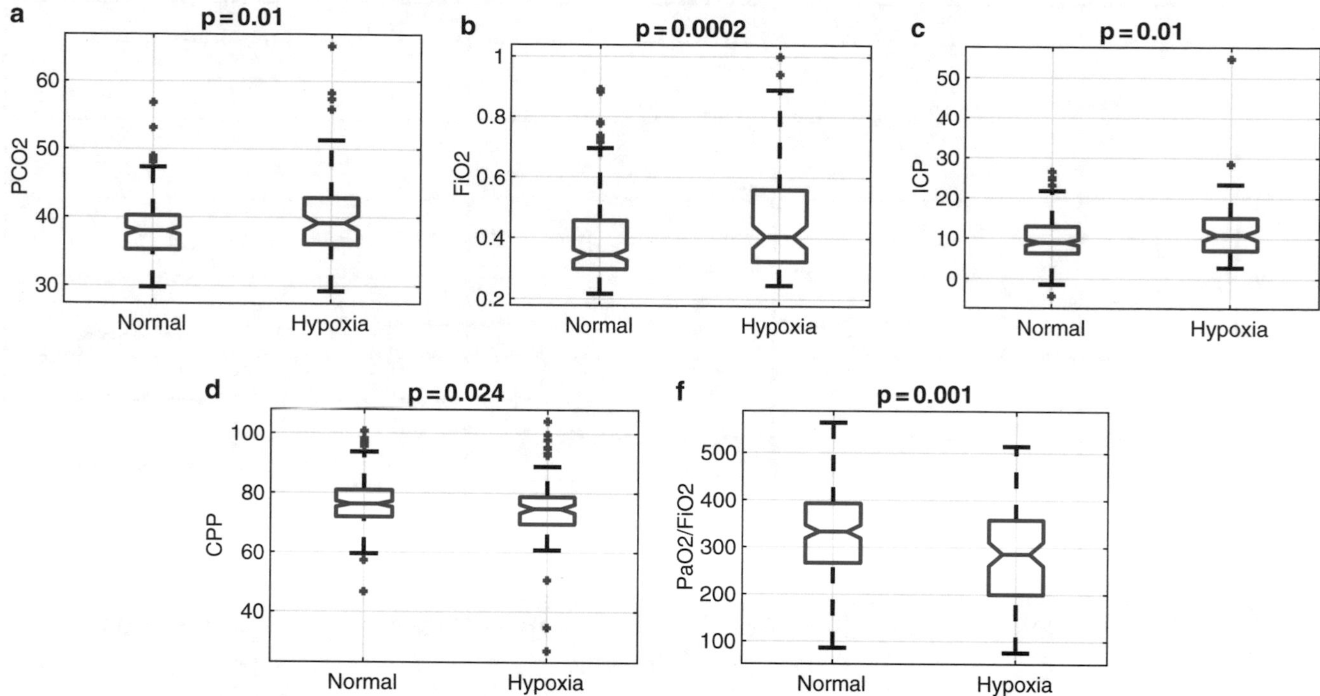

Fig. 2 Box plots of values of the variables that showed significant differences between normoxia and hypoxia. (**a**) Partial pressure of carbon dioxide in arterial blood (PCO_2). (**b**) Fraction of inspired oxygen (FiO_2). (**c**) Intracranial pressure (ICP). (**d**) Cerebral perfusion pressure (CPP). (**e**) PF ratio (the ratio between the partial arterial oxygenation pressure (PaO_2) and the fraction of inspired oxygen)

nificant differences between hypoxia and normoxia. Use of each of these variables resulted in accuracy of <60% in detection of hypoxia. However, with use of a combination of all of these five variables in a support vector machine classifier, accuracy of 70% was achieved in detection of hypoxia.

After adjustment for PCO_2, CPP, Temp and Hb, the results of implementing a multivariable forward step regression model revealed strong and independent correlations between $PbtO_2$ and the PF ratio, and between $PbtO_2$ and PaO_2, with adjusted p values of <0.001 for both correlations.

Figure 3 demonstrates box plots for $PbtO_2$ according to four different ranges of PF ratios: $PF \leq 100$, $100 < PF \leq 200$, $200 < PF \leq 330$, and $PF > 330$. The median $PbtO_2$ value for episodes with $PF > 330$ (median 27.4 mmHg, interquartile range (IQR) 20.3–35.1) was significantly greater than those for episodes with $200 < PF \leq 330$ (median 24.3 mmHg, IQR 18.5–30.9), those for episodes with $100 < PF \leq 200$ (median 20.3 mmHg, IQR 14.6–24.2) and those for episodes with $PF \leq 100$ (median 14.4 mmHg, IQR 6–22.5), with p values of <0.03 for all comparisons.

Finally, after adjustment for ICP, age, sex and the GCS score, we found that a $PF \leq 330$ was indeed an independent risk factor for compromised $PbtO_2$, with an adjusted odds ratio of 1.94 (95% confidence interval 1.12–3.34) and a p value of 0.02.

Discussion

The pathophysiology of brain tissue oxygenation is complicated and is dependent on several factors, including oxygen delivery (cerebral blood flow), arterial oxygen content, oxygen diffusion from the capillary into the mitochondria and mitochondrial oxygen consumption, Hb and CPP. Studies have shown that after TBI, patients who will not survive have lower $PbtO_2$ values [6–8].

$PbtO_2$ depends on ventilatory parameters and systemic oxygenation. There is further evidence showing a strong correlation between $PbtO_2$ and FiO_2, and a relationship between $PbtO_2$ and PaO_2 [8–10]. In patients with acute respiratory distress syndrome (ARDS), the PF ratio beyond 24 h, while the patient is on standard ventilator settings, is an appropriate tool to ensure correct categorization of patients with ARDS by disease severity [6]. Most patients with severe TBI normally require mechanical ventilatory support, and lung injury very often coexists in head injury as a result of polytrauma. In these settings, FiO_2 can be controlled easily but PaO_2 may be variable; therefore, variations in PaO_2 and FiO_2—and consequently the PF ratio—would have an effect on $PbtO_2$ [10]. Indeed, our correlation analysis results showed that there was a significant correlation between $PbtO_2$ and the PF ratio, and our independent association analysis revealed that the PF ratio was

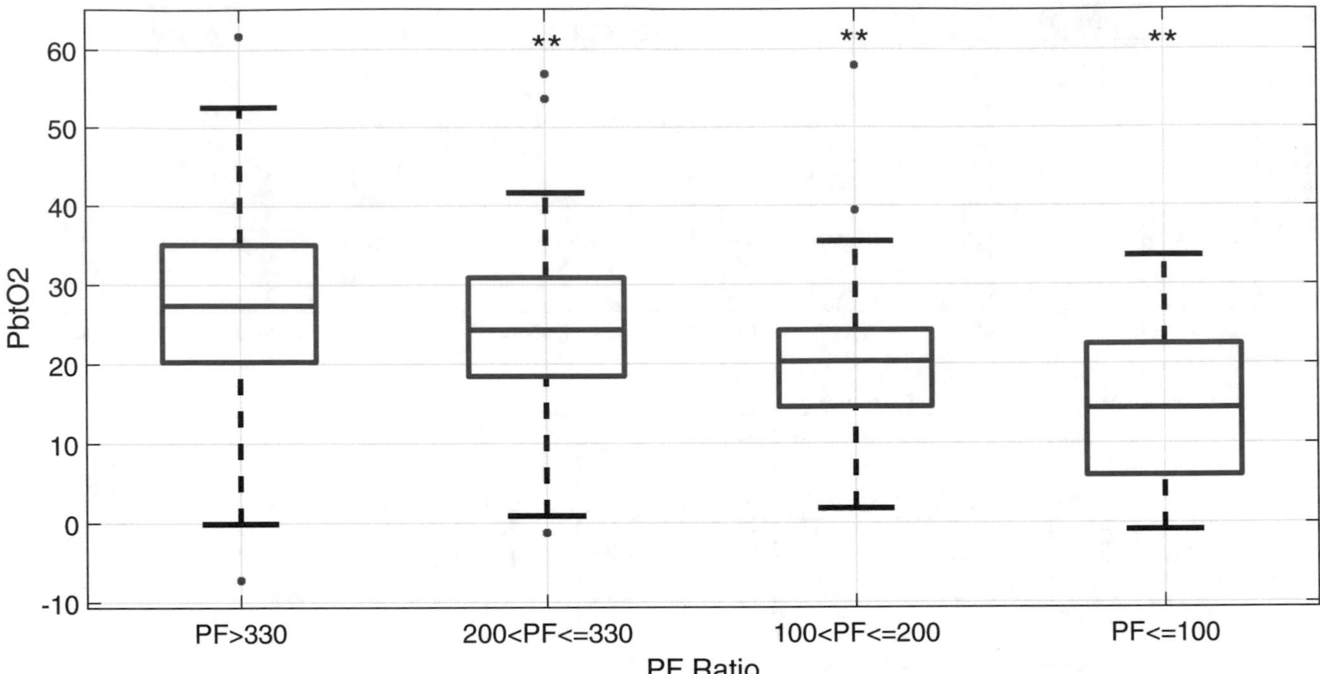

Fig. 3 Box plots of brain tissue oxygen tension ($PbtO_2$) values for four ranges of values of the PF ratio (the ratio between the partial arterial oxygenation pressure and the fraction of inspired oxygen). $**p < 0.03$ for comparison with samples obtained at a PF ratio of >330

independently correlated with $PbtO_2$ after adjustment for confounding factors. As a result, it may be better to implement the absolute $PbtO_2$ while also considering the PF ratio.

Conclusion

Our results confirm the importance of ventilator management and strategies in brain-injured patients in order to optimize cerebral oxygenation and prevent secondary brain damage. In patients with TBI, lung-protective strategies are often used to prevent brain hypoxia, and the PF ratio may reflect the severity of injury and the possible outcome.

Conflict of Interest **The authors declare that they have no conflict of interest.**

References

1. Lee S, Kim S, Kim C, Park S, Park J, Yeo M (2012) Prediction of outcome after traumatic brain injury using clinical and neuroimaging variables. J Clin Neurol 8(3):224
2. MRC CRASH Trial Collaborators, Perel P, Arango M, Clayton T, Edwards P, Komolafe E, Poccock S, Roberts I, Shakur H, Steyerberg E, Yutthakasemsunt S (2008) Predicting outcome after traumatic brain injury: practical prognostic models based on large cohort of international patients. BMJ 336(7641):425–429. https://doi.org/10.1136/bmj.39461.643438.25
3. Steyerberg EW, Mushkudiani N, Perel P, Butcher I, Lu J et al (2008) Predicting outcome after traumatic brain injury: development and international validation of prognostic scores based on admission characteristics. PLoS Med 5(8):e165
4. Maloney-Wilensky E, Gracias V, Itkin A, Hoffman K, Bloom S, Yang W et al (2009) Brain tissue oxygen and outcome after severe traumatic brain injury: a systematic review. Crit Care Med 37(6):2057–2063
5. Nangunoori R, Maloney-Wilensky E, Stiefel M, Park S, Kofke WA, Levine J et al (2011) Brain tissue oxygen–based therapy and outcome after severe traumatic brain injury: a systematic literature review. Neurocrit Care 17(1):131–138
6. Oddo M, Lavine JM, Mackenzie L, Frangos S, Feihl F (2011) Brain hypoxia is associated with short term outcome after severe traumatic brain injury independently of intracranial hypertension and low cerebral perfusion pressure. Neurosurgery 69(5):1037–1045. https://doi.org/10.1227/NEU.0b013e3182287ca7
7. Narotam PK, Morrison JF, Nathoo N (2009) Brain tissue oxygen monitoring in traumatic brain injury and major trauma: outcome analysis of a brain tissue oxygen–directed therapy. J Neurosurg 111(4):672–682. https://doi.org/10.3171/2009.4.JNS081150
8. Chang J, Youn T, Benson D, Mattick H, Andrade N, Harper C et al (2009) Physiologic and functional outcome correlates of brain tissue hypoxia in traumatic brain injury. Crit Care Med 37(1):283–290
9. Carney N, Totten AM, O'Reilly C, Ullman JS, Hawryluk GW, Bell MJ, Bratton SL, Chesnut R, Harris OA, Kissoon N, Rubiano AM, Shutter L, Tasker RC, Vavilala MS, Wilberger J, Wright DW, Ghajar J (2017) Guidelines for the management of severe traumatic brain injury, fourth edition. Neurosurgery 80(1):6–15. https://doi.org/10.1227/NEU.0000000000001432
10. Wang L (ed) (2005) Support vector machines: theory and applications. Springer, Berlin

Comparison of Two Intracranial Pressure Calculation Methods and Their Effects on the Mean Intracranial Pressure and Intracranial Pressure Dose

Ka Hing Chu, Erta Beqiri, Marek Czosnyka, and Peter Smielewski

Introduction

Traumatic brain injury (TBI) is a common cerebral pathology affecting more than 50 million people every year. Acute head trauma can be followed by swelling of the brain (secondary damage), which causes the pressure within the cranial cavity (intracranial pressure (ICP)) to increase, as the brain is surrounded by a rigid skull. This rise in ICP can cause secondary damage to the brain, partly because it disrupts cerebral perfusion, resulting in ischaemia and hypoxia [1]. In a head-injured patient, ICP is a vital quantity to monitor. It not only provides information about secondary damage to the brain but also provides an indication of the physiological state of the brain (such as compliance and elastance), and clinical decisions can be made on the basis of the ICP level to ensure adequate cerebral perfusion [2]. It is common to have ICP above 20 mmHg after head trauma, and efforts are made to stabilise it below this level.

It is believed that the clinical outcome of a patient with TBI is significantly influenced by his or her mean ICP and ICP dose. The ICP dose is defined as the area under the curve (AUC) of an ICP–time graph that exceeds a certain threshold (20 mmHg in this study); it is considered to be a more informative parameter than the mean ICP when describing secondary brain damage, as it describes both the extent and the duration of the insult [3].

Commonly, in a critical care unit, ICP is recorded on hourly basis even when electronic record systems are used. Two methods can be used to report such hourly values: the hour-averaged ICP (which is available only when electronic record systems are used, as they are configured to return these values) and, more often (possibly because of continuing use of paper-based nursing charts), the end-hour ICP. The former method averages the ICP over the whole hour, while the latter reports a point measurement of the mean ICP at the end of each hour. The end-hour ICP is naturally a more practical option when bedside monitoring values are entered into nursing charts manually [4]. However, the significance of under-sampling of the true ICP variability with end-hour reporting, which entirely misses an hour's worth of variability in ICP at each reporting time point, has not been fully examined. Previously, Zanier et al. compared digital hour-averaged ICP measurements with manually recorded end-hour ICP measurements, including the number of episodes of high ICP (HICP, where ICP is above 20 mmHg) and the percentage of time when HICP was present [4]. Our study, on the other hand, investigated the mean ICP and ICP dose obtained using hour-averaged ICP and digital end-hour ICP (which averages the ICP in the final minute of every hour), and thus the difference in predictive power for patient mortality.

Methods

A retrospective data analysis was conducted using high-frequency ICP monitoring data. The raw ICP data were obtained using ICM+ software (Cambridge Enterprise Ltd., Cambridge, UK); they were recorded with digital data transfer or digitised by analogue/digital (A/D) converters

K. H. Chu (✉) · M. Czosnyka · P. Smielewski
Brain Physics Laboratory, Division of Neurosurgery, Department of Clinical Neurosciences, University of Cambridge, Cambridge, UK
e-mail: khc42@cam.ac.uk

E. Beqiri
Brain Physics Laboratory, Division of Neurosurgery, Department of Clinical Neurosciences, University of Cambridge, Cambridge, UK

Department of Physiology and Transplantation, Milan University, Milan, Italy

https://doi.org/10.1007/978-3-030-59436-7_7,

(DT9801; Data Translation, Marlboro, MA, USA) and sampled at a frequency of at least 50 Hz [5]. The age, sex, injury severity (assessed as the Glasgow Coma Scale (GCS) score) and status at discharge (assessed as the Glasgow Outcome Scale (GOS) score) were also included for each recording; the data were fully anonymised. This study examined the ICP data of 1060 patients admitted with TBI to the Neurocritical Care Unit (NCCU) at Addenbrooke's Hospital (Cambridge, UK) during the period from 1993 to 2017.

Data Processing

Using the 'batch export' function of ICM+, the end-hour ICP and hour-averaged ICP time series for each patient were created automatically. Each patient's mean ICP and ICP dose were calculated using both methods; the ICP dose was estimated using the trapezoidal method, which modelled the AUC as a series of rectangles and summed up their areas.

Statistical Analysis

The patients were first dichotomised by mortality (as 244 patients died), and the average mean ICP and ICP dose of each group were calculated. The correlation coefficient (r) between the end-hour and hour-averaged mean ICP values was then evaluated for each patient, and the average correlation of all patients was obtained. After that, the coefficient of determination (r^2) between the methods was calculated for each patient, and an estimate of the average proportion of the variance that was unexplained (i.e. missed) by the end-hour values (calculated as $1 - r^2$) of all patients was thus found. With use of a Student's t test, the mean ICP and ICP dose values yielded by both calculation methods were compared between the patient group that survived and the group that died. In addition, a t test comparing the two methods was also performed within each group. The Bland–Altman method was used to illustrate the difference between the two methods.

Results

The mean age of the patients was 38 ± 17.2 years (range 3–89), and 827 of the 1010 patients were male (78.0%). The GCS score ranged from 3 to 15, and the GOS score ranged from 1 to 5. The average correlation between the end-hour and hour-averaged mean ICP values was 0.747, and the average relative ICP variance missed by end-of-hour measurement was 40.49%. The mean ICP and ICP dose averaged with the two calculation methods did not differ significantly. The Student's t test gave similar results, but it also suggested that in both calculation methods, the mean ICP and ICP dose values were significantly higher in the group of patients who died. The t test performed on the ICP dose to compare the two methods within the group that survived showed that $t = 1.82$, which almost reached significance ($p < 0.07$). Table 1 lists the mean ICP and ICP dose averaged for both patient groups and both calculation methods, and the results of the Student's t test. Figure 1 shows Bland–Altman plots for the mean ICP and ICP dose. For the mean ICP, the mean difference (shown by a solid line) was 0.015 mmHg and the limits of agreement (shown by dotted lines) were 1.10 and −1.07. For the ICP dose, the mean difference was 21.52 mmHg h and the limits of agreement were 102.04 and −59.00.

Discussion

As expected, both the mean ICP and ICP dose values were significantly higher for patients who died than for those who survived. In the Bland–Altman plots, the narrower limits of agreement for the mean ICP implied less uncertainty and hence a more reliable analysis than in the case of ICP dose. The mean ICP values calculated using end-hour and hour-averaged methods were moderately correlated. Despite that, the end-hour method missed a substantial amount (40.49%) of the dynamic variability in ICP. Statistically, the relationships with the outcomes of the two methods did not differ significantly from each other. This may suggest that the end-hour ICP is a suitable method to assess the clinical outcome of TBI patients. However, this analysis was performed by

Table 1 Mean intracranial pressure (ICP) and ICP dose (± standard error) in both patient groups and with both calculation methods, and results of the Student's t test between patient groups

		Mean ICP			ICP dose		
Method.	Patient status	Mean (mmHg)	t Test value	p Value	Mean (mmHg h)	t Test value	p Value
End-hour	Died	20.9 ± 0.9	6.92	$<1 \times 10^{-10}$	352 ± 36	5.93	$<1 \times 10^{-8}$
	Survived	14.2 ± 0.2			132 ± 9		
Hour-averaged	Died	20.8 ± 0.9	6.89	$<1 \times 10^{-10}$	335 ± 35	6.18	$<1 \times 10^{-8}$
	Survived	14.3 ± 0.2			109 ± 9		

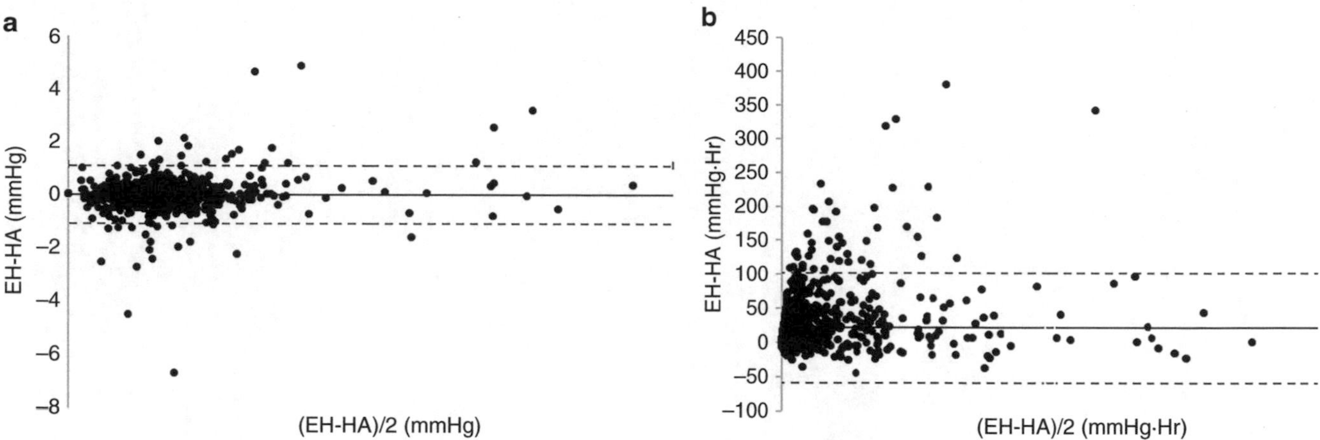

Fig. 1 Bland–Altman plots. In each plot, the mean difference is shown by a solid line and the limits of agreement are shown by dotted lines. (**a**) Mean intracranial pressure (ICP). (**b**) ICP dose. EH end-hour method, HA hour-averaged method

averaging patient measurements so that individual differences between the methods could be smoothed out. In particular, the relatively low *p* value in the *t* test performed on the ICP dose within the group that survived meant that the end-hour method was almost significantly different from the hour-averaged method. Therefore, the results did not indicate that one can make clinical decisions with confidence on the basis of individual end-hour mean ICP or ICP dose measurements during the management of TBI patients.

Acknowledgments M. Czosnyka is supported by the National Institute for Health Research (NIHR), Cambridge Biomedical Research Centre, Cambridge, UK.

Conflict of Interest: **ICM+ software is licensed by Cambridge Enterprise Ltd. (Cambridge, UK) (https://icmplus.neurosurg.cam.ac.uk). M. Czosnyka and P. Smielewski have a financial interest in a fraction of the licensing fee.**

References

1. Maas AIR, Menon DK, Adelson PD et al (2017) Traumatic brain injury: integrated approaches to improve prevention, clinical care, and research. Lancet Neurol 16(12):987–1048. https://doi.org/10.1016/S1474-4422(17)30371-X
2. Wells A, Smielewski P, Trivedi R, Hutchinson P (2020) Intracranial pressure monitoring in head injury. In: Whitfield P, Welbourne J, Thomas E, Summers F, Whyte M, Hutchinson P (eds) Traumatic brain injury: a multidisciplinary approach. Cambridge University Press, Cambridge, pp 110–131. https://doi.org/10.1017/9781108355247.013
3. Vik A, Nag T, Fredriksli OA, Skandsen T, Moen KG, Schirmer-Mikalsen K, Manley GT (2008) Relationship of "dose" of intracranial hypertension to outcome in severe traumatic brain injury. J Neurosurg 109(4):678–684. https://doi.org/10.3171/JNS/2008/109/10/0678
4. Zanier ER, Ortolano F, Ghisoni L, Colombo A, Losappio S, Stocchetti N (2007) Intracranial pressure monitoring in intensive care: clinical advantages of a computerized system over manual recording. Crit Care 11(1):R7. https://doi.org/10.1186/cc5155
5. Zeiler FA, Donnelly J, Menon DK, Smielewski P, Hutchinson PJA, Czosnyka M (2018) A description of a new continuous physiological index in traumatic brain injury using the correlation between pulse amplitude of intracranial pressure and cerebral perfusion pressure. J Neurotrauma 35(7):963–974. https://doi.org/10.1089/neu.2017.5241

External Hydrocephalus After Traumatic Brain Injury: Retrospective Study of 102 Patients

Laurent Gergelé, Romain Manet, A. Kolias, Marek Czosnyka, A. Lalou, Peter Smielewski, Peter J. Hutchinson, and Zofia H. Czosnyka

Introduction

External hydrocephalus (EH) has been described extensively in the paediatric population [1, 2], but there have been very few published reports on it in brain-injured adult patients, and this entity is probably not well known and is underestimated. In adults, EH refers to impairment of extra-axial cerebrospinal fluid (CSF) flow with enlargement of the subarachnoid space (SAS) concomitant to raised intracranial pressure (ICP) [3, 4] and alteration of CSF dynamics [5] but without ventriculomegaly. Occurrence of subarachnoid haemorrhage is probably a significant cause of EH. EH should not be confused with a subdural hygroma (Fig. 1), which is primarily caused by a vacuum effect on CSF precipitated by atrophic brain sinking without raised ICP [6]. In our practice, we regularly encounter patients with intracranial hypertension and imaging signs of EH. The aim of this study was to describe the incidence and consequences of EH in an adult population with traumatic brain injury (TBI).

L. Gergelé (✉)
Intensive Care Unit, Ramsay Santél, Hôpital Privé de la Loire, Saint Etienne, France

Brain Physics Laboratory, Division of Neurosurgery, Department of Clinical Neuroscience, Addenbrooke's Hospital, University of Cambridge, Cambridge, UK

R. Manet
Department of Neurosurgery B, Hôpital P. Wertheimer, Hospices Civiles de Lyon, Lyon, France

A. Kolias · M. Czosnyka · A. Lalou · P. Smielewski
P. J. Hutchinson · Z. H. Czosnyka
Brain Physics Laboratory, Division of Neurosurgery, Department of Clinical Neuroscience, Addenbrooke's Hospital, University of Cambridge, Cambridge, UK

Materials and Methods

A retrospective analysis was done of TBI patients admitted to Cambridge University Hospital (Cambridge, UK) between February 2014 and January 2017. The inclusion criteria were TBI requiring intensive care unit (ICU) admission with ICP monitoring and at least three CT scans within the first 21 days. Patients who underwent craniectomy were excluded. An individual SAS assessment was performed on each CT scan by two independent investigators (LG and RM). EH was diagnosed when SAS was assessed as being dilated or increased between two successive CT scans despite a context of intracranial hypertension. Both investigators had to agree for the diagnosis to be definitive. Data on demographics, the global Glasgow Coma Scale (GCS) score (especially the motor score (M score) component), TBI mechanism (a fall, motor vehicle collision, strike or other mechanism) and several CT scan severity scores (the Marshall, Helsinki, Stockholm and Rotterdam scores) were collected at admission to describe the population. The duration of mechanic ventilation, the incidence of tracheostomy and the duration of the ICU stay were also recorded to assess the impact of EH on the short-term patient course. We also assessed the long-term consequences of EH with use of the 6-month Glasgow Outcome Scale (GOS) and Glasgow Outcome Scale Extended (GOS-E) scores. The ICP data were analysed with ICM+ software (Cambridge Enterprise, Cambridge, UK). The effects of EH on the ICP course after TBI were assessed by measurement of the mean ICP in the 48 h before and after diagnosis of EH. We also checked the ICP course and several markers of brain compliance (the ICP amplitude, pulsatility, and compensatory reserve index (RAP)). The EH group was compared with the non-EH group to assess the consequences of development of EH on short- and long-term TBI evolution.

B. Depreitere et al. (eds.), *Intracranial Pressure and Neuromonitoring XVII*, Acta Neurochirurgica Supplement 131,
https://doi.org/10.1007/978-3-030-59436-7_8,

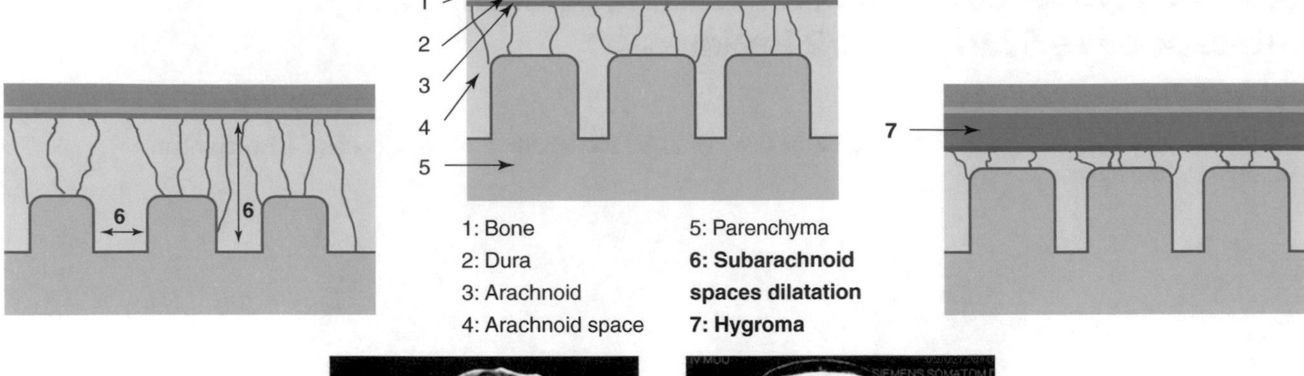

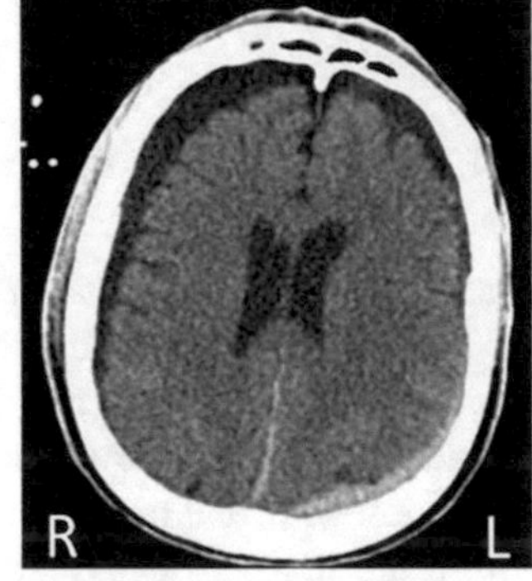

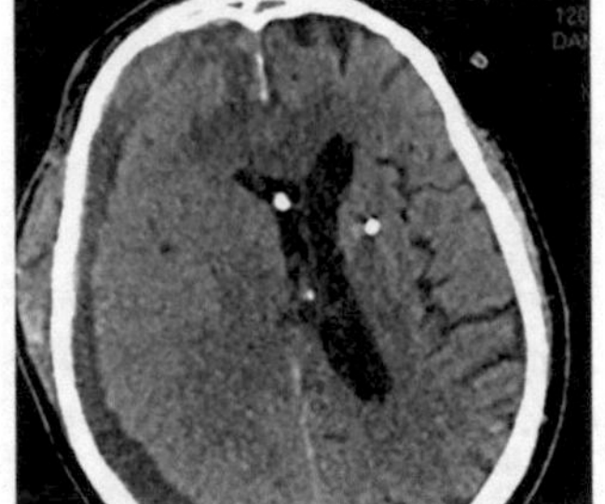

SIEMENS SOMATOM
Right Hygroma:
New space between dura and arachnoid with CSF draining and decreasing of subarachnoid spaces
R
L

Fig. 1 Difference between external hydrocephalus and a subdural hygroma. In patients with external hydrocephalus (in the subarachnoid spaces), the cerebrospinal fluid (CSF) diffuses in a physiological space, whereas in patients with a hygroma, CSF collects in a 'new' subdural space. Tears in the arachnoid membrane can probably explain mixed situations that are not described in this figure. (Reproduced from Gergelé et al. [7], with permission)

Results

During the study period, 143 patients met the study inclusion criteria. Of these, 41 patients were excluded after undergoing a craniectomy; thus, 102 patients were included in the final analysis, and 31 of them (30.4%) developed EH.

The mean time to development of EH after TBI was 2.98 ± 2.4 days. The patients in the EH group were slightly older than those in the non-EH group. The clinical severity, expressed by the global GCS score and its M score component, was equivalent in both groups. The Marshall and Rotterdam CT scan scores did not differ. The other CT scan scores were worse in the EH group. Post-traumatic subarachnoid haemorrhage plays an important part in the Helsinki and Stockholm scores, which explains the significant differences in these scores between the two groups. Indeed, the part of the Stockholm score that describes traumatic subarachnoid haemorrhage (t-SAH) was significantly higher in the EH group (Table 1).

In univariate analysis, risk factors for EH development were the patient's age and t-SAH score. In multivariate analysis, only the t-SAH score remained an independent risk factor for development of EH after TBI. A Stockholm t-SAH CT scan score of ≤2 was protective against EH, with an odds ratio 0.285 [0.105; 0.712] p<0.01.

Table 1 Principal characteristics of patients with and without external hydrocephalus (EH) in this study

	EH group ($N = 31$)[a]	Non-EH group ($N = 71$)[a]	*P* value
Age (years)	51.7 ± 17.2	44.1 ± 18.4	0.048
Female/male ratio (*n*)	5/26	19/52	NS
Global GCS score	8.1 ± 3.4	8.4 ± 4.0	NS
GCS M score component	3.8 ± 1.9	4.0 ± 1.7	NS
Marshall CT scan score	3.2 ± 1.5	3.3 ± 1.5	NS
Rotterdam CT scan score	3.4 ± 0.9	3.2 ± 1.1	NS
Helsinki CT scan score	4.1 ± 3.4	2.9 ± 1.2	0.041
Stockholm CT scan score	2.9 ± 1.2	1.5 ± 1.3	<0.001
Stockholm CT t-SAH score	3.8 ± 1.5	2.2 ± 1.7	<0.001

CT computed tomography, *GCS* Glasgow Coma Scale, *M score* motor score, *NS* nonsignificant, *t-SAH* traumatic subarachnoid haemorrhage
[a]The values are expressed as mean ± standard deviation except for the female/male ratio

Table 2 Short-term and long-term evolution of patients with and without external hydrocephalus (EH) in this study

	EH group ($N = 31$)[a]	Non-EH group ($N = 71$)[a]	P value
Duration of mechanical ventilation (days)	19.4 ± 11.4	12.5 ± 10.8	0.02
Duration of ICU stay (days)	26.6 ± 12.9	18.1 ± 13.7	0.008
CT/MRI scanning within the first 21 days (n)	6.1 ± 2.1	4.7 ± 3.2	0.024
Tracheostomy (n%)	17/54,8	23/32,4%	0.033
Secondary CSF shunt in survivors (%)	17.4	1.8	0.018
Secondary ventricular dilation (%)	58	14	<0.01
GOS score	3.5 ± 1.3	3.5 ± 1.6	NS
GOS score in survivors	3.9 ± 0.8	4.2 ± 0.9	NS
GOS-E score	4.2 ± 2.1	4.7 ± 2.8	NS
GOS-E score in survivors	4.6 ± 1.8	5.9 ± 2.0	0.0096

CSF cerebrospinal fluid, *CT* computed tomography, *GOS* Glasgow Outcome Scale, *GOS-E* Glasgow Outcome Scale Extended, *ICU* intensive care unit, *MRI* magnetic resonance imaging, *NS* nonsignificant
[a]The values are expressed as mean ± standard deviation except for those expressed as a percentage

The patients in the EH group had a longer duration of mechanical ventilation (19.4 versus 12.5 days), were more likely to have a tracheostomy (54,8% versus 32,43%) and had a longer ICU stay (26.6 versus 18.1 days, $P = 0.002$) (Table 2). When we considered the survivors, those in the EH group had a worse long-term outcome (mean GOS-E score 4.6 versus 5.9, $P = 0.031$) and were more likely to have secondary hydrocephalus requiring management with shunting (17.4% versus 1.8%, OR 7.1).

Data for analysis of the ICP course for 48 h before and after diagnosis of EH were available for only eight patients. In this small EH subgroup, the mean ICP was higher after diagnosis of EH (14.7 ± 5.5 mmHg) than before it (8.1 ± 1.6 mmHg, $P = 0.0018$).

Discussion

In our analysis of SAS volumes after severe TBI, we found that 30.4% of EH cases had significant clinical consequences. The EH group had a worse course in the ICU (a longer duration of mechanical ventilation, a longer ICU stay, more CT/MRI scans and a higher incidence of tracheostomy). The EH group also had a worse long-term prognosis, with higher incidence rates of ventricular dilatation and secondary hydrocephalus requiring a shunt, and a worse GOS-E score in survivors.

The incidence of EH in the current series was coherent with rates of EH previously observed after aneurysmal haemorrhage. Yoshimoto et al. reported that 38% of patients with aneurysmal SAH developed EH 8 [8]. Despite its high incidence, there is definitely underreporting of this problem in the literature and thus in the medical population, which is likely a consequence of the difficulty of diagnosing EH. Although the CSF in the SAS is not easily visible, particularly in the cortical sulci, it still represents an important volume. A 2-mm increase in the thickness of the CSF layer surrounding the brain represents an inflation of the total CSF volume of more than 100 mL and may explain difficulties in controlling ICP [3, 9]. However, such a 2-mm increase can be difficult to diagnose visually; hence, it requires very accurate analysis of CT scans. As a result, in TBI patients with raised ICP, abnormal brain compliance or difficulty in waking up, CT scans must be checked carefully for signs of EH. Several signs of EH that may be observed on CT scans have been described previously: frontal extra-axial fluid collection, inter-hemispheric CSF accumulation, abnormally wide cortical sulci, an abnormally large Sylvian fissure and large basal cisterns [3, 4]. While these signs can help the physician to recognise EH, its diagnosis may still remain a challenging problem. The most helpful approach is to compare consecutive CT scan images in order to detect subtle changes in SAS size and particularly changes in CSF thickness in the cortical sulci.

The confusion between EH and hygroma represents an additional challenge, which has been emphasised in all publications on adult EH. The differentiation is important because CSF drainage is the treatment of choice for EH, whereas drainage would exacerbate a hygroma. Figure 1 summarises the differences between EH and hygroma. In addition to CT scan considerations, ICP has been proposed as a means to differentiate between EH and hygroma after TBI. Huh et al. analysed ICP before removing an extra-axial collection diagnosed after TBI. They found higher ICP in patients with EH than in those with a subdural hygroma (21.7 versus 7.7 mmHg) [6]. In our study, we also observed an increase in ICP after development of EH.

We found that the presence and severity of SAH was the main risk factor for development of EH after TBI. This finding supports the pathophysiological hypothesis that EH is caused by arachnoid villus obstruction due to the presence of blood. Depending on the quantity of blood in the subarachnoid space, and depending on patient factors, EH can take a couple of days to develop. In our series, we found that EH developed at an interval of about 3 days after TBI. This could probably partly explain the secondary increase in ICP we observed after day 4, which has previously been described in 25% of TBI patients [10].

The main limitation of our study was in the visual assessment of SAS size. To increase accuracy, we used a double CT scan reading by two investigators. However, to further improve accuracy, automated CSF volume calculation may be helpful to avoid misdiagnosis or over-diagnosis of EH.

Despite comparable characteristics on admission, the EH group definitely had worse short-term and long-term outcomes. However, EH can be treated easily by CSF drainage [3]. Therefore, we propose to carefully check SAS changes in patients in whom ICP increases secondarily few days after the accident.

Conclusion

EH is frequent and has significant clinical consequences. As it is difficult to diagnose, we propose to develop automated repeated CT scan analyses to help clinicians diagnose EH and differentiate it from a subdural hygroma. This is even more important, since EH can be treated easily by CSF drainage.

Acknowledgments M. Czosnyka is supported by the National Institute for Health Research (NIHR), Cambridge Biomedical Research Centre, Cambridge, UK.

Dr. Benjamin Singh (ActiFS Laboratory, Saint Etienne, France) provided assistance with English editing of this manuscript.

Conflict of Interest: **ICM+ software is licensed by Cambridge Enterprise Ltd. (Cambridge, UK) (https://icmplus.neurosurg.cam.ac.uk). P. Smielewski and M. Czosnyka have a financial interest in a fraction of the licensing fee.**

References

1. Fingarson AK, Ryan ME, McLone SG, Bregman C, Flaherty EG (2017) Enlarged subarachnoid spaces and intracranial hemorrhage in children with accidental head trauma. J Neurosurg Pediatr 19(2):254–258
2. Zahl SM, Egge A, Helseth E, Wester K (2011) Benign external hydrocephalus: a review, with emphasis on management. Neurosurg Rev 34(4):417–432
3. Manet R, Payen J-F, Guerin R, Martinez O, Hautefeuille S, Francony G, Gergelé L (2017) Using external lumbar CSF drainage to treat communicating external hydrocephalus in adult patients after acute traumatic or non-traumatic brain injury. Acta Neurochir 159(10):2003–2009
4. Maytal J, Alvarez LA, Elkin CM, Shinnar S (1987) External hydrocephalus: radiologic spectrum and differentiation from cerebral atrophy. AJR Am J Roentgenol 148(6):1223–1230
5. Marmarou A, Foda MA, Bandoh K, Yoshihara M, Yamamoto T, Tsuji O, Zasler N, Ward JD, Young HF (1996) Posttraumatic ventriculomegaly: hydrocephalus or atrophy? A new approach for diagnosis using CSF dynamics. J Neurosurg 85(6):1026–1035
6. Huh P-W, Yoo D-S, Cho K-S, Park C-K, Kang S-G, Park Y-S, Kim D-S, Kim M-C (2006) Diagnostic method for differentiating external hydrocephalus from simple subdural hygroma. J Neurosurg 105(1):65–70. https://doi.org/10.3171/jns.2006.105.1.65
7. Geregelé L, Baledent O, Manet R, Lalou A, Barszcz S, Kasprowicz M, Smielewski P, Pickard JD, Czosnyka M (2019) Dynamics of cerebrospinal fluid: from theoretical models to clinical applications. In: Miller K (ed) Biomechanics of the brain, 2nd edn. Springer, Cham, pp 181–214
8. Yoshimoto Y, Wakai S, Hamano M (1998) External hydrocephalus after aneurysm surgery: paradoxical response to ventricular shunting. J Neurosurg 88(3):485–489
9. Rekate HL, Nadkarni TD, Wallace D (2008) The importance of the cortical subarachnoid space in understanding hydrocephalus. J Neurosurg Pediatr 2(1):1–11
10. Stocchetti N, Colombo A, Ortolano F, Videtta W, Marchesi R, Longhi L, Zanier ER (2007) Time course of intracranial hypertension after traumatic brain injury. J Neurotrauma 24(8):1339–1346

Analysis of Cardio-Cerebral Crosstalk Events in an Adult Cohort from the CENTER-TBI Study

Giovanna Maria Dimitri, Erta Beqiri, Marek Czosnyka, Ari Ercole, Peter Smielewski, Pietro Lio, and CENTER-TBI High Resolution Substudy Participants and Investigators

Introduction

Treatment and management of traumatic brain injury (TBI) remains a leading research priority in clinical practice, with TBI being a worldwide cause of death and disabilities [1, 2]. Although there is a focus on brain-monitoring information such as the intracranial pressure (ICP), importance should also be given to the interaction between the brain and the heart. Previous research in this field has shown the presence of bidirectional causality between ICP, the mean arterial pressure (MAP) and the heart rate (HR) in a 24-h period post-TBI, and has linked this to the mortality rate [3].

This interest in the interaction between the brain's and the heart's homeostatic processes is, in fact, part of a wide field of research that has been developed in the last few years [4]. The physiological coupling between the two systems has been shown to be an important signal and biomarker for pathological and traumatic events [4].

The senior authors Peter Smielewski and Pietro Lio contributed equally to this work.

CENTER-TBI High Resolution Substudy Participants and Investigators

G. M. Dimitri (✉) · P. Lio
Computer Laboratory, University of Cambridge, Cambridge, UK
e-mail: gmd43@cl.cam.ac.uk

E. Beqiri
Brain Physics Laboratory, Division of Neurosurgery, Department of Clinical Neuroscience, University of Cambridge, Cambridge, UK

Department of Anaesthesia, University of Cambridge, Cambridge, UK

Department of Physiology and Transplantation, Milan University, Milan, Italy

M. Czosnyka · A. Ercole · P. Smielewski
Brain Physics Laboratory, Division of Neurosurgery, Department of Clinical Neuroscience, University of Cambridge, Cambridge, UK

In our previous study of paediatric patients, we observed the presence of simultaneous onsets of transient increases in ICP and HR, and we related the number of such events to patient outcomes [5]. In this chapter, we present an extension of that work to an adult cohort from the Collaborative European NeuroTrauma Effectiveness Research in TBI (CENTER-TBI) study to explore the relationship between cardio-cerebral crosstalks (CC) behaviour and patient outcomes.

Data Set

The data used for the present analysis were collected from a subset cohort of the CENTER-TBI study, a consortium established in 2011 with the goal of improving classification and treatment of patients with TBI [6]. The data were collected in accordance with national or local regulatory ethics requirements. The CENTER-TBI study (supported by European Commission grant number 602150) was conducted in accordance with European regulations where applicable and the relevant regulations in the countries where the recruiting sites were based. Among those regulations are laws regarding privacy, data protection and human material, and guidance documents related to clinical studies (for example, the International Council for Harmonisation of Technical Requirements for Pharmaceuticals for Human Use (ICH) Harmonised Tripartite Guideline for Good Clinical Practice (CPMP/ICH/135/95) and the World Medical Association's Declaration of Helsinki, titled 'Ethical Principles for Medical Research Involving Human Subjects'). Informed consent was obtained from patients and/or their legal representatives/next of kin, in accordance with local regulations, for recruitment of all patients into the CENTER-TBI core data set and documented in the electronic case report form (e-CRF).

As part of the recruitment process, demographic and clinical data were collected prospectively, together with intensive care unit (ICU) monitoring information. ICP data were

B. Depreitere et al. (eds.), *Intracranial Pressure and Neuromonitoring XVII*, Acta Neurochirurgica Supplement 131,
https://doi.org/10.1007/978-3-030-59436-7_9, © Springer Nature Switzerland AG 2021

collected via an intraparenchymal strain gauge probe (Codman ICP MicroSensor, Codman & Shurtleff, Raynham, MA, USA), a parenchymal fibre-optic pressure sensor (Camino ICP Monitor, Integra Life Sciences, Plainsboro, NJ, USA; https://www.integralife.com/) or an external ventricular drain. The signals were recorded through digital data transfer or alternatively digitized using an analogue/digital (A/D) converter (DT9801, Data Translation, Marlboro, MA, USA), where appropriate, sampled at a frequency of 100 Hz or higher, using ICM+ software (Cambridge Enterprise Ltd., Cambridge, UK; http://icmplus.neurosurg.cam.ac.uk) or a Moberg CNS Monitor (Moberg Research, Ambler, PA, USA). For the purpose of the present study, 271 patients from the CENTER-TBI high-resolution subcohort were screened. Only patients without an external ventricular drain and with both good-quality data and outcome data available at the time of the analysis ($N = 226$) were included in this analysis. ICP and HR waveforms were processed with ICM+ software [7]. Demographic data as per version 1.0 were retrieved. The outcome variable we considered in the present analysis was a binary variable indicating patient mortality.

Methods

High-resolution waveforms were partially cleaned manually to remove larger sections of invalid data, and partially cleaned automatically to exclude non-physiological transient events such as arterial line–flushing periods. The waveforms were then down-sampled to 0.1 Hz by coarse graining using a 10-s moving average filter. For each patient, the whole monitored period was considered.

We then used our own sliding window approach to detect the presence of CC events in the 0.1-Hz time series, as had been done in our previous paediatric cohort study [5]. Briefly, the algorithm considered 10-min subwindows of observations and if simultaneous increases of at least 20% in ICP and HR occurred with respect to the minimum ICP and HR values in the time windows, then a CC event was detected (Fig. 1).

Since the total length of the recordings varied between patients, we normalized the number of CC events per patient by dividing it by the total number of data points in the time series.

We denominated the normalized CC measure *Ct_np*. This measure was the ratio between the absolute number of observations and the total length of the time series. For subsequent statistical analysis, the patient cohort was split into a mortality group (patients who died) and a non-mortality group (patients who survived) and the normalized counts of CC events were compared between the groups. The point biserial correlation coefficient [8] between the number of CC events and mortality was then computed.

Results

The analysis included 180 male and 46 female patients. The age range was 16–85 (mean 47) years. The raw number of CC events detected was, on average, 50 per patient, with a large standard deviation of 58. The distribution of the number of normalized CC events per patient is shown in Fig. 2. We then computed the point biserial correlation coefficient between the new variable and mortality, obtaining a point biserial correlation coefficient of −0.13. A box plot chart of

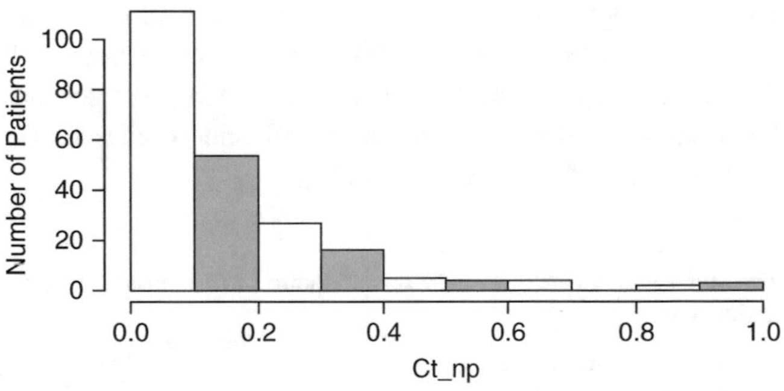

Fig. 2 Distribution of normalized cardio-cerebral crosstalk events per patient in the adult cohort

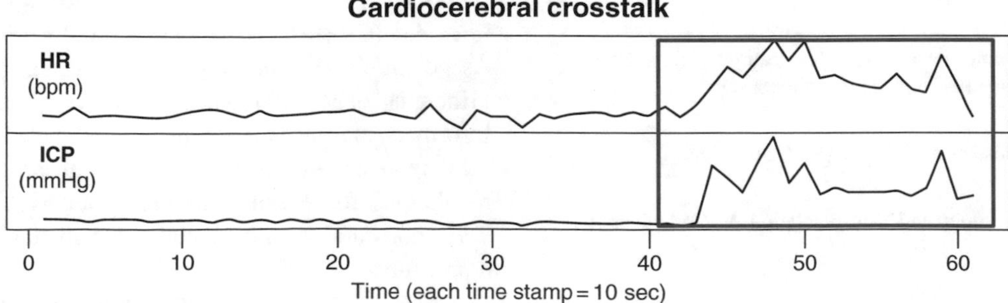

Fig. 1 Presence of cardio-cerebral crosstalk events (highlighted with a *blue square*) in 10-min observations of the heart rate (HR; measured in beats/min (bpm)) and intracranial pressure (ICP; measured in mmHg) in one patient in our cohort. Each timestamp on the *x*-axis corresponds to 10 s of observations

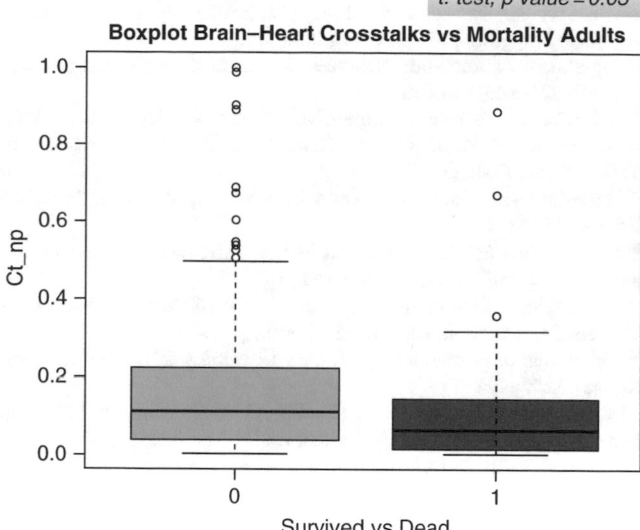

Fig. 3 Box plot showing the distribution of cardio-cerebral crosstalk events and mortality in the cohort analysed. The box plot shows a larger number of crosstalk events in the survivors. The Welch two-sample *t* test of the two vectors of crosstalk events in the two groups of dead and surviving patients yielded a significant *p* value of 0.03

mortality with respect to the distribution of the number of normalized CC events is shown in Fig. 3.

The median value of *Ct_np* in the case of mortality was 0.064, while in the case of non-mortality it corresponded to 0.11, as shown in the figure. Moreover, in Fig. 3, we can also see the resulting *p* value from the Welch two-sample *t* test between the two vectors of *Ct_np* (in the cases of mortality and non-mortality). The Welch two-sample *t* test was chosen because of its greater reliability with unequal sample sizes. The test returned a significant *p* value of 0.03, therefore exhibiting a significant difference between the *Ct_np* distributions in the cases of mortality and non-mortality. This finding was interesting, as it confirmed our previous findings in the paediatric cohort [5]. At the same time, it showed slightly different behaviour. In fact, although the correlation was slightly weaker than that observed in the paediatric cohort (in which the point biserial correlation coefficient value was −0.30), the negative sign of the correlation was replicated.

Discussion and Conclusion

In this work, we have presented a computational workflow in which we first computed the presence of events of simultaneous increases in ICP and HR, and then we related this phenomenon to mortality in patients with TBI. The quantification of the number of CC events was pursued using the sliding window algorithm proposed by Dimitri et al. [5]. Here, simultaneous subwindows of 10-min observations of ICP and HR were considered and a CC was detected if increases of at least 20% in ICP and HR occurred with respect to the minimum ICP and HR values in the time windows. The values of 10 min and a 20% increase were retained in this work so that it would be comparable with our previous paediatric study.

We are aware that identification of only such events of simultaneous increases may be a limitation of the present study. However, we leave to future work the investigation of different time window sizes in which such CC events may be detected. Analysis of the CC vectors for the cases of mortality and non-mortality also yielded interesting results. First of all, from the Welch two-sample *t* test, a significant *p* value of 0.03 was detected, showing a significant difference between the two cases of mortality and non-mortality when CC distributions were considered. No significant difference in the number of CC events between sexes was found. The CC events were then related to patient mortality, and we detected consistency with the results previously obtained in the paediatric cohort. The negative direction of the correlation between mortality and the number of CC events was retained between the two cohorts. However, the adult cohort from the CENTER-TBI study presented a lower correlation value (−0.13) than that observed in the paediatric cohort (−0.30). In both cases, however, the more CC events occurred, the better the patient outcome was. This is an interesting finding, as it sheds more light on healthy cardiovascular interactions between the brain and the heart [5]. This study could be enriched along many different paths; these represent limitations of the study and future directions for the work presented. The parameters of the sliding window algorithm could be varied according to different clinical hypothesis to be tested—for example, the size of the time windows considered in the sliding window algorithm, as well as the percentage increase with respect to the minimum ICP and HR values in the time windows. Moreover, more variables (such as the mean ICP, cerebral autoregulation, Glasgow Coma Scale score and age) could be included in multivariate modelling of the system.

Acknowledgments This study was supported by a European Union Seventh Framework Program grant (number 602150) for the Collaborative European NeuroTrauma Effectiveness Research in Traumatic Brain Injury (CENTER-TBI) study.

CENTER-TBI High Resolution (HR ICU) Substudy Participants and Investigators: Audny Anke[1], Ronny Beer[2], Bo-Michael Bellander[3], Andras Buki[5], Manuel Cabeleira[6], Marco Carbonara[7], Arturo Chieregato[4], Giuseppe Citerio[8,9], Endre Czeiter[10], Bart Depreitere[11], Shirin Frisvold[13], Raimund Helbok[2], Stefan Jankowski[14], Danile Kondziella[15], Lars-Owe Koskinen[16], Ana Kowark[17], David K. Menon[12], Geert Meyfroidt[18], Kirsten Moeller[19], David Nelson[3], Anna Piippo-Karjalainen[20], Andreea Radoi[21], Arminas Ragauskas[22], Rahul Raj[20], Jonathan Rhodes[23], Saulius Rocka[22], Rolf Rossaint[17], Juan Sahuquillo[21],

Oliver Sakowitz[24,25], Nino Stocchetti[26], Nina Sundström[27], Riikka Takala[28], Tomas Tamosuitis[29], Olli Tenovuo[30], Peter Vajkoczy[31], Alessia Vargiolu[8], Rimantas Vilcinis[32], Stefan Wolf[33], Alexander Younsi[25], Frederick A. Zeiler[12,34]

[1]Department of Physical Medicine and Rehabilitation, University Hospital Northern Norway, Tromso, Norway
[2]Department of Neurology, Neurological Intensive Care Unit, Medical University of Innsbruck, Innsbruck, Austria
[3]Department of Neurosurgery & Anesthesia & Intensive Care Medicine, Karolinska University Hospital, Stockholm, Sweden
[4]NeuroIntensive Care, Niguarda Hospital, Milan, Italy
[5]Department of Neurosurgery, Medical School, University of Pécs; and Neurotrauma Research Group, János Szentágothai Research Centre, University of Pécs, Pécs, Hungary
[6]Brain Physics Lab, Division of Neurosurgery, Dept of Clinical Neurosciences, University of Cambridge, Addenbrooke's Hospital, Cambridge, UK
[7]Neuro ICU, Fondazione IRCCS Cà Granda Ospedale Maggiore Policlinico, Milan, Italy
[8]NeuroIntensive Care Unit, Department of Anesthesia & Intensive Care, ASST di Monza, Monza, Italy
[9]School of Medicine and Surgery, Università Milano Bicocca, Milano, Italy
[10]Department of Neurosurgery, University of Pécs; MTA-PTE Clinical Neuroscience MR Research Group and János Szentágothai Research Centre, University of Pécs; and Hungarian Brain Research Program (grant number KTIA 13 NAP-A-II/8), Pécs, Hungary
[11]Department of Neurosurgery, University Hospitals Leuven, Leuven, Belgium
[12]Division of Anaesthesia, University of Cambridge, Addenbrooke's Hospital, Cambridge, UK
[13]Department of Anesthesiology and Intensive Care, University Hospital Northern Norway, Tromso, Norway
[14]Neurointensive Care, Sheffield Teaching Hospitals NHS Foundation Trust, Sheffield, UK
[15]Departments of Neurology, Clinical Neurophysiology and Neuroanesthesiology, Region Hovedstaden Rigshospitalet, Copenhagen, Denmark
[16]Department of Clinical Neuroscience, Neurosurgery, Umeå University, Umeå, Sweden
[17]Department of Anaesthesiology, University Hospital of Aachen, Aachen, Germany
[18]Intensive Care Medicine, University Hospitals Leuven, Leuven, Belgium
[19]Department of Neuroanesthesiology, Region Hovedstaden Rigshospitalet, Copenhagen, Denmark
[20]Helsinki University Central Hospital, Helsinki, Finland
[21]Department of Neurosurgery, Vall d'Hebron University Hospital, Barcelona, Spain
[22]Department of Neurosurgery, Kaunas University of Technology and Vilnius University, Vilnius, Lithuania
[23]Department of Anaesthesia, Critical Care & Pain Medicine, NHS Lothian & University of Edinburgh, Edinburgh, UK
[24]Klinik für Neurochirurgie, Klinikum Ludwigsburg, Ludwigsburg, Germany
[25]Department of Neurosurgery, University Hospital Heidelberg, Heidelberg, Germany
[26]Department of Pathophysiology and Transplantation, Milan University; and Neuroscience ICU, Fondazione IRCCS Cà Granda Ospedale Maggiore Policlinico, Milano, Italy
[27]Department of Radiation Sciences, Biomedical Engineering, Umeå University, Umeå, Sweden
[28]Perioperative Services, Intensive Care Medicine and Pain Management, Turku University Central Hospital and University of Turku, Turku, Finland
[29]Neuro-intensive Care Unit, Kaunas University of Health Sciences, Kaunas, Lithuania
[30]Rehabilitation and Brain Trauma, Turku University Central Hospital and University of Turku, Turku, Finland
[31]Neurologie, Neurochirurgie und Psychiatrie, Charité – Universitätsmedizin Berlin, Berlin, Germany
[32]Department of Neurosurgery, Kaunas University of Health Sciences, Kaunas, Lithuania
[33]Department of Neurosurgery, Charité – Universitätsmedizin Berlin; corporate member of Freie Universität Berlin; Humboldt-Universität zu Berlin; and Berlin Institute of Health, Berlin, Germany
[34]Section of Neurosurgery, Department of Surgery, Rady Faculty of Health Sciences, University of Manitoba, Winnipeg, MB, Canada

References

1. Czosnyka M, Pickard JD (2004) Monitoring and interpretation of intracranial pressure. J Neurol Neurosurg Psychiatry 75(6):813–821
2. Hu X, Xu P, Scalzo F, Vespa P, Bergsneider M (2009) Morphological clustering and analysis of continuous intracranial pressure. IEEE Trans Biomed Eng 56(3):696–705
3. Gao L, Smielewski P, Czosnyka M, Ercole A (2017) Early asymmetric cardio-cerebral causality and outcome after severe traumatic brain injury. J Neurotrauma 34(19):2743–2752
4. Valenza G, Toschi N, Barbieri R (2016) Uncovering brain–heart information through advanced signal and image processing. Phil Trans R Soc A 374:20160020. https://doi.org/10.1098/rsta.2016.0020
5. Dimitri GM, Agrawal S, Young A, Donnelly J, Liu X, Smielewski P, Hutchinson P, Czosnyka M, Lio' P, Haubrich C (2018) Simultaneous transients of intracranial pressure and heart rate in traumatic brain injury: methods of analysis. In: Heldt T (ed) Intracranial pressure & neuromonitoring XVI. Springer, Cham, pp 147–151
6. Maas AI, Menon DK, Steyerberg EW, Citerio G, Lecky F, Manley GT, Hill S, Legrand V, Sorgner A (2014) Collaborative European Neurotrauma Effectiveness Research in Traumatic Brain Injury (CENTER-TBI): a prospective longitudinal observational study. Neurosurgery 76(1):67–80
7. Smielewski P, Czosnyka M, Steiner L, Belestri M, Piechnik S, Pickard JD (2005) ICM+: software for on-line analysis of bedside monitoring data after severe head trauma. In: Poon WS, Avezaat CJJ, Chan M, Czosnyka M, Goh K, Hutchinson PJA, Katayama Y, Lam JMK, Marmarou A, Ng SCP, Pickard JD (eds) Intracranial pressure and brain monitoring XII. Springer, Vienna, pp. 43–49
8. Linacre J, Rasch G (2008) The expected value of a point–biserial (or similar) correlation. Rasch MeasureTrans 22(1):1154

Cerebrovascular Consequences of Elevated Intracranial Pressure After Traumatic Brain Injury

Leanne Alexis Calviello, Frederick A. Zeiler, Joseph Donnelly, András Czigler, Andrea Lavinio, Peter J. Hutchinson, Marek Czosnyka, and Peter Smielewski

Introduction

Intracranial pressure (ICP) is a reference pressure for cerebral blood flow (CBF). It is well documented that elevated ICP (>20 mmHg) after TBI increases the risk of a worse outcome independently of low cerebral perfusion pressure (CPP) or the severity of the primary injury [1]. However, the outcome cannot be predicted on the basis of ICP alone. It has been shown that the impact of the insults from intracranial hypertension depends heavily on other factors, including CPP and the state of hemodynamic homeostasis [2]. These mechanisms work to protect the brain against the secondary brain damage brought about by pathological processes unfolding during the first few days following acute brain trauma that could lead to severe brain swelling. It is now widely accepted in the neurocritical care community that routine measurement of ICP should, if possible, be augmented by other modalities reflecting CBF, such as the cerebral oxygen partial tension ($PbtO_2$) or the velocity of blood in the arteries comprising the circle of Willis (using transcranial Doppler ultrasound (TCD)). With appropriate software tools, these modalities can also provide clinicians with further information about the state of the cerebrovascular system, from either cerebrovascular impedance or the critical closing pressure (CrCP), the latter providing indications of arterial blood pressure ischemic thresholds [3]. Individually, these various indices of cerebral hemodynamics have been previously studied in a population of TBI patients, with well-established associations with outcome [4]. What is missing is a more conceptual picture of what happens to those indices when ICP is significantly elevated. Therefore, this study examined the effects of intracranial hypertension on cerebral autoregulation and on other cerebrovascular properties in patients with TBI by comparing two distinctive groups of patients: one group with significantly elevated ICP and another group with normal ICP. It aimed to provide a clear description of the differences in the physiology/pathophysiology of cerebral hemodynamics in those two groups and their resulting consequences for patient outcome.

Materials and Methods

For this analysis, we used a data set acquired from patients with severe TBI monitored in the Neurosciences Critical Care Unit (NCCU) at Addenbrooke's Hospital, Cambridge, UK ($N = 1023$), with continuous recordings of ICP and arterial blood pressure (ABP). From this data set of over 1000 patients, we selected 517 patients with, on average, elevated ICP (>23 mmHg) or normal ICP (<15 mmHg). The value of 23 mmHg is a critical level of ICP from the standpoint of differentiation between survival and mortality, whereas 15 mmHg is a consensus-accepted threshold for normal ICP.

The senior authors Marek Czosnyka and Peter Smielewski contributed equally to this work.

L. A. Calviello · J. Donnelly · P. J. Hutchinson · M. Czosnyka
P. Smielewski (✉)
Division of Neurosurgery, Department of Clinical Neurosciences, University of Cambridge, Cambridge, UK
e-mail: ps10011@cam.ac.uk

F. A. Zeiler
Division of Anesthesia, University of Cambridge, Cambridge, UK

Department of Surgery, Rady Faculty of Health Sciences, University of Manitoba, Winnipeg, MB, Canada

A. Czigler
Department of Neurosurgery, University of Pécs, Pécs, Hungary

A. Lavinio
Division of Anesthesia, Department of Medicine, Addenbrooke's Hospital, Cambridge, UK

B. Depreitere et al. (eds.), *Intracranial Pressure and Neuromonitoring XVII*, Acta Neurochirurgica Supplement 131,
https://doi.org/10.1007/978-3-030-59436-7_10,

All patients were sedated with a mixture of propofol, fentanyl, and midazolam, and mechanically ventilated. Seventy-five percent of patients presented with an admission Glasgow Coma Scale (GCS) score of <9 and were treated with a graded management protocol aiming to keep CPP above 60–70 mmHg and ICP at <20 mmHg. Six-month Glasgow Outcome Scale (GOS) data were collected for all of these patients. ABP was monitored invasively from the radial artery via pressure monitoring kits (Baxter Healthcare, Deerfield, IL, USA). ICP was monitored with invasive intraparenchymal probes equipped with strain gauge sensors (Codman & Shurtleff, Raynham, MA, USA, or Camino Laboratories, San Diego, CA, USA) inserted predominantly into the right frontal lobe. A subpopulation of patients (n = 109) had $PbtO_2$ monitoring via invasive parenchymal monitoring, typically placed in the right frontal lobe. These monitors were co-inserted with ICP monitors via a bolt. $PbtO_2$ monitoring was conducted with a Licox probe (Licox Brain Oxygen Monitoring System, Integra LifeSciences, Plainsboro, NJ, USA). Finally, in 193 patients, TCD assessment of middle cerebral artery (MCA) cerebral blood flow velocity (CBFV) was conducted via a Doppler-Box (Compumedics, Singen, Germany) or Neuroguard (Medasonic, Fremont, CA, USA) on the side of the ICP microtransducer placement, or on the opposite side if the TCD signal window was better there. The data were recorded digitally at a minimum of 100 Hz using ICM+® software (https://icmplus.neurosurg.cam.ac.uk) or, before 2003, at 50 Hz, using its predecessors ICM and WREC (Warsaw University of Technology, Warsaw, Poland). The early data sets did not include full raw data recordings; in those patients, only a subset of the calculated indices was available for analysis, with no possibility of recalculation. Post-acquisition, the data were further processed using ICM+ software where raw data were available. Signal artifacts were removed either manually or by using automated detection criteria. CPP was calculated as the difference between the mean ABP and ICP signals.

Tables 1 and 2 present various secondary indices that were calculated using a sliding window approach (with a calculation update rate of 1 min, whereas the window length, and thus the window overlap, varied depending on the index, and this is specified in the tables). Table 1 lists the parameters that were extracted from ICP and ABP signals alone and thus were present in the whole cohort of analyzed patients. Table 2 lists all of the TCD-derived parameters, which were present only in a subset of patients. The statistical significance of differences between the normal- and elevated-ICP groups was determined via the Mann–Whitney U test, with an alpha value of 0.05. Given that this analysis was an exploration of multimodal defined cerebrovascular parameters during normal ICP and intracranial hypertension (i.e., ICP >23 mmHg), we elected to not correct for multiple comparisons, in keeping with the methods used in other physiological exploratory studies.

This study was conducted as a retrospective analysis of a prospectively maintained database cohort, in which high-frequency monitoring data had been archived. Monitoring of brain modalities was conducted as a part of standard NCCU patient care, using an anonymized database of physiological monitoring variables in neurocritical care. Patient outcome data were extracted from hospital records and fully anonymized; no data on patient identifiers were available, and thus no separate ethical approval nor formal patient or proxy consent was sought.

Table 1 Lists of metrics extracted from ICP and ABP waveforms alone, and thus present in the whole cohort of analysed patients, calculated using a sliding window approach. Actual length (duration) of the sliding window (termed calculation window) is provided. For all the calculations the sliding windows were moved by 1 min, at a time, thus introducing a varying level of overlap

Index	Description	Calculation window [s]
PRx	Pressure reactivity index [5]	300
HR	Heart rate	60
AMP	Fundamental amplitude of pulse wave of ICP	60
SLOW	Amplitude of slow waves of ICP	1200
PAx	Pulse amplitude index (correlation between AMP and mean ABP) [6]	300
RAC	Correlation between AMP and CPP [7]	300

CPP cerebral perfusion pressure

Table 2 Lists of metrics extracted from TCD waveforms, and thus present only in a subset of analysed patients, calculated using a sliding window approach. Actual length (duration) of the sliding window (termed calculation window) is provided. For all the calculations the sliding windows were moved by 1 min, at a time, thus introducing a varying level of overlap

Index	Description	Calculation window [s]
Mx	Mean flow index (coefficient of correlation between CBFV and CPP) [8]	300
CrCP	Critical closing pressure (ABP at which blood flow ceases) [3]	60
DCM	Diastolic closing margin (= diastolic ABP – CrCP) [3]	60
sPI	Spectral pulsatility index (F1/CBFVm)	60
ARI	Autoregulation index (transfer function-based grading index) [8]	300

ABP arterial blood pressure, *CBFV* cerebral blood flow velocity, *CBFVm* mean CBFV, *CPP* cerebral perfusion pressure, *F1* fundamental pulse amplitude of CBFV

Results

Examples of selected recorded cerebrovascular variables are provided in Figs. 1, 2, and 3. They include the short-term elevation of ICP provoked by the cerebrovascular vasodilatory cascade, causing a temporary increase in ICP—a plateau wave (Fig. 1). The second example features refractory intracranial hypertension associated with malignant brain edema (Fig. 2). The third presents a temporary rise in ICP driven by an increase in CBFV; this may have been attributable to an increase in either the partial pressure of carbon dioxide ($PaCO_2$) or brain metabolism (Fig. 3).

The results of the analysis are detailed in Table 3, which lists demographic data as well as the mean values of each of the measured or calculated parameters stratified by ICP group (elevated versus normal). Most of the studied parameters differed significantly between the two groups, except for the GCS score, heart rate, amplitude of slow waves and—somewhat surprisingly—$PbtO_2$, though the sample was small. Not only were the outcomes (measured by the GOS) highly significantly different in the two groups, but also the median GOS score in the elevated-ICP group was 1 (a fatal outcome), whereas the score in the normal-ICP group was 4 (moderate disability).

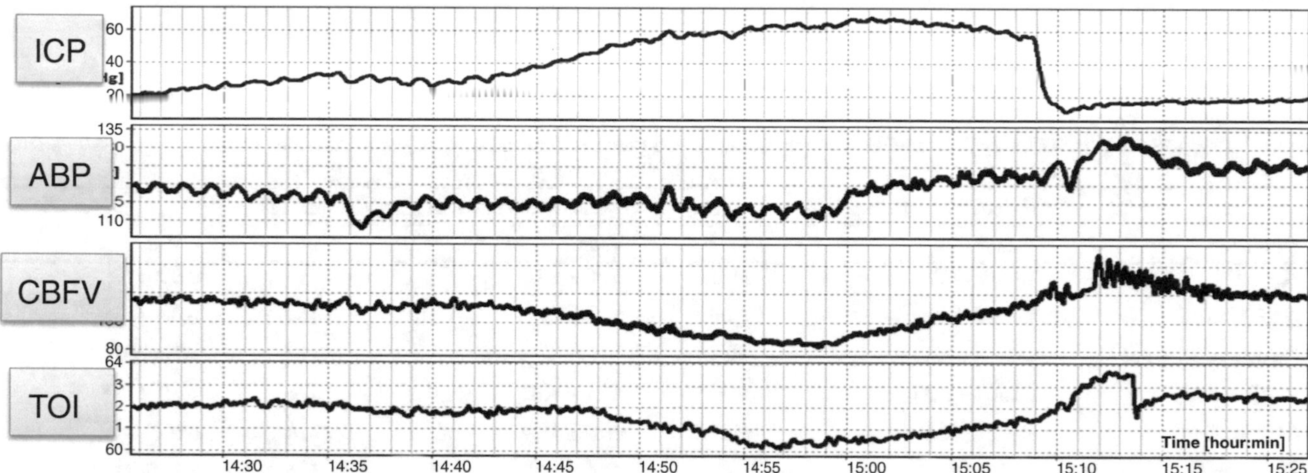

Fig. 1 A plateau wave of ICP and decreasing CPP. This is an example of when CBFV decreases due to failing autoregulation. Brain oxygen saturation measured using near-infrared spectroscopy (TOI) decreases, indicating a similar response in cerebral blood flow. This elevation in ICP occurred over 15 min and was managed by nursing intervention (vasoconstriction via a short term increase in arterial blood pressure)

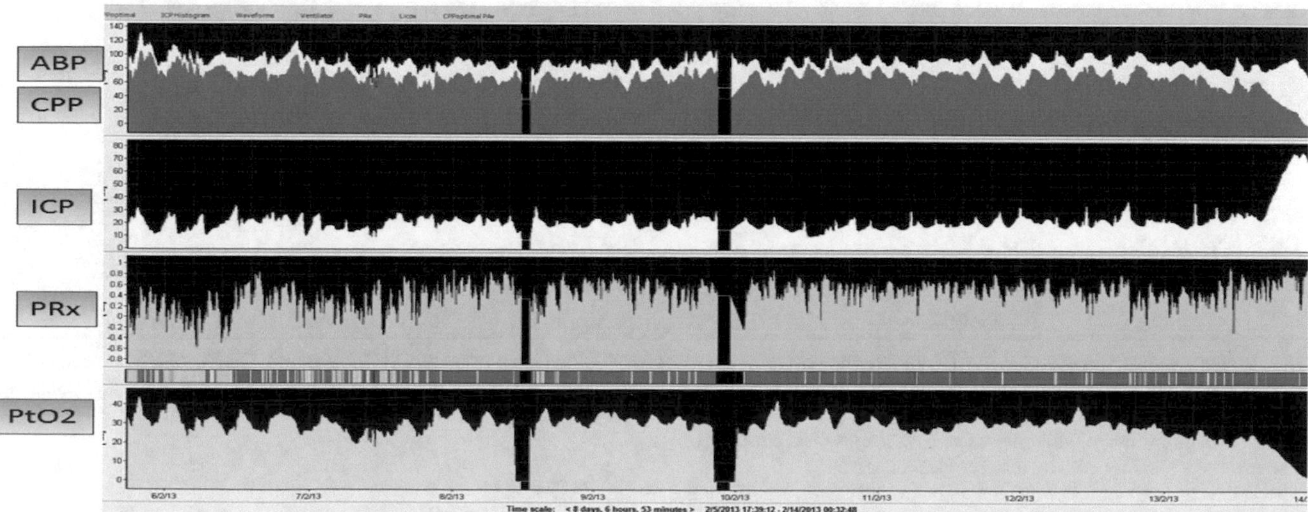

Fig. 2 Refractory intracranial hypertension. Note the persistent, and total loss of pressure reactivity PRx (solid red line) preceding the terminal increase in ICP and decrease in $PbtO_2$

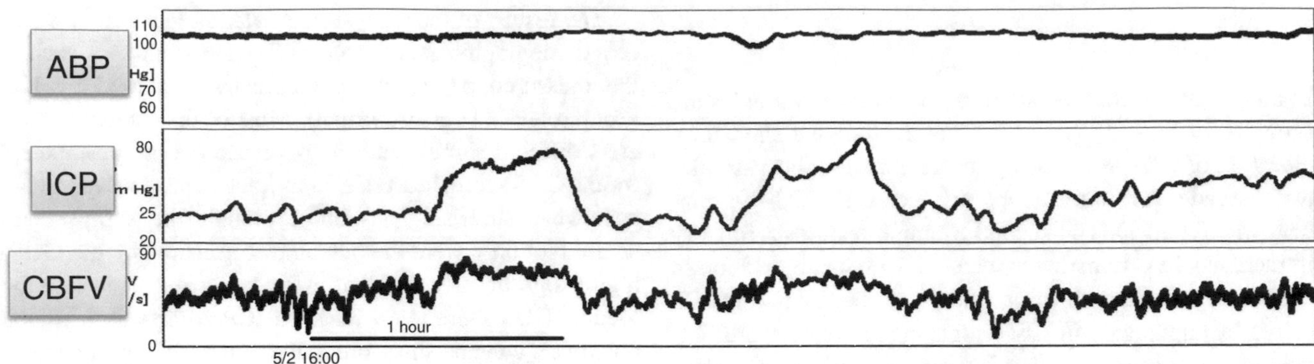

Fig. 3 Deep ICP waves related to the increase in cerebral blood flow and therefore cerebral blood volume. This effect can be observed quite frequently after TBI. Note that the change in CBFV is not caused by intracranial hypertension, but that intracranial hypertension is secondary to the rise in cerebral blood volume

Table 3 Comparison of cerebral hemodynamic parameters stratified by normal and elevated levels of intracranial pressure (ICP) in both the intermittently measured cohort (a smaller sample of patients in whom parameters derived from transcranial Doppler ultrasound were measured) and the long-term ICP/ABP/PbtO$_2$ (intracranial pressure/arterial blood pressure/cerebral oxygen partial tension) cohort (i.e., the whole study sample)

	Patients with normal ICP (<15 mmHg)		Patients with elevated ICP (>23 mmHg)		
Parameter	Value[b]	*n*[c]	Value[b]	*n*[c]	*p* Value[a]
Age [y]	39.0 ± 17.2	401	34.0 ± 15.5	116	0.0065**
GCS score	7.0 ± 3.4	396	6.4 ± 3.3	104	0.089
Median GOS score	4.0	401	1.0	116	<0.00001****
ICP [mmHg]	10.504 ± 3.21	401	31.1 ± 9.22	116	<0.0001***
CPP [mmHg]	80.52 ± 10.2	401	66.9 ± 13.9	116	0****
ABP [mmHg]	91.3 ± 10.1	401	97.6 ± 12.2	116	<0.001**
HR [beats/min]	80.6 ± 16.1	401	83.7 ± 16.0	105	0.16
PbtO$_2$ [mmHg]	30.14 ± 19.8	99	24.9 ± 45.0	10	0.15
PRx	0.07 ± 0.15	334	0.2 ± 0.24	66	<0.001***
PAx	−0.12 ± 0.17	334	0.41 ± 0.17	66	<0.0001***
RAC	−0.252 ± 0.24	223	−0.118 ± 0.26	38	0.0076**
AMP [mmHg]	1.44 ± 0.86	394	2.63 ± 1.6	110	0****
SLOW [mmHg]	1.28 ± 2.52	63	1.13 ± 1.28	85	0.63
CBFVd/CBFVm	0.61 ± 0.067	127	0.57 ± 0.089	66	0.0056**
Mx	−0.015 ± 0.29	127	0.13 ± 0.31	66	0.0019**
ARI	4.36 ± 1.51	101	3.44 ± 1.36	52	<0.0001***
CrCP [mmHg]	36.8 ± 8.32	109	53.7 ± 9.8	56	0****
DCM [mmHg]	28.0 ± 6.5	109	19.5 ± 7.4	56	<0.0001***
sPI	0.3 ± 0.08	127	0.36 ± 0.096	66	0.0014**

AMP fundamental frequency of ICP, *ARI* autoregulation index, *CBFV* cerebral blood flow velocity, *CBFVd* diastolic CBFV, *CBFVm* mean CBFV, *CPP* cerebral perfusion pressure, *CrCP* critical closing pressure, *DCM* diastolic closing margin, *GCS* Glasgow Coma Scale, *GOS* Glasgow Outcome Scale, *HR* heart rate, *Mx* mean flow index, *PAx* pulse amplitude index, *PRx* pressure reactivity index, *RAC* correlation between AMP and CPP, *SLOW* amplitude of slow waves of ICP, *sPI* spectral pulsatility index

[a]The asterisks visually convey the significance levels

[b]The values are expressed as mean ± standard deviation, except for the median GOS score

[c]The *n* values differ because data for some parameters were unavailable in the early cohort of patients without full raw data recordings

Discussion

Elevated ICP significantly affects healthy cerebrovascular dynamic function. Both the invasive, continuously measured and derived parameters and the noninvasive but intermittently measured and derived TCD-based parameters reflected physiological variability with respect to patient subgroups. It was determined that ABP was higher in patients with elevated ICP, resulting either from natural fluctuations in cerebral blood volume attributable to vasodilation or from administration of vasopressors to stabilize patients with TBI. In patients with intact cerebral autoregulation, slow waves in ABP and ICP are inversely related, as blood pressure changes affect the cerebral blood volume via reactive cerebral vasodilation/vasoconstriction, which, in turn, drives swings in ICP in the opposite direction. With high ICP, this vasoactive capacity is lost as the vascular bed become pressure passive, and ICP passively follows ABP. This is reflected in the pressure reactivity index (PRx; the coefficient of correlation between the mean ABP and ICP) [5], which was significantly higher (representing pressure passivity) in the elevated-ICP group. However, strictly speaking, this index is a measure not of CBF autoregulation but, rather, of vasoreactive capacity.

For more direct assessment of flow regulation, one must consider transmission of arterial pressure to CBF. This can be accomplished with TCD and indices such as the mean flow index (Mx; the coefficient of correlation between the cerebral perfusion pressure (CPP) and flow velocity) or some form of analysis of the transfer function between ABP and FV [8]. In our analysis, both Mx and the transfer function–derived autoregulation index (ARI) showed significantly greater degrees of impairment in patients with elevated ICP, consistent with the loss of vasoreactivity.

The blood flow velocity waveform was significantly affected in patients with intracranial hypertension. In particular, the diastolic portion of the flow velocity pulse waveform was markedly decreased relative to the mean velocity. Compared with those patients who had normal ICP, patients with elevated ICP had a much higher CrCP (the value of ABP at which CBF ceases) and a lower diastolic closing margin (DCM; the difference between the diastolic ABP and CrCP), making it more likely for them to exhibit episodes of zero diastolic flow (when ABP falls below DCM). This state, if sustained, precedes imminent hypoxia and brain death [3], which is consistent with the high mortality found in the elevated-ICP group. Continuous, long-term monitoring of these parameters is clearly desirable in patients with TBI and may soon be possible with the emergence of robotic TCD probes [9].

The indices PAx (the pressure amplitude index—the correlation between the pulse amplitude of the ICP waveform, AMP, and mean ABP) and RAC (the correlation between AMP and CPP) can also identify the effects of ICP on cerebral hemodynamics in a way closely related to PRx but, in theory, less dependent on the pressure/volume curve. As PAx is the correlation between the AMP and mean ABP, it has been argued that transmission of the arterial pulse to the ICP pulse is modulated by the vascular tone, which is, in turn, affected by the mean ABP, and that this mechanism helps to overcome issues with high pressure/volume compliance [6]. RAC goes one step further and relates the pulse amplitude not to ABP but to CPP (so, in effect, to both ABP and ICP, making it a fusion of the autoregulatory index, PAx, and the compensatory reserve index (RAP)) [7]. In our data set, patients with elevated ICP exhibited significantly higher PAx and RAC values than those with normal ICP. As RAC is particularly sensitive to both ICP and CPP, its potential for individualizing both has been noted [10, 11].

Some limitations of this study must be mentioned. The study was somewhat limited by our arbitrary categorization of "normal" versus "elevated" ICP thresholds on the basis of grand mean values of ICP and the potential ramifications of this effect for our statistical reporting when assigning our patients to subgroups. Not all parameters were available for all of the data sets, and the number of patients assigned to each ICP group varied with each parameter and thus they were all generally unevenly distributed between the two groups. Given these issues, we limited ourselves to the univariate analysis approach and chose not to correct for multiple comparisons, in keeping with the methods used in other physiological exploratory studies.

Conclusion

Elevated intracranial pressure severely affects cerebral hemodynamics. Vascular reactivity and cerebral blood flow autoregulation break down, and the critical closing pressure becomes dangerously close to the mean arterial blood pressure, threatening cessation of cerebral blood flow during the diastolic phase. Combined, these effects accompanying severe intracranial hypertension lead to more than a twofold increase in mortality.

Conflict of Interest **Marek Czosnyka and Peter Smielewski both have a financial interest in a portion of ICM+ licensing fees. Frederick Zeiler has received salary support for dedicated research time, during which this project was completed. His research program is supported by the University of Manitoba through its Thorlakson Chair in Surgical Research Establishment Fund, Vice-President (Research and International) (VPRI) Research Investment Fund (RIF), and Rudy Falk Clinician–Scientist Professorship. Peter Hutchinson is supported by the National Institute for Health Research (NIHR) (Research Professorship, Cambridge Biomedical Research Centre) and the Global Health Research Group in Neurotrauma.**

References

1. Balestreri M, Czosnyka M, Hutchinson P, Steiner LA, Hiler M, Smielewski P, Pickard JD (2006) Impact of intracranial pressure and cerebral perfusion pressure on severe disability and mortality after head injury. Neurocrit Care 4(1):8–13. https://doi.org/10.1385/NCC:4:1:008
2. Güiza F, Depreitere B, Piper I et al (2015) Visualizing the pressure and time burden of intracranial hypertension in adult and paediatric traumatic brain injury. Intensive Care Med 41(6):1067–1076
3. Varsos GV, Richards HK, Kasprowicz M, Reinhard M, Smielewski P, Brady KM, Pickard JD, Czosnyka M (2014) Cessation of diastolic cerebral blood flow velocity: the role of critical closing pressure. Neurocrit Care 20(1):40–48
4. Varsos GV, Budohoski KP, Kolias AG, Liu X, Smielewski P, Varsos VG, Hutchinson PJ, Pickard JD, Czosnyka M (2014) Relationship of vascular wall tension and autoregulation following traumatic brain injury. Neurocrit Care 21(2):266–274
5. Czosnyka M, Smielewski P, Kirkpatrick P, Laing RJ, Menon D, Pickard JD (1997) Continuous assessment of the cerebral vasomotor reactivity in head injury. Neurosurgery 41(1):11–19
6. Liu X, Czosnyka M, Donnelly J, Budohoski KP, Varsos GV, Nasr N, Brady KM, Reinhard M, Hutchinson PJ, Smielewski P (2015) Comparison of frequency and time domain methods of assessment of cerebral autoregulation in traumatic brain injury. J Cereb Blood Flow Metab 35(2):248–256. https://doi.org/10.1038/jcbfm.2014.192
7. Zeiler FA, Smielewski P, Donnelly J, Czosnyka M, Menon DK, Ercole A (2018) Estimating pressure reactivity using non-invasive Doppler-based systolic flow index. J Neurotrauma 35(14):1559–1568
8. Aries MJH, Czosnyka M, Budohoski KP, Kolias AG, Radolovich DK, Lavinio A, Pickard JD, Smielewski P (2012) Continuous monitoring of cerebrovascular reactivity using pulse waveform of intracranial pressure. Neurocrit Care 17(1):67–76
9. Zeiler FA, Donnelly J, Menon DK, Smielewski P, Hutchinson PJA, Czosnyka M (2018) A description of a new continuous physiological index in traumatic brain injury using the correlation between pulse amplitude of intracranial pressure and cerebral perfusion pressure. J Neurotrauma 35(7):963–974
10. Zeiler FA, Donnelly J, Smielewski P, Menon DK, Hutchinson PJ, Czosnyka M (2018) Critical thresholds of intracranial pressure–derived continuous cerebrovascular reactivity indices for outcome prediction in noncraniectomized patients with traumatic brain injury. J Neurotrauma 35(10):1107–1115. https://doi.org/10.1089/neu.2017.5472
11. Zeiler FA, Ercole A, Cabeleira M, Carbonara M, Stocchetti N, Menon DK, Smielewski P, Czosnyka M (2019) Comparison of performance of different optimal cerebral perfusion pressure parameters for outcome prediction in adult traumatic brain injury: a Collaborative European NeuroTrauma Effectiveness Research in Traumatic Brain Injury (CENTER-TBI) study. J Neurotrauma 36(10):1505–1517. https://doi.org/10.1089/neu.2018.6182

Part II

Neuromonitoring and Management in Adult Nontraumatic Brain Injury

Assessment of Cerebral Autoregulation in the Perifocal Zone of a Chronic Subdural Hematoma

Svetlana Trofimova, Alex Trofimov, Antony Dubrovin, Darya Agarkova, Ksenia Trofimova, Michael Dobrzeniecki, Ann Zorkova, and Denis E. Bragin

Introduction

A chronic subdural hematoma (CSDH) is a common neurosurgical disease characterized by formation of a capsule around a subdural hemorrhage, causing local compression of cerebral tissue [1]. The risk factors for CSDH development are age, alcoholism, use of anticoagulants, and coagulopathy, and the patients at highest risk of CSDH development are elderly patients who have had a nonsevere traumatic brain injury (TBI) [2]. Key factors determining the course and clinical outcome of a CSDH are the reactions of the microcirculation bed in the underlying region of the cerebral cortex—the so-called perifocal zone [3]. The results of a few investigations of the state of global and local cortical perfusion, as well as investigations of the state of autoregulation in this zone, have been contradictory. Commonly, cerebral blood flow is measured by xenon-enhanced and perfusion computed tomography (PCT). However, imperfections in the existing software for cerebral perfusion quantification during CT scanning [4] lead to contradictory results. At the same time, the introduction of CT algorithms that exclude voxels with blood flow in the cortical vessels has made it possible to assess the state of pial blood flow in the region of interest without an admixture of large-vessel flow data [5]. Thus, it is now possible to assess cerebral blood flow and the autoregulation status in the perifocal zone of a CSDH, which is worth pursuing because the available knowledge of conservative treatment modalities for a CSDH is sparse and is based on small case series and low-grade evidence [6].

S. Trofimova · A. Trofimov (✉) · A. Dubrovin · D. Agarkova
K. Trofimova · M. Dobrzeniecki · A. Zorkova
Department of Neurosurgery, Privolzhsky Research Medical University, Nizhniy Novgorod, Russia

D. E. Bragin
Lovelace Biomedical Research Institute, Albuquerque, NM, USA

Department of Neurosurgery, University of New Mexico School of Medicine, Albuquerque, NM, USA

The purpose of this work was to study cerebral microcirculation and autoregulation in the perifocal CSDH zone on the basis of analysis of PCT to understand the mechanisms of CSDH development.

Materials and Methods

This retrospective, observational, nonrandomized, single-center study was conducted as an analysis of a prospectively maintained database cohort (2016–2018) and included patients in the subacute stage of severe polytrauma and head injury. The study protocol was reviewed and approved by the institutional ethics committee and conformed to the standards of the Declaration of Helsinki. All patients gave informed consent to participate in the study. Twenty patients with a CSDH after polytrauma (between January 2016 and July 2018) were included in the study. The inclusion criteria were (1) a CSDH on CT or magnetic resonance scans, (2) an indication for surgery, (3) signed informed consent to participate in the study, and (4) a baseline PCT scan. We excluded patients who (1) were younger than 16 years, (2) had a bilateral CSDH, (3) had a serum blood creatinine level >120 mmol/L, or (4) had acute deterioration necessitating decompressive craniotomy. The study was performed under an approved institutional review board guideline as part of a multicenter study of the results of conservative and surgical CSDH treatment in the chronic stage of a concomitant TBI.

All patients underwent craniotomy with a burr hole under navigation by a SINA App (Sina Intraoperative Neurosurgical Assist). The cavity of the CSDH was washed out with a warm isotonic saline solution. A drainage catheter (Pleurofix®, B. Braun, Melsungen, Germany) was placed in the cavity of the CSDH for 48 days. All patients underwent PCT within the first day before surgery. It was performed on a Philips Ingenuity CT® scanner (Philips

B. Depreitere et al. (eds.), *Intracranial Pressure and Neuromonitoring XVII*, Acta Neurochirurgica Supplement 131,
https://doi.org/10.1007/978-3-030-59436-7_11,

Medical Systems, Cleveland, OH, USA). We used the following scan parameters: 160-mm coverage on the *z*-axis, 80 kV, 150 mA, effective dose 3.3 mSv, slice thickness 5 mm, and collimation 64 × 0.625 mm. The total acquisition time was 60 s (30 consecutive spiral acquisitions of 2 s each). Fifty milliliters of Ultravist 370 (Bayer Pharma, Berlin, Germany) was injected intravenously through a 20 G catheter by an automatic syringe injector (Medrad Stellant, Bayer HealthCare, Whippany, NJ, USA). CTP data were processed using a Philips Ingenuity Core workstation (2013, v.3.5.5.25007; Philips Healthcare, Amsterdam, the Netherlands). First, the arterial input function was detected automatically by using a cluster analysis algorithm. This arterial input function was subsequently used with the Bayesian probabilistic method to generate the perfusion parametric maps. Color-coded perfusion maps were produced to describe cerebral perfusion: cerebral blood flow (CBF), cerebral blood volume (CBV), the mean transit time (MTT), and the time to the peak concentration of contrast (TTP). The same PCT data were assessed quantitatively in the cortical brain region beneath the CSDH (zone 1) and in the corresponding contralateral brain hemisphere (zone 2) without and with use of a perfusion calculation mode excluding vascular voxels ("remote vessels" (RVs)) in the first and second analysis methods, respectively. Quantitative perfusion indices, including CBF, were calculated on a voxel-wise basis and were used to generate color-coded maps. The voxels with CBF >100 mL/100 g/min or CBV >8 mL/100 g were assumed to contain vessels and removed from the perfusion map [7]. Statistical analysis was performed using a paired Student's *t* test. The data were expressed as mean ± standard deviation. *P* values of <0.05 were considered statistically significant.

Results

The sex distribution had a male predominance (8 women and 12 men). The mean age was 54.7 ± 15.6 (range 17–87) years. The CSDH was mainly located in the left hemisphere (in 11 patients). The average volume of the CSDH was 84.2 ± 12.4 (range 55–113) cm^3. The mean midline shift was 9.1 ± 1.2 (range 7–12) mm. The level of wakefulness according to the Glasgow Coma Score was 13.1 ± 0.5 (range 10–15), and the Markwalder level was 1.8 ± 0.5 (range 0–3). The acquired and analyzed data are summarized in Table 1. Comparison with normal values for perfusion indices [9] in zone 1 in the calculation algorithm with flow in the cortical vessels (in the first analysis method) showed significant ($P < 0.01$) increases in CBV and CBF, and no significant increases in MTT and TTP ($P > 0.01$). However, when vascular voxels were excluded by the RV mode (in the second analysis method), the comparison of perfusion parameters in zone 1 with normal values showed nonsignificant changes ($P > 0.01$). In zone 2 (on the contralateral side), the comparison with normal values for perfusion indices in the first analysis method revealed statistically significant increases in CBV and CBF ($P < 0.01$), but the changes in MTT and TTP were nonsig-

Table 1 Data on the analyzed parameters

		CBF (mL/100 g × min)	CBV (mL/100 g)	TTP (s)	MTT (s)
1	First analysis method (zone 1 without RVs)	148.97 ± 32.98	10.98 ± 2.79	28.58 ± 0.79	4.23 ± 0.63
2	First analysis method (zone 2 without RVs)	123.15 ± 29.51	9.28 ± 2.25	27.72 ± 1.17	4.61 ± 0.77
3	Second analysis method (zone 1 with RVs)	87.97 ± 15.95	5.57 ± 0.91	26.45 ± 0.81	3.14 ± 0.59
4	Second analysis method (zone 2 with RVs)	74.88 ± 21.02	5.14 ± 0.76	28.06 ± 1.28	4.11 ± 0.85
5	Normal values [8]	64.02 ± 0.6	4.6 ± 0.8	–	4.3 ± 0.8
P values for comparisons					
1 versus 2		0.011	0.041	0.521	0.532
1 versus 3		<0.001*	<0.001*	0.702	0.004*
2 versus 4		0.002*	<0.001*	0.704	0.049
3 versus 4		0.047	0.091	0.192	0.321

CBF cerebral blood flow, *CBV* cerebral blood volume, *MTT* mean transit time, *RVs* remote vessels, *TTP* time to peak concentration of contrast
*Significant difference ($p < 0.01$)

nificant. At the same time, use of the second analysis method showed no significant changes in perfusion parameters ($P > 0.01$) in zone 2.

Discussion

The main property of the brain circulation—cerebral autoregulation—is the ability to maintain constant cerebral perfusion under fluctuating mean arterial and intracranial pressure [10]. It was previously noted that indicators of cerebral perfusion and the state of autoregulation are in close interdependence, and that microvasculature perfusion disorders result from damage to the autoregulation mechanisms [8, 11]. It has been proposed that a CSDH disrupts the mechanisms of CBF autoregulation, as is evident in cerebral microcirculation disorders with development of congestion and hyperperfusion syndromes. Thus, there is a fair increase in CBV in comparison with the symmetrical zones in the opposite hemisphere, while the time characteristics do not change significantly, which corresponds to congestion and hyperperfusion patterns and indicates a cerebral autoregulation disorder [1, 3]. Nevertheless, these findings, as well as the fact that the studies were carried out without using algorithms, appear to be the basis for critical comments on this work. In our study, we used a CT analysis algorithm that excluded pixels from large vessels, thus enabling us to adequately assess perfusion in the pial bed of the perifocal zone of the CSDH. We think that we can use the second algorithm in the *intact* hemisphere because microcirculation in this area is also abnormal in patients with a CSDH. Microcirculatory disturbances in the intact hemisphere are probably caused by venous drainage failure and intracranial hypertension. This belief is based on results reported by other investigators [1, 3]. Our data prove the stability of microvasculature perfusion in the CSDH perifocal zone and, consequently, preserved CBF autoregulation in patients with such pathology. Hyperemia and hyperperfusion in the perifocal zone of the CSDH, which have been described in previous studies [3], do not affect the microcirculation, as no pial perfusion disorders were observed. A possible reason for development of such syndromes in the perifocal zone could be formation of de novo blood vessels in the capsule, with development of an over-capillary shunting phenomenon, causing an increase in blood flow. In practice, our results show that the onset of foci of local cerebral hyperperfusion not affecting the pial bed direction is probably an early marker of de novo angiogenesis in capsule formation with development of brain compression [12]. Clarification of this statement could be the basis for early diagnosis of compression formation on the basis of detection of the characteristic features of cerebral perfusion.

It should be noted that our study had some methodological limitations, the main one being the impossibility of dynamic noninvasive assessment of the state of perfusion in the perihematomal area without PCT rescanning. Moreover, considering the characteristics of our study design, we were unable to assess the perfusion characteristics of the perifocal zone in patients with a bilateral CSDH or in patients with a CSDH in a decompensated state. Both of these issues require further study.

Conclusion

Detection of hyperemia and hyperperfusion in the perifocal zone of a CSDH is associated with changes in blood flow and blood supply at the level of resistive and capacitive vessels, and does not affect the capillary bed. The perfusion indices of blood flow in the perifocal zone of the CSDH show no significant differences from those in the symmetrical zone of the contralateral hemisphere. The maintenance of microcirculatory blood flow perfusion reflects preservation of CBF autoregulation in patients with a CSDH. Exclusion of large vessels from analysis of the microcirculation is more suitable for evaluation of CBF status in patients with a CSDH.

Acknowledgments Denis Bragin was supported by National Institutes of Health grant number R01NS112808-01. Alex Trofimov was supported by a grant-in-aid for exploratory research from the Privolzhsky Research Medical University.

Conflict of Interest: **The authors declare that they have no conflict of interest.**

References

1. Aries MJ, Budohoski K (2013) Cerebral perfusion in chronic subdural hematoma. J Neurotrauma 19:1680–1680
2. Akgun B, Cakin H, Ozturk S (2018) Evaluation of cortical brain parenchyma by diffusion and perfusion MRI before and after chronic subdural hematoma surgery. Turk Neurosurg 28(3):405–409
3. Slotty PJ, Kamp MA, Steige H (2012) Cerebral perfusion in chronic subdural hematoma. J Neurotrauma 30:347–351
4. Omura T, Fukushima Y, Yoshikawa G (2019) Cerebral hyperperfusion syndrome after a burr hole drainage surgery for chronic subdural hematoma. World Neurosurg S1878-8750(18):32923–32921. https://doi.org/10.1016/j.wneu.2018.12.100
5. Campbell BC, Christensen S, Levi CR, Desmond PM, Donnan GA, Davis SM, Parsons MW (2011) Cerebral blood flow is the optimal CT perfusion parameter for assessing infarct core. Stroke 42(12):3435–3440. https://doi.org/10.1161/STROKEAHA.111.618355
6. Soleman J, Nocera F, Mariani L (2017) The conservative and pharmacological management of chronic subdural haematoma. Swiss Med Wkly 147:w14398. https://doi.org/10.4414/smw.2017.14398

7. Miles K, Eastwood JD, Konig M (eds) (2007) Multidetector computed tomography in cerebrovascular disease: CT perfusion imaging. Informa, Abingdon
8. Almenawer SA, Farrokhyar F, Hong C (2014) Chronic subdural hematoma management: a systematic review and meta-analysis of 34829 patients. Ann Surg 259(3):449–457
9. Tanioka S, Sato Y, Tsuda K, Niwa S, Suzuki H (2017) Prolonged cerebral hyperperfusion and subcortical low intensity on fluid-attenuated inversion recovery images: unusual manifestation after removal of organized chronic subdural hematoma. World Neurosurg 101:812.e1–812.e4. https://doi.org/10.1016/j.wneu.2017.03.089
10. Mehta V, Harward SC, Sankey EW (2018) Evidence based diagnosis and management of chronic subdural hematoma: a review of the literature. J Clin Neurosci 50:7–15
11. Bivard A, Levi C, Krishnamurthy V, Hislop-Jambrich J, Salazar P, Jackson B, Davis S, Parsons M (2014) Defining acute ischemic stroke tissue pathophysiology with whole brain CT perfusion. J Neuroradiol 41(5):307–315. https://doi.org/10.1016/j.neurad.2013.11.006
12. Hong HJ, Kim YJ, Yi HJ (2009) Role of angiogenic growth factors and inflammatory cytokine on recurrence of chronic subdural hematoma. Surg Neurol 71:161–166

Noninvasive Intracranial Pressure Monitoring in Chronic Stroke Patients with Sedentary Behavior: A Pilot Study

Gabriela Nagai Ocamoto, Deusdedit Lineu Spavieri Junior, Jean Alex Matos Ribeiro, Gustavo Henrique Frigieri Vilela, Aparecida Maria Catai, and Thiago Luiz Russo

Introduction

Monitoring of intracranial pressure (ICP) as a clinical parameter is a practice adopted by the health team during the first hours of a stroke in order to guide treatment and achieve better neurological outcomes. Monitoring of absolute values and ICP waveforms provides crucial information about intracranial dynamics and brain compliance [1]. The ICP waveforms P1, P2, and P3 correspond to the percussion wave, tidal wave, and dicrotic wave, respectively. Normal brain compliance is represented by the P1 value being higher than the P2 value. However, poor brain compliance is related to the P2 value being higher than the P1 value [2]. During the acute phase of stroke, impairment of brain compliance and a marked reduction in cerebral blood flow (CBF) signifies a worse prognosis [3, 4]. Commonly, after a stroke, people have chronic disabilities, which can permanently affect their function, activity, and participation in society [5].

After a stroke, most patients tend to adopt sedentary behavior, regardless of their functional ability [6]. The large amount of sedentary time increases the risks of cardiovascular diseases and recurrent stroke [7]. Studies have shown that prolonged time spent in sedentary behavior (e.g., sitting time) leads to a reduction in CBF in different populations, such as healthy desk workers [8] and the elderly [9].

Advances in noninvasive ICP-monitoring technology and the growing number of noninvasive ICP-monitoring devices have create the possibility to monitor ICP in a variety of environments and at the chronic stage of stroke. In this context, this study aimed to verify if there is a relationship between cerebral compliance and sedentary behavior during the chronic stage of stroke, using a noninvasive ICP-monitoring device. The study hypothesized that in patients who were in the chronic phase of stroke, the fewer steps they walked each day and the more time they spent being inactive each day, the more impaired their cerebral compliance would be.

Materials and Methods

Participants

Eight patients from São Carlos, Brazil, participated in this pilot study. All patients presented moderate sensory motor impairment (assessed using the Fugl-Meyer Assessment Scale) and met the following inclusion criteria: (1) hemiparesis caused by a stroke in the middle cerebral artery; (2) being in the chronic phase, at least 6 months poststroke; (3) a Mini–Mental State Examination score between 26 and 30, depending on the educational level; and (4) ability to complete the experimental protocol. The exclusion criteria were (1) more than one stroke episode; (2) bilateral stroke; (3) any pre-existing neurological disorder; and (4) severe heart, lung, or kidney disease. Before data collection, patients signed a written consent form explaining the protocol. All experimental procedures complied with the requirements of the ethics committee at the Federal University of São Carlos (ethical approval number 80457317.0.0000.5504). Table 1 presents the demographic and functional characteristics of the included patients.

Physical Activity Monitoring

The time spent in walking activities was recorded using an activity monitor, and the patients also completed an activity questionnaire. Each patient used a StepWatch Activity

G. Nagai Ocamoto · J. A. Matos Ribeiro · A. M. Catai
T. L. Russo (✉)
Department of Physical Therapy, Federal University of São Carlos-UFSCar, São Carlos, São Paulo, Brazil
e-mail: russo@ufscar.br

D. L. Spavieri Junior · G. H. Frigieri Vilela
Brain4Care Health Technology, São Carlos, São Paulo, Brazil

B. Depreitere et al. (eds.), *Intracranial Pressure and Neuromonitoring XVII*, Acta Neurochirurgica Supplement 131,
https://doi.org/10.1007/978-3-030-59436-7_12,

Monitor™ (SAM) placed on the nonparetic ankle for 7 days continuously except during bathing, showering, or swimming. After 7 days of SAM use, the patients answered the International Physical Activity Questionnaire to verify the correspondent activities recorded by the SAM, focusing on data regarding the number of steps walked and the time spent in inactivity.

Intracranial Pressure Monitoring

Before the ICP assessment, the patients were asked to avoid ingesting food and drinks that would cause any stimulation (i.e., caffeine) for at least 12 h. The noninvasive intracranial pressure (niICP) device Brain4Care® (a strain gauge) monitored their ICP waveforms continuously during a postural change maneuver involving 15 min spent in a supine position and 15 min in an orthostatic position. The niICP sensor was placed over the ipsilesional hemisphere at the electroencephalography position C5 or C6, depending on the side of the injury. A sample of the ICP data collection is presented in Fig. 1.

Table 1 Patient characteristicss [$N = 8$]

Characteristic	Number
Male/female ratio (*n*/*n*)	7/1
Age (years)[a]	56.67 ± 10.46
Body mass index[a]	26.29 ± 3.10
Type of stroke: ischemic/hemorrhagic (*n*/*n*)	3/5
Lesioned hemisphere: right/left (*n*/*n*)	4/4
Fugl-Meyer total score[a]	162.17 ± 33.40

[a]The values are expressed as mean ± standard deviation

Statistical Analysis

Spearman's correlation coefficient was used to analyze the P2/P1 ratio, the number of steps walked, and the data on time spent in inactivity. The level of significance was taken as $p < 0.05$. Statistical analysis was performed using SPSS software version 17.0 (SPSS, Chicago, IL, USA), and the level of significance was taken as $p \leq 0.05$.

Results

In the supine and orthostatic positions, the P2/P1 ratios were 0.84 ± 0.14 and 0.98 ± 0.17. The percentage of time spent in inactivity was 71 ± 11%, and the number of steps walked per day was 4220 ± 2239. We found a high positive correlation ($r = 0.881$, $p = 0.004$) between the P2/P1 ratio and the percentage of time spent in inactivity (Fig. 2). No correlation was observed between the P2/P1 ratio and the number of steps walked per day ($p = 0.183$).

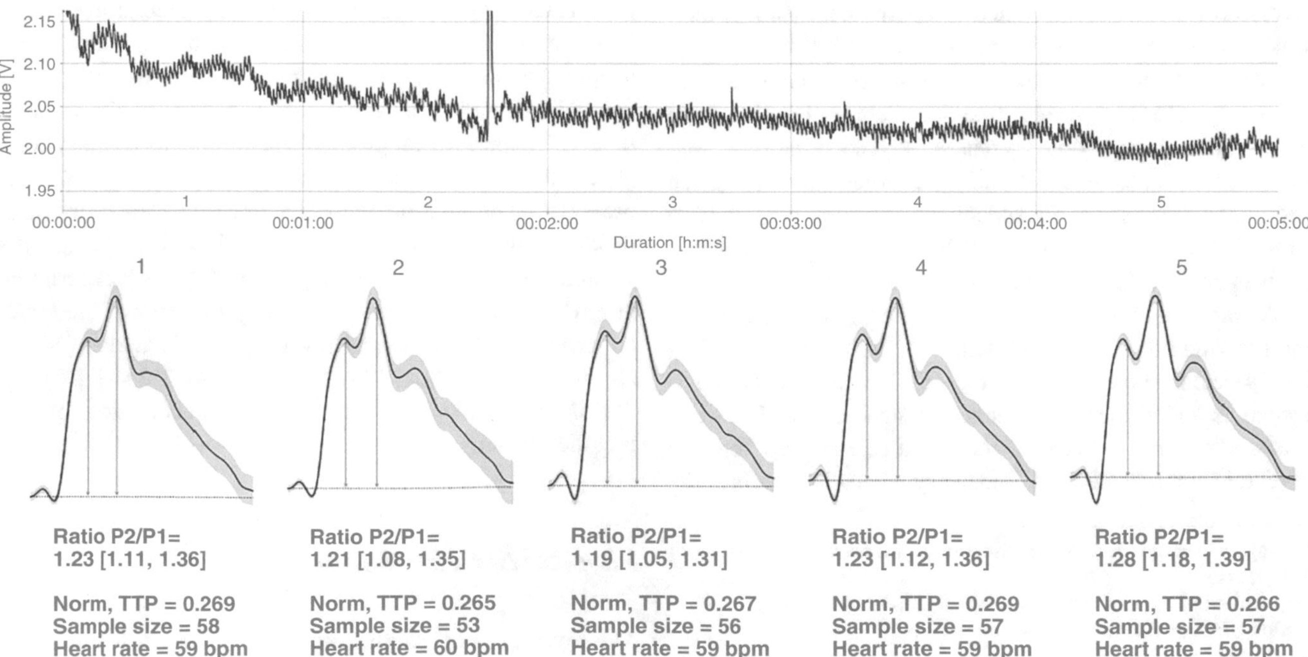

Fig. 1 Sample of intracranial pressure (ICP) data collection during a postural maneuver. *Bpm* beats/min, *P1* systolic peak, *P2* tidal peak, *Norm. TTP* normalized time to peak

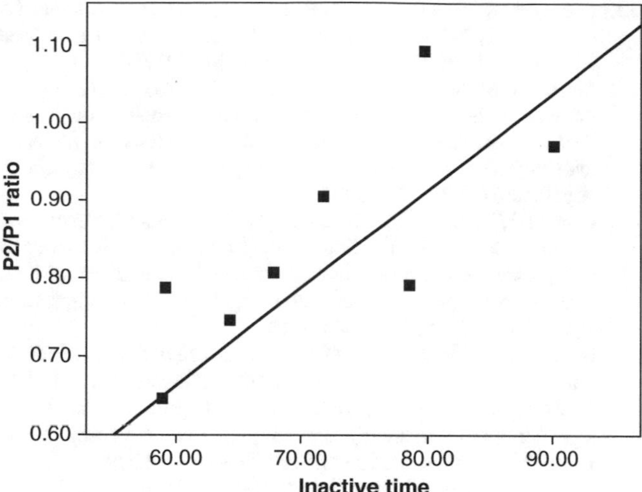

Fig. 2 Correlation between the P2/P1 ratio and the percentage of time spent in inactivity

Discussion

This study provided new perspectives for use of noninvasive techniques to assess ICP outside critical care—more precisely, during the late stage of a stroke. The findings of the study demonstrate that people in the chronic stage of stroke who spend prolonged time in inactivity present a higher P2/P1 ratio in their ICP waveforms, suggesting reduced cerebral compliance. Although no normal range has been established for P2/P1 ratio values provided by noninvasive measurement techniques, an increase in the P2/P1 ratio could be associated with decreased brain compliance.

Considering the reduction in cerebral compliance we observed, these findings could be associated with impairment of cerebral autoregulation. Aoi et al. (2012) showed that brain atrophy and functional recovery in stroke patients depend on dynamic cerebral autoregulation and perfusion adaptation [10]. According to the literature, autoregulation can be impaired as a result of a stroke. One of the causes of an alteration in autoregulation may be chronic hypertension [11].

In the past, guidelines and taskforces have suggested that sedentary behavior is a risk factor associated with noncommunicable diseases, cardiovascular diseases, and stroke [12]. Thus, the possibility of monitoring ICP during the chronic stage of a stroke and during sedentary behavior could provide new insights into risk management and new perspectives on assessment.

The noninvasive method used in the present study enabled continuous assessment of the ICP waveform peaks P1, P2, and P3 during the monitoring period. This method has previously been validated and described in other neurological conditions [13–15]. If the P2 value equals or slightly exceeds the P1 value, this characterizes potentially pathological morphology showing evidence of a decrease in intracranial compliance [16].

This study had a few limitations: the sample size was small; there was no control group; and the device used to monitor ICP provided values only in millivolts, not in millimeters of mercury. Despite these limitations, the findings still provide an insight into how the function of cerebral compliance is impaired during the chronic phase of a stroke.

Conclusion

This preliminary study showed a correlation between sedentary behavior and a decrease in cerebral compliance. Thus, monitoring of intracranial pressure during the late stage of a stroke could guide the clinician's treatment to reduce sedentary behavior and the risks of recurrent stroke and cardiovascular diseases.

Acknowledgments This study was supported by the Fundação de Amparo à Pesquisa do Estado de São Paulo (FAPESP) through scholarship grant number 2017/22173-5 and by the Coordenação de Aperfeiçoamento de Pessoal de Nível Superior (CAPES) (finance code 001).

Conflict of Interest: **Brain4Care Health Technology provided the noninvasive devices used in this project for research purposes. Gabriela Nagai Ocamoto, Jean Alex Matos Ribeiro, Aparecida Maria Catai, and Thiago Luiz Russo have no financial interests related to Brain4Care Health Technology. Deusdedit Lineu Spavieri Junior and Gustavo Henrique Frigieri Vilela have received financial support from Brain4Care Health Technology.**

References

1. Abraham M, Singhal V (2015) Intracranial pressure monitoring. J Neuroanaesth Crit Care 2(3):193–203. https://doi.org/10.4103/2348-0548.165039
2. Tasneem N, Samaniego EA, Pieper C, Leira EC, Adams HP, Hasan D et al (2017) Brain multimodality monitoring: a new tool in neurocritical care of comatose patients. Crit Care Res Pract 2017:6097265. https://doi.org/10.1155/2017/6097265
3. Donnelly J, Budohoski KP, Smielewski P, Czosnyka M (2016) Regulation of the cerebral circulation: bedside assessment and clinical implications. Crit Care 20:129. https://doi.org/10.1186/s13054-016-1293-6
4. Salinet ASM, Silva NCC, Caldas J, de Azevedo DS, de-Lima-Oliveira M, Nogueira RC et al (2018) Impaired cerebral autoregulation and neurovascular coupling in middle cerebral artery stroke: influence of severity? J Cereb Blood Flow Metab 39(11):2277–2285. https://doi.org/10.1177/0271678X18794835
5. Hatem SM, Saussez G, Faille M, Prist V, Zhang X, Dispa D et al (2016) Rehabilitation of motor function after stroke: a multiple systematic review focused on techniques to stimulate upper extremity recovery. Front Hum Neurosci 10:442. https://doi.org/10.3389/fnhum.2016.00442

6. Tieges Z, Mead G, Allerhand M, Duncan F, van Wijck F, Fitzsimons C et al (2015) Sedentary behavior in the first year after stroke: a longitudinal cohort study with objective measures. Arch Phys Med Rehabil 96(1):15–23. https://doi.org/10.1016/j.apmr.2014.08.015
7. Hendrickx W, Riveros C, Askim T, Bussmann JBJ, Callisaya ML, Chastin SFM et al (2019) Identifying factors associated with sedentary time after stroke: secondary analysis of pooled data from nine primary studies. Top Stroke Rehabil 26(5):327–334. https://doi.org/10.1080/10749357.2019.1601419
8. Carter SE, Draijer R, Holder SM, Brown L, Thijssen DHJ, Hopkins ND (2018) Regular walking breaks prevent the decline in cerebral blood flow associated with prolonged sitting. J Appl Physiol 125:790–798. https://doi.org/10.1152/japplphysiol.00310.2018
9. Zlatar ZZ, Hays CC, Mestre Z, Campbell LM, Meloy MJ, Bangen KJ et al (2019) Dose-dependent association of accelerometer-measured physical activity and sedentary time with brain perfusion in aging. Exp Gerontol 110679:125. https://doi.org/10.1016/j.exger.2019.110679
10. Aoi MC, Tzung-Lo M, Selim M, Olufsen MS, Novak V (2012) Impaired cerebral autoregulation is associated with brain atrophy and worse functional status in chronic ischemic stroke. PLoS One 7(10):e46794. https://doi.org/10.1371/journal.pone.0046794
11. Aires MJH, Elting JW, Keyser JD, Kremer BPH, Vroomen PCAJ (2010) Cerebral autoregulation in stroke. Stroke 41:2697–2704. https://doi.org/10.1161/STROKEAHA.110.594168
12. González K, Fuentes J, Márquez JL (2017) Physical inactivity, sedentary behavior and chronic diseases. Korean J Fam Med 38(3):111–115. https://doi.org/10.4082/kjfm.2017.38.3.111
13. Ballestero MFM, Frigieri G, Cabella BCT, Oliveira SM, Oliveira RS (2017) Prediction of intracranial hypertension through noninvasive intracranial pressure waveform analysis in pediatric hydrocephalus. Childs Nerv Syst 33(9):1517–1524. https://doi.org/10.1007/s00381-017-3475-1
14. Cabella B, Vilela GHF, Mascarenhas S, Czosnyka M, Smielewski P, Dias C et al (2016) Validation of a new noninvasive intracranial pressure monitoring method by direct comparison with an invasive technique. Acta Neurochir Suppl 122:93–96. https://doi.org/10.1007/978-3-319-22533-3_18
15. Frigieri G, Andrade RAP, Dias C Jr, Spavieri DL, Brunelli R, Cardim DA, Wang CC, Verzola RMM, Mascarenhas S (2018) Analysis of a non-invasive intracranial pressure monitoring in patients with traumatic brain injury. Acta Neurochir Suppl 126:107–110. https://doi.org/10.1007/978-3-319-65798-1_23
16. Nucci CG, Bonis PD, Mangiola A, Santini P, Sciandrone M, Risi A et al (2016) Intracranial pressure wave morphological classification: automated analysis and clinical validation. Acta Neurochir 158(3):581–588. https://doi.org/10.1007/s00701-015-2672-5

Use of Clustering to Investigate Changes in Intracranial Pressure Waveform Morphology in Patients with Ventriculitis

Murad Megjhani, Kalijah Terilli, Aaron Kaplan, Brendan K. Wallace, Ayham Alkhachroum, Xiao Hu, and Soojin Park

Introduction

External ventricular drains (EVDs) are widely used to control hydrocephalus, with roughly 37,000 patients a year receiving EVDs in the USA alone, generating in-hospital charges of $151,672 per patient, or US$5.6 billion a year [1]. EVDs are frequently complicated by ventriculitis, an infection of the ventricular system. Penetration into the central nervous system (CNS) with ventriculostomy can introduce infectious species into the cerebrospinal fluid (CSF), which acts as a reservoir for microbiota. The infection can lead to inflammation of the arachnoid villi, decreasing CSF outflow and instigating hydrocephalus [2]. Up to 22% of patients with EVDs develop ventriculitis [3]. The Centers for Disease Control guidelines define ventriculitis by combinations of clinical features such as fever, headache, or meningeal signs (neck stiffness, photophobia), laboratory test features such as elevations in the CSF white blood cell count and protein level, a decreased CSF glucose level, and a CSF culture that is positive for an organism [4]. A negative CSF Gram stain does not exclude the presence of ventriculitis [5, 6]. Patients with certain conditions such as subarachnoid hemorrhage (SAH) or intraventricular hemorrhage (IVH) are at increased risk of ventriculitis [7].

Delays in implementing proper antimicrobial therapy for infections are associated with increases in mortality [7], so neurocritical care units commonly institute periodic or responsive (to fever) drawing of CSF from EVDs to send away for culturing and other laboratory studies [8]. The longer an EVD remains indwelling, the higher the risk of ventriculitis, with the rate of infection ranging from 6.3 to 10.4 infections per 1000 EVD-days [9]. The frequency of drawing fluid samples from the EVD is, in itself, another risk factor. One study showed a 5% decrease in the rate of ventriculitis in patients sampled every 3 days versus daily [10], and another study found a significant increase in the risk of infection with both daily and alternate-day sampling regimens in comparison with sampling 1–2 times per week [11]. Imaging and laboratory test characteristics can also identify ventriculitis. Magnetic resonance imaging has shown promise in small studies, where intraventricular debris and pus on fluid attenuation inversion recovery (FLAIR) imaging and choroid plexitis on T-1 imaging were sensitive for ventriculitis [12]. Serum procalcitonin, a marker of bacterial pneumonia, has shown utility in distinguishing bacterial meningitis from viral meningitis, and early high serum procalcitonin concentrations were predictive of bacterial ventriculitis in a study of 36 patients with EVDs [13]. However, neither serum nor CSF procalcitonin have proven able to differentiate between fevers of infectious or noninfectious etiology, making procalcitonin a poor noninvasive predictor [14, 15]. One study showed a significant increase in CSF red blood cell counts in culture-positive ventriculitis, though this was shown to be neither sensitive nor specific and is confounded by concurrent hemorrhage [16]. Furthermore, any detection system that relies on assaying CSF still requires periodic draws, thus negating the hypothetical advantages of another method of detection.

We made clinical observations of blunted single-peak waveforms in patients with ventriculitis. Understanding that ICP waveforms should reflect the changing poroelastic property of the parenchyma, we hypothesized that the temporal dynamics of intracranial pressure waveforms could reveal a pathological change in compliance in patients developing ventriculitis.

M. Megjhani · K. Terilli · A. Alkhachroum · S. Park (✉)
Division of Hospitalist and Critical Care Neurology, Department of Neurology, Columbia University Irving Medical Center, New York, NY, USA
e-mail: spark@columbia.edu

A. Kaplan · B. K. Wallace
Columbia University Vagelos College of Physicians and Surgeons, New York, NY, USA

X. Hu
Division of Physiological Nursing, School of Nursing, University of California San Francisco, San Francisco, CA, USA

B. Depreitere et al. (eds.), *Intracranial Pressure and Neuromonitoring XVII*, Acta Neurochirurgica Supplement 131,
https://doi.org/10.1007/978-3-030-59436-7_13,

Materials and Methods

Study Population and Data Collection

We studied consecutive patients with EVDs who were prospectively enrolled in a hemorrhage outcomes study from 2006 to 2018. The study was approved by the Columbia University Medical Center institutional review board. In each case, written informed consent was obtained from the patient or a surrogate.

Physiological data for the duration of the intensive care unit stay were acquired using a high-resolution acquisition system (BedMasterEX, Excel Medical Electronics, Jupiter, FL, USA) from General Electric Solar 8000i monitors (Port Washington, NY, USA; 2006–2013) at 240 Hz (waveforms) or Philips Intellivue MP70/MX800 monitors (Amsterdam, the Netherlands; 2013–present) at 125 Hz (waveforms). We converted the proprietary file format (STP) defined by BedMasterEx into the Hierarchical Data Format, version 5 (HDF5; 1997–2018; http://www.hdfgroup.org/HDF5/), which is specifically designed to store and efficiently organize large quantities of data.

Outcome Definition

Given the uncertainty around the clinical diagnosis of definite ventriculitis, we limited the outcome in our cohort to culture-positive ventriculitis [4, 17].

Data Analysis

Using wavelet analysis [18], we extracted uninterrupted segments of ICP waveforms. We extracted dominant pulses from continuous high-resolution data, using a validated technique, morphological clustering analysis of intracranial pressure (MOCAIP) [19]. Then we applied hierarchical k-means clustering, using the dynamic time warping (DTW) distance to obtain morphologically similar groupings [20]. DTW is an algorithm for measuring similarity between two temporal sequences, which may vary in speed. Metaclusters were categorized for broad comparison by clinician consensus and labeled as compliant (three peaks), noncompliant (one peak), and artifactual groups. Finally, we compared the distribution of these metaclusters before, during, and after the diagnosis of definite ventriculitis.

Statistical Analysis

We used a chi-squared test of independence to compare the distribution of the metaclusters before, during, and after ventriculitis, and we used change point analysis [21] to identify significant changes in the distribution leading to ventriculitis.

Results

Consecutive patients (N = 1653) were prospectively enrolled in a hemorrhage outcomes study from 2006 to 2018. Of these, 435 patients (26%) required EVDs, and 76 (17.5% of those with EVDs) had ventriculitis. Nineteen patients (25% of those with ventriculitis) showed culture-positive CSF and were included in the present analysis. Of these, nine patients had enough physiological data recorded for analysis.

We extracted 275,911 dominant pulses from 459.9 h of EVD data. Of these, 112,898 pulses (40.9%) occurred before culture positivity, 41,300 pulses (15.0%) occurred during culture positivity, and 121,713 pulses (44.1%) occurred after it. K-means identified 20 clusters, which were further grouped into metaclusters: tri–/biphasic, single-peak, and artifactual waveforms. Prior to ventriculitis, 61.8% of dominant pulses were tri–/biphasic; this percentage reduced to 22.6% during ventriculitis and 28.4% after it ($p < 0.0001$) (Fig. 1a, b).

Change point analysis [21] with 99% confidence showed a significant change in the distribution of the metaclusters 1 day before the cultures that revealed ventriculitis were sent away for analysis (Fig. 1c, d).

Discussion

There is a compelling need for identification of ventriculitis that does not rely on CSF sampling. We analyzed ICP waveforms before, during, and after adjudication of ventriculitis. We found significant differences in the distribution of the morphologies of the ICP waveforms. Using change point analysis, we further identified that there was a significant difference in the distribution of the cluster 1 day before the cultures that revealed ventriculitis were sent away for analysis. The distribution of ICP waveform morphology changes significantly prior to the clinical diagnosis of ventriculitis and may be a potential biomarker.

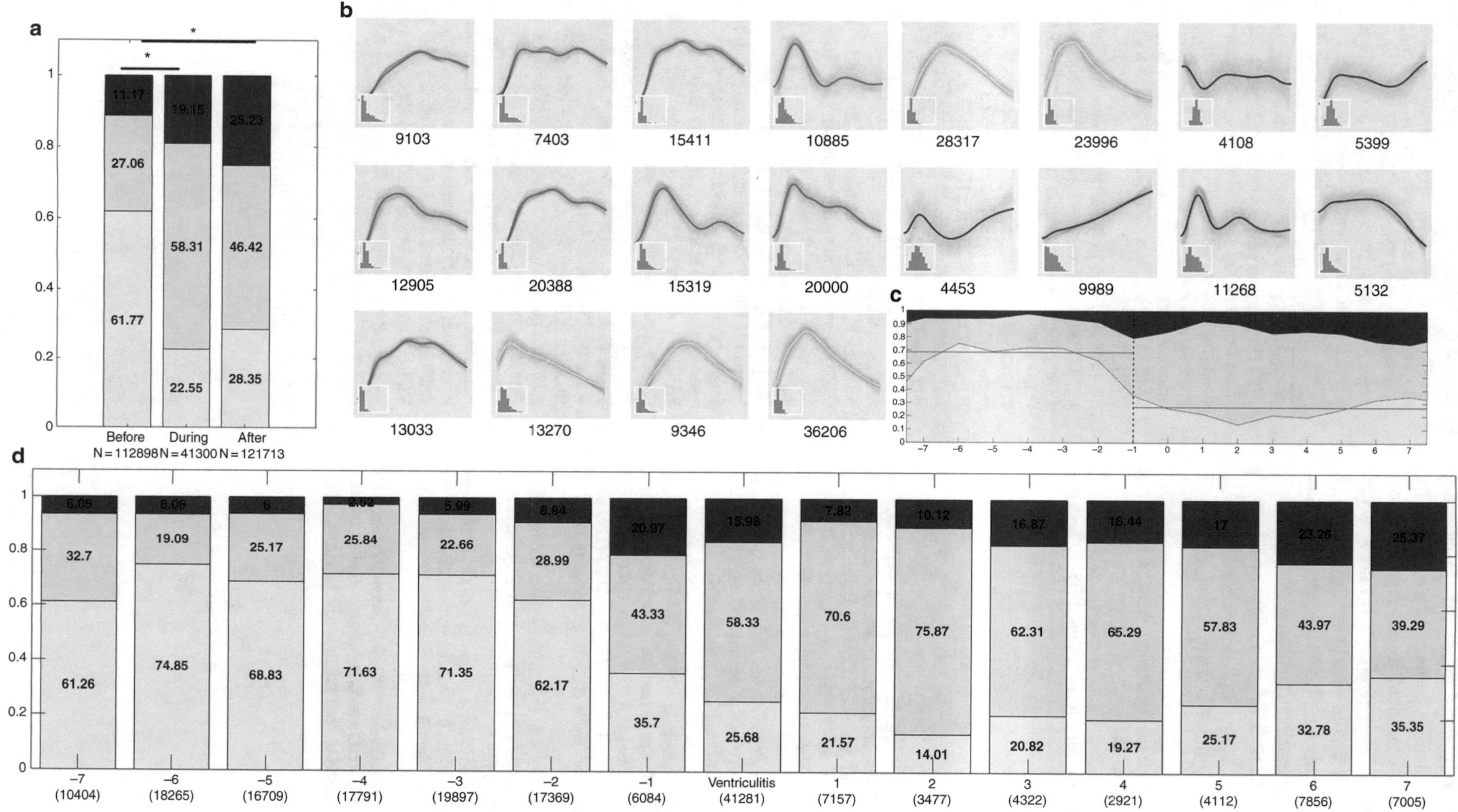

Fig. 1 Changes in the distribution of intracranial pressure tri–/biphasic (*green*), single-peak (*yellow*), and artifactual (*red*) waveforms. (**a**) Cumulative changes before, during, and after ventriculitis; an *asterisk* denotes a significant change ($p < 0.0001$). (**b**) The top 20 metaclusters; the *inset* in each graph indicates the dynamic time warping distance to the centroid of each waveform. (**c**) Change point analysis (in days) indicating that there is a change in the distribution of the waveforms at least 1 day before the diagnosis of ventriculitis. (**d**) Changes in the distribution of clusters over time (in days) before and after ventriculitis

This study had the following limitations: (1) the study cohort included only ventriculitis patients, and a comparison with matched controls is warranted in order to create any predictive models; and (2) to generalize this finding across different institutions, further validation using external data is required. In our future work, we plan to address these challenges by comparing our ventriculitis cohort with a matched control group, in order to develop predictive models using ICP waveform dynamics as a biomarker for ventriculitis. Additionally, an external validation study is under way.

Acknowledgments Soojin Park is supported by National Institutes of Health grant number K01 ES026833.

Conflict of Interest **The authors have no conflicts of interest to declare.**

References

1. Rosenbaum BP, Vadera S, Kelly ML, Kshettry VR, Weil RJ (2014) Ventriculostomy: frequency, length of stay and in-hospital mortality in the United States of America, 1988–2010. J Clin Neurosci 21(4):623–632. https://doi.org/10.1016/j.jocn.2013.09.001
2. Salmon JH (1972) Ventriculitis complicating meningitis. Am J Dis Child 124(1):35–40
3. Lewis A, Wahlster S, Karinja S, Czeisler BM, Kimberly WT, Lord AS (2016) Ventriculostomy-related infections: the performance of different definitions for diagnosing infection. Br J Neurosurg 30(1):49–56
4. Horan TC, Andrus M, Dudeck MA (2008) CDC/NHSN surveillance definition of health care–associated infection and criteria for specific types of infections in the acute care setting [published correction appears in Am J Infect Control 2008;36(9):655]. Am J Infect Control 36(5):309–332. https://doi.org/10.1016/j.ajic.2008.03.002
5. Kim HI, Kim SW, Park GY et al (2012) The causes and treatment outcomes of 91 patients with adult nosocomial meningitis. Korean J Intern Med 27(2):171–179
6. Tunkel AR, Hasbun R, Bhimraj A et al (2017) 2017 Infectious Diseases Society of America's clinical practice guidelines for healthcare-associated ventriculitis and meningitis. Clin Infect Dis 64(6):e34–e65
7. Aronin SI, Peduzzi P, Quagliarello VJ (1998) Community-acquired bacterial meningitis: risk stratification for adverse clinical outcome and effect of antibiotic timing. Ann Intern Med 129(11):862–869
8. Halpern C, Grady M (2015) Neurosurgury. In: Brunicardi FC, Andersen DK, Billiar TR, Dunn DL, Hunter JG, Matthews JB, Pollock RE (eds) Schwartz's principles of surgery, 10th edn. McGraw-Hill, New York, pp 1733–1734
9. Hagel S, Bruns T, Pletz M, Engel C, Kalff R, Ewald C (2014) External ventricular drain infections: risk factors and outcome. Interdiscip Perspect Infect Dis 2014:708531. https://doi.org/10.1155/2014/708531
10. Williams TA, Leslie GD, Dobb GJ, Roberts B, van Heerden PV (2011) Decrease in proven ventriculitis by reducing the frequency of cerebrospinal fluid sampling from extraventricular drains. J Neurosurg 115(5):1040–1046
11. Jamjoom AA, Joannides AJ, Poon MT-C et al (2018) Prospective, multicentre study of external ventricular drainage–related infections in the UK and Ireland. J Neurol Neurosurg Psychiatry 89(2):120–126
12. Fujikawa A, Tsuchiya K, Honya K, Nitatori T (2006) Comparison of MRI sequences to detect ventriculitis. AJR Am J Roentgenol 187(4):1048–1053. https://doi.org/10.2214/AJR.04.1923
13. Omar AS, ElShawarby A, Singh R (2015) Early monitoring of ventriculostomy-related infections with procalcitonin in patients with ventricular drains. J Clin Monit Comput 29(6):759–765. https://doi.org/10.1007/s10877-015-9663-1
14. Halvorson K, Shah S, Fehnel C et al (2017) Procalcitonin is a poor predictor of non-infectious fever in the neurocritical care unit. Neurocrit Care 27(2):237–241. https://doi.org/10.1007/s12028-016-0337-8
15. Martinez R, Gaul C, Buchfelder M, Erbguth F, Tschaikowsky K (2002) Serum procalcitonin monitoring for differential diagnosis of ventriculitis in adult intensive care patients. Intensive Care Med 28(2):208–210. https://doi.org/10.1007/s00134-001-1176-3
16. Hoogmoed J, van de Beek D, Coert BA, Horn J, Vandertop WP, Verbaan D (2017) Clinical and laboratory characteristics for the diagnosis of bacterial ventriculitis after aneurysmal subarachnoid hemorrhage. Neurocrit Care 26(3):362–370
17. Walti LN, Conen A, Coward J, Jost GF, Trampuz A (2013) Characteristics of infections associated with external ventricular drains of cerebrospinal fluid. J Inf Secur 66(5):424–431
18. Strang G, Nguyen T (1996) Wavelets and filter banks, 2nd edn. Wellesley-Cambridge, Cambridge
19. Hu X, Xu P, Scalzo F, Vespa P, Bergsneider M (2009) Morphological clustering and analysis of continuous intracranial pressure. IEEE Trans Biomed Eng 56(3):696–705
20. Niennattrakul V, Ratanamahatana CA (2007) On clustering multimedia time series data using k-means and dynamic time warping. Presented at the 2007 International Conference on Multimedia and Ubiquitous Engineering (MUE'07), Seoul, pp 26–28
21. Killick R, Eckley I, Haynes K (2019) Changepoint: an R package for changepoint analysis. R package version 1.1.5. http://CRAN.R-project.org/package=changepoint.

Perioperative Dynamics of Intracranial B-waves of Blood Flow Velocity in the Basal Cerebral Arteries in Patients with Brain Arteriovenous Malformation

Vladimir Semenyutin, Vugar Aliev, Grigory Panuntsev, and Andreas Patzak

Introduction

B-waves were first observed by Lundberg [1] in intracranial pressure (ICP) monitoring as regular oscillations in ICP at frequencies of 0.5–2 waves/min (8–30 mHz). The exact cause of their occurrence is not entirely clear. There are different physiological and pathophysiological factors that are considered sources of this phenomenon: primary slow rhythmic changes in the partial pressure of arterial CO_2 (related to the respiration rhythm), changes in systemic blood pressure (BP), and cerebral perfusion pressure [2–4]. Various classifications and subgroups of B-waves in ICP based on their amplitude, types of waveform, and rate of occurrencehave been proposed for correct identification and interpretation of possible mechanisms that can generate these fluctuations. With the introduction of transcranial Doppler ultrasound (TCD) into clinical practice, similar patterns of slow waves have been found in the spectrum of linear blood flow velocity (BFV) in the basal cerebral arteries in both healthy individuals and patients with a severe head injury, hydrocephalus, a ruptured cerebral aneurysm, or a hypertensive intracerebral hemorrhage [5–8]. Nevertheless, it is still debatable which of the B-waves (of ICP or BFV) is the surrogate and which one is the original. Newell et al. [5] simultaneously recorded TCD and ICP signals in artificially ventilated patients with a severe head injury and demonstrated high coherence of both parameters within the range of B-waves. However, B-waves of BFV preceded B-waves of ICP and were independent of any change in arterial or cerebral perfusion pressure, as well as respiration and end-tidal CO_2 pressure. These findings, supported by those of other experimental and clinical studies, underpin the most acceptable vasogenic theory of the origin of intracranial B-waves [9–13]. According to this theory, intracranial B-waves are induced by periodic changes (dilation and constriction) of small regulating arteries in the cerebral microcirculation, with a frequency of 8–30 mHz. Hence, one can conclude that cerebral blood flow is a basic parameter where intracranial B-waves initially occur. From this point of view, it would be more correct to define B-waves in ICP as a surrogate, whereas B-waves in BFV in the basal cerebral arteries, for obvious reasons, are considered to be the first derivative of a similar fluctuation in cerebral blood flow.

It is still unknown whether slow vasogenic activity with such a periodicity reflects the functional state of either myogenic or neurogenic mechanisms (with an intrinsic brain stem pacemaker) of cerebral blood flow regulation. Moreover, there is no agreement about the prognostic and diagnostic value of intracranial B-waves. Some authors insist that TCD B-waves often occur in healthy individuals and that their disappearance highly correlates with impaired cerebral autoregulation (CA) and poor outcomes in various pathological conditions [2, 10]. Other investigators suggest that increased B-wave amplitude in ICP and BFV is the result of intracranial hypertension and low compliance, as well as cerebral hypoperfusion [5, 8, 9].

The cerebral circulation system in patients with brain arteriovenous malformation (AVM) is commonly characterized by impaired autoregulation on the affected side, which is due to pathological arteriovenous shunting [14, 15]. However, there are no data clarifying the relationship between B-waves of BFV in the basal arteries and this type of compromised cerebral hemodynamics without evident signs of intracranial hypertension.

V. Semenyutin (✉) · G. Panuntsev
Laboratory of Brain Circulation Pathology, Russian Polenov Neurosurgical Institute of the Almazov National Medical Research Centre, Saint Petersburg, Russia

V. Aliev
Laboratory of Brain Circulation Pathology, Russian Polenov Neurosurgical Institute of the Almazov National Medical Research Centre, Saint Petersburg, Russia

2nd Department of Neurosurgery, Municipal Hospital of Saint Martyr Elizabeth, Saint Petersburg, Russia

A. Patzak
Johannes-Mueller Institute of Vegetative Physiology University Hospital Charité, Humboldt University of Berlin, Berlin, Germany

B. Depreitere et al. (eds.), *Intracranial Pressure and Neuromonitoring XVII*, Acta Neurochirurgica Supplement 131,
https://doi.org/10.1007/978-3-030-59436-7_14,

The aim of this study was to evaluate the amplitude of BFV within the range of B-waves (BWA) in patients with AVM before and after endovascular intervention.

Materials and Methods

The design of the study was approved by the local ethical standards committee of the Almazov National Medical Research Centre, in accordance with the 1975 Declaration of Helsinki (and as revised in 1983). The study procedures were performed after written informed consent was obtained from the patients or their legal representatives.

We retrospectively examined a cohort of 38 patients with brain AVM who were admitted to the neurovascular department of the Russian Polenov Neurosurgical Institute for endovascular management. The main demographic and clinical characteristics of the patients are presented in Table 1. The patients were studied and operated on beyond the stage of hemorrhagic and epileptic symptoms. The type of AVM located in one of the hemispheres of the brain was classified in accordance with the Spetzler–Martin Grading Scale [16]. AVMs were embolized with either an adhesive agent (n-butyl-2-cyanoacrylate; Hystoacryl) or a nonadhesive agent (Onyx) through afferent vessels originating from the middle cerebral artery (MCA) and/or the anterior cerebral artery (ACA) [17]. Clinical assessment was performed according to the Modified Rankin Scale (mRs) prior to and after the endovascular intervention [18]. All patients had standard perioperative computer tomography (CT) imaging of the brain, Doppler ultrasound of the precerebral and cerebral arteries, and evaluation of CA.

Table 1 Demographic and clinical characteristics of patients with a supratentorial arteriovenous malformation (AVM)

Characteristic	Value
Age (years)[a]	38 ± 11
Male/female ratio (*n*/*n*)	20/18
Type of AVM according to the Spetzler–Martin scale (*n*)	
I–II	9
III	18
IV–V	11
Manifestation of hemorrhage/epileptic seizure (*n*/*n*)	21/17
Radicality of AVM embolization (*n*)	
75–100%	10
50–75%	16
50%	12
Shunt flow index: preoperative/postoperative (ml/min)[a]	564 ± 115/346 ± 96[*]
Modified Rankin scale score: preoperative/postoperative[a]	1.3 ± 0.6/1.1 ± 0.4

[a]The values are expressed as mean ± standard deviation
[*]$p < 0.05$

The patients underwent ultrasound assessment of the precerebral arteries, using the Vivid E ultrasound system (GE Healthcare, Chicago, IL, USA) with a multifrequency linear transducer (4–12 MHz). The benefits of duplex scanning for assessment of the radicality of AVM embolization on the basis of shunting blood flow dynamics before and after the procedure have been demonstrated previously [15].

CA measurements were performed with both a cuff test [19, 20] and transfer function analysis (TFA) [21, 22]. The subjects were in a supine position with 30° elevation of the upper body while breathing at a rate of 6 breaths/min. The end-tidal partial pressure of CO_2, measured with a Novametrix Tidal Wave capnograph (Philips Medical Systems, Eindhoven, the Netherlands) corresponded to normocapnia (36–38 mmHg). BFV in the main basal cerebral arteries was insonated through the temporal bone window at a depth of 50–60 mm with a 2-MHz probe fixed on a headframe. BP was registered continuously via a servocontrolled finger photoplethysmograph (CNAP Monitor 500 HD, CNSystems Medizintechnik, Graz, Austria) with the subject's hand position at the heart level. BP recording was transmitted through the analogue input channel of a MultiDop X system block into the monitoring module of DWL software.

For TFA, the data segments were inspected visually and edited for artifacts and ectopy. Only steady state data were digitized and stored on a hard disk in universal ASC files in DWL software for further offline CA assessment. While TFA was performed, the spectral amplitudes of BP and BFV, the phase shift (PS), and the coherence coefficient were calculated in a specifically selected range of systemic Mayer waves (M-waves, 80–120 mHz). This frequency band commonly reflects periodic fluctuations in BP and is more informative for assessment of the myogenic component of the cerebrovascular response than high-frequency oscillations. According to the high-pass filter model, the pressure–flow relation between the input (BP) and output (BFV) signals is characterized by a positive PS (0.8–1.2 rad). In the case of impaired autoregulation, the passing capacity of the filter for slow waves increases; therefore, the PS between both parameters reduces, even to zero. Coherence between 0 and 1 reflects a linear relation between BP and BFV. To ensure the greatest reliability of PS values for further statistical analysis, they were estimated only at frequencies that exhibited coherence >0.6 and maximum M-wave amplitude in BP. Additionally, the spectral amplitudes of BP and BFV were also calculated within the range of slow B-waves (8–30 mHz). TFA was performed with the commercially available data acquisition software Statistica for Windows version 7 (StatSoft, Tulsa, OK, USA) in the "time series and forecasting" module.

Descriptive statistics were used to describe the patients' demographic characteristics and clinical, angiographic, ultrasound, and TFA data. A paired Student's t test was used to estimate the significance of CA changes after AVM embolization. Parametric data were expressed as mean ± standard deviation, and values of $p < 0.05$ were considered statistically significant.

Results

Among 38 patients with brain AVM, 21 manifested with intracranial hemorrhage and 17 with epileptic seizures. Nevertheless, none of them had any clinical or CT/MRI (magnetic resonance imaging) markers of intracranial hypertension at the time of admission, examination, and endovascular intervention. The mean mRs value prior to intervention was 1.3 ± 0.6 and indicated slight or insignificant disability (Table 1). AVMs located in one of the hemispheres and supplied with a feeding artery originated from the unilateral MCA and/or ACA.

In patients with a type I–II of AVM, according to the Spetzler–Martin scale (n = 9), embolization in one or two sessions led to elimination of up to 75–100% of the initial size of the pathological arteriovenous lesion from the circulation. In cases of AVM type III (n = 18) or type IV–V (9) on the Spetzler–Martin scale, because the AVM was located in a functionally important area or was bigger (more than 3 cm in size), the first session of endovascular intervention was significantly less effective. The original size of the AVM was reduced by 50–75% in 16 cases and by no more than 50% in 12 cases. No early postoperative neurological complications nor complications at the time of hospital discharge (7–10 days after the procedure) were observed in our study. The postoperative mean mRs value increased to 1.3 ± 0.6 but nonreliably (Table 1).

Ultrasound examinations were performed 1–3 days prior to intervention, as well as on the third day after it. The shunt flow index prior to intervention in all 38 patients was 564 ± 115 ml/min and reliably correlated ($p < 0.01$) with the type of AVM according to the Spetzler–Martin scale. After embolization, the shunt flow index decreased remarkably to 292 ± 76 ml/min but remained high mainly because the patients had an AVM of type IV–V gradation and it was only partly embolized. In patients with a type I–II of AVM, shunt flow index was zero postoperatively (Table 1).

Perioperative dynamics of BP, BFV, and autoregulation parameters before and after AVM embolization are presented in Table 2. Initial TCD patterns in the basal cerebral arteries on the affected side showed pathological arteriovenous shunting through the AVM. The mean BFV values were 142 ± 49 cm/s on the AVM side and 71 ± 14 cm/s contralaterally. The pulsatility indices were 0.49 ± 0.13 and 0.87 ± 0.14, respectively. Moreover, a reliable decrease in the CA rate on the AVM side was noted (autoregulation index (ARI) 1.2 ± 0.8, PS 0.2 ± 0.1 rad) in comparison with the contralateral side (ARI 5.8 ± 1.5, PS 0.9 ± 0.2 rad). As for BWA, it was significantly greater ($p < 0.01$) on the AVM side (4.5 ± 2.7 cm/c) than on the contralateral side (2.2 ± 1.4 cm/s). These asymmetrical changes in BFV within the B-wave range appeared under stable recordings of BP, end-tidal CO_2 pressure, and the respiration rhythm, without any slow fluctuations at the same frequency.

Figure 1 illustrates the results of a perioperative examination of a patient with a left frontal lobe AVM (type III according to the Spetzler–Martin scale), which manifested with a headache and epileptic seizure. There were no symptoms of intracranial hypertension in the patient's medical history or in the neurological examination at the time of admission. Preoperative BFV values in the left MCA showed the presence of pathological arteriovenous shunting. A cuff test and TFA indicated CA impairment on the affected side (ARI 1, PS 0.21 rad). BWA in the left MCA (3.8 cm/s) was considerably greater than that in the right MCA (2.2 cm/s). On the third day after safe and total AVM embolization, the BFV and pulsatility index on the side of the lesion normalized and the CA parameters reached

Table 2 Dynamics of blood pressure, blood flow velocity, and autoregulation parameters before/after embolization in 38 patients with a supratentorial arteriovenous malformation (AVM)

Variable	Ipsilateral side	Contralateral side
Blood flow velocity in the basal artery (cm/s)	142 ± 49/101 ± 23*	71 ± 14/68 ± 12
Pulsatility index	0.49 ± 0.13/0.69 ± 0.11*	0.87 ± 0.14/0.86 ± 0.14
Phase shift (rad)[a]	0.2 ± 0.1/0.6 ± 0.1*	0.9 ± 0.2/0.9 ± 0.1
Autoregulation index (cuff test)	1.2 ± 0.8/3.6 ± 1.6*	5.8 ± 1.5/5.7 ± 1.4
B-wave amplitude of blood flow velocity (cm/s)	4.5 ± 2.7/2.7 ± 1.8*	2.2 ± 1.4/2.0 ± 0.5
Blood pressure (mmHg)	89 ± 10/85 ± 12	

The values are expressed as mean ± standard deviation before/after embolization

[a]Phase shift between M-waves of blood pressure and blood flow velocity

*$p < 0.05$

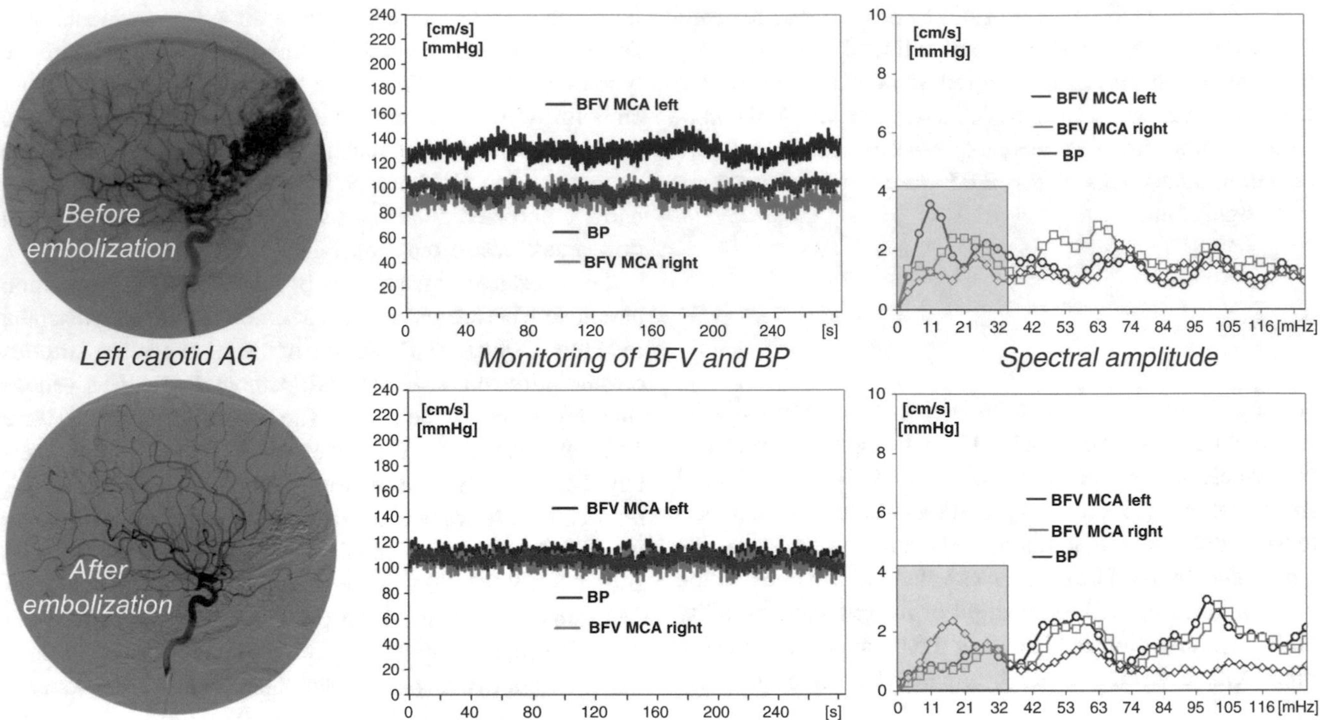

Fig. 1 Results of examination of a 41-year-old man with an arteriovenous malformation (AVM) in the left frontal lobe of the brain. Afferent vessels originate from the left middle cerebral artery (MCA). *From left to right:* left carotid angiogram, multichannel monitoring of blood pressure (BP) and blood flow velocity (BFV) in the MCA over a period of 280 s, and amplitude spectra within the low-frequency range. *From top to bottom:* before and 3 days after total (up to 100%) embolization. The *blue area* comprises the range of intracranial B-waves in an amplitude spectrum analysis

normal values (ARI 4, PS 0.8 rad). The postoperative BWA values in both MCAs were almost identical and less than 2 cm/s.

Moreover, 10 out of the 38 patients (six type IV–V and four type III according to the Spetzler–Martin scale) had greater BWA (exceeding 3 cm/s (4.7 ± 1.1 cm/s)) on the AVM side ($p < 0.01$) than the other 28 patients. There were no reliable differences between the two subgroups in terms of BFV, BP, ARI, and PS on the AVM side. After embolization, there were reliable increases ($p < 0.01$) in the CA rate (ARI 3.6 ± 1.9, PS 0.5 ± 0.2 rad) and decreases in BWA on the AVM side (2.7 ± 1.8 cm/s) in the whole cohort.

Figure 2 illustrates the results achieved in a patient with a left temporal lobe AVM (type IV according to the Spetzler–Martin scale) and no symptoms of intracranial hypertension. Along with TCD patterns of shunting and severe CA impairment, there was also an extremely large BWA (13 cm/s) with a period of more than 2 min. On the third day after the first session of partial embolization (of up to 30% of the lesion), BFV in the left MCA remained high and CA did not improve substantially. Of note, BWA decreased but was still greater than that on the contralateral side. There were no postoperative neurological complications.

Discussion

Intrinsic CA impairment in the basal cerebral arteries, which are involved in AVM feeding, can be due to cerebral hypoperfusion and "steal" in the perinidal area. Sato et al. [23] discovered the presence of abnormally enlarged capillaries (up to 7 mm in diameter) in the brain adjacent to the AVM nidus. The so-called perinidal dilated capillary network, with its inherent pathomorphological features and their functional disability, may potentially reflect the real state of autoregulation under conditions of cerebral hypoperfusion and inadequate collateral circulation. However, in practice, it is quite difficult to preoperatively differentiate true negative results of CA assessment from false negative ones, particularly in AVM type III–V, because of high shunting through AVM. In such cases, baseline low CA indices on the affected side reflect the inability for regulation in the afferent vessels of the AVM and its network as a result of their morphologically determined low resistance. Actually, CA assessment is most informative after total embolization of the AVM, when the perfusion pressure has normalized, and we can detect the real state of CA after intervention and predict the risk of possible hemorrhagic complications.

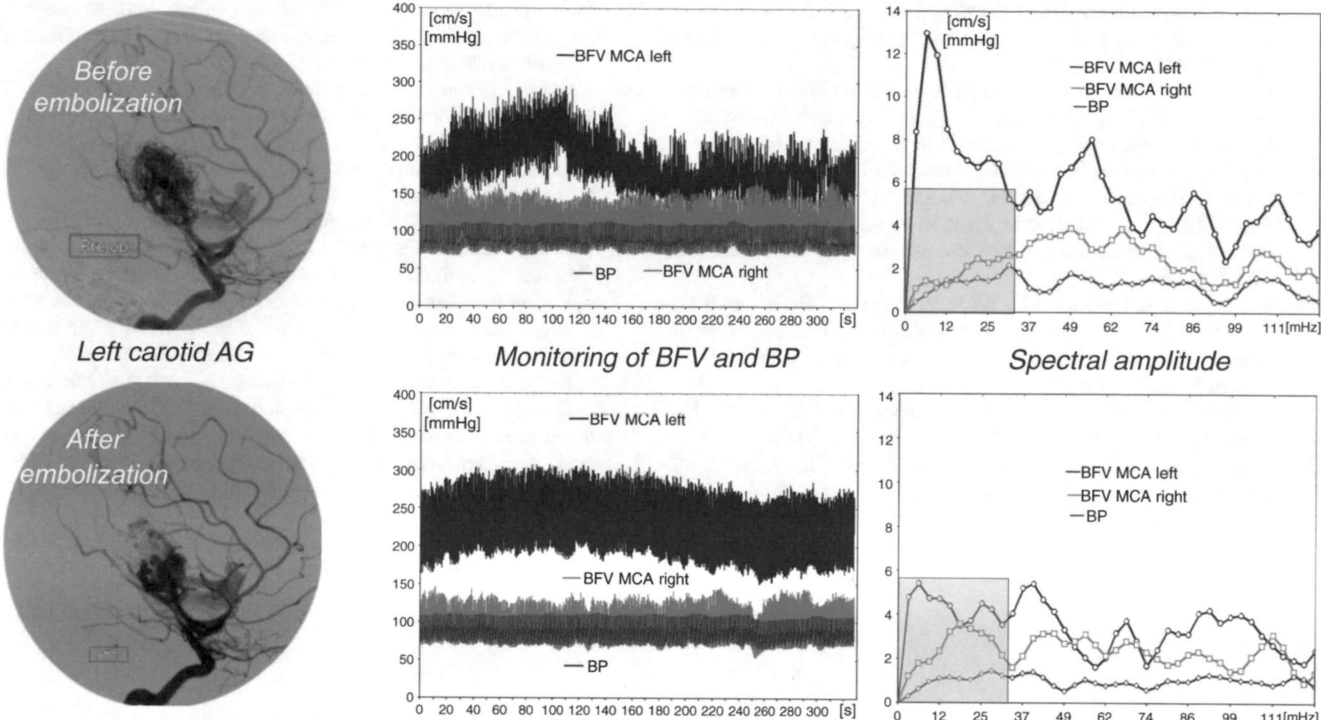

Fig. 2 Results of examination of a 31-year-old man with an arteriovenous malformation (AVM) in the left temporal lobe of the brain. Afferent vessels originate from the left middle cerebral artery (MCA). *From left to right:* left carotid angiogram, multichannel monitoring of blood pressure (BP) and blood flow velocity (BFV) in the MCA over a period of 280 s, and amplitude spectra within the low-frequency range. *From top to bottom:* before and 3 days after partial (up to 30%) embolization

A significantly increased BWA of BFV not induced by fluctuations in BP prior to endovascular treatment may be due to additional neurogenic vasodilation of pial arteries in the perinidal zone of the AVM when the perfusion pressure is quite low. This assumption is supported by a reduction in BWA in BFV in the basal cerebral arteries on the affected side even after partial AVM embolization. Further research is needed to establish the reasons for this phenomenon and the interrelation between myogenic and neurogenic components of regulation. Along with CA assessment in patients with an AVM in the brain, it might provide a useful tool for evaluation of the treatment strategy and prognostication of the risk of hemorrhage in the patient's natural course and after endovascular interventions.

Acknowledgments This study was supported by grant number 19-29-01190/19 from the Russian Foundation for Basic Research (RFBR).

References

1. Lundberg N (1960) Continuous recording and control of ventricular fluid pressure in neurosurgical practice. Acta Psychiatr Scand Suppl 36(149):1–193
2. Balestreri M, Czosnyka M, Steiner LA, Schmidt EA, Smielewski P, Matta B, Pickard JD, Robertson CS, Dunn LT, Chambers IR (2004) Intracranial hypertension: what additional information can be derived from ICP waveform after head injury? Acta Neurochir 146:131–141
3. Spiegelberg A, Preus M, Kurtcuoglu V (2016) B-waves revisited. Interdiscip Neurosurg 6:13–17. https://doi.org/10.1016/j.inat.2016.03.004
4. Martinez-Tejada I, Arum A, Wilhjelm J, Juhler M, Andresen M (2019) B waves: a systematic review of terminology, characteristics and analysis methods. Fluids Barriers CNS 16(1):33. https://doi.org/10.1186/s12987-019-0153-6
5. Newell D, Aaslid R, Stooss R, Reulen HJ (1992) The relationship of blood flow velocity fluctuations to intracranial pressure B waves. J Neurosurg 76:415–421
6. Lavinio A, Menon DK (2011) Intracranial pressure: why we monitor it, how to monitor it, what to do with the number and what's the future? Curr Opin Anesthesiol 24:117–123
7. Lalou DA, Donnelly J, Czosnyka M, Nabbanja E, Garnett M, Pickard JD, Czosnyka Z (2015) Are B-waves of intracranial pressure suppressed by general anesthesia? Fluid Barrier CNS 12:63
8. Lang EW, Diehl RR, Timmermann L, Baron R, Deusch G, Mehdorn HM, Zunker P (1999) Spontaneous oscillations of arterial blood pressure, cerebral and peripheral blood flow in healthy and comatose subjects. Neurol Res 21:665–669
9. Semenyutin V, Aliev V, Nikitin P, Kozlov A (2005) The intracranial B-waves' amplitude as prognostication criterion of neurological complications in neuroendovascular interventions. Acta Neurochir 94:53–58
10. Droste DW, Krauss JK, Berger W, Schuler E, Brown MM (2009) Rhythmic oscillations with a wavelength of 0.5–2 min in transcranial Doppler recordings. Acta Neurol Scand 90:99–104
11. Auer L, Sayama I (1983) Intracranial pressure oscillations (B-waves) caused by oscillations in cerebrovascular volume. Acta Neurochir 68:93–100

12. Zhang R, Zuckerman JH, Giller CA, Levine BD (1998) Transfer function analysis of dynamic cerebral autoregulation in humans. Am J Phys 274:233–241
13. Schytz HW, Hansson A, Phillip D, Selb J, Boas DA, Iversen HK, Ashina M (2010) Spontaneous low-frequency oscillations in cerebral vessels: applications in carotid artery disease and ischemic stroke. J Stroke Cerebrovasc Dis 19:465–474
14. Diehl R, Henkes H, Nahser H, Kühne D, Berlit P (1994) Blood flow velocity and vasomotor reactivity in patients with arteriovenous malformations: a transcranial Doppler study. Stroke 25:1574–1580
15. Semenyutin V, Panuntsev G, Aliev V, Patzak A, Pechiborsch D, Kozlov A (2014) Capability of cerebral autoregulation assessment in arteriovenous malformations perinidal zone. Int J Clin Neurosci Mental Health 1:119–126
16. Spetzler RF, Martin NA (1986) A proposed grading system for arteriovenous malformations. J Neurosurg 65:476–483
17. Derdeyn C, Zipfel G, Albuquerque F, Cooke D, Feldmann E, Sheehan J, Torner J (2017) Management of brain arteriovenous malformations: a scientific statement for healthcare professionals from the American Heart Association/American Stroke Association. Stroke 48:200–224
18. Banks JL, Marotta CA (2007) Outcomes validity and reliability of the modified Rankin scale: implications for stroke clinical trials: a literature review and synthesis. Stroke 38:1091–1096
19. Aaslid R, Lindegaard KF, Sorteberg W, Nornes H (1989) Cerebral autoregulation dynamics in humans. Stroke 20:45–52
20. Tiecks F, Lam A, Aaslid R, Newell D (1995) Comparison of static and dynamic cerebral autoregulation measurements. Stroke 26:1014–1019
21. Claassen JA, Meel-van den Abeelen AS, Simpson DM, Panerai RB, International Cerebral Autoregulation Research Network (CARNet) (2016) Transfer function analysis of dynamic cerebral autoregulation: a white paper from the International Cerebral Autoregulation Research Network. J Cereb Blood Flow Metab 36(4):665–680. https://doi.org/10.1177/0271678X15626425
22. Semenyutin V, Asaturyan G, Nikiforova A, Aliev V, Panuntsev G, Iblyaminov V, Savello A, Patzak A (2017) Predictive value of dynamic cerebral autoregulation assessment in surgical management of patients with high-grade carotid artery stenosis. Front Physiol 8:872. https://doi.org/10.3389/fphys.2017.00872
23. Sato S, Kodama N, Sasaki T, Matsumoto M, Ishikawa T (2004) Perinidal dilated capillary networks in cerebral arteriovenous malformations. Neurosurgery 54:163–168

Part III

Neuromonitoring and Management in Adult Mixed Brain Injury Populations

Effects of Hyperthermia on Intracranial Pressure and Cerebral Autoregulation in Patients with an Acute Brain Injury

Andrey Oshorov, Anastasya Baranich, Alexander Polupan, Alexander Sychev, Ivan Savin, and Alexander Potapov

Introduction

Hyperthermia (an increased temperature of the "body core" above 38.30 °C) is considered a risk factor for secondary brain damage, regardless of the etiology of the primary damage (cerebral ischemia, traumatic brain injury, subarachnoid hemorrhage, etc.) [1–5]. The frequency of hyperthermia in neurointensive care units varies from 30% to 60% [3–8] and is associated with a prolonged duration of hospitalization, adverse outcomes, and high mortality [4, 5, 8–10].

The existing temperature gradient between the "core" of the body and the brain [11] explains the importance of direct measurement of cerebral temperature in patients with acute cerebral damage, and it is recommended to measure the temperature in the bladder or esophagus [4] for early diagnosis of hyperthermia [12].

The aim of this study was to estimate the effects of hyperthermia on intracranial pressure (ICP) dynamics and ICP dependence on cerebral autoregulation (CA), measured by the pressure reactivity index (PRx).

Materials and Methods

The study used data from multimodal monitoring of eight patients with acute brain injuries of various etiologies: three patients with a severe traumatic brain injury (TBI), three patients with a subarachnoid hemorrhage (SAH) due to rupture of a cerebral aneurysm (Hunt and Hess grade 3, Fisher grade 3), one patient with a gunshot wound to the head, and one patient who had undergone resection of a metastasis in the cerebral hemisphere. The average age of the patients was 53 (range 18–72) years. Six of the eight patients were female.

All patients were admitted to the neurointensive care unit 1 day (range 0–5 days) after the insult and had negative neurological status dynamics, cerebral edema, and signs of intracranial hypertension according to computed tomography (CT). The patients were treated with a standard local protocol, including mechanical ventilation and monitoring of ICP, cerebral perfusion pressure (CPP), and PRx.

ICP measurement was provided by a Neurovent-P-Temp sensor (Raumedic, Helmbrechts, Germany) combined with a temperature probe. The intraparenchymal sensor was installed at a depth of 2–2.5 cm at Kocher's point. Invasive arterial blood pressure monitoring was performed by a radial artery cannula. CPP was considered as the difference between the average blood pressure and the average ICP. All patients were monitored for partial expiratory CO_2 pressure ($EtCO_2$) by a mainstream CO_2 sensor (Philips Healthcare, Andover, MA, USA). The core body temperature was measured in the bladder by a Foley catheter combined with a thermistor (Smith Medical ASD, Dublin, OH, USA). Hyperthermia was defined as an increase in brain temperature above 38.3 °C.

All parameters were displayed on a Philips MP40 monitor. PRx was calculated by ICM+ software (Cambridge, UK). PRx is a linear correlation coefficient between 40 consecutive averaged measurements of mean arterial pressure and mean intracranial pressure with 5-s increments. PRx values <0 were considered to signify intact autoregulation, while PRx values ≥0 signified loss of autoregulation.

Statistica version 10.0 software (StatSoft, Tulsa, OK, USA) was used for statistical data analysis of parametric and nonparametric criteria. The median values and quartiles of each of the analyzed parameters were used because of the abnormal distribution of the variables.

A. Oshorov (✉) · A. Potapov
Burdenko Neurosurgical Institute, Moscow, Russia

A. Baranich · A. Polupan · A. Sychev · I. Savin
Neurosurgical Intensive Care Department, Burdenko Neurosurgical Institute, Moscow, Russia

B. Depreitere et al. (eds.), *Intracranial Pressure and Neuromonitoring XVII*, Acta Neurochirurgica Supplement 131,
https://doi.org/10.1007/978-3-030-59436-7_15, © Springer Nature Switzerland AG 2021

Results

Thirty-three episodes of an increase in cerebral temperature from 37.8 [quartiles 37.6–38] to 38.9 [quartiles 38.3–39.6] °C were detected. The cerebral temperature delta as a difference between median cerebral temperature before and during hyperthermia$_{(max-min)}$ was 1.2 [quartiles 0.5–2.6] °C.

Analysis of monitored parameters during development of cerebral hyperthermia (blood pressure, CPP, ICP, PRx, $EtCO_2$, and heart rate) revealed a significant change only in ICP, which increased by 6 [quartiles 3–11] mmHg ($p < 0.01$). The Spearman's rank correlation coefficient between brain temperature and ICP was 0.11 ($t(N-2)$, $p < 0.01$).

The dependence of ICP dynamics on the initial value is shown in Table 1.

Before development of hyperthermia, ICP was within normal ranges in 25 observations (76%), with a median value of 11 [8–16] mmHg, while in eight observations (24%), ICP was moderately elevated, with a median value of 23 [22–25] mmHg (Table 1). During progression of hyperthermia, elevated ICP was found in 13 instances (52%) where it was initially normal, with a median value of 24 [22–28] mmHg, while further progression of intracranial hypertension occurred in all eight instances (100%) where ICP was initially elevated (Table 1), and the ICP value increased significantly to 31 [27–32] mmHg ($p < 0.01$).

According to the PRx, CA was intact in 17 observations (52%) and impaired in 16 (48%) (Table 2). CA became impaired in almost half (47%) of the instances where it was initially intact, whereas it recovered in half (50%) of the instances where it was initially impaired (Table 2). Thus, the total numbers of observations with intact and impaired CA remained the same (17 (52%) and 16 (48%), respectively, $p > 0.05$)).

Analysis of ICP dependence on the initial CA state during hyperthermia revealed that the number of episodes of elevated ICP increased by 41% in instances where CA was initially intact but ICP was above 20 mmHg and by 38% in instances where it was initially impaired and ICP was above 20 mmHg ($p > 0.05$) (Table 3). Thus, an increase in ICP during hyperthermia occurred both in instances with intact CA and in instances with impaired CA.

Table 1 Dynamics of intracranial pressure (ICP) during development of cerebral hyperthermia, depending on the initial ICP

$N = 33$ observations (100%) Median 14 [10–20] mmHg		
$ICP_1 \leq 20$ mmHg: $N = 25$ (76%) Median 11 [8–16] mmHg		$ICP_1 > 20$ mmHg: $N = 8$ (24%) Median 23 [22–25] mmHg
$ICP_2 \leq 20$ mmHg: $N = 12$ (48%) Median 13 [10–16] mmHg	$ICP_2 > 20$ mmHg: $N = 13$ (52%) Median 24 [22–28] mmHg	$ICP_2 > 20$ mmHg: $N = 8$ (100%) Median 31 [27–32] mmHg

The values shown in square brackets are quartiles ranges
ICP_1 intracranial pressure before hyperthermia, *ICP_2* intracranial pressure during hyperthermia, *N* number of observations

Discussion

The existing literature data describing the effects of hyperthermia on ICP are controversial. Some researchers believe there is a direct linear relationship between the brain temperature and ICP, and that development of hyperthermia is thus accompanied by an increase in ICP and progression of brain edema [13–15]. Other researchers believe there is no correlation between the brain temperature and ICP [12].

In our study, we did not attempt to analyze the correlation between cerebral temperature and ICP for the entire monitoring period; however, their correlation during hyperthermia was analyzed. We compared the monitoring parameter values prior to hyperthermia with those during hyperthermia. According to our data, ICP parameters changed significantly only with development of cerebral hyperthermia above 38.3 °C. Changes in parameters such as the blood pressure, CPP, $EtCO_2$, heart rate, and PRx were bidirectional and nonsignificant, whereas the ICP value increased significantly during hyperthermia by 6 [quartiles 3–11] mmHg ($p < 0.05$).

Cerebral temperature measurement is considered a more accurate method for temperature monitoring in patients with

Table 2 Dynamics of autoregulation (as shown by the pressure reactivity index (PRx)) during development of cerebral hyperthermia

$N = 33$ observations (100%) Median − 0.01 [range quartiles −0.15 to 0.09]			
$PRx_1 < 0$: $N = 17$ (52%)		$PRx_1 \geq 0$: $N = 16$ (48%)	
$PRx_2 < 0$: $N = 9$ (53%)	$PRx_2 \geq 0$: $N = 8$ (47%)	$PRx_2 < 0$: $N = 8$ (50%)	$PRx_2 \geq 0$: $N = 8$ (50%)

N number of observations, *PRx < 0* intact autoregulation, *PRx ≥ 0* impaired autoregulation, *PRx_1* pressure reactivity index before hyperthermia, *PRx_2* pressure reactivity index during hyperthermia. The values shown in square brackets are quartiles

Table 3 Dynamics of intracranial pressure (ICP) during development of cerebral hyperthermia, depending on the initial autoregulation status (as shown by the pressure reactivity index (PRx)) and the initial ICP

$N = 33$ observations (100%)			
Intact autoregulation, PRx < 0: $N = 17$		Impaired autoregulation, PRx ≥ 0: $N = 16$	
$ICP_1 < 20$ mmHg: $N = 14$ (82%)	$ICP_1 \geq 20$ mmHg: $N = 3$ (18%)	$ICP_1 < 20$ mmHg: $N = 11$ (69%)	$ICP_1 \geq 20$ mmHg: $N = 5$ (31%)
$ICP_2 < 20$ mmHg: $N = 7$ (41%)	$ICP_2 \geq 20$ mmHg: $N = 10$ (59%)	$ICP_2 < 20$ mmHg: $N = 5$ (31%)	$ICP_2 \geq 20$ mmHg: $N = 11$ (69%)

ICP_1 intracranial pressure before hyperthermia, *ICP_2* intracranial pressure during hyperthermia, *N* number of observations

acute cerebral pathology, since cerebral hyperthermia is associated with secondary brain damage [16, 17].

The detrimental effects of hyperthermia could be explained by increases in the release of glutamate (excitotoxicity) [18], free radicals, and products of lipid peroxidation [19]; blood–brain barrier permeability; the severity of brain edema [20]; and protein degradation [21].

Development of secondary brain damage during hyperthermia can be assessed using the dynamics of the neurological status, changes in neuromonitoring parameters (such as ICP), and cerebral temperature monitoring, which directly indicates the probability of secondary brain damage [11, 12, 14–17].

In our study, we decided to diagnose hyperthermia by measuring the cerebral temperature, thus minimizing any controversy that could arise from the temperature gradient between the brain and the "core" [11, 12, 15]. In this chapter, we do not discuss the difference between hyperthermia and fever, because that was not the purpose of our study. It should be noted that we defined hyperthermia as an increase in cerebral temperature above 38.3 °C.

All patients included in the analysis had signs of cerebral edema on CT scanning, and in 24% of instances, ICP was already increased ICP (Table 1). These two facts may explain the increase in ICP due to the development of hyperthermia. In addition, in almost half of all instances (48%), CA was impaired according to the PRx (Table 2).

We excluded the increase in blood carbon dioxide (CO_2) stress because we did not observe a significant increase in $EtCO_2$ in the presence of hyperthermia. In our work, we did not evaluate brain metabolism, but it is known from the literature that hyperthermia leads to increases in brain metabolism and brain tissue oxygen consumption, which, through perfusion–metabolic coupling, cause a rise in the cerebral blood volume and, as a consequence, ICP elevation [13, 22].

Thus, analysis of the monitored parameters revealed that development of cerebral hyperthermia was accompanied by significant changes only in ICP. CA impairment during hyperthermia was observed in 47% of instances where it was initially intact and in 50% of those where it was initially impaired. A possible explanation for the autoregulatory response recovery phenomenon is increases in arterial blood pressure and CPP.

Conclusion

In this study, cerebral hyperthermia was associated with development of intracranial hypertension in 52% of instances where ICP was initially normal and further progression of intracranial hypertension in all instances where ICP was initially elevated. The cerebral hyperthermia–associated increase in ICP was not associated with impaired cerebral autoregulation.

Conflict of Interest **The authors declare that they have no conflict of interest.**

References

1. Badjatia N (2011) Fever control in the NICU: is there still a simpler and cheaper solution? Neurocrit Care 15(3):373–374
2. Fernandez A, Schmidt JM, Claassen J, Pavlicova M, Huddleston D, Kreiter KT, Ostapkovich ND, Kowalski RG, Parra A, Connolly ES, Mayer SA (2007) Fever after subarachnoid hemorrhage: risk factors and impact on outcome. Neurology 68(13):1013–1019
3. Hajat C, Hajat S, Sharma P (2000) Effects of poststroke pyrexia on stroke outcome: a meta-analysis of studies in patients. Stroke 31(2):410–414
4. Madden LK, Hill M, May TL, Human T, Guanci MM, Jacobi J, Moreda MV, Badjatia N (2017) The implementation of targeted temperature management: an evidence-based guideline from the Neurocritical Care Society. Neurocrit Care 27(3):468–487
5. Scaravilli V, Tinchero G, Citerio G, Participants in the International Multi-Disciplinary Consensus Conference on the Critical Care Management of Subarachnoid Hemorrhage (2011) Fever management in SAH. Neurocrit Care 15(2):287–294
6. Andrews PJD, Verma V, Healy M, Lavinio A, Curtis C, Reddy U, Andrzejowski J, Foulkes A, Canestrini S (2018) Targeted temperature management in patients with intracerebral haemorrhage, subarachnoid haemorrhage, or acute ischaemic stroke: consensus recommendations. Br J Anaesth 121(4):768–775
7. Niven DJ, Laupland KB (2016) Pyrexia: aetiology in the ICU. Crit Care 20:247. https://doi.org/10.1186/s13054-016-1406-2
8. Greer DM, Funk SE, Reaven NL, Ouzounelli M, Uman GC (2008) Impact of fever on outcome in patients with stroke and neurologic injury: a comprehensive meta-analysis. Stroke 39(11):3029–3035
9. Prasad K, Krishnan PR (2010) Fever is associated with doubling of odds of short-term mortality in ischemic stroke: an updated meta-analysis. Acta Neurol Scand 122(6):404–408
10. Springer MV, Schmidt JM, Wartenberg KE, Frontera JA, Badjatia N, Mayer SA (2009) Predictors of global cognitive impairment 1 year after subarachnoid hemorrhage. Neurosurgery 65(6):1043–1050
11. Childs C, Lunn KW (2013) Clinical review: brain–body temperature differences in adults with severe traumatic brain injury. Crit Care 17(2):222
12. Huschak G, Hoell T, Wiegel M, Hohaus C, Stuttmann R, Meisel HJ, Mast H (2008) Does brain temperature correlate with intracranial pressure? J Neurosurg Anesthesiol 20(2):105–109
13. Nyholm L, Howells T, Lewén A, Hillered L, Enblad P (2017) The influence of hyperthermia on intracranial pressure, cerebral oximetry and cerebral metabolism in traumatic brain injury. Ups J Med Sci 122(3):177–184
14. Rossi S, Zanier ER, Mauri I, Columbo A, Stocchetti N (2001) Brain temperature, body core temperature, and intracranial pressure in acute cerebral damage. J Neurol Neurosurg Psychiatry 71(4):448–454
15. Stocchetti N, Rossi S, Zanier ER, Colombo A, Beretta L, Citerio G (2002) Pyrexia in head-injured patients admitted to intensive care. Intensive Care Med 28(11):1555–1562
16. Busto R, Dietrich WD, Globus MY, Ginsberg MD (1989) The importance of brain temperature in cerebral ischemic injury. Stroke 20(8):1113–1114

17. Mellergard P, Nordstrom CH (1991) Intracerebral temperature in neurosurgical patients. Neurosurgery 28:709–713
18. Takagi K, Ginsberg MD, Globus MY, Martinez E, Busto R (1994) Effect of hyperthermia on glutamate release in ischemic penumbra after middle cerebral artery occlusion in rats. Am J Phys 267:H1770–H1776
19. Globus MY, Busto R, Lin B, Schnippering H, Ginsberg MD (1995) Detection of free radical activity during transient global ischemia and recirculation: effects of intraischemic brain temperature modulation. J Neurochem 65:1250–1256
20. Clasen RA, Pandolfi S, Laing I, Casey D Jr (1974) Experimental study of relation of fever to cerebral edema. J Neurosurg 41:576–581
21. Morimoto T, Ginsberg MD, Dietrich WD, Zhao W (1997) Hyperthermia enhances spectrin breakdown in transient focal cerebral ischemia. Brain Res 746:43–51
22. Kiyatkin EA (2018) Brain temperature: from physiology and pharmacology to neuropathology. Handb Clin Neurol 157:483–504

A Comparative Study of the Effects of Early Versus Late Cranioplasty on Cognitive Function

Carla B. Rynkowski, Chiara Robba, Ricardo Vigolo de Oliveira, Rodrigo Fabretti, Thais Malickovski Rodrigues, Angelos G. Kolias, Guilherme Finger, Marek Czosnyka, and Marino Muxfeldt Bianchin

Introduction

Cranioplasty (CP) after decompressive craniectomy (DC) can improve cerebral blood flow (CBF), cerebrospinal fluid (CSF) hydrodynamics, and cerebral metabolism [1–5], thus leading to improvements in neurological functions. It was previously standard practice to perform CP around 3–6 months after DC (which is now considered delayed CP) in order to reduce postcranioplasty infection rates and the need for cerebrospinal fluid diversion [6–8]. However, recent studies have suggested that neurological outcomes are better when early CP is applied (as soon as brain swelling disappears), without reproducing those complications [9–13]. Therefore, there is still uncertainty about how late CP can affect neurological status. The aim of this study was to evaluate if we could still detect neurological recovery in those patients submitted to late CP longer than 6 months after DC.

Methods

This was an observational cohort study including patients who underwent CP at a neurosurgery tertiary hospital between January 2015 and April 2018. The study was approved by the local research ethics committee, and informed consent was obtained from all participants. The study included adult patients aged ≥18 years who had undergone a large decompressive craniectomy (for a cranial defect area >125 cm^2 calculated by computed tomography (CT)). For the purpose of the analysis, patients were classified as having early CP if the interval between DC and CP was ≤6 months and late CP if this interval was >6 months.

The primary outcome was the cognitive status assessed using the Addenbrooke's Cognitive Examination Revised (ACE-R), evaluated 1 day before CP, 3 days after CP, and within 90 days after CP. The secondary outcomes were the Mini–Mental State Examination (MMSE) score, Barthel Index (BI) score, and Modified Rankin Scale (mRS) score, evaluated 1 day before and 90 days after CP. The ACE-R was checked with a Brazilian version previously adapted and

C. B. Rynkowski (✉)
Graduate Program in Medical Science, Universidade Federal do Rio Grande do Sul, Porto Alegre, Brazil

Adult Critical Care Unit, Hospital Cristo Redentor, Porto Alegre, Brazil

C. Robba
Department of Anaesthesia and Intensive Care, San Martino Policlinico Hospital, IRCCS for Oncology, Genoa, Italy

R. V. de Oliveira · R. Fabretti
Psychology Department, Hospital Cristo Redentor, Porto Alegre, Brazil

T. M. Rodrigues
Graduate Program, Medical School, Universidade Luterana do Brasil, São José, Brazil

A. G. Kolias
Neurosurgical Division, Department of Clinical Neurosciences, University of Cambridge, Cambridge, UK

NIHR Global Health Research Group on Neurotrauma, University of Cambridge, Cambridge, UK

G. Finger
Department of Neurosurgery, Hospital Cristo Redentor, Porto Alegre, Brazil

M. Czosnyka
Neurosurgical Division, Department of Clinical Neurosciences, University of Cambridge, Cambridge, UK

M. M. Bianchin
Graduate Program in Medical Science, Universidade Federal do Rio Grande do Sul, Porto Alegre, Brazil

B.R.A.I.N., Division of Neurology, Hospital de Clínicas de Poro Alegre, Porto Alegre, Brazil

B. Depreitere et al. (eds.), *Intracranial Pressure and Neuromonitoring XVII*, Acta Neurochirurgica Supplement 131, https://doi.org/10.1007/978-3-030-59436-7_16,

tested in patients with cognitive compromise [14, 15]. The neuropsychological evaluations were carried out by the same trained team of a neurosurgeon, a neurointensivist, and a psychologist.

Results

Over the study period, 51 patients were included in the study. The average age was 33.4 ± 12.2 years, and most patients (66%) were male. The indications for DC were traumatic brain injury (TBI) in 73% (37/51), subarachnoid hemorrhage (SAH) in 10% (5/51), intracerebral hemorrhage in 8% (4/51), stroke in 6% (3/51), and a noninfiltrating tumor in 4% (2/51). The mean (± standard deviation (SD)) time between DC and CP was 93.2 ± 32.08 days in the early-CP group and 608.36 ± 485.39 in the late-CP group (Table 1).

We observed general increments in the cognitive and functional scale scores 90 days after CP, especially in the late-CP group (Table 2). ACE-R was the only cognitive scale also tested 3 days after CP, and the scores increased from the time point before CP to 3 days after CP in both the late-CP group (51 ± 28.94 versus 53.1 ± 30.39 points, $P = 0.016$) and the early-CP group (41.6 ± 32.89 versus 44.6 ± 33.47 points, $P = 0.199$). However, only in the late-CP group did the MMSE score increase from the time point before CP to 90 days after it (18.54 ± 1.51 versus 20.34 ± 1.50, $P = 0.003$) (Table 2).

Considering functional status, the mRS score increased from the time point before CP to 90 days after it in both the early-CP group (2.45 ± 0.47 versus 1.67 ± 0.54, $P = 0.0001$) and the late-CP group (2.07 ± 0.22 versus 1.74 ± 0.20, $P = 0.015$), but only the late-CP group increased their BI scores from the time point before CP to 90 days after it (79.84 ± 4.66 versus 85.62 ± 4.10, $P = 0.028$).

Discussion

Our results are only partially in agreement with those of previous studies, which showed better results with early CP in terms of functional status [10, 11, 16]. In fact, surprisingly,

Table 1 Baseline characteristics of patients undergoing early and late cranioplasty (CP)

	Overall	Early CP	Late CP	*P* value
Patients [*n* (%)]	51 (100)	9 (18)	42 (82)	
Reason for DC [*n* (%)]				0.45
TBI	37 (72)	7	30	
SAH	5 (10)	2	3	
ICH	4 (8)	0	4	
Stroke	3 (6)	0	3	
Tumor	2 (4)	0	2	
Age [years; mean ± SD]	33.4 ± 12.2	32.78 ± 14.41	33.62 ± 11.86	0.853
Male sex [*n* (%)]	33 (66.6)	6 (66.7)	31 (73.8)	0.692
Time between DC and CP [days; mean ± SD]	399 ± 480	93.2 ± 32.08	608.36 ± 485.39	
DC location [*n* (%)]				0.669
Right DC	21 (40)	4 (44.4)	17 (40.4)	
Left DC	27 (54)	5 (55.6)	22 (52.4)	
Bifrontal DC	3 (6)	0	3 (7.2)	
Cognition before CP [mean ± SD]				
ACE-R score	48.47 ± 4.94	35.17 ± 33.37	51.97 ± 28	0.287
MMSE score	18.87 ± 9.64	20.5 ± 10.78	24.09 ± 7.32	0.464
Functionality before CP [mean ± SD]				
BI score	79.32 ± 30.14	71 ± 44.21	80.63 ± 28.10	0.659
mRS score	2.16 ± 1.50	2.63 ± 1.5	2.07 ± 1.5	0.345

A paired-samples Student's *t* test was applied for these comparisons

ACE-R Addenbrooke's Cognitive Examination Revised, *BI* Barthel Index, *DC* decompressive craniectomy, *ICH* intracranial hemorrhage, *MMSE* Mini–Mental State Examination, *mRS* Modified Rankin Scale, *SAH* subarachnoid hemorrhage, *SD* standard deviation, *TBI* traumatic brain injury

Table 2 Global neurological assessment of patients undergoing early and late cranioplasty (CP)

	Overall			Early CP			Late CP		
	Before CP [mean ± SD]	90 days after CP [mean ± SD]	*P* value	Before CP [mean ± SD]	90 days after CP [mean ± SD]	*P* value	Before CP [mean ± SD]	90 days after CP [mean ± SD]	*P* value
ACE-R score	49.66 ± 29.20	56.89 ± 30.22	**0.009**	41.60 ± 32.89	49.60 ± 31.17	**0.009**	51 ± 28.94	58.10 ± 30.46	**0.0001**
MMSE score	18.87 ± 9.64	19.73 ± 9.16	**0.008**	20.66 ± 3.53	22.06 ± 3.38	0.468	18.54 ± 1.51	20.34 ± 1.50	**0.003**
BI score	79.32 ± 30.14	86.08 ± 24.94	**0.022**	71 ± 44.21	79.07 ± 12.05	0.608	80.63 ± 28.1	85.62 ± 4.10	**0.028**
mRS score	2.16 ± 1.5	1.76 ± 1.37	**0.0001**	2.45 ± 0.47	1.67 ± 0.54	**0.0001**	2.07 ± 0.22	1.74 ± 0.20	**0.015**

A paired-samples Student's *t* test was applied for these comparisons. Significant *P* values are shown in bold text
ACE-R Addenbrooke's Cognitive Examination Revised, *BI* Barthel Index, *MMSE* Mini–Mental State Examination, *mRS* Modified Rankin Scale, *SD* standard deviation

we observed cognitive improvement in the late-CP group. The cognitive improvement occurred very early, just 3 days after CP, even in the late-CP group, reinforcing a possible mechanical effect of CP. Moreover, cognitive improvement in the late-CP group occurred in both aggregated and more detailed cognitive scales. Like our study, the study by Corallo et al. considered 6 months as the interval between early and late CP after DC and observed that cognitive improvement was similar in both the early- and late-CP groups [7]. Songara et al. demonstrated better cognitive function results when CP was performed up to 3 months after DC [13]. In a recent systematic review, Cola et al. stated that cognition tends to improve as soon as CP is performed [12]. We could perhaps attribute the differences in our results, compared with those of the other studies, to the heterogeneity of etiologies of DC in our study cohort.

Our study had the following limitations. First, we could not perform a complex and larger neuropsychological appraisal of the patients. Second, we could not determine the effects of a shorter interval between DC and CP, because the timing of CP was dependent on the scheduling for this procedure in the local public health system? evaluations of cerebral blood flow and intracranial pressure with noninvasive methods would have added important information about the effects of cranioplasty [12, 17–19] but were not performed.

Conclusion

Our study emphasizes the importance of CP in the improvement of neurological function. According to our results, even late CP can favorably improve neurological status.

Conflict of Interest: **The authors have no conflict of interest to declare.**

References

1. Chibbaro S, Vallee F, Beccaria K, Poczos P, Makiese O, Fricia M, Vicaut E (2013) The impact of early cranioplasty on cerebral blood flow and its correlation with neurological and cognitive outcome. Prospective multicentre study on 24 patients. Rev Neurol (Paris) 169(3):240–248. https://doi.org/10.1016/j.neurol.2012.06.016
2. Fodstad H, Love JA, Ekstedt J, Fridén H, Liliequist B (1984) Effect of cranioplasty on cerebrospinal fluid hydrodynamics in patients with the syndrome of the trephined. Acta Neurochir 70(1–2):21–30
3. Lazaridis C, Czosnyka M (2012) Cerebral blood flow, brain tissue oxygen, and metabolic effects of decompressive craniectomy. Neurocrit Care 16(3):478–484. https://doi.org/10.1007/s12028-012-9685-1
4. Parichay PJ, Khanapure K, Joshi KC, Aniruddha TJ, Sandhya M, Hegde AS (2017) Clinical and radiological assessment of cerebral hemodynamics after cranioplasty for decompressive craniectomy—a clinical study. J Clin Neurosci 42:97–101. https://doi.org/10.1016/j.jocn.2017.04.005
5. Winkler PA, Stummer W, Linke R, Krishnan KG, Tatsch K (2000) The influence of cranioplasty on postural blood flow regulation, cerebrovascular reserve capacity, and cerebral glucose metabolism. Neurosurg Focus 8(1):1–9
6. Beauchamp KM, Kashuk J, Moore EE (2010) Cranioplasty after postinjury decompressive craniectomy: is timing of the essence? J Trauma 69:270–274. https://doi.org/10.1097/TA.0b013e3181e491c2
7. Corallo F, De Cola MC, Lo Buono V, Marra A, De Luca R, Trinchera A, Calabro RS (2017) Early vs late cranioplasty: what is better? Int J Neurosci 127(8):688–693. https://doi.org/10.1080/00207454.2016.1235045
8. Thavarajah D, Lacy P, Hussein A, Sugar A (2012) The minimum time for cranioplasty insertion from craniectomy is six months to reduce risk of infection—a case series of 82 patients. Br J Neurosurg 26(1):78–80. https://doi.org/10.3109/02688697.2011.603850
9. De Cola MC, Corallo F, Pria D, Lo Buono V, Calabro RS (2018) Timing for cranioplasty to improve neurological outcome: a systematic review. Brain Behav 8:e1106. https://doi.org/10.1002/brb3.1106
10. Kim BW, Kim TU, Hyun JK (2017) Effects of early cranioplasty on the restoration of cognitive and functional impairments. Ann Rehabil Med 41(3):354–361. https://doi.org/10.5535/arm.2017.41.3.354

11. Nasi D, Dobran M, Di Rienzo A, di Somma L, Gladi M, Moriconi E, Iacoangeli M (2018) Decompressive craniectomy for traumatic brain injury: the role of cranioplasty and hydrocephalus on outcome. World Neurosurg 116:e543–e549. https://doi.org/10.1016/j.wneu.2018.05.028
12. Song J, Liu M, Mo X, Du H, Huang H, Xu GZ (2014) Beneficial impact of early cranioplasty in patients with decompressive craniectomy: evidence from transcranial Doppler ultrasonography. Acta Neurochir 156(1):193–198
13. Songara A, Gupta R, Jain N, Rege S, Masand R (2016) Early cranioplasty in patients with posttraumatic decompressive craniectomy and its correlation with changes in cerebral perfusion parameters and neurocognitive outcome. World Neurosurg 94:303–308
14. Carvalho VA, Barbosa MT, Caramelli P (2010) Brazilian version of the Addenbrooke Cognitive Examination—Revised in the diagnosis of mild Alzheimer disease. Cogn Behav Neurol 23(1):8–13. https://doi.org/10.1097/WNN.0b013e3181c5e2e5
15. Carvalho VA, Caramelli P (2007) Brazilian adaptation of the Addenbrooke's Cognitive Examination—Revised (ACE-R). Dement Neuropsychol 1(2):212–216
16. Yang NR, Song J, Yoon KW, Seo EK (2018) How early can we perform cranioplasty for traumatic brain injury after decompressive craniectomy? A retrospective multicenter study. World Neurosurg 110:e160–e167. https://doi.org/10.1016/2017.10.117
17. Paredes I, Castaño AM, Cepeda S, Alén JAF, Salvador E, Millán JM, Lagares A (2016) The effect of cranioplasty on cerebral hemodynamics as measured by perfusion computed tomography and Doppler ultrasonography. J Neurotrauma 33(17):1586–1597
18. Robba C, Cardim D, Tajsic T, Pietersen J, Bulman M, Rasulo F, Czosnyka M (2018) Non-invasive intracranial pressure assessment in brain injured patients using ultrasound-based methods. Acta Neurochir Suppl 126:69–73. https://doi.org/10.1007/978-3-319-65798-1_15
19. Robba C, Goffi A, Geeraerts T, Cardim D, Via G, Czosnyka M, Citerio G (2019) Brain ultrasonography: methodology, basic and advanced principles and clinical applications: a narrative review. Intensive Care Med 45(7):913–927. https://doi.org/10.1007/s00134-019-05610-4

Effects of Cranioplasty After Decompressive Craniectomy on Neurological Function and Cerebral Hemodynamics in Traumatic Versus Nontraumatic Brain Injury

Carla B. Rynkowski, Chiara Robba, Melina Loreto, Ana Carolina Wickert Theisen, Angelos G. Kolias, Guilherme Finger, Marek Czosnyka, and Marino Muxfeldt Bianchin

Introduction

In patients who have undergone a decompressive craniectomy (DC), cranioplasty (CP) can potentially improve neurological symptoms and cerebral blood flow (CBF) [1–5]. However, the literature is lacking regarding those improvements in patients with different etiologies of DC. The aim of this study was to investigate the effects of CP on neurological status and cerebral hemodynamics in patients with and without TBI.

Methods

This was a prospective observational study at a single center in a middle-income country. It included patients who underwent CP after DC between January 2015 and April 2018. The study was approved by the local research ethics committee, and informed consent was obtained from all participants.

Adult patients (aged ≥18 years) who had undergone a large DC (for a cranial defect area >125 cm² calculated by computed tomography (CT) on a GE workstation with Advantage Workstation version 4.4 software) were included in the study. The exclusion criteria were absence of informed consent, CP performed to correct a small or moderate scalp defect, and the need to remove the cranial prosthesis because of infection or rejection. CBF was studied by transcranial Doppler ultrasound (TCD), analyzing the mean velocity (MV) of flow in the ipsilateral and contralateral middle cerebral arteries. The neurological status was checked using the Mini–Mental State Examination (MMSE), Barthel Index (BI), and modified Rankin Scale (mRS). All evaluations were performed 1 day before CP and again 90 days after it. The patients were grouped as TBI patients and non-TBI patients.

Results

Of the 51 patients included in the study, 37 had TBI and 14 did not. The TBI group was younger (28.86 ± 9.71 versus 45.64 ± 9.55 years, $P = 0.0001$), with a greater proportion of men than the non-TBI group (31 versus 6, $P = 0.011$) (Table 1).

C. B. Rynkowski (✉)
Graduate Program in Medical Science, Universidade Federal do Rio Grande do Sul, Porto Alegre, Brazil

Adult Critical Care Unit, Hospital Cristo Redentor, Porto Alegre, Brazil

C. Robba
Department of Anaesthesia and Intensive Care, San Martino Policlinico Hospital, IRCCS for Oncology, Genoa, Italy

M. Loreto
Adult Critical Care Unit, Hospital Divina Providência, Porto Alegre, Brazil

A. C. W. Theisen
Graduate Program, Medical School, Universidade Luterana do Brasil, Canoas, Brazil

A. G. Kolias
Neurosurgical Division, Department of Clinical Neurosciences, University of Cambridge, Cambridge, UK

NIHR Global Health Research Group on Neurotrauma, University of Cambridge, Cambridge, UK

G. Finger
Department of Neurosurgery, Hospital Cristo Redentor, Porto Alegre, Brazil

M. Czosnyka
Neurosurgical Division, Department of Clinical Neurosciences, University of Cambridge, Cambridge, UK

M. M. Bianchin
Graduate Program in Medical Science, Universidade Federal do Rio Grande do Sul, Porto Alegre, Brazil

B.R.A.I.N., Division of Neurology, Hospital de Clínicas de Poro Alegre, Porto Alegre, Brazil

B. Depreitere et al. (eds.), *Intracranial Pressure and Neuromonitoring XVII*, Acta Neurochirurgica Supplement 131, https://doi.org/10.1007/978-3-030-59436-7_17,

In both groups, there was an improvement in MMSE and mRS scores 90 days after CP. However, BI scores increased only in non-TBI patients (Table 2).

In TBI and non-TBI patients, the MV of blood flow before CP was lower in the middle cerebral artery ipsilateral to the cranial defect than in the contralateral one (Table 3). In the TBI group, there was an increase in MV in the ipsilateral artery from the time point before CP to 90 days after it (34.24 ± 11.02 versus 42.14 ± 10.19 cm/s, P = 0.0001). However, in non-TBI patients, the MV in that artery did not change over that time.

Table 1 Baseline characteristics of patients with and without traumatic brain injury (TBI) undergoing cranioplasty (CP) after decompressive craniectomy

	Overall	TBI group	Non-TBI group	*P* value
Patients [*n* (%)]	51 (100)	37 (73)	14 (27)	
Reason for DC [*n* (%)]				
TBI		37 (72)		
SAH			5 (10)	
ICH			4 (8)	
Stroke			3 (6)	
Tumor			2 (4)	
Age [years; mean ± SD]	33.4 ± 12.2	28.86 ± 9.71	45.64 ± 9.55	**0.0001**
Male sex [*n* (%)]	33 (66.6)	31 (83.7)	6 (42.8)	**0.011**
Time between DC and CP [months; mean ± SD]	13.3 ± 16.07	16.84 ± 16.56	18.31 ± 15.23	0.774
MMSE score before CP [mean ± SD]	18.87 ± 9.64	22.90 ± 8.37	25.40 ± 6.29	0.394
BI score before CP [mean ± SD]	79.32 ± 30.14	84.62 ± 27.85	66.82 ± 32.96	0.101
mRS score before CP [mean ± SD]	2.16 ± 1.50	1.86 ± 1.53	2.45 ± 1.75	0.299

A paired-samples Student's *t* test was applied for these comparisons. Significant *P* values are shown in bold text
BI Barthel Index, *DC* decompressive craniectomy, *ICH* intracerebral hemorrhage, *MMSE* Mini–Mental State Examination, *mRS* Modified Rankin Scale, *SAH* subarachnoid hemorrhage, *SD* standard deviation

Table 2 Global neurological assessment of patients with and without traumatic brain injury (TBI) undergoing cranioplasty (CP)

	TBI group			Non-TBI group		
	Before CP	90 days after CP	*P* value	Before CP	90 days after CP	*P* value
MMSE score [mean ± SD]	19.31 ± 9.65	20.13 ± 8.84	**0.028**	17.6 ± 10.01	18.63 ± 10.32	**0.002**
BI score [mean ± SD]	84.61 ± 27.85	83.57 ± 27.14	0.416	66.81 ± 32.96	93.88 ± 14.95	**0.015**
mRS score [mean ± SD]	2 ± 1.43	1.59 ± 1.38	**0.005**	2.61 ± 1.66	2.07 ± 1.38	**0.048**

A paired-samples Student's *t* test was applied for these comparisons. Significant *P* values are shown in bold text
With regard to the MMSE, BI, and mRS scores, there was no significant difference between the TBI and non-TBI groups before CP (P = 0.394, P = 0.101, and P = 0.299, respectively) or after CP (P = 0.592, P = 0.886, and P = 0.258, respectively)
BI Barthel Index, *MMSE* Mini–Mental State Examination, *mRS* Modified Rankin Scale, *SD* standard deviation

Table 3 Mean velocity (MV) of blood flow in the middle cerebral arteries ipsilateral and contralateral to the cranial defect in patients with and without traumatic brain injury (TBI) undergoing cranioplasty (CP)

	TBI group			Non-TBI group		
	Before CP	90 days after CP	*P* value	Before CP	90 days after CP	*P* value
Ipsilateral MV [cm/s; mean ± SD]	34.24 ± 11.22[a]	42.14 ± 10.19[b]	**0.0001**	33.12 ± 11.87[a]	32.90 ± 10.40[b]	1
Contralateral MV [cm/s; mean ± SD]	48.89 ± 16.11	43.06 ± 13.68	0.145	44.08 ± 12.41	44.06 ± 17.71	1
P value	**0.0001**	0.680		**0.0001**	**0.0001**	

A paired-samples Student's *t* test was applied for these comparisons. Significant *P* values are shown in bold text
SD standard deviation
[a]Before CP, both TBI patients and non-TBI patients had low MV values in the ipsilateral middle cerebral artery (34.24 ± 11.22 versus 33.12 ± 11.87 cm/s, P = 0.764)
[b]Ninety days after CP, TBI patients had higher MV values in the ipsilateral middle cerebral artery than non-TBI patients (42.14 ± 2.01 versus 32.90 ± 3.30 cm/s, P = 0.017)

Discussion

This was a prospective study of patients with DC of different etiologies who underwent CP. In our cohort, TBI patients were younger than non-TBI patients, and a greater proportion of them were men. These differences reflected the characteristics of the TBI population [6]. Moreover, in this study population, CP was generally performed at a late stage (about 1 year after DC), which could be attributed to the characteristics of the local public health system.

Neurological improvement after CP, including both cognition and functional status, has previously been described in TBI patients [7–11]. Our study confirms those previous findings and also provides further insights regarding the outcomes of non-TBI patients after DC. Even considering the small sample of diverse etiologies of DC in non-TBI patients, we observed global neurological recovery, reinforcing the contribution of CP to neurological outcomes.

Considering cerebral hemodynamics, we observed an initial asymmetry between the hemispheres. Before CP, both TBI patients and non-TBI patients had lower blood flow in the middle cerebral artery ipsilateral to the cranial defect than in the contralateral one. This initial asymmetry represents the impact of a cranial defect on the uncovered brain, as has previously been reported [12–14], even with different methods being used to evaluate CBF [5, 15].

After CP, TBI patients had a comparative increase in MV in the middle cerebral artery ipsilateral to the cranial defect. Comparing CBF evaluation in both groups before and 90 days after CP, we found that initially low CBF persisted after CP for longer in non-TBI patients than in TBI patients. In a similar study using TCD, Kuo et al. observed no CBF improvement in the hemisphere ipsilateral to the cranial defect in TBI and non-TBI patients, maybe because the patient numbers in that study were small [16]. In another study that included TBI patients evaluated with TCD, Ergodan et al. did observe an increment in CBF in the hemisphere ipsilateral to the cranial defect [12]. Therefore, further research in larger cohorts is needed to evaluate CBF changes in TBI versus other causes of DC to verify our findings [17].

Another option to explore intracerebral hemodynamics would be use of ultrasonography of the optic nerve sheath diameter, which is a safe method for noninvasive estimation of intracranial pressure [18–23]. It could complement TCD and contribute to better understanding of cerebral hemodynamics before and after CP.

Our study had the following limitations. First, because of logistical and financial constraints, we could not apply specialized and complex neurological evaluations. Second, our non-TBI patients presented a mix of different etiologies that may have resulted in particular differences in the parameters that were evaluated.

Conclusion After CP, there is an improvement in both functional outcome and cognitive function in both TBI and non-TBI patients, but only TBI patients have an increment in CBF velocity after CP.

Conflict of Interest: **The authors have no conflict of interest to declare.**

References

1. Chibbaro S, Vallee F, Beccaria K, Poczos P, Makiese O, Fricia M, Vicaut E (2013) The impact of early cranioplasty on cerebral blood flow and its correlation with neurological and cognitive outcome: prospective multicentre study on 24 patients. Rev Neurol (Paris) 169(3):240–248. https://doi.org/10.1016/j.neurol.2012.06.016
2. Fodstad H, Love JA, Ekstedt J, Fridén H, Liliequist B (1984) Effect of cranioplasty on cerebrospinal fluid hydrodynamics in patients with the syndrome of the trephined. Acta Neurochir 70(1–2):21–30
3. Lazaridis C, Czosnyka M (2012) Cerebral blood flow, brain tissue oxygen, and metabolic effects of decompressive craniectomy. Neurocrit Care 16(3):478–484. https://doi.org/10.1007/s12028-012-9685-1
4. Parichay PJ, Khanapure K, Joshi KC, Aniruddha TJ, Sandhya M, Hegde AS (2017) Clinical and radiological assessment of cerebral hemodynamics after cranioplasty for decompressive craniectomy—a clinical study. J Clin Neurosci 42:97–101. https://doi.org/10.1016/j.jocn.2017.04.005
5. Winkler PA, Stummer W, Linke R, Krishnan KG, Tatsch K (2000) The influence of cranioplasty on postural blood flow regulation, cerebrovascular reserve capacity, and cerebral glucose metabolism. Neurosurg Focus 8(1):1–9
6. Bonow RH, Barber J, Temkin NR, Videtta W, Rondina C, Petroni G, Lujan S, Alanis V, La Fuente G, Lavadenz A, Merida R, Jibaja M, Gonzáles L, Falcao A, Romero R, Dikmen S, Pridgeon J, Chesnut RM, Global Neurotrauma Research Group (2018) The outcome of severe traumatic brain injury in Latin America. World Neurosurg 111:e82–e90. https://doi.org/10.1016/j.wneu.2017.11.171
7. Chibbaro S, Di Rocco F, Mirone G, Fricia M, Makiese O, Di Emidio P, Bresson D (2011) Decompressive craniectomy and early cranioplasty for the management of severe head injury: a prospective multicenter study on 147 patients. World Neurosurg 75(3–4):558–562. https://doi.org/10.1016/j.wneu.2010.10.020
8. Corallo F, De Cola MC, Lo Buono V, Marra A, De Luca R, Trinchera A, Calabro RS (2017) Early vs late cranioplasty: what is better? Int J Neurosci 127(8):688–693. https://doi.org/10.1080/00207454.2016.1235045
9. Jasey N, Ward I, Lequerica A, Chiaravalloti ND (2018) The therapeutic value of cranioplasty in individuals with brain injury. Brain Inj 32(3):318–324. https://doi.org/10.1080/02699052.2017.1419283
10. Kim BW, Kim TU, Hyun JK (2017) Effects of early cranioplasty on the restoration of cognitive and functional impairments. Ann Rehabil Med 41(3):354–361. https://doi.org/10.5535/arm.2017.41.3.354
11. Posti JP, Yli-Olli M, Heiskanen L, Aitasalo KMJ, Rinne J, Vuorinen V, Piitulainen JM (2018) Cranioplasty after severe traumatic brain injury: effects of trauma and patient recovery on cranioplasty outcome. Front Neurol 9:223. https://doi.org/10.3389/fneur.2018.00223
12. Erdogan E, Düz B, Kocaoglu M, Izci Y, Sirin S, Timurkaynak E (2003) The effect of cranioplasty on cerebral hemodynamics:

evaluation with transcranial Doppler sonography. Neurol India 51(4):479
13. Song J, Liu M, Mo X, Du H, Huang H, Xu GZ (2014) Beneficial impact of early cranioplasty in patients with decompressive craniectomy: evidence from transcranial Doppler ultrasonography. Acta Neurochir 156(1):193–198. https://doi.org/10.1007/s00701-013-1908-5
14. Yoshida K, Furuse M, Izawa A, Iizima N, Kuchiwaki H, Inao S (1996) Dynamics of cerebral blood flow and metabolism in patients with cranioplasty as evaluated by 133Xe CT and 31P magnetic resonance spectroscopy. J Neurol Neurosurg Psychiatry 61(2):166–171
15. Paredes I, Castano AM, Cepeda S, Alen JA, Salvador E, Millan JM, Lagares A (2016) The effect of cranioplasty on cerebral hemodynamics as measured by perfusion computed tomography and Doppler ultrasonography. J Neurotrauma 33(17):1586–1597. https://doi.org/10.1089/neu.2015.4261
16. Kuo JR, Wang CC, Chio CC, Cheng TJ (2004) Neurological improvement after cranioplasty—analysis by transcranial Doppler ultrasonography. J Clin Neurosci 11(5):486–489. https://doi.org/10.1016/j.jocn.2003.06.005
17. Halani SH, Chu JK, Malcolm JG, Rindler RS, Allen JW, Grossberg JA, Ahmad FU (2017) Effects of cranioplasty on cerebral blood flow following decompressive craniectomy: a systematic review of the literature. Neurosurgery 81(2):204–216. https://doi.org/10.1093/neuros/nyx054
18. Robba C, Bacigaluppi S, Cardim D, Donnelly J, Bertuccio A, Czosnyka M (2016) Non-invasive assessment of intracranial pressure. Acta Neurol Scand 134(1):4–21. https://doi.org/10.1111/ane.12527
19. Robba C, Cardim D, Tajsic T, Pietersen J, Bulman M, Rasulo F, Czosnyka M (2018) Non-invasive intracranial pressure assessment in brain injured patients using ultrasound-based methods. Acta Neurochir Suppl 126:69–73. https://doi.org/10.1007/978-3-319-65798-1_15
20. Robba C, Donnelly J, Cardim D, Tajsic T, Cabeleira M, Citerio G, Pelosi P, Smielewski P, Hutchinson P, Menon DK, Czosnyka M (2019) Optic nerve sheath diameter ultrasonography at admission as a predictor of intracranial hypertension in traumatic brain injured patients: a prospective observational study. J Neurosurg 8:1–7
21. Robba C, Goffi A, Geeraerts T, Cardim D, Via G, Czosnyka M, Citerio G (2019) Brain ultrasonography: methodology, basic and advanced principles and clinical applications. A narrative review. Intensive Care Med 45(7):913–927. https://doi.org/10.1007/s00134-019-05610-4
22. Robba C, Santori G, Czosnyka M, Corradi F, Bragazzi N, Padayachy L, Citerio G (2018) Optic nerve sheath diameter measured sonographically as non-invasive estimator of intracranial pressure: a systematic review and meta-analysis. Intensive Care Med 44(8):1284–1294. https://doi.org/10.1007/s00134-018-5305-7
23. Schreiber M, Robba C, Cardim D, Tajsic T, Pietersen J, Bulman M, Czosnyka M (2017) Ultrasound non-invasive measurement of intracranial pressure in neurointensive care: a prospective observational study. PLoS Med 14(7):e1002356. https://doi.org/10.1371/journal.pmed.1002356

Brain Multimodal Monitoring in Severe Acute Brain Injury: Is It Relevant to Patient Outcome and Mortality?

Elisabete Monteiro, António Ferreira, Edite Mendes, Cláudia Camila Dias, Marek Czosnyka, José Artur Paiva, and Celeste Dias

Introduction

The primary focus of neurocritical care is early detection and prevention of secondary brain injury because the impact of the primary lesion is often irreversible [1]. Thus, advanced multimodal monitoring (MMM) of the brain has been recommended as an important tool to manage severe acute brain injury in intensive care units (ICUs). MMM allows simultaneous and continuous assessment of cerebral hemodynamics, oxygenation, and metabolism, providing an individualized approach at the bedside [2]. MMM should be done in a continuous way so as not to overlook clinically significant events. Data should be collected simultaneously, time synchronized, and displayed in an integrated fashion [2] to provide targeted individualized care. MMM of the brain includes monitoring provided by different devices, including intracranial pressure (ICP), cerebral perfusion pressure (CPP), cerebral oximetry with near-infrared spectroscopy (NIRS), brain tissue oxygen partial pressure ($pbtO_2$), and cerebral blood flow (CBF) evaluated by transcranial Doppler ultrasonography and/or by thermal diffusion flowmetry.

Use of the pressure reactivity index (PRx) for continuous assessment of autoregulation and optimal CPP [3] is the fulcrum of MMM and is feasible at the bedside [4]. Impaired autoregulation leads to secondary injury and is an independent predictor of a fatal outcome following acute brain injury (ABI) [4]. Although there are retrospective published data on the association between cerebral autoregulation and acute brain injury outcomes [5–8], suggesting that preserved autoregulation leads to a better prognosis, there is a lack of robust evidence that use of MMM (including PRx) and treatment by a dedicated team contributes to better outcomes. Outcomes at ICU discharge, 28 days, 3 months, and 6 months can be assessed with use of the Glasgow Outcome Scale (GOS). A GOS score of 1 means death, a score of 2 means a persistent vegetative state, a score of 3 means severe disability, a score of 4 means moderate disability, and a score of 5 means good recovery [9].

The aim of this study was to determine if MMM has implications for mortality and outcomes in patients with severe acute brain injury—namely, severe aneurysmal subarachnoid hemorrhage (SAH) or severe traumatic brain injury (TBI).

Materials and Methods

Patient Selection

This study included all patients admitted with a diagnosis of severe aneurysmal SAH or severe TBI to two general ICUs and one neurocritical care ICU (level III) in the same intensive care department at Centro Hospitalar Universitário São João between March 2014 and December 2016. Severity was defined by clinical evaluation and the decision to manage the patient with level III care. A total of 389 patients were included in the study.

Patients less than 18 years old, pregnant females, and patients with expected survival of <3 days were excluded. The research ethics committee at Centro Hospitalar Universitário São João approved the study protocol and data collection.

E. Monteiro (✉) · A. Ferreira · E. Mendes · J. A. Paiva · C. Dias
Department of Intensive Care Medicine, Centro Hospitalar e Universitário São João, Porto, Portugal

C. C. Dias
Faculdade de Medicina da Universidade do Porto MEDCIDS—Departamento de Medicina da Comunidade, Informação e Decisão em Saúde e CINTESIS—Centro de Investigação em Tecnologias e em Serviços de Saúde, Porto, Portugal

M. Czosnyka
Brain Physics Laboratory, Division of Neurosurgery, Department of Clinical Neurosciences, University of Cambridge, Cambridge, UK

B. Depreitere et al. (eds.), *Intracranial Pressure and Neuromonitoring XVII*, Acta Neurochirurgica Supplement 131,
https://doi.org/10.1007/978-3-030-59436-7_18,

Data Collection

Patient files were reviewed retrospectively, and data on several demographic and clinical variables were recorded—namely, the patient's age, sex, Glasgow Coma Scale score at ictus and at hospital admission, pupillary response at admission, blood glucose level, blood pressure (absence or presence of hypotension, defined as systolic arterial blood pressure <90 mmHg), oxygenation (absence or presence of hypoxemia with peripheral oxygen saturation (SpO_2) of <90%), and the presence or absence of seizures. Disease severity and mortality prediction on admission were calculated by use of the Simplified Acute Physiology Score (SAPS II). For SAH, other scales of severity were also used: the Hunt and Hess Scale, the Fisher Scale [10], and the World Federation of Neurological Surgeons (WFNS) Grading Scale [11, 12].

With regard to systemic monitoring, all patients were managed with a Philips Intellivue multiparameter monitor, which allowed continuous bedside acquisition of electrocardiographic, heart rate, respiratory rate, invasive arterial blood pressure, pulse oximetry, and end-tidal CO_2 data. With regard to MMM of the brain [4], ICP wave, CPP, NIRS, $pbtO_2$, and CBF data were recorded. For evaluation of autoregulation, PRx was continuously calculated at the bedside, using ICM+ software. PRx was calculated as the Pearson coefficient between 30 consecutive 10-s averaged values of arterial blood pressure (ABP) and corresponding ICP signals. A positive correlation between ABP and ICP at a low frequency indicates passive cerebral vessels and impaired autoregulation. A zero or negative correlation indicates intact autoregulation [5]. The optimal CPP is the CPP value with the lowest associated PRx value. Outcomes at ICU discharge, 28 days, 3 months, and 6 months were assessed with use of the GOS.

Statistical Analysis

Continuous variable data were expressed as mean values with standard deviations or medians and 25th–75th percentile ranges. Categorical variable data were presented as numbers (n) and percentages (%). The GOS score was dichotomized into a poor outcome (GOS score $\leq$ 3) and a good outcome (GOS score > 3), and comparative analysis was performed for all patients and also separately for the two subgroups of patients with TBI and SAH. When a hypothesis about continuous variables was being tested, nonparametric Mann–Whitney or Kruskall–Wallis tests were used, as appropriate, taking into account normality assumptions and the number of groups compared. When a hypothesis about categorical variables was being tested, a χ^2 test and a Fisher's exact test were used, as appropriate. To gain more thorough understanding of the factors associated with a poor outcome and mortality (dependent variables), univariate and multivariate logistic regression modeling was used with sex, age, glycemia, hypotension, and the Glasgow Coma Scale at first aid and the kind of ICU (general versus NeuroCritical) as independent variables.

The significance level used was 0.05. Statistical analyses was performed using SPSS version 24.0 software.

Results

The total studied population consisted of 389 patients: 95 with SAH and 294 with TBI. The overall median age was 61 (17–97) years; the median ages were 64 years in patients with SAH and 60 years in those with TBI. The ICU lengths of stay (LOSs) for SAH and TBI were 12 (6–28) and 15 (8–23) days, respectively, and the hospital LOSs were 29 (18–52) and 30 (17–49) days, respectively, with no statistical differences between the two groups. The SAPS II score was 44 in patients with SAH and 32 in those with TBI ($P < 0.0001$). There were no differences between SAH and TBI in terms of the pupillary response at hospital admission. With regard to hypoxia, 29 patients with TBI versus only 3 with SAH presented SpO2 values <90% ($P = 0.039$). Hypotension was also more frequent in TBI patients than in SAH patients (12.6% versus 4.2%, $P = 0.021$). In terms of metabolic control, 39.8% of TBI patients versus 23.2% of SAH were hyperglycemic and 57.1% of TBI patients versus 68.4% of SAH patients were normoglycemic ($P = 0.003$).

With regard to outcomes at ICU discharge, 47.4% of patients with SAH had a poor outcome, compared with 77.1% of those with TBI ($P < 0.001$). Good outcomes were recorded in 55.3% of patients with SAH versus 31.6% of those with TBI at 28 days ($P < 0.001$), 74.7% versus 50.2% at 3 months ($P < 0.001$), and 81% versus 56.5% at 6 months ($P < 0.001$) (Table 1).

Of the 259 males, 221 had TBI and 38 had SAH; of the 130 females, 73 had TBI and 57 had SAH.

A second analysis was done in which two different groups were compared: group 1, comprising 69 patients managed with MMM and use of PRx; and group 2, comprising 320 patients managed without MMM in either a general ICU or the NCCU.

In this comparison of the above groups, there were no differences in age, sex, ICU LOS, or hospital LOS. The median Glasgow Coma Scale (GCS) scores at hospital admission were 4 (3–12) in group 1 versus 8 (3–13) in group 2 ($P = 0.050$). The median SAPS II scores were 40 (29–49) in group 1 versus 43 (33–55) in group 2 ($P = 0.047$) (Table 2).

Table 1 Demographic and clinical variables, outcome, and survival in subarachnoid hemorrhage (SAH) and traumatic brain injury (TBI) patients

	SAH (*n* = 95)	TBI (*n* = 294)	*P* value[a]
Male sex [*n* (%)]	38 (40)	221 (75)	**<0.001**[b]
Age [years; median (P25–P75)]	64 (43–78)	60 (48–75)	0.530[c]
Length of stay [days; median (P25–P75)]			
In ICU	12 (6–28)	15 (8–23)	0.807[c]
In hospital	29 (18–52)	30 (17–49)	0.704[c]
SAPS II score [median (P25–P75)]	32 (24–48)	44 (37–55)	**<0.001**[c]
Mortality adjusted for the SAPS II score [%; median (P25–P75)]	14 (6–44)	33 (20–56)	**<0.001**[c]
Treatment location [*n* (%)]			**<0.001**[b]
Neurocritical care unit	77 (81)	160 (55)	
UCIPU: General ICU 1	7 (7)	60 (20)	
UCIPG: General ICU 2	11 (12)	74 (25)	
Poor outcome [*n* (%)][d]			
In ICU	45 (47)	226 (77)	**<0.001**[b]
At 28 days	38 (45)	171 (68)	**<0.001**[b]
At 3 months	20 (25)	107 (50)	**<0.001**[b]
At 6 months	15 (19)	87 (43)	**<0.001**[b]
Mortality [*n* (%)][e]			
In ICU	14 (15)	51 (17)	0.545[b]
At 28 days	11 (13)	47 (19)	0.217[b]
At 3 months	11 (14)	51 (24)	0.068[b]
At 6 months	11 (14)	50 (25)	**0.044**[b]

ICU intensive care unit, *P25* 25th percentile, *P75* 75th percentile, *SAPS II* Simplified Acute Physiology Score
[a]Significant *P* values are shown in bold text
[b]χ^2 test
[c]Kruskall–Wallis test
[d]Poor outcome: Glasgow Outcome Scale score between 1 and 3
[e]Mortality: Glasgow Outcome Scale score of 1

With regard to outcomes, good outcomes were seen in 59% of group 1 versus 24% of group 2 at ICU discharge, 65% versus 30% at 28 days, and 77% versus 51% at 3 months ($P < 0.001$ at all three times of evaluation). At 6 months, good outcomes were seen in 78% of group 1 versus 59% of group 2 ($P = 0.005$).

The mortality rates were 7% in group 1 versus 19% in group 2 at ICU discharge ($P = 0.020$), 7% versus 20% at 28 days ($P = 0.013$), 9% versus 25% at 3 months ($P = 0.008$), and 13% versus 25% at 6 months ($P = 0.039$).

When outcomes were adjusted for injury severity (evaluated by SAPS II) with poor outcome as a dependent variable, the odds ratios were 0.215 at ICU discharge ($P < 0.001$), 0.234 at 28 days ($P < 0.001$), 0.338 at 3 months ($P < 0.001$), and 0.474 at 6 months ($P = 0.044$). Thus, the differences between groups 1 and 2 persisted despite adjustment for injury severity.

Table 2 Comparison between subarachnoid hemorrhage (SAH) and traumatic brain injury (TBI) patients managed with and without multimodal monitoring (MMM) of the brain

	With MMM (*n* = 69)	Without MMM (*n* = 320)	*P* value[a]
Male sex [*n* (%)]	45 (18)	214 (83)	0.791[b]
Age [years; median (P25–P75)]	58 (41–69)	63 (49–79)	0.057[c]
Length of stay [days; median (P25–P75)]			
In ICU	23 (15–29)	13 (7–22)	<0.001[c]
In hospital	41 (26–67)	26 (16–47)	**<0.001**[c]
SAPS II score [median (P25–P75)]	40 (29–49)	43 (33–55)	**0.047**[c]
SAPS II mortality [%; median (P25–P75)]	25 (11–44)	31 (16–58)	**0.049**[c]
GCS at first aid: local [median (P25–P75)]	10 (6–14)	12 (7–14)	0.409[c]
GCS score: hospital [median (P25–P75)]	4 (3–12)	8 (3–13)	0.050[c]
Injury [*n* (%)]			0.057[b]
SAH	23 (33)	72 (23)	
TBI	46 (67)	248 (73)	
Hypoxia [*n* (%)]	0 (0)	32 (10)	**0.006**[b]
Hypotension [*n* (%)]	1 (1)	40 (13)	**0.007**[b]
Glycemia [*n* (%)]			**0.144**[b]
Normoglycemia	44 (64)	189 (59)	
Hypoglycemia	0 (0)	17 (5)	
Hyperglycemia	25 (36)	114 (36)	
Poor outcome [*n* (%)][d]			
In ICU	28 (41)	243 (76)	**<0.001**[b]
At 28 days	24 (35)	185 (70)	**<0.001**[b]
At 3 months	15 (23)	112 (49)	**<0.001**[b]
At 6 months	14 (22)	88 (41)	**0.005**[b]
Mortality [*n* (%)][e]			
In ICU	5 (7)	60 (19)	**0.020**[b]
At 28 days	5 (7)	53 (20)	**0.013**[b]
At 3 months	6 (9)	56 (25)	**0.008**[b]
At 6 months	8 (13)	53 (25)	**0.039**[b]

GCC Glasgow Coma Scale, *ICU* intensive care unit, *P25* 25th percentile, *P75* 75th percentile, *SAPS II* Simplified Acute Physiology Score
[a]Significant *P* values are shown in bold text
[b]χ^2 test
[c]Mann–Whitney test
[d]Poor outcome: Glasgow Outcome Scale score between 1 and 3
[e]Mortality: Glasgow Outcome Scale score of 1

However, when mortality was adjusted for the SAPS II score, there were no significant differences between groups 1 and 2.

Discussion

Our comparison between TBI and SAH confirmed our clinical and subjective perceptions that at baseline, TBI patients are more severely injured; in fact, they had higher SAPS II scores and higher rates of hypoxemia and hypotension. Although there were no differences in mortality between these two groups until 6 months (at which stage, mortality was higher in TBI patients), their outcomes were clearly different, and patients with SAH had better outcomes than those with TBI. We hypothesized that this might depend on the initial insult and inability to promptly revert causes of secondary lesions, such as hypoperfusion and hypoxemia, since the initial diagnosis (either TBI or SAH) did not limit or direct the type of monitoring used in each patient. Another hypothesis was that if MMM was used in patients with acute brain injury, their prognoses would be better. For that reason, we analyzed two different groups on the basis of use or nonuse of MMM. Despite statistical differences between the two groups at baseline, when the results were adjusted for severity scores, outcomes were better in patients who received MMM (including use of PRx). Whether this benefit arose from use of all of the monitoring devices together or from use of one device in particular warrants further investigation.

Conclusion

Despite the limitations of a small population ($n = 389$), our study showed that use of MMM was beneficial. Outcomes at all points of evaluation were better in patients managed with MMM. Regarding mortality the group with MMM had lower mortality rates. Use of a dedicated team to manage patients with acute brain lesions may contribute to improve outcomes and reduce mortality. However, this work warrants further validation, preferably in a multicenter, randomized, controlled study.

Conflict of Interest **The authors have no conflicts of interest.**

References

1. Roh D, Soojin P (2016) Brain multimodality monitoring: updated perspectives. Curr Neurol Neurosci Rep 16(6):56. https://doi.org/10.1007/s11910-016-0659-0
2. Citerio G, Oddo M, Taccone F (2015) Recommendations for the use of multimodal monitoring in the neurointensive care unit. Curr Opin Crit Care 21:113–119
3. Smith M (2018) Multimodality neuromonitoring in adult traumatic brain injury. Anesthesiology 128:401–415. https://doi.org/10.1097/ALN.0000000000001885
4. Dias C, Silva MJ, Pereira E, Monteiro E, Maia I, Barbosa S, Silva S, Honrado T, Cerejo A, Aries M, Smielewski P, Paiva JA, Czosnyka M (2015) Optimal cerebral perfusion pressure management at bedside: a single-center pilot study. Neurocrit Care 23(1):92–102. https://doi.org/10.1007/s12028-014-0103-8
5. Aries M, Czosnyka M, Budohoski P, Steiner L, Lavinio A, Kolias A, Hutchinson P, Brady K, Menon D, Pickard J, Smielewski P (2012) Continuous determination of optimal cerebral perfusion pressure in traumatic brain injury. Crit Care Med 40(8):2456–2463. https://doi.org/10.1097/CCM.0b013e3182514eb6
6. Rasulo FA, Girardini A, Lavinio A et al (2012) Are optimal cerebral perfusion pressure and cerebrovascular autoregulation related to long-term outcome in patients with aneurysmal subarachnoid hemorrhage? J Neurosurg Anesthesiol 24(1):3–8
7. Stein SC, Georgoff P, Meghan S, Mirza KL, El Falaky OM (2010) Relationship of aggressive monitoring and treatment to improved outcomes in severe traumatic brain injury. J Neurosurg 112(5):1105–1112
8. Czosnyka M, Balestreri M, Steiner L et al (2005) Age, intracranial pressure, autoregulation, and outcome after brain trauma. J Neurosurg 102(3):450–454
9. Jennett B (1975) Assessment of outcome after severe brain damage: a practical scale. Lancet 305:480–484
10. Fisher CM, Kistler JP, Davis JM (1980) Relation of cerebral vasospasm to subarachnoid hemorrhage visualized by computerized tomographic scanning. Neurosurgery 6(1):1–9
11. Drake C (1988) Report of the World Federation of Neurological Surgeons Committee on a universal subarachnoid hemorrhage grading scale. J Neurosurg 68(6):985–986
12. Lagares A, Gómez PA, Lobato RD, Alén JF, Alday R, Campollo J (2001) Prognostic factors on hospital admission after spontaneous subarachnoid haemorrhage. Acta Neurochir 143:665–672

Long-Term Outcome After Decompressive Craniectomy in a Developing Country

Carla B. Rynkowski, Luciano Silveira Basso, Angelos G. Kolias, and Marino Muxfeldt Bianchin

Introduction

Decompressive craniectomy (DC) is an important tool for control of intracranial hypertension [1]. It can reduce mortality but may increase the number of survivors in a vegetative state [2, 3]. The functional outcome after DC is dependent on accurate evaluation of the indications for it, and it should not be performed in patients with a poor prognosis [4, 5].

Data on outcomes after DC usually come from high-income countries [2, 3]. It is possible that the profile of patients who undergo DC, as well as their conditions, are different in other countries [6]. In this study, we investigated the long-term functional outcome of patients who underwent DC at a tertiary neurosurgery hospital in a middle-income country. The aim of the study was to evaluate the outcome after DC in patients with different pathologies in a middle-income country.

Materials and Methods

This was a prospective observational study of patients undergoing DC in a single tertiary hospital in southern Brazil between January 2015 and December 2018. All patients undergoing DC in the hospital during that period were included, whether it was primary or secondary DC and regardless of the etiology. A Glasgow Outcome Scale (GOS) score of 4 or 5 at 6 months after DC was considered a favorable outcome.

When the lesion was limited to one cerebral hemisphere, unilateral hemicraniectomy was performed. For bilateral or frontal lesions, bifrontal craniectomy was chosen. The surgical technique used was similar to that described by Ragel et al. [7], with minimal adaptations. In our service, we usually perform watertight closure duraplasty with pericranium. Patients receiving intracranial pressure (ICP) monitoring were treated for intracranial hypertension when the ICP was ≥22 mmHg, sustained for ≥5 min.

Statistical analysis was performed using SPSS version 20 software. We considered probability values lower than 5% ($P < 0.05$) as statistically significant. Quantitative data were expressed as mean ± standard deviation. Categorical data were expressed as frequency and percentage. A Student's t test was used for quantitative variables, and a χ^2 test was used for nominal variables. Logistic regression analysis was performed to determine independent risk factors for an unfavorable clinical outcome (GOS scores of 1, 2, or 3) at 6-month follow-up. The study was approved by the local institutional ethical committee.

Results

In our sample, 125 patients underwent DC in this 4-year period. Most of our patients (57.6% (72/125)) underwent DC because of a traumatic brain injury (TBI) (Table 1). The mean age was 45.18 ± 19.6 years, and 71% were men. The mean initial Glasgow Coma Scale (GCS) score was 7.8 ± 3.6. The mean lengths of stay were 16.1 ± 12.7 days in the intensive care unit (ICU) and 40.3 ± 48.3 days in the hospital. Primary DC represented 89.6% of cases (112/125). Left-side hemicraniectomy was the most frequently performed

C. B. Rynkowski (✉)
Adult Critical Care Unit, Hospital Cristo Redentor, Porto Alegre, Brazil

L. S. Basso
Department of Neurosurgery, Hospital Cristo Redentor, Porto Alegre, Brazil

A. G. Kolias
Neurosurgical Division, Department of Clinical Neurosciences, University of Cambridge, Cambridge, UK

M. M. Bianchin
B.R.A.I.N., Division of Neurology, Hospital de Clínicas de Porto Alegre, Porto Alegre, Brazil

B. Depreitere et al. (eds.), *Intracranial Pressure and Neuromonitoring XVII*, Acta Neurochirurgica Supplement 131, https://doi.org/10.1007/978-3-030-59436-7_19,

Table 1 Patient characteristics and outcome assessment analysis

Parameter	Overall	Outcome Favorable[a]	Unfavorable[b]	*P* value[c]
Patients [*n* (%)]	125 (100)	35 (28)	90 (72)	
Reason for DC [*n* (%)]				0.597
TBI	72 (57.6)	21 (65.6)	51 (54.8)	
Stroke	27 (21.6)	5 (15.6)	22 (23.6)	
ICH, SAH, or AVM	24 (19.2)	6 (18.7)	18 (19.3)	
Age [years; mean ± SD]	45.18 ± 19.6	33.3 ± 16.2	49.7 ± 18.9	**0.0001**
Male sex [*n* (%)]	87 (71)	22 (68.7)	65 (69.8)	0.470
Initial GCS score [mean ± SD]	7.83 ± 3.6	8.75 ± 3.54	7.5 ± 3.6	**0.046**
Length of stay [days; mean ± SD]				
In ICU	16.1 ± 12.7	18.21 ± 8.3	15.4 ± 13.8	**0.041**
In hospital	40.4 ± 48.3	39.5 ± 17.3	40.5 ± 55.5	**0.013**
ICP monitoring [*n* (%)]				
Before DC	11 (8.8)	2 (6.2)	9 (9.67)	0.726
After DC	38 (30.4)	10 (31.2)	20 (30.1)	0.563

AVM arteriovenous malformation, *DC* decompressive craniectomy, *GCS* Glasgow Coma Scale, *ICH* intracranial hemorrhage, *ICP* intracranial pressure, *ICU* intensive care unit, *SAH* subarachnoid hemorrhage, *SD* standard deviation, *TBI* traumatic brain injury
[a]Glasgow Outcome Scale score: 4 or 5
[b]Glasgow Outcome Scale score: 1, 2, or 3
[c]Significant *P* values are shown in bold text

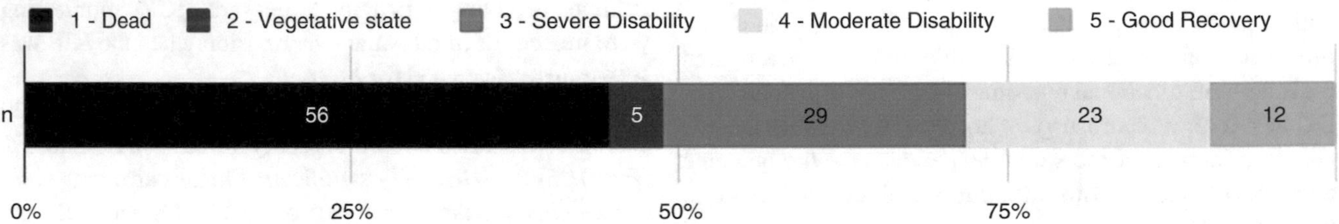

Fig. 1 Glasgow Outcome Scale (GOS) scores 6 months after decompressive craniectomy

procedure (49.6%), followed by right-side hemicraniectomy (45.6%) and bifrontal craniectomy (4.8%).

The hospital mortality rate was 44.8% (56/125). Among survivors, 50.7% (35/69) had a favorable outcome (with a GOS score of 4 or 5) 6 months after DC (Fig. 1). After multivariate analysis (which also included sex and the reasons for DC), a lower initial GCS score (7.5 ± 3.6 versus 8.8 ± 3.5 points, $P = 0.007$) and older age (49.7 ± 18.9 versus 33.3 ± 16.2 years, $P = 0.0001$) were associated with an unfavorable outcome (with a GOS score of 1, 2, or 3) (Table 1). Patients with an unfavorable outcome also had greater lengths of stay in the ICU and in the hospital (Table 1).

Discussion

In our study, the in-hospital mortality rate after DC was around 45%. Half of the survivors had a favorable outcome 6 months after DC.

This in-hospital mortality rate after DC was greater than those previously reported from centers in high-income countries (which are around 20% even for TBI and for malignant brain infarction (MBI)) but lower than those reported from low-income world regions (60–70%) [2, 8, 9]. It must be noted that our sample consisted of patients treated at a neurosurgical referral center in a middle-income country. Unfortunately, there are still few data available regarding the profiles of patients undergoing DC in places other than high-income countries [9, 10]. Although it is focused only on patients with TBI, we hope that the Global Neurotrauma Outcomes Study (GNOS)—a multicenter study of TBI patients undergoing emergency neurosurgery—will provide comprehensive information about the particulars of DC in low-income countries [11].

Generally, the most common indications for DC are TBI and MBI. Although half of our patients had TBI, the other had a mix of different etiologies (Table 1). This aspect might have contributed to the outcomes we observed. The incidence of TBI is higher in low- and middle-income countries, and the associated mortality rate is also higher than those observed in high-income countries—an important factor that needs to be considered when assessing worldwide mortality associated with DC [10, 12]. The outcome after DC is dependent on many factors such as those related to the surgical technique, the neurosurgeon's expertise, the time to the procedure, the initial etiology and severity of the case, the patient's age, the time to cranioplasty (CP), and the conditions for rehabilitation after DC [8, 13]. Like previously published research, our study also found that older age and a poor initial neurological status (as shown by a lower Glasgow Coma Scale score) were associated with an unfavorable outcome [9, 10, 13]. We also observed greater lengths of stay in the ICU and in the hospital among patients with an unfavorable outcome. These results can, of course, be explained by a predictably longer hospital stay for patients whose clinical and neurological conditions are the most severe.

The timing of DC has a direct impact on the outcome because it is related to the duration and severity of brain injury before the procedure. If DC is performed too late, it can be futile and not save otherwise possibly recoverable brain tissue. Although it is focused only on patients with TBI could save the patient's life but with an increased likelihood of an unfavorable outcome [2, 3]. However, it can be difficult to precisely estimate what proportion of recommendations for DC are late or ill-advised. The perspective of neurological recovery after brain injury is also an important ethical aspect to be considered in decision making about the timing of DC [5].

An important point to take into account, considering recovery after DC, is the effect of cranioplasty. In addition to enhancing cerebral hemodynamics and metabolism, CP leads to functional and global neurological improvements [14–16]. In our sample, unfortunately, CP was performed at a late stage and no patient underwent CP within 6 months. These data reinforce the importance of DC not only as a procedure that saves lives but also as a procedure that can offer a favorable outcome for survivors of a severe brain injury [17]. We hypothesize that if our patients could have access to early CP and perhaps better rehabilitation protocols, we would observe better outcomes.

Conclusion

DC has an important role to play in improving the outcome of patients with a severe brain injury. This procedure can be performed with considerable success even in parts of the world with poor medical resources, and it has a major impact on the survival and prognosis of these patients.

Conflict of Interest **The authors have no conflict of interest to declare.**

References

1. Carney N, Totten AM, O'Reilly C, Ullman JS, Hawryluk GW, Bell MJ, Bratton SL, Chesnut R, Harris OA, Kissoon N, Rubiano AM, Shutter L, Tasker RC, Vavilala MS, Wilberger J, Wright DW, Ghajar J (2017) Guidelines for the management of severe traumatic brain injury, fourth edition. Neurosurgery 80(1):6–15. https://doi.org/10.1227/NEU.0000000000001432
2. Cooper DJ, Rosenfeld JV, Murray L, Arabi YM, Davies AR, D'Urso P et al (2011) Decompressive craniectomy in diffuse traumatic brain injury. N Engl J Med 364:1493–1502
3. Hutchinson PJ, Kolias AG, Timofeev IS, Corteen EA, Czosnyka M, Timothy J et al (2016) Trial of decompressive craniectomy for traumatic intracranial hypertension. N Engl J Med 375:1119–1130
4. Hutchinson PJ, Kolias AG, Tajsic T, Adeleye A, Aklilu AT, Apriawan T, Bajamal AH, Barthélemy EJ, Devi BI, Bhat D et al (2019) Consensus statement from the International Consensus Meeting on the Role of Decompressive Craniectomy in the Management of Traumatic Brain Injury: consensus statement. Acta Neurochir 161(7):1261–1274. https://doi.org/10.1007/s00701-019-03936-y
5. Kwan K, Schneider J, Ullman JS (2019) Chapter 12: decompressive craniectomy: long term outcome and ethical considerations. Front Neurol 10:876. https://doi.org/10.3389/fneur.2019.00876
6. Laghari AA, Bari ME, Waqas M, Ahmed SI, Nathani KR, Moazzam W (2018) Outcome of decompressive craniectomy in traumatic closed head injury. Asian J Neurosurg 13(4):1053–1056
7. Ragel BT, Klimo P Jr, Martin JE, Teff RJ, Bakken HE, Armonda RA (2010) Wartime decompressive craniectomy: technique and lessons learned. Neurosurg Focus 28(5):E2
8. Champeaux C, Weller J (2019) Long-term survival after decompressive craniectomy for malignant brain infarction: a 10-year nationwide study. Neurocrit Care 32(2):522–531. https://doi.org/10.1007/s12028-019-00774-9
9. Kaushal A, Bindra A, Kumar A, Goyal K, Kumar N, Rath GP, Gupta D (2019) Long term outcome in survivors of decompressive craniectomy following severe traumatic brain injury. Asian J Neurosurg 14(1):52–57
10. Bonow RH, Barber J, Temkin NR, Videtta W, Rondina C, Petroni G, Lujan S, Alanis V, La Fuente G, Lavadenz A, Merida R, Jibaja M, Gonzáles L, Falcao A, Romero R, Dikmen S, Pridgeon J, Chesnut RM, Global Neurotrauma Research Group (2018) The outcome of severe traumatic brain injury in Latin America. World Neurosurg 111:e82–e90
11. Kolias AG, Rubiano AM, Figaji A, Servadei F, Hutchinson PJ (2019) Traumatic brain injury: global collaboration for a global challenge. Lancet Neurol 18(2):136–137
12. Roozenbeek B, Maas AI, Menon DK (2013) Changing patterns in the epidemiology of traumatic brain injury. Nat Rev Neurol 9(4):231–236
13. Morgalla MH, Will BE, Roser F, Tatagiba M (2008) Do long-term results justify decompressive craniectomy after severe traumatic brain injury? J Neurosurg 109(4):685–690
14. Chibbaro S, Vallee F, Beccaria K, Poczos P, Makiese O, Fricia M, Mateo J, Gobron C, Guichard JP, Romano A, Levy B, George B,

Vicaut E (2013) The impact of early cranioplasty on cerebral blood flow and its correlation with neurological and cognitive outcome: prospective multicentre study on 24 patients. Rev Neurol (Paris) 169(3):240–248
15. De Cola MC, Corallo F, Pria D, Lo Buono V, Calabrò RS (2018) Timing for cranioplasty to improve neurological outcome: a systematic review. Brain Behav 8(11):e01106
16. Fodstad H, Love JA, Ekstedt J, Fridén H, Liliequist B (1984) Effect of cranioplasty on cerebrospinal fluid hydrodynamics in patients with the syndrome of the trephined. Acta Neurochir 70(1–2):21–30
17. Stevens RD, Shoykhet M, Cadena R (2015) Emergency neurological life support: intracranial hypertension and herniation. Neurocrit Care 23(Suppl 2):S76–S82. https://doi.org/10.1007/s12028-015-0168-z

Predictors of Successful Extubation in Neurocritical Care Patients

Walter Videtta, Jeanette Vallejos, Gisela Roda, Hugo Collazos, Nico Naccarelli, Alex Tamayo, Noelia Calderón, Ariadna Bairaclioti, Martín Yoshida, Gabriel Vandaele, Ruth Toloza, Juan Quartino, Pablo Dunne, Maria G. Rodríguez, Marcos A. Teheran Wilches, Jhimmy J. Morales Vasquez, Brenda L. Fernandez Fernandez, and On Behalf of the Merlo ICU Research Group

Introduction

In neurocritical care patients, delayed extubation is associated with a longer duration of hospital stay, a higher incidence of pneumonia associated with mechanical ventilation, and increased mortality [1]. Few previous studies have established the success of extubation in patients with acute neurological pathology. There is also no available evidence to support use of particular variables that—with a reasonable margin of safety—can predict the success of extubation in this population. Neurocritical care patients commonly require mechanical ventilation (MV) and monitoring in an intensive care unit (ICU) [1]. The reasons for failed extubation in brain-injured patients are poorly understood [2, 3]. A low Glasgow Coma Scale (GCS) score, inability to follow commands, and airway reflexes may be independent of each other [4]. Delayed extubation in neurocritical care patients is associated with an increased length of stay (LOS) in the ICU, a higher incidence of ventilator-associated pneumonia (VAP), and a worse outcome, without decreasing the risk of extubation failure [4, 5]. There is no evidence available to support the use of certain variables over others as predictors of successful extubation in these patients.

Materials and Methods

During a 30-month study period, 34 neurocritical care patients aged ≥18 years who required MV for ≥48 h were included in this prospective, observational cohort study. The study excluded patients in whom tracheostomy was performed before the first extubation attempt.

The study protocol was approved by the ethics committee at Hospital Municipal Eva Perón de Merlo. A written consent form was signed by each patient's surrogate. For each patient, we recorded data on demographic characteristics, the acute neurological disorder, the motor component of the GCS score (mGCS), the Acute Physiology and Chronic Health Evaluation II (APACHE II) score, the Sequential Organ Failure Assessment (SOFA) score, the length of stay (LOS) in the ICU, the duration of MV, the Airway Care Score (ACS), and the outcome. Patients undergoing extubation were categorized by its success or failure.

Successful extubation was defined as weaning and absence of ventilatory support for ≥7 days [6]. Univariate analysis was performed. Spearman's ρ was used to quantify the association between the studied predictors and successful extubation. To identify independent prognostic variables, multiple regression analysis was performed, and *P* values of ≤0.05 were considered significant. For analysis of continuous variables, the Mann–Whitney *U* test was applied. To ascertain the association between age and success or failure of extubation, Spearman's ρ was used. A χ^2 test was used for analysis of nominal variables. Statistical analysis was performed using IBM SPSS Statistics version 21 software.

On Behalf of the Merlo ICU Research Group

W. Videtta (✉) · J. Quartino · P. Dunne · M. G. Rodríguez
Adult ICU Hospital Municipal Eva Perón de Merlo, Buenos Aires, Argentina

Universidad Nacional del Oeste, Merlo, Buenos, Argentina

J. Vallejos · M. A. T. Wilches · B. L. F. Fernandez
Adult ICU Hospital Municipal Eva Perón de Merlo, Buenos Aires, Argentina

Hospital Paroissien, San Justo, Argentina

G. Roda
Universidad Nacional del Oeste, Merlo, Buenos, Argentina

Unidad Asistencial Doctor César Milstein, INSSJP, CABA, Merlo, Argentina

H. Collazos · N. Naccarelli · A. Tamayo · N. Calderón · A. Bairaclioti
M. Yoshida · G. Vandaele · R. Toloza · J. J. M. Vasquez
Adult ICU Hospital Municipal Eva Perón de Merlo, Buenos Aires, Argentina

B. Depreitere et al. (eds.), *Intracranial Pressure and Neuromonitoring XVII*, Acta Neurochirurgica Supplement 131,
https://doi.org/10.1007/978-3-030-59436-7_20,

Results

During the 30-month study period, 82 patients were admitted. After exclusion of 48 patients (of whom 25 died before extubation, 17 underwent tracheostomy, 4 had missing data, and 2 self-extubated), 34 patients underwent planned extubation. A total of 34 patients were included in the study: 21 (61.8%) with a traumatic brain injury (TBI), 7 (20.6%) with an ischemic stroke, 2 (5.9%) with a subarachnoid hemorrhage, 2 (5.9%) with meningitis, 1 (2.9%) with status epilepticus, and 1 (2.9%) with a brain tumor. Twenty-five of the 34 patients (73.5%) achieved successful extubation. None of them required reintubation within 7 days. The rate of extubation failure was 26.5% (9/34). Table 1 shows the patients' demographic data. Table 2 shows the results of univariate analysis of extubation success or failure and clinical demographic data. The following variables had no impact on the success or failure of extubation: the duration of MV, APACHE II score, mGCS score, SOFA score, mechanical ventilation, airway occlusion pressure/maximum inspiratory pressure (P 0.1/PIMax), LOS in ICU, and ACS. To identify independent prognostic variables, multiple regression analysis was performed, in which P values of ≤0.05 were considered significant. For analysis of continuous variables, a Mann–Whitney U test was applied; the results are shown in Table 2. None of the variables that were evaluated in relation to the success or failure of extubation showed statistical significance, except for the variable of age. The only factor independently associated with successful extubation was age <42.5 years ($Z = -2.014$, $P < 0.044$ with a wide confidence interval). To understand the association between age and the success or failure of extubation, Spearman's ρ was used ($r = 0.351$, $P < 0.042$). The value of 42.5 corresponded to the cutoff point found in the decision tree procedure with application of the random forest method, which established that there was a greater probability of successful extubation when the patient's age was less than 42.5 years; if this is not the case, other variables such as the APACHE II score, LOS in the ICU, and use of vasopressors must be taken into account.

Of the patients in this study, those whose extubation was successful had been mechanically ventilated for 9.08 ± 4.42 days and those whose extubation failed had been mechanically ventilated for 17.33 ± 20.26 days, but the difference between these two groups was not significant.

An mGCS score of >4 was not associated with successful extubation; the scores in patients with successful versus failed extubation were 5.64 versus 5.56.

Table 1 Variable description according to predictor of success or failure of extubation

	Success/failure					
	Success			Failure		
	Mean	Standard deviation	Median	Mean	Standard deviation	Median
Age	39.72	16.43	42.00	51.67	11.74	51.00
APACHE	19.32	7.62	22.00	20.22	4.74	21.00
SOFA	6.20	2.55	6.00	6.11	3.41	6.00
MV duration (days)	9.08	4.42	9.00	17.33	20.16	10.00
ICU length of stay (days)	19.40	15.91	13.00	28.33	20.54	25.00
Glasgow Coma Scale (motor)	5.64	0.49	6.00	5.56	0.53	6.00
PVA	5.28	1.37	5.00	4.78	1.48	5.00
P01/PIMAx	0.03	0.03	0.02	0.03	0.02	0.03

Table 2 Statistical tests

Test statistic[a]								
	Age	APACHE	SOFA	MV duration (days)	ICU LOS	GCS (Motor)	PVA	P01/ PIMAx
Mann–Whitney U	61,000	111,000	111,500	93,500	72,000	103,000	90,500	95,500
Wilcoxon W	386,000	436,000	156,500	418,500	397,000	148,000	135,500	420,500
Z	−2.014	−0.059	−0.039	−0.744	−1.584	−0.440	−0.883	−0.664
Bilateral asymptotic significance	0.044	0.953	0.969	0.457	0.113	0.660	0.377	0.507
Exact significance [2*(undateral significance)]	.045[b]	.969[b]	.969[b]	.465[b]	.120[b]	.730[b]	.397[b]	.514[b]

[a]Grouping variable success failure
[b]Not corrected for draws

Discussion

Age was identified as an independent factor associated with successful extubation. In our study, the cutoff point for age was 42.5 years, which was slightly above the age of 40 years identified in other studies focusing on prediction of the success of extubation in brain-injured patients [7]. Age has previously been identified as a risk factor for failure of extubation in non-neurological patients >65 years old [8]. Physicians should consider the patient's age when considering extubation in brain-injured patients >42.5 years old.

In our study, the duration of MV was greater in patients with extubation failure. This was in accordance with the findings of other studies in the literature [9].

In previous studies, the lowest mGCS score was associated with an increased risk of extubation failure [10, 11], whereas the highest mGCS score was associated with successful extubation [12].

The rate of extubation failure in our study was 26.5%. This rate was in accordance with those previously described in the literature, with reported rates of 20–40% in neurocritical care patients. Some studies have reported lower failure rates of 6–16% in different populations with use of different definitions [2, 7, 9, 11].

Our study had many limitations, including its small sample size, its observational nature, and the fact that it included patients treated at only one center.

Conclusion

In the population we studied, the only significant predictor of the success or failure of extubation was the patient's age: the lower the age, the greater the chance of successful extubation, with a cutoff point of 42.5 years. In brain-injured patients above this age, physicians should consider other clinical variables when deciding whether to attempt extubation. These findings need to be validated in larger patient cohorts.

Conflict of Interest **The authors have no conflict of interest to declare.**

References

1. Lazaridis C, DeSantis SM, McLawhorn M, Krishna V (2012) Liberation of neurosurgical patients from mechanical ventilation and tracheostomy in neurocritical care. J Crit Care 27:417e.1–417e.8
2. Karanjia N, Nordquist D, Stevens R et al (2011) A clinical description of extubation failure in patients with primary brain injury. Neurocrit Care 15:4–12
3. Ko R, Ramos L, Chalela JA (2009) Conventional weaning parameters do not predict extubation failure in neurocritical care patients. Neurocrit Care 10:269–273
4. King CS, Moores LK, Epstein SK (2010) Should patients be able to follow commands prior to extubation? Respir Care 55:56–65
5. Coplin WM, Pierson DJ, Cooley KD, Newell DW, Rubenfeld GD (2000) Implications of extubation delay in brain-injured patients meeting standard weaning criteria. Am J Respir Crit Care Med 161:1530–1536
6. Béduneau G, Pham T, Schortgen F, Piquilloud L, Zogheib E, Jonas M, Grelon F, Runge I, Terzi N, Grangé S, Barberet G, Guitard PG, Frat JP, Constan A, Chretien JM, Mancebo J, Merçat A, Richard JM, Brochard L, WIND (Weaning According to a New Definition) Study Group and the REVA (Réseau Européen de Recherche en Ventilation Artificielle) Network (2017) Epidemiology of weaning outcome according to a new definition: the WIND study. Am J Respir Crit Care Med 195(6):772–783. https://doi.org/10.1164/rccm.201602-0320OC
7. Asehnoune K, Seguin P, Lasocki S, Roquilly A, Delater A, Gros A, Denou F, Mahé PJ, Nesseler N, Demeure-Dit-Latte D, Launey Y, Lakhal K, Rozec B, Mallédant Y, Sébille V, Jaber S, Le Thuaut A, Feuillet F, Cinotti R, ATLANREA Group (2017) Extubation success prediction in a multicentric cohort of patients with severe brain injury. Anesthesiology 127:338–346
8. Thille AW, Harrois A, Schortgen F, Brun-Buisson C, Brochard L (2011) Outcomes of extubation failure in medical intensive care unit patients. Crit Care Med 39:2612–2618
9. Dos Reis HFC, Gomes-Neto M, Almeida MLO, da Silva MF, Guedes LBA, Martinez BP, de Seixas Rocha M (2017) Development of a risk score to predict extubation failure in patients with traumatic brain injury. J Crit Care 42:218–222
10. Mokhlesi B, Tulaimat A, Gluckman TJ, Wang Y, Evans AT, Corbridge TC (2007) Predicting extubation failure after successful completion of a spontaneous breathing trial. Respir Care 52:1710–1717
11. Vidotto MC, Sogame LC, Calciolari CC, Nascimento OA, Jardim JR (2008) The prediction of extubation success of postoperative neurosurgical patients using frequency–tidal volume ratios. Neurocrit Care 9:83–89
12. Namen AM, Ely EW, Tatter SB, Case LD, Lucia MA, Smith A et al (2001) Predictors of successful extubation in neurosurgical patients. Am J Respir Crit Care Med 163(3):658–664

Part IV

Neuromonitoring and Management in the Pediatric Population

Impaired Autoregulation Following Resuscitation Correlates with Outcome in Pediatric Patients: A Pilot Study

Julian Zipfel, Konstantin L. Hockel, Ines Gerbig, Ellen Heimberg, Martin U. Schuhmann, and Felix Neunhoeffer

Introduction

We recently showed that the duration of autoregulation impairment correlates with the neurological outcome in children and adolescents with a traumatic brain injury (TBI) [1]. The current pilot study investigated whether similar mechanisms and relations exist in nontraumatic hypoxic–ischemic brain injury following resuscitation. As in TBI, cerebral hypoperfusion (which eventually leads to secondary brain damage) is a well-described brain insult during resuscitation and a leading cause of an unfavorable outcome [2]. It has been suggested that changes in cerebral blood flow after cardiac arrest and the initial resuscitation are the primary reasons for ischemic–hypoxic brain injury [3]. However, secondary damage during the first days in ICU is at least as likely to happen and needs to be detected and prevented.

Thus, we have established a postresuscitation care protocol for children who are intubated and sedated postresuscitation and likely to sustain a low-flow brain injury, which includes insertion of a sensor for intracranial pressure (ICP) measurement. Measurement and (if needed) lowering of ICP alone might not be sufficient to prevent secondary brain damage. Maintenance of adequate—preferably optimal—cerebral perfusion pressure (CPP) is of crucial importance in addition to reduction of high ICP. Guidelines for CPP management following TBI define a wide range of CPP thresholds between 40 and 65 mmHg. As yet, there are no guidelines that specifically address management of CPP in ischemic–hypoxic brain injury.

To optimize cerebral perfusion, CPP can be managed and adapted individually, and this includes use of cerebrovascular autoregulation data—mainly the so-called pressure reactivity index (PRx), which is calculated as the correlation index of ICP and arterial blood pressure, as described previously [4, 5]. In TBI, PRx has been validated as a marker of cerebrovascular reactivity [5]. It can predict an unfavorable neurological outcome and allows definition of individual thresholds for CPP [6–8]. This is true in both adult and pediatric patients [9–12]. We previously showed that independent assessment and management of cerebral autoregulation is feasible in pediatric patients with TBI and that a longer duration of autoregulation impairment is strongly correlated with an unfavorable outcome [1].

The current pilot study investigated the value of cerebrovascular autoregulation monitoring in pediatric patients after resuscitation with clinically significant low-flow time.

Materials and Methods

The study included pediatric patients postresuscitation and with clinical indices of significant cerebral low-flow time (e.g., intermittently dilated pupils). At our institution, these children underwent initial cranial computed tomography (CT) and placement of a right frontal intraparenchymal pressure transducer into the white matter at a depth of 3 cm within hours after admission, as soon as coagulation was normalized. Blood pressure, ICP, and CPP measurements were actively managed to determine and maintain an optimal CPP (CPPopt), using the correlation index of arterial blood

Martin Schuhmann and Felix Neunhoeffer contributed equally to this work.

J. Zipfel (✉) · M. U. Schuhmann
Division of Pediatric Neurosurgery, Department of Neurosurgery, University Hospital of Tuebingen, Tuebingen, Germany
e-mail: julian.zipfel@med.uni-tuebingen.de

K. L. Hockel
Division of Pediatric Neurosurgery, Department of Neurosurgery, University Hospital of Tuebingen, Tuebingen, Germany

Department of Spine Surgery, Isar Klinikum, Munich, Germany

I. Gerbig · E. Heimberg · F. Neunhoeffer
Pediatric Intensive Care Unit, University Children's Hospital of Tuebingen, Tuebingen, Germany

B. Depreitere et al. (eds.), *Intracranial Pressure and Neuromonitoring XVII*, Acta Neurochirurgica Supplement 131,
https://doi.org/10.1007/978-3-030-59436-7_21,

pressure (ABP) and ICP—PRx—as an indicative factor, as has been described previously in patients with TBI [6]. Outcomes were scored clinically via use of the Glasgow Outcome Scale (GOS) at discharge (GOS0) and at 3 months (GOS3). Before discharge to rehabilitation, all children underwent cerebral magnetic resonance imaging (MRI) to detect or rule out visible areas of cerebral ischemia.

An overview of patient characteristics and causes of cardiac arrest can be seen in Table 1. All patients were intubated and mechanically ventilated, and analgosedation was initiated immediately.

On the basis of their GOS scores, patients were dichotomized into favorable outcomes (with a GOS score of 4–5) and unfavorable outcomes (with a GOS score of 2–3). Arterial blood pressure was monitored continuously and referenced to the level of the foramen of Monro. Monitoring parameters were digitally sampled via use of ICM+ software (Cambridge Enterprise, Cambridge, UK). CPP and PRx were calculated as described previously [5]. In the final analysis, the mean ICP, MAP [mean arterial pressure], CPP, and PRx values were calculated for the entire treatment period. The patients' mean overall ICP, CPP, and PRx values were evaluated against their outcomes. In addition, the monitoring period was segmented into 1-h intervals for each patient. For each 1-h interval, the mean ICP, CPP, and PRx values were calculated and used to calculate the "dose" of each parameter according to thresholds.

The mean PRx values were calculated for each CPP bin as the mean of means for the entire cohort. On the basis of similar thresholds in the literature, a PRx above 0.2 was defined as impaired cerebrovascular reactivity, whereas a PRx below 0 clearly signified intact autoregulation. For each patient, the durations of PRx values above 0.2, between 0 and 0.2, and below 0 were evaluated as absolute time (hours) and calculated as percentages of the total monitoring time. The respective time and percentage values were then dichotomized into the favorable and unfavorable outcome groups. With regard to ICP thresholds, we assumed that ICP values above 20 mmHg were critically elevated and those below 15 mmHg were normal. Consecutively, the percentages of the monitoring time with ICP values above 20 mmHg, between 15 and 20 mmHg, and below 15 mmHg were calculated and dichotomized into the favorable and unfavorable outcome groups.

Results

Eleven children were included in the study. The mean age was 5 years and 3 months (range 1 month to 15 years). The most frequent cause of circulatory arrest in our cohort was drowning (36.3%), followed by hypoxia (18.2%) and other reasons for hypotonia. Six of the eleven patients had undergone prolonged preclinical cardiopulmonary resuscitation (CPR) for >30 min (with the exact duration often being undetermined). In-hospital CPR lasted between 5 and 40 min. Three children died within 24 h: two of them already had a "black brain" on their initial CT scan, signifying the most severe hypoxic–ischemic brain damage; the third received an ICP transducer. Of the eight survivors, three had an unfavorable outcome (with a GOS score of 2–3) and five had a favorable outcome (with a GOS score of 4–5). The overall ABP, ICP, CPP, and PRx values did not differ significantly between the two groups. There was a trend toward higher ICP and higher PRx values in the unfavorable outcome group. Table 2 summarizes the basic and overall monitoring data. The PRx/CPP plots were dichotomized into the favorable and unfavorable outcome groups.

Table 1 Overview of patient characteristics and causes of cardiac arrest

					GOS score	
Patient number	Age (months)	Mechanism of cardiac arrest	Duration of CPR (min)	Monitoring time (h)	At hospital discharge	At 3 months
1	3	Septic shock	>60	144	2	2
2	40	Unclear	>60	84	2	2
3	58	Hypoxia	5	182	1	1
4	4	Hypotonia	>60	52	1	1
5	23	Drowning	30	186	4	5
6	64	Drowning	?	114	5	5
7	122	Hemorrhagic shock	>60?	134	5	5
8	180	Hypoxia	40	19	1	1
9	51	Hypotonia	>60	113	3	3
10	14	Drowning	10	111	5	5
11	132	Drowning	>60	110	5	5

CPR cardiopulmonary resuscitation, *GOS* glasgow outcome scale

Table 2 Overview of basic and overall monitoring data in patients with favorable and unfavorable outcomes

	Patient outcome[a]		
	Unfavorable [GOS score 2–3]	Favorable [GOS score 4–5]	*P* value
Age (months)	56 ± 65.07	71 ± 54.6	0.692
Duration of CPR (min)	47.5 ± 22.30	40 ± 24.49	0.629
ABP (mmHg)	74.93 ± 12.98	73.46 ± 7.07	0.826
ICP (mmHg)	21.21 ± 22.40	7.86 ± 1.20	0.220
CPP (mmHg)	53.63 ± 15.74	65.60 ± 7.83	0.158
PRx	0.19 ± 0.06	−0.5 ± 0.43	0.247

ABP arterial blood pressure, *CPP* cerebral perfusion pressure, *CPR* cardiopulmonary resuscitation, *GOS* Glasgow Outcome Scale, *ICP* intracranial pressure, *PRx* pressure reactivity index
[a]The values are expressed as mean ± standard deviation

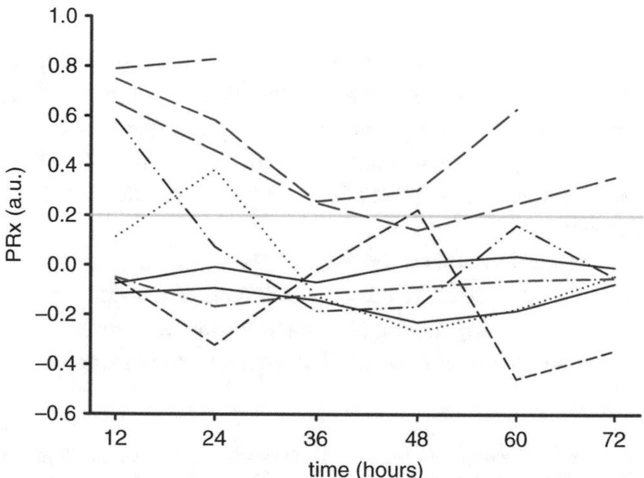

Fig. 1 Individual mean pressure reactivity index (PRx) course over the first 72 h of monitoring. Children with an unfavorable outcome are shown in *red*. One child with functional autoregulation and an unfavorable outcome had basal ganglia ischemia but no signs of ischemia in the cortex

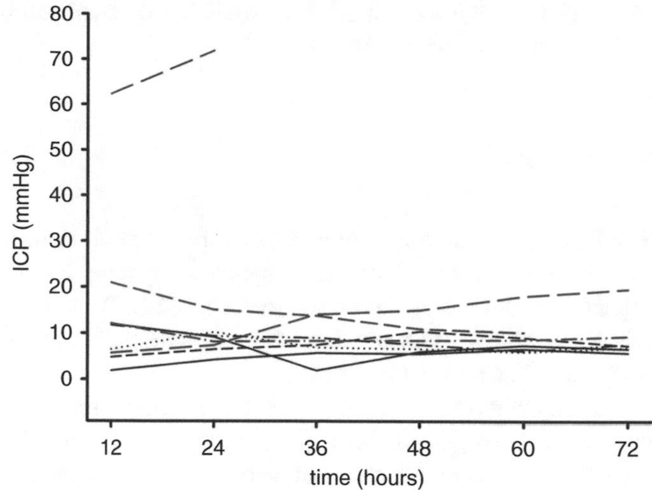

Fig. 2 Individual mean intracranial pressure (ICP) course over the first 72 h of monitoring. Children with an unfavorable outcome are shown in *red*. One child with extremely high initial ICP died within the first 24 h

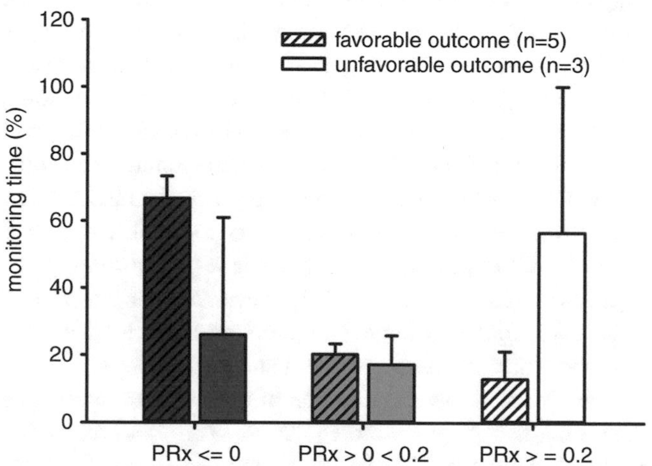

Fig. 3 Percentage of monitoring time during the first 72 h in children with a favorable outcome ($n = 5$) and in those with an unfavorable outcome ($n = 3$)

The initial PRx value in the three children with a GOS score of 1 was significantly higher than those in the rest of the cohort (0.55 (standard error 0.03) versus −0.10 (standard error 0.14), $P < 0.001$), predicting irreversible generalized brain injury without significantly different ICP or CPP values (Fig. 1). Only in one child (who started with a PRx value of >0.2) did treatment efforts lead to restoration of autoregulation, and the outcome was favorable. A PRx value of ≤0.2 was associated with a favorable outcome in all except one child ($P = 0.06$). This patient had severe but limited ischemia in the region of the basal ganglia; therefore, the good autoregulation parameters did not correlate with the child's unfavorable neurological outcome. On their MRI scans, all children with a GOS score of 2–3 had areas with signal changes compatible with ischemic brain tissue.

Furthermore, in the first 72 h, the survivors' ICP and CPP values calculated from the 1-h bins did not differ between the favorable and unfavorable outcome groups and thus carried no predictive value. One child with severely disturbed autoregulation and a PRx value of >0.2 had significantly higher initial mean ICP levels than the rest of the cohort (72.03 versus 59.00 mmHg, $P < 0.001$). Subsequently, this child's ICP could not be reduced and autoregulation control was not restored; thus, hypoxic–ischemic brain death was inevitable (Fig. 2).

Most importantly, the relative dose of PRx ≥0.2 was significantly higher in children with an unfavorable outcome (60% versus 18%, $P < 0.001$) (Fig. 3). Conversely, the relative dose of PRx <0 was associated with a favorable outcome (70% versus 25%, $P = 0.06$). The durations of PRx values between 0 and 0.2 did not differ between the favorable and unfavorable outcome groups.

Discussion

The literature on autoregulation after cardiac arrest is sparse and is mainly focused on adult patients. In most cases, impairment of autoregulation was detected [13]. We add to this limited body of knowledge with our findings from this pilot study in a pediatric cohort.

Initially compromised cerebrovascular reactivity seems to be an adverse prognostic factor [14], and this was also true in our cohort. We demonstrated that a dose of poor autoregulation within the first 72 h is likely to be associated with an unfavorable outcome. Prognostic signs of insult severity are initially poor autoregulation plus inability to restore autoregulation despite active attempts to determine and reach/maintain CPPopt. A further finding from these data is that limited brain ischemia, especially in the basal ganglia, is unlikely to be detected by global autoregulation monitoring via an intraparenchymal ICP transducer. Thus, functional overall autoregulation according to the PRx value may still result in an individually well explained unfavorable outcome. This is congruent with our experience in TBI: that initially poor autoregulation and inability to quickly restore it by active CPPopt-guided treatment is a prognostic sign of grave initial insult severity [1]. However, further prospective data in a sufficiently large patient cohort are needed to support these new findings and our ensuing hypothesis.

We observed that the duration of a PRx value lower than 0, as a marker of intact autoregulation, was associated with a favorable outcome. This has also been shown previously in adults [15].

Interestingly, we saw no prognostic implication of ICP levels in our cohort of survivors. This observation supports our current hypothesis that the postresuscitation ICP value alone is, instead, a discriminant between early death—in which severe initial hypoxic–ischemic brain damage results in early uncontrollable ICP rises and brain death—and survival.

PRx and CPPopt values in the first 3 days, which can be calculated only with ICP data and use of dedicated software, seem to predict whether the outcome will be favorable or unfavorable. Most importantly, by enabling CPP to be optimized and avoiding significant secondary brain damage, they may enable a better outcome to be achieved for patients in whom secondary damage due to secondary ischemia could still "flip the coin" toward an unfavorable outcome.

It must be assumed that cerebrovascular reactivity of the precapillary resistance vessels, which is a dynamic phenomenon, is not static but changing over the course of time and treatment in the ICU [16]. This is why the overall monitoring data (over the total monitoring time) did not show significant differences between the outcome groups in our study, yet assessment of hourly and daily dynamics of autoregulation was able to do so. Consequently, continuous bedside monitoring should be performed that allows the treating team to display not only the current status of CPP, PRX, and CPPopt but also the trends and developments during the chosen time intervals.

Conclusion

The PRx threshold for evaluating autoregulation status and its correlation with outcomes have not been defined precisely in children on the basis of large cohort studies. Like our TBI cohort study, the current pilot study showed that an hourly mean PRx value that remained above 0.2 continuously for more than 24 h was associated with an unfavorable outcome in 100% of cases. Thus, we are confident that larger cohort studies will confirm that a PRx dose >0.2 for the first 24 h is a negative prognostic marker of outcome, whereas a PRx dose <0 for the first 24 h is a positive prognostic marker of outcome.

The results of this pilot study also suggest that insertion of an ICP bolt postresuscitation is a beneficial act that enables detection of early fatal cases, has the potential to optimize treatment of survivors, and helps to predict the outcome after 72 h.

Conflict of Interest **On behalf of all authors, the corresponding author states that there is no conflict of interest.**

References

1. Hockel K, Diedler J, Neunhoeffer F, Heimberg E, Nagel C, Schuhmann MU (2017) Time spent with impaired autoregulation is linked with outcome in severe infant/paediatric traumatic brain injury. Acta Neurochir 159(11):2053–2061
2. Vavilala MS, Bowen A, Lam AM, Uffman JC, Powell J, Winn HR et al (2003) Blood pressure and outcome after severe pediatric traumatic brain injury. J Trauma 55(6):1039–1044
3. van den Brule JMD, van der Hoeven JG, Hoedemaekers CWE (2018) Cerebral perfusion and cerebral autoregulation after cardiac arrest. Biomed Res Int 2018:4143636
4. Brain Trauma Foundation; American Association of Neurological Surgeons; Congress of Neurological Surgeons; Joint Section on Neurotrauma and Critical Care, AANS/CNS, Bratton SL, Chestnut RM, Ghajar J, et al (2007) Guidelines for the management of severe traumatic brain injury. IX. Cerebral perfusion thresholds. J Neurotrauma 24(Suppl 1):S59–S64
5. Czosnyka M, Smielewski P, Kirkpatrick P, Laing RJ, Menon D, Pickard JD (1997) Continuous assessment of the cerebral vasomotor reactivity in head injury. Neurosurgery 41(1):11–17; discussion 17–19

6. Aries MJ, Czosnyka M, Budohoski KP, Steiner LA, Lavinio A, Kolias AG et al (2012) Continuous determination of optimal cerebral perfusion pressure in traumatic brain injury. Crit Care Med 40(8):2456–2463
7. Figaji AA, Zwane E, Fieggen AG, Argent AC, Le Roux PD, Siesjo P et al (2009) Pressure autoregulation, intracranial pressure, and brain tissue oxygenation in children with severe traumatic brain injury. J Neurosurg Pediatr 4(5):420–428
8. Sorrentino E, Diedler J, Kasprowicz M, Budohoski KP, Haubrich C, Smielewski P et al (2012) Critical thresholds for cerebrovascular reactivity after traumatic brain injury. Neurocrit Care 16(2):258–266
9. Brady KM, Shaffner DH, Lee JK, Easley RB, Smielewski P, Czosnyka M et al (2009) Continuous monitoring of cerebrovascular pressure reactivity after traumatic brain injury in children. Pediatrics 124(6):e1205–e1212
10. Lewis PM, Czosnyka M, Carter BG, Rosenfeld JV, Paul E, Singhal N et al (2015) Cerebrovascular pressure reactivity in children with traumatic brain injury. Pediatr Crit Care Med 16(8):739–749
11. Nagel C, Diedler J, Gerbig I, Heimberg E, Schuhmann MU, Hockel K (2016) State of cerebrovascular autoregulation correlates with outcome in severe infant/pediatric traumatic brain injury. Acta Neurochir Suppl 122:239–244
12. Young AM, Donnelly J, Czosnyka M, Jalloh I, Liu X, Aries MJ et al (2016) Continuous multimodality monitoring in children after traumatic brain injury—preliminary experience. PLoS One 11(3):e0148817
13. Sundgreen C, Larsen FS, Herzog TM, Knudsen GM, Boesgaard S, Aldershvile J (2001) Autoregulation of cerebral blood flow in patients resuscitated from cardiac arrest. Stroke 32(1):128–132
14. Iordanova B, Li L, Clark RSB, Manole MD (2017) Alterations in cerebral blood flow after resuscitation from cardiac arrest. Front Pediatr 5:174
15. Lovett ME, Maa T, Chung MG, O'Brien NF (2018) Cerebral blood flow velocity and autoregulation in paediatric patients following a global hypoxic–ischaemic insult. Resuscitation 126:191–196
16. Tontisirin N, Armstead W, Waitayawinyu P, Moore A, Udomphorn Y, Zimmerman JJ et al (2007) Change in cerebral autoregulation as a function of time in children after severe traumatic brain injury: a case series. Childs Nerv Syst 23(10):1163–1169

Brain Biomarkers in Children After Mild and Severe Traumatic Brain Injury

Elena G. Sorokina, Zhanna B. Semenova, Valentin P. Reutov, Elena N. Arsenieva, Olga V. Karaseva, Andrey P. Fisenko, Leonid M. Roshal, and Vsevolod G. Pinelis

Introduction

Traumatic brain injury (TBI) has been a leading pathology for many years, causing huge social and material damage in society [1]. The search for informative markers of brain damage remains an important challenge for predicting the outcome and treatment of children with TBI. The diagnostic capabilities of magnetic resonance imaging (MRI) and computed tomography (CT) are limited by high capital costs and often do not provide information that can predict the consequences and outcome of TBI, particularly in mild TBI (mTBI) [2, 3]. Many mTBI diagnoses go undetected because of the subtlety of the initial neurological deficit [4]. Problems in the search for adequate brain markers include the need for neuromarkers that reflect the earliest response of the brain and lesions preceding development of secondary damage after TBI. Secondary damage includes excessive release of the excitatory amino acid glutamate (Glu) in the synaptic gap and development of a cascade of excitotoxic reactions, including increased proteolytic enzyme activity, lipid and protein peroxidation, membrane degradation, and mitochondrial de-energization and energy collapse, all of which contribute to neuronal cell death [5, 6]. Many reviews have focused on the pathogenesis of TBI, but the roles of the immune system and oxidative stress remain underestimated [7, 8]. Oxidative stress and damage to glutamate receptors (GluR), with development of an autoimmune response to fragments of GluR, play important roles in the pathological chain of reactions to secondary brain injury [9, 10]. Along with traditional neuromarkers (S100b and neuron-specific enolase (NSE)), brain injury markers such as antibodies (aAb) to GluR, their degradation products (peptides), nitric oxide (NO), and its product 3-nitrotyrosine (NT) may be useful for understanding of TBI pathogenesis and may indicate development of hypoxia and neuroinflammation [11].

E. G. Sorokina (✉) · E. N. Arsenieva · A. P. Fisenko · V. G. Pinelis
National Medical Research Center for Children's Health, Moscow, Russia
e-mail: sorokelena@mail.ru

Z. B. Semenova · O. V. Karaseva · L. M. Roshal
Research Institute for Emergency Pediatric Surgery and Traumatology, Moscow, Russia

V. P. Reutov
Institute of Higher Nervous Activity and Neurophysiology of Russian Academy of Sciences, Moscow, Russia

Materials and Methods

In this study, the severity of TBI in 159 children aged >3 years was evaluated on the basis of the Glasgow Coma Scale score (GCS), and the children were divided into the following groups: mTBI (GCS 14–15; 100 children), moderate TBI (mdTBI) (GCS 9–13; 25 children), and severe TBI (sTBI) (GCS <9; 34 children). The outcomes of TBI were evaluated according to the Glasgow Outcome Scale score (GOS): full recovery (GOS 5), moderate disability (GOS 4), high disability (GOS 3), vegetative status (GOS 2), and death (GOS 1). Venous blood samples were investigated on days 1–2, as were the dynamics during the first 2 weeks after TBI. Biomarker levels in blood serum or plasma were determined with an enzyme-linked immunosorbent assay (ELISA) and colorimetric methods: S100b and NSE (CanAg), 3-nitrotyrosine (Hycult Biotech), and the αII-spectrin breakdown product SBDP145 (Cusabio Biotech). Nitrogen oxide (NOx) was measured as "nitrites and nitrates" in plasma (Calbiochem, R&D Systems). The levels of antibodies to NR2(NMDA) and GluR1(AMPA) and NR2 and AMPA peptides of GluR were measured using a method developed by Dambinova et al. [12, 13]. For control values and calculations, we used data on the upper limits of normal marker ranges prescribed by developers and our own data from children without neurological pathology. Statistical evaluation of the data was carried out using Statistica version 6 (StatSoft) and Excel (Microsoft)

B. Depreitere et al. (eds.), *Intracranial Pressure and Neuromonitoring XVII*, Acta Neurochirurgica Supplement 131,
https://doi.org/10.1007/978-3-030-59436-7_22,

software. Differences between parameters were compared by means of a Kruskal–Wallis analysis of variance (ANOVA). *P* values of <0.05 were considered significant and represented as means ± standard errors of the means. Graphics were processed using Prism software (GraphPad).

Results

In the first 2 days, almost all of the children had increases in serum levels of NSE and S100b. In the following days, decreases in these proteins were observed in those with GOS 3, 4, and 5, whereas further increases in their levels was observed in those with a lethal outcome (GOS 1) (Table 1).

We found that immediately after TBI, there was an increase in the level of nitrites and nitrates (NOx); the more severe the damage, the higher the plasma level of these NO metabolites (Table 2). We also noted the appearance of the protein nitrosation product NT in the plasma of children with TBI. At the onset of mTBI, 25% of the children developed a measurable NT level. The highest NT level was found in children with a lethal outcome of combined TBI (the NT level reached 1890 nmol/L in mdTBI and 8101 nmol/L in sTBI).

In the first 2 days, we also detected traces of SBDP145 in the plasma of children with mTBI (0.036 ± 0.012 ng/mL) and mdTBI (0.119 ± 0.023 ng/mL).

Figure 1a, b, c, d presents a more visual demonstration of the levels of antibodies to NR2(NMDA) and peptides, and shows individual data for children with mTBI. The level of antibodies to NR2(NMDA) in 91% of children with mTBI immediately after injury was 2.8 times that in children with mdTBI (GOS 3, 4) and was several times the upper limit of the normal range (Table 2, Fig. 1a). A similar pattern was observed in children with sTBI with different outcomes: the lowest level of antibodies to NR2(NMDA) on the first day after sTBI was found in children with the worst prognosis (GOS 1), and the highest level was found in the group with good recovery (GOS 5) (Fig. 1b). The level of NR2 peptides exceeded the upper limit of the normal range in only 14% of children with mTBI, and this difference versus the normal values was not significant (Fig. 1c). Conversely, the level of AMPA peptides exceeded the upper limit of the normal range in 91% of children with mTBI (Fig. 1d).

The opposite pattern of changes was shown for antibodies to GluR1(AMPA). Children with mdTBI had a higher initial level of antibodies to GluR1(AMPA) and a lower level of AMPA peptides than patients with mTBI. Thus, the more severe the TBI, the lower the blood level of antibodies to NR2(NMDA) and the higher the level of antibodies to (GluR1)AMPA on the first day.

Table 1 S100b and NSE levels in blood serum samples collected from children during the first 15 days after a traumatic brain injury (TBI)

Severity of TBI	Outcome	Time after TBI, days	Level, μg/L[a] S100b [ULN <0.125 μg/L]	NSE [ULN <13.0 μg/L]
Mild: GCS 14–15		1	0.25 ± 0.04*	19.07 ± 4.86*
		2–3	0.08 ± 0.01	9.41 ± 2.02
	GOS 5 (*n* = 65)	5–7	0.05 ± 0.01	5.71 ± 0.57
		10–15	0.04 ± 0.01	7.42 ± 0.90
Moderate: GCS 9–13	GOS 5 (*n* = 19)	1	0.23 ± 0.044*	20.08 ± 5.01*
		2–3	0.13 ± 0.020	7.42 ± 0.91
		10–15	0.08 ± 0.03	6.52 ± 0.05
	GOS 3, 4 (*n* = 6)	1	0.26 ± 0.09*	22.52 ± 6.01*
		2–3	0.15 ± 0.06	4.9 ± 1.68
		10–14	0.12 ± 0.05	6.87 ± 1.27
Severe: GCS <9	GOS 5 (*n* = 7)	1	0.30 ± 0.10*	24.11 ± 8.7*
		2–3	0.08 ± 0.02	5.35 ± 0.60
		5–7	0.06 ± 0.02	7.44 ± 1.60
		10–15	0.04 ± 0.01	6.90 ± 1.50
	GOS 3, 4 (*n* = 14)	1	0.32 ± 0.09*	26.0 ± 7.70*
		2–3	0.20 ± 0.08	6.30 ± 0.62
		5–7	0.12 ± 0.05	11.3 ± 5.37
		10–15	0.06 ± 0.01	7.43 ± 1.03
	GOS 2 (*n* = 5)	1	0.35 ± 0.15*	28.4 ± 21.2*
		2–3	0.06 ± 0.03	8.4 ± 1.20
		5–10	0.04 ± 0.01	6.5 ± 0.87
		15–75	0.04 ± 0.03	7.27 ± 0.72
	GOS 1 (*n* = 8)	1	0.50 ± 0.29*	25.0 ± 10.0*
		2–3	0.83 ± 0.39*	39.0 ± 17.0*
		5–7	0.98 ± 0.30*	42.9 ± 17.0*
		10–15	0.56 ± 0.30*	23.0 ± 10.0*

GCS Glasgow coma scale score, *GOS* Glasgow outcome scale score, *ULN* upper limit of the normal range

[a]The data are expressed as mean ± standard error of the mean

*Significant difference versus control values ($P < 0.05$)

Discussion

S100b protein and NSE are generally accepted biochemical markers of brain damage. S100b protein is considered a glial protein, predominantly localized in astrocytes, and appears to be involved in signal transduction, energy metabolism, and many other processes, especially through regulation of protein phosphorylation [14, 15]. At nanomole concentrations, S100b stimulates neurite outgrowth and enhances neuron survival; in contrast, micromole levels of extracellular S100b in vitro may have deleterious effects [1, 3]. NSE is a dimer of the cytoplasmic isoenzyme glycolytic enolase,

Table 2 Metabolic products of NO and antibodies to GluR in blood samples collected from children during the first 1–2 days after a traumatic brain injury (TBI)

	Severity of TBI					
	Mild: GCS 15 ($n = 35$)		Moderate: GCS 9–13 ($n = 21$)		Severe: GCS <9 ($n = 29$)	
Biomarker in blood serum or plasma	Level[a]	Outcome	Level[a]	Outcome	Level[a]	Outcome
NOx (nitrites and nitrates), μmol/L plasma [ULN 10 ± 5 μmol/L]	–	–	–	–	176 ± 45[*,**]	GOS 1
	–	–	40 ± 7[*,**]	GOS 3, 4	69 ± 7[*,**]	GOS 3, 4
	19 ± 2	GOS 5	23 ± 6[*]	GOS 5	25 ± 6[*]	GOS 5
3-Nitrotyrosine, nmol/L plasma [ULN 0 nmol/L][b]	–	–	–	–	52–2799	GOS 1
	–	–	–	–	7–42	GOS 2
	–	–	23–759	GOS 3, 4	24–2265	GOS 3, 4
	0–70	GOS 5	0–27	GOS 5	13–28	GOS 5
NR2(NMDA) antibodies, ng/mL serum [ULN <2.0 ng/mL]	–	–	–	–	2.75 ± 1.01[**]	GOS 1
	–	–	4.57 ± 0.54[*,**]	GOS 3, 4	6.38 ± 1.32[*,**]	GOS 3, 4
	13.13 ± 1.58[*]	GOS 5	7.85 ± 1.95[*,**]	GOS 5	10.04 ± 2.34[*]	GOS 5
GluR1(AMPA) antibodies, ng/mL serum [ULN <1.5 ng/mL]	–	–	2.34 ± 0.55[*,**]	GOS 3, 4	–	–
	0.64 ± 0.14	GOS 5	1.45 ± 0.79	GOS 5	–	–
NR2 peptides, ng/mL plasma [ULN <0.5 ng/mL]	0.58 ± 0.32	GOS 5	0.38 ± 0.15	GOS 5	–	–
AMPA peptides, ng/mL plasma [ULN <0.4 ng/mL]	1.49 ± 0.19[*]	GOS 5	0.70 ± 0.24	GOS 5	–	–

GCS Glasgow Coma Scale score, *GOS* Glasgow Outcome Scale score, *NOx* nitrogen oxide, *ULN* upper limit of the normal range
[a]The values are expressed as the mean ± standard error of the mean, except for 3-nitrotyrosine values, which are expressed as the range
[b]The 3-nitrotyrosine values in the moderate and severe TBI groups cover only the first 7 days after the injury
[*]Significant difference versus control values
[**]Significant difference versus values in mild TBI ($P < 0.05$)
–not available

localized in central and peripheral neurons, as well as in neuroendocrine cells [4, 16].

Our results showed that blood levels of the brain injury markers S100b and NSE during the first 2 days after TBI did not have a strong correlation with the severity of brain injury. Our data were supported by the research of Sedaghat and Notopoulos, who found that the S100b level correlated with CT scanning data in only 30% of cases [17]. Kleindienst and Ross reported that in 48% of children with mTBI without cognitive impairment, there was an increase in the serum level of S100b [18], which most likely indicated participation of this protein in adaptive processes developing in response to stress. We found that NSE and S100b levels increased immediately after injury regardless of the severity of TBI, but in cases with a favorable outcome, the levels of both markers decreased to normal within the first 3 days. The maximum S100b protein and NSE levels were observed in children with a lethal outcome of TBI (GOS 1), who had high levels of these proteins throughout the posttraumatic period.

The central excitotoxic roles of GluR and NO in hypoxia are known [10], but there have been very few clinical studies on these aspects of TBI pathogenesis [19–21]. Our determination of markers of GluR and their degradation products, together with NO metabolites and nitrotyrosine as a marker of protein nitrosation, was an attempt to assess the development of oxidative stress and the neuroimmunological response to hypoxia. NO has multiple effects and, in different concentrations, plays both protective and damaging roles. Similar dual effects of NO can be observed in the fact that with a small increase, NO can activate the immune system and reduce the excitotoxicity of Glu, but at high levels, NO suppresses the immune response, promotes protein nitrosation, and enhances the damaging effect of Glu [20, 22]. Tisdall et al. [21] showed that in cases of lethal TBI, NOx content in the brain extracellular fluid reached 150 μmol/L in the first 48 h. We also obtained data showing that children with a negative outcome of severe TBI have high levels of NOx and NT soon after the initial injury, which correlates with a decrease in adenosine triphosphate (ATP) content in lymphocytes [23]. At the same time, NO inhalation prevents secondary damage in TBI [24].

Posttraumatic brain injury may be based on immunological mechanisms that sometimes ameliorate the course of TBI and sometimes cause additional damage to brain tissue with development of edema [25, 26]. The appearance in the blood of

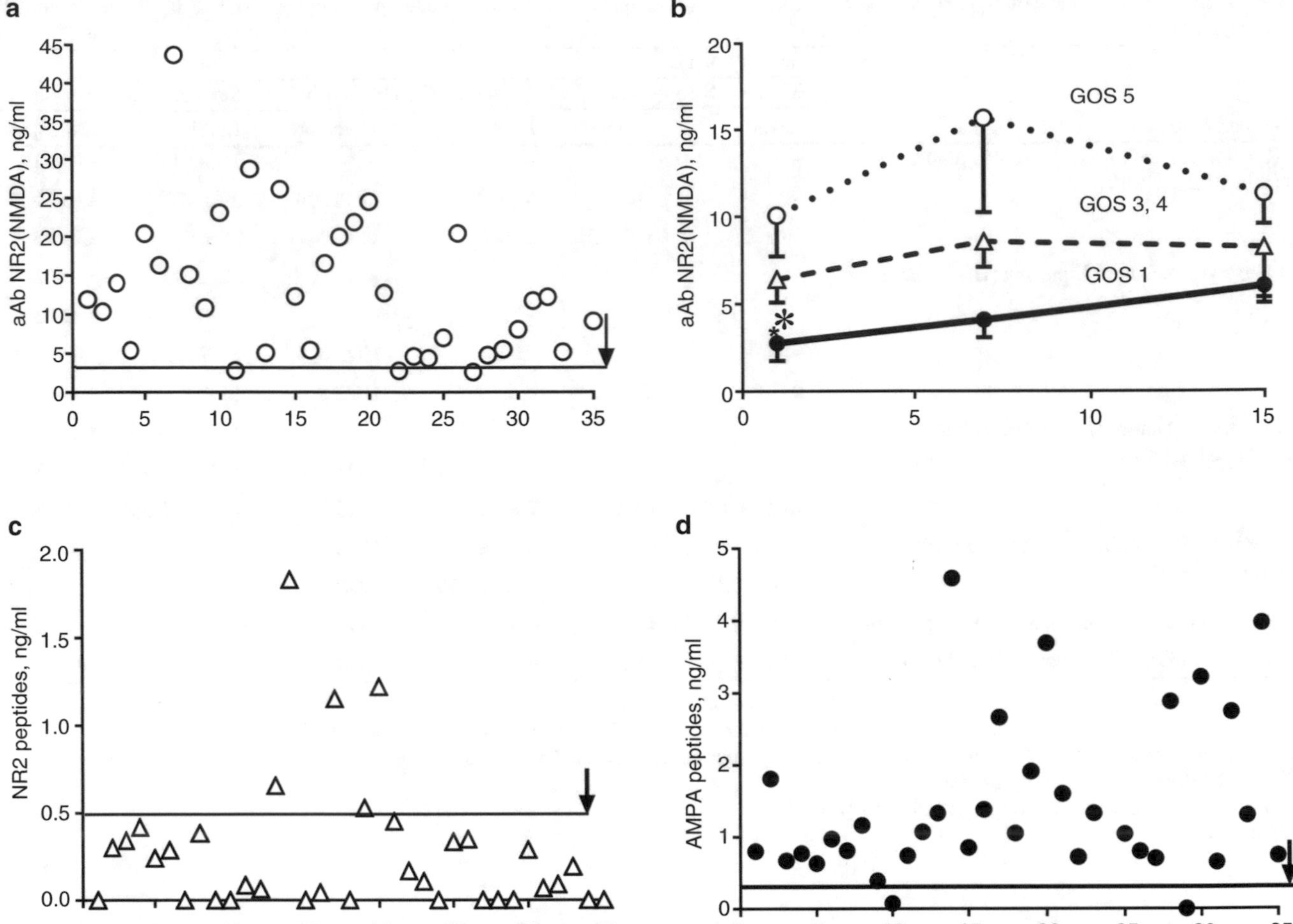

Fig. 1 NR2(NMDA) antibodies and degradation products of GluR—NR2 and AMPA peptides—in the blood of children with a traumatic brain injury (TBI). (**a, c, d**) Individual data from 35 children with mild TBI. (**b**) Days after brain injury. (**a**) NR2(NMDA) antibody level on the first day after mild TBI. (**b**) Dynamics of NR2(NMDA) antibodies in children after severe TBI with different Glasgow Outcome Scale scores (GOS). (**c, d**) NR2 and AMPA peptide levels in blood plasma samples from children with mild TBI. $^{*}P < 0.05$ for the difference between GOS 1 and GOS 5; a *vertical arrow* indicates the upper limit of the normal range

antibodies to functionally important brain structures, including GluR, indicates their activation. In this case, the increase in the pool of these antibodies should be preceded by the appearance in the blood of the degradation products of these receptors (at the N-terminal site of GluR)—peptides. On the basis of the dual roles of different antibodies [27], it can be assumed that early appearance of antibodies to excitotoxic receptors can reduce their activity and weaken the development of a further cascade of damage. We noted that in cases of mTBI, there was a significant increase in the level of antibodies to NR2(NMDA), while the level of peptides of these receptors in the blood remained within normal limits. These data indicated the existence of mechanisms aimed at early protection of NMDA GluR from development of a cascade of excitotoxic damage. It is possible that with more severe brain damage in sTBI, this mechanism does not work and the level of antibodies to NR2(NMDA) does not increase at the onset of TBI. An adverse outcome of sTBI—especially death—was associated with the lowest level of antibodies to NR2(NMDA) on the first 2 days after the initial injury. The question arises: how can the body react so early to brain damage? Such an early response is most likely associated with activation of innate immunity. The detected significant increase in antibodies to NR2(NMDA) on the first 2 days after mTBI indicated rapid secretion of immunoglobulins by innate-like B-lymphocytes. Activation of such lymphocytes can produce tissue breakdown products—DAMPs (danger-associated molecular patterns)—as well as mediators of activated microglia cells, which, in turn, are stimulated by nitric oxide, the concentration of which increases with mTBI. We demonstrated such a stimulatory effect of subphysiological concentrations of NO in an experiment in which injection of the NO-generated agent $NaNO_2$ to rats led to a rapid increase in the level of antibodies to GluR content in the blood as early as 1 h after administration, and the increase was significant after 24 h [28].

We found no increase in the level of antibodies to GluR1(AMPA), while the AMPA peptide level was found to be increased in 91% of children with mTBI. The development of methods for peptide determination and the establishment of the preferred localization of GluR in brain structures indicate a significant presence of NMDA GluR in neurovascular units and AMPA GluR in axonal structures [11]. A high level of AMPA peptides and the appearance of SBDP145 in the blood may be early signs of diffuse axonal injury in children with mTBI. As a rule, children with mTBI have a very short stay in the hospital but, as a result of underestimation of the severity of their condition, they may later have complications in the form of headaches and a decrease in mental abilities. The questions of the regulation of neuroimmune relationships are quite difficult to address, and we are not yet able to explain all of the data. However, we can assume that NO and its products are involved in the immune response and that nitrosative stress accompanies TBI [23]. We suggest that the opposite characters of the NR2(NMDA) antibody level on the first 2 days of mild and moderate versus severe TBI may be associated with an important mechanism aimed at protecting neurons from Glu excitotoxicity.

Acknowledgments The authors thank Professor G. A. Ignatieva for valuable tips in discussing the results of this work.

This work was supported by the Russian Ministry of Health (grant number AAA-A19-119012590190-6 injury).

Conflict of Interest **The authors have no conflict of interest.**

References

1. Hergenroeder GW, Redell JB, Moore AN, Dash PK (2008) Biomarkers in the clinical diagnosis and management of traumatic brain injury. Mol Diagn Ther 12:347–358
2. Beamont A, Gennarelli T (2006) CT prediction of contusion evolution after closed head injury: the role of pericontusional edema. Acta Neurochir Suppl 96:30–32
3. Mechtler LL, Dhadtri KK, Crutchfield KE (2014) Advanced neuroimaging of mild traumatic brain injury. Neurol Clin 32:31–58
4. Guzel E, Kemaloglu S, Ceviz A, Kaplan A (2008) Serum neuronspecific enolase as a predictor of short-term outcome and its correlation with Glasgow Coma Scale in traumatic brain injury. Neurosurg Rev 31:439–444
5. Algattas H, Jason H (2014) Traumatic brain injury pathophysiology and treatments: early, intermediate, and late phases post-injury. Int J Mol Sci 15:309–341
6. Pearn ML, Niesman IR, Egawa J, Sawada A, Almenar A, Shah SB, Duckworth J, Head BP (2017) Pathophysiology associated with traumatic brain injury: current treatments and potential novel therapeutics. Cell Mol Neurobiol 37:571–585
7. Kumar A, Loane DJ (2012) Neuroinflammation after traumatic brain injury: opportunities for therapeutic intervention. Brain Behav Immun 26:1191–1201
8. Needham EJ, Helmy A, Zanier ER, Jones JL, Coles AJ, Menon DK (2019) The immunological response to traumatic brain injury. J Neuroimmunol 332:112–125. https://doi.org/10.1016/j.jneuroim.2019.04.005
9. Arent AM, de Souza LF, Walz R, Dafre AL (2014) Perspectives on molecular biomarkers of oxidative stress and antioxidant strategies in traumatic brain injury. Biomed Res Int 2014:723060. https://doi.org/10.1155/2014/723060
10. Reutov VP, Samosudova NV, Sorokina EG (2019) A model of glutamate neurotoxicity and mechanisms of the development of the typical pathological process. Biophysics 64:233–250. https://doi.org/10.1134/S0006350919020143
11. Dambinova SA (2012) Neurodegradomics: the source of biomarkers for mild traumatic brain injury. In: Dambinova SA, Hayes RL, Wang KW (eds) Biomarkers for TBI. RSC Publishing, London, pp 66–86
12. Dambinova SA, Bettermann K, Glynn T, Tews M, Olson D, Weissman JD, Sowell RL (2012) Diagnostic potential of the NMDA receptor peptide assay for acute ischemic stroke. PLoS One 7(7):e42362. https://doi.org/10.1371/journal.pone.0042362
13. Dambinova SA, Khounteev GA, Izykenova GA, Zavolokov IG, Ilyukhina AY, Skoromets AA (2003) Blood test detecting autoantibodies to N-methyl-D-aspartate neuroreceptors for evaluation of patients with transient ischemic attack and stroke. Clin Chem 49:1752–1762
14. Donato R (2001) S100: a multigenic family of calcium-modulated proteins of EF-hand type with intracellular and extracellular functional roles. Int J Biochem Cell Biol 33:637–668
15. Rothermundt M, Peters M, Prehn JHM, Arolt V (2003) S100b in brain damage and neurodegeneration. Microsc Res Tech 6:614–632
16. Berger R, Adelson P, Dulani T, Cassidy L, Kochanek P (2005) Serum neuron-specific enolase, S100b, and myelin basic protein concentrations after inflicted and noninflicted traumatic brain injury in children. J Neurosurg 103:61–68
17. Sedaghat F, Notopoulos A (2008) S100 protein family and its application in clinical practice. Hippokratia 12:198–204
18. Kleindienst A, Ross BM (2006) A critical analysis of the role of the neurotrophic protein S100b in acute brain injury. J Neurotrauma 23:1185–1200
19. Carpenter KLH, Timofeev I, Al-Rawi PG, Menon DK, Pickard JD, Hutchinson PJ (2008) Nitric oxide in acute brain injury: a pilot study of NOx concentrations in human brain microdialysates and their relationship with energy metabolism. Acta Neurochir Suppl 102:207–213
20. Sorokina EG, Semenova ZB, Bazarnaya NA, Meshcheryakov SV, Reutov VP, Goryunova AV, Pinelis VG, Granstrem OK, Roshal LM (2009) Autoantibodies to glutamate receptors and products of nitric oxide metabolism in serum in children in the acute phase of craniocerebral trauma. Neurosci Behav Physiol 39:329–334
21. Tisdall MM, Konrad R, Kitchen ND, Smith M, Petzold A (2013) The prognostic value of brain extracellular fluid nitric oxide. Metabolites after traumatic brain injury. Neurocrit Care 19:65–68
22. Bal-Price A, Brown GC (2001) Inflammatory neurodegeneration mediated by nitric oxide from activated glia-inhibiting neuronal respiration, causing glutamate release and excitotoxicity. J Neurosci 21:6480–6491
23. Zakirov RS, Sorokina EG, Karaseva OV, Semenova ZB, Petrichuk SV, Roshal LM, Pinelis VG (2015) Peripheral blood lymphocytes mitochondrial function in children with traumatic brain injury [in Russian]. Vestn Ross Akad Med Nauk 6:710–717. https://doi.org/10.15690/vramn568
24. Terpolilli NA, Kim S-W, Thal SC, Kuebler WM, Plesnila N (2013) Inhaled nitric oxide reduces secondary brain damage after traumatic brain injury in mice. J Cereb Blood Flow Metab 33:311–318
25. Gannushkina IV (1974) Immunological aspects of trauma and vascular brain lesions [in Russian]. Meditsina, Moscow
26. Smith RM, Giannoudis PV (1998) Trauma and immune response. J R Soc Med 91:417–420
27. Archelos JJ, Hartung HP (2000) Pathogenic role of autoantibodies in neurological diseases. Trends Nerosci 23:317–327
28. Sorokina EG, Reutov VP, Granstrem OK, Fadyukova OE, Obrezchikova MN, Krushinsky AL, Kuzenkov VS, Koshelev VB, Dambinova SA, Pinelis VG (2003) A possible role of nitric oxide in damage of glutamate receptors in epilepsy. Vesti Nats Acad Navuk Belarusi Ser Med-Biol Nauk 1:18–22

Decompressive Craniectomy for Traumatic Intracranial Hypertension in Children

Zhanna B. Semenova, Semen Meshcheryakov, Valery Lukyanov, and Sergey Arsenyev

Introduction

Control of intracranial pressure (ICP) is important in the management of severe traumatic brain injury (TBI) in both adults and children [1, 2]. Intracranial hypertension occurs in 80% of patients with severe TBI, and in a third of them, it determines an adverse outcome.

Patients with ICP ≤20 mmHg have a lower mortality rate and a better recovery [1, 3].

To control ICP, step-by-step therapies are used (hypothermia, sedation, moderate hypocapnia, intravenous mannitol, barbiturates, and hyperventilation). Decompressive craniectomy has been suggested as a last resort to reduce intractable ICP, but this surgical treatment remains a controversial procedure because of its invasiveness and lack of clearly defined indications, the absence of an established surgical technique, the variability of its outcomes, and the significant risk of complications [3–8].

In the modern literature, there are insufficient data for recommendations on DC in children, and so pediatric neurosurgeons use recommendations for adults to make decisions about DC in children. There have been a few publications on mortality and functional outcomes after DC in pediatric populations, but they are not used to support recommendations. These studies differed in their criteria for DC, the DC methods used, and their initial parameters [3, 9–12]. In assessing the effectiveness of DC for severe TBI, it is important to correlate neuromonitoring data and other important physiological and clinical variables with outcomes. From this point of view, it is very important to identify clinical variables that will help predict an adverse outcome.

The aim of this study was to identify risk factors for unfavorable outcomes after DC in children with severe TBI.

Z. B. Semenova (✉) · S. Meshcheryakov · V. Lukyanov · S. Arsenyev
Clinical and Research Institute of Emergency Pediatric Surgery and Trauma, Moscow, Russia

Materials and Methods

The study population consisted of 287 children admitted to our hospital with severe TBI, 169 of whom had ICP monitoring. They were treated in accordance with contemporary guidelines and a modern management protocol for severe TBI [1, 3].

Over a period of 6 months, we followed up 64 patients who had undergone DC for intractable intracranial hypertension. The results were evaluated by use of the Glasgow Outcome Scale (GOS). All patients had secondary DC and demonstrated displacement or a threat of displacement of the brain stem, together with progressive obliteration of the parasellar and interpeduncular cisterns on computed tomography (CT) scans prior to surgery. The indication for frontotemporoparietal DC was lateral dislocation (in 34 patients) and the indication for bifrontal DC was axial dislocation (in 30 patients).

The GCS score at admission, the interval between the injury and hospital admission, transportation and management before admission, CT scans (at admission and during the hospital stay), and data from neuromonitoring (ICP, cerebral perfusion pressure (CPP), and the energy of process (E^2) value) were analyzed. E^2 is the sum of the square of the average ICP value and the square of process dispersion: E^2 (ICP) = M (ICP)^2 + STD (ICP)^2 [3].

The patients' mean age was 10.8 ± 4.8 years, and the majority (58%) had concomitant injuries. They were evaluated with the Injury Severity Score (ISS). The ISS in our series was 28.3 ± 10.2.

Traffic accidents were the main cause of injury (70%), followed by falls (18%), violence (8%), and other causes (4%).

Most of these patients (n = 46) were transferred from other hospitals where they had stayed for several hours or days after the injury. Only 18 were admitted directly from the injury site to our hospital.

B. Depreitere et al. (eds.), *Intracranial Pressure and Neuromonitoring XVII*, Acta Neurochirurgica Supplement 131,
https://doi.org/10.1007/978-3-030-59436-7_23,

The patients were divided into two subgroups on the basis of the time between the injury and admission to our hospital: (1) within the first 24 h (49 patients) and (2) during a later period (14 patients). The mean GCS score at admission was 6 ± 2.

CT scans were performed at admission in all cases. In addition, CT scans were repeated in cases of deterioration of neurological status or sustained elevation of ICP above 20 mmHg. Subsequent CT images were divided qualitatively into three categories: (a) improved, (b) equal, and (c) worse.

The imaging results were discussed by a team (including neurosurgeons, radiologists, and pediatric intensivists) to decide on the treatment strategy. Most patients (52.5%) had a Marshall Classification score of 3.

ICP monitoring was performed in 56 cases (87.5%). High ICP was treated by normothermia, sedation, hypertonic saline, etc. followed by barbiturates and moderate hypothermia. DC was viewed as a last resort to reduce ICP. The indication for urgent DC (in eight patients without ICP monitoring) was dislocation syndrome.

For better analysis of variations in ICP (its dynamics and intensity), the E^2 value was used.

Treatment results were evaluated after 6 months, using the GOS.

The information was processed using Statistica version 6 software (StatSoft) and SPSS version 17 software. A χ^2 nonparametric test of goodness of fit was used to evaluate the relationship between two variables. Values of $P \leq 0.05$ were considered statistically significant.

Results

There was good recovery at 6 months (with a GOS score of 4–5) in 45.3% of cases and severe disability in 31.0% of cases (with a GOS score of 3); the GOS score was 1–2 in 23.4% of cases.

On the basis of binary logistic regression, significant factors that were predictive of an unfavorable outcome after DC in children with refractory intracranial hypertension were selected (Table 1). These significant factors were the GCS score, ICP, combined trauma, the state of the pupils, pupil reactivity, and displacement of the median brain structures by more than 5 mm.

According to the classification table (Table 2), the percentage of correct prediction of outcomes after DC was 97.7%, which indicated the statistical significance of the mathematical model for outcomes. Receiver operating characteristic (ROC) curves demonstrated the degree of influence of the selected factors on outcomes (Table 3). GCS and ICP had the highest area under the curve (AUC) values (Fig. 1).

Table 2 Classification according to the Glasgow Outcome Scale (GOS) score

		Predicted		
		F33_b		
Observed		0	1	Percentage correct
GOS	0	32	1	97.0
	1	0	10	100.0
Overall percentage				97.7

Table 3 Area under the receiver operating characteristic curve of factors predicting an unfavorable outcome after decompressive craniotomy

Test result variable	Area	Standard error	Asymptotic significance	Asymptotic 95% confidence interval: Lower bound	Upper bound
F11	0.858	0.079	0.001	0.686	1.000
F15	0.839	0.060	0.001	0.722	0.957
F17_2	0.632	0.093	0.211	0.449	0.815
F18	0.730	0.094	0.029	0.546	0.915
F20	0.788	0.068	0.006	0.655	0.921
F22	0.605	0.110	0.321	0.389	0.820

F11 value of intracranial pressure, *F15* Glasgow Coma Scale score, *F17* type of injury (isolated/combined), *F18* pupils, *F20* pupil reactivity, *F22* midline shift.

Table 1 Variables in the logistic regression equation for predictive unfavorable features

Variable	B	Standard error	Wald	Degrees of freedom	Significance	Exp (B)	95% confidence limits for EXP (B): Lower	Upper
F11	0.044	0.086	0.266	1	0.606	1.045	0.884	1.236
F18	10.305	8.401	1.504	1	0.220	29875.133	0.002	4.233E+11
F20	31.653	5628.645	0.000	1	0.996	5.581E+13	0.000	
F15*	2.453	3.011	0.664	1	0.415	11.624	0.032	4247.424
F17_2	10.617	8.456	1.576	1	0.209	40810.688	0.003	6.439E+11
F22	−2.274E+00	1.747	1.693	1	0.193	0.103	0.003	3.162
Constant	−9.699E+01	11257.394	0.000	1	0.993	7.549E−43		

F11 value of intracranial pressure, *F15** value calculated using the formula F11 = 15 – Glasgow Coma Scale score, *F17* type of injury (isolated/combined), *F18* pupils, *F20* pupil reactivity, *F22* midline shift

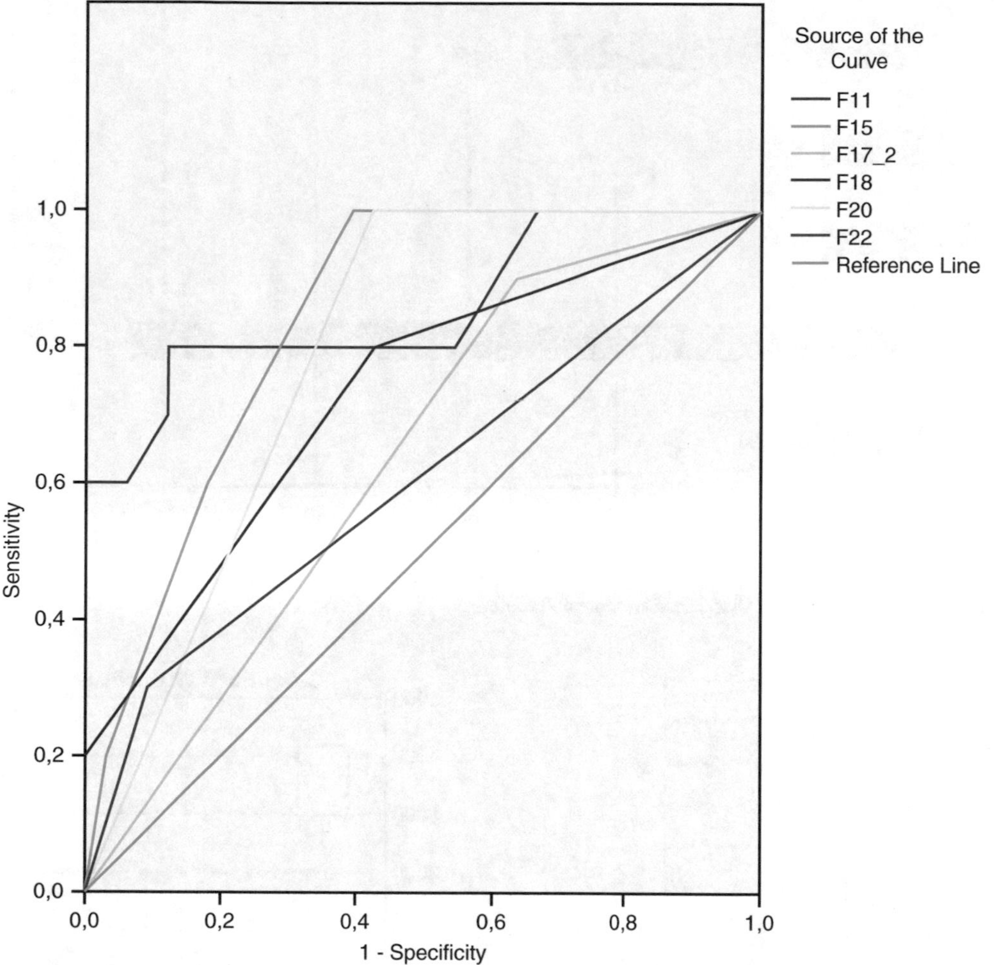

Fig. 1 Receiver operating characteristic (ROC) curve of prognostic factors for an unfavorable outcome after decompressive craniectomy (DC). *F11* intracranial pressure (ICP) value, *F15* Glasgow Coma Scale (GCS) score, *F17* type of injury (isolated/combined), *F18* pupils, *F20* pupil reactivity, *F22* midline shift

In addition, we compared what influence different clinical variables—including use of ICP monitoring, the Marshall Classification score, pupillary status, and multiplicity of ICP rises—had on outcomes. There was no statistical difference in outcomes between patients with and without ICP monitoring. When outcomes were compared on the basis of Marshall Classification scores, the highest percentage of mortality was seen in the group with a Marshall Classification score of 3 (Fig. 2). There were no statistical differences in outcomes on the basis of multiplicity of ICP elevations (up to two times and more than two times). Patients with dilated, unreactive pupils had a GOS score of −1 ($P \leq 0.05$) (Fig. 3).

ICP and its derivatives proved to be the most sensitive predictors of outcomes after DC. Patients who had ICP >40 mmHg showed unfavorable outcomes (Fig. 4). In addition, we investigated the E^2 parameter, a quantitative indicator that reflects the process of oscillation or dispersion more objectively [13]. Statistical differences in outcomes were revealed on the basis of the dynamics and intensity of ICP (Fig. 5).

All surviving patients underwent early reconstruction of the skull defect (30–55 days after surgery). Eight patients received a ventriculoperitoneal shunt (VPS) because of post-traumatic hydrocephalus. Six months later, 69% of survivors had good recovery (with a GOS score of 4–5).

Discussion

Almost two decades ago, Taylor et al. [14] published the results of a randomized trial of very early decompressive craniectomy in children with TBI and sustained intracranial hypertension. However, the efficacy of DC is still debated. Two randomized trials of DC in adults have been published: the Decompressive Craniectomy (DECRA) study and the Randomised Evaluation of Surgery with Craniectomy for Uncontrollable Elevation of Intracranial Pressure (RESCUEicp) trial [4, 9]. The DECRA study demonstrated that outcomes were worse in patients managed surgically

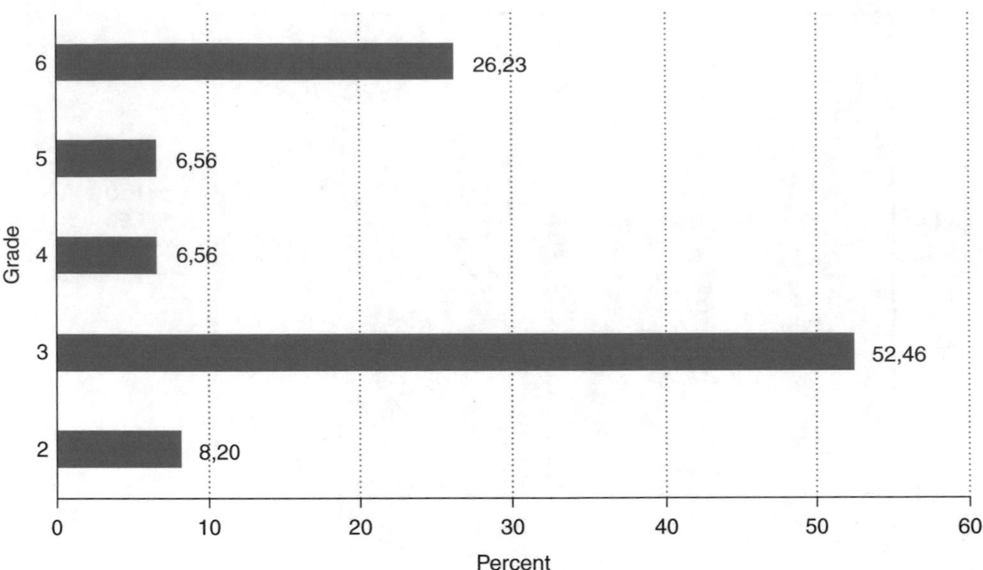

Fig. 2 Relationship between the Marshall Classification score and mortality

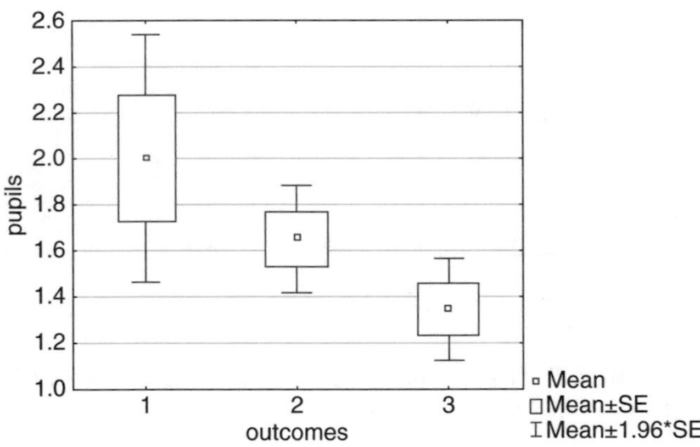

Fig. 3 Relationship between pupil size and outcomes. *1* good recovery (Glasgow Outcome Scale (GOS) score 4–5), *2* severe disability (GOS score 3), *3* unfavorable result (GOS score 1–2)

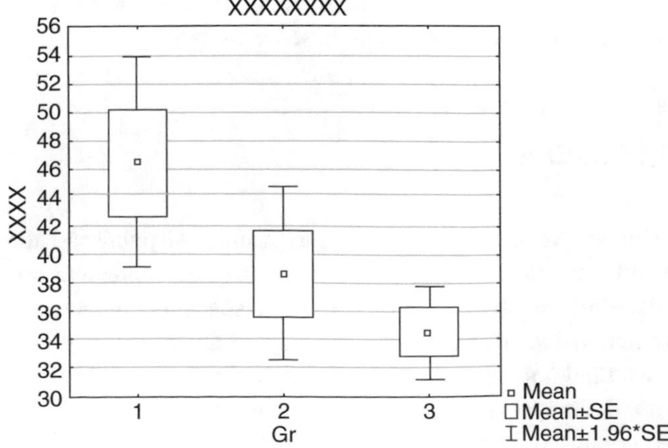

Fig. 4 Relationship between intracranial pressure and outcomes. *1* unfavorable result (Glasgow Outcome Scale (GOS) score 1–2), *2* severe disability (GOS score 3), *3* good recovery (GOS score 4–5)

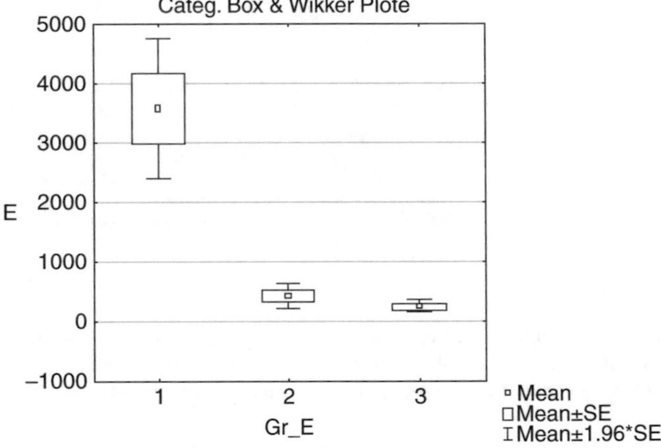

Fig. 5 Relationship between energy of process (E^2) and outcomes. *1* unfavorable result (Glasgow Outcome Score (GOS) 1–2), *2* severe disability (GOS score 3), 3 good recovery (GOS score 4–5)

than in those managed medically. According to the RESCUEicp trial results at 6 months, DC resulted in lower mortality but higher rates of vegetative state, lower severe disability, and upper severe disability than medical care. Randomized studies in children would be very difficult to conduct, because of the small numbers of patients. Most reported series in children have been small and observational. Some of these studies did not find a significant difference in results between patients treated with DC and those treated medically [6, 14, 15]. Others reported that the average GOS score at 6 months after TBI was higher in patients treated with DC [2, 12, 16]. Modern guidelines on adult TBI recommend DC as a third-tier option for refractory high ICP (values of >20 mmHg). For young children, these values need to be clarified [4, 11, 16–18].

According to our data, outcomes after DC are affected by the severity of the primary injury and clinical manifestations of dislocation syndrome. GCS remains the primary clinical indicator of the severity of primary brain damage. In our series, patients with a low GCS score (≤5) had an unfavorable outcome (11 patients had a GCS score of 3–5 and four had a GCS score of 6–8). Dilated, unreactive pupils were another clinical predictor of an unfavorable outcome ($P \leq 0.05$). In addition, CT scan findings are also important for outcome prediction: patients with a Marshall Classification score of 3 had the most unfavorable outcomes. This was the group of patients in whom cisterns were compressed or completely effaced. The combination of low GCS scores, wide pupils, and a Marshall Classification score of 3 in the absence of basal cisterns significantly reduced patient survival.

Some researchers have concluded that ICP is the main predictor of outcomes after severe TBI [4, 7, 13, 17]. Our study confirms this observation. As the debate on the efficacy of DC, ICP thresholds, and the duration of intracranial hypertension continues, use of the additional parameter E^2 may be helpful. This quantitative indicator objectively reflects fluctuations in ICP. It is easy to register it through the ICP monitor or to extract it from the ICP time series over a specified period of time. The standard deviation can yield a complete picture of variations in ICP. Therefore, we find it useful as another tool for deciding on the need for DC.

Conclusion

Outcomes after DC are largely determined by the severity of the primary injury and the occurrence of secondary complications. DC falls into the category of preventive surgery and may be an effective method for controlling dislocation syndrome; however, its effectiveness is doubtful for patients with brain herniation.

References

1. Gallardo AJL, Pérez DA, Pazos MM, Caraguay GPV, Criales GMO et al (2018) Decompressive craniectomy in pediatric severe head trauma. Int J Pediatr Res 4:033
2. Rubiano AM, Villarreal W, Hakim EJ et al (2009) Early decompressive craniectomy for neurotrauma: an institutional experience. Ulus Travma Acil Cerrahi Derg 15(1):28–38
3. Kochanek PM, Tasker RC, Carney N, Totten AM, Adelson PD et al (2019) Guidelines for the management of pediatric severe traumatic brain injury, third edition: update of the Brain Trauma Foundation guidelines. Pediatr Crit Care Med 20(3S Suppl 1):S1–S82
4. Cooper DJ, Rosenfeld JV, Murray L et al (2011) Decompressive craniectomy in diffuse traumatic brain injury. N Engl J Med 364:1493–1502. https://doi.org/10.1056/NEJMoa1102077
5. Figaji AA, Fieggen AG, Argent A et al (2006) Surgical treatment for "brain compartment syndrome" in children with severe head injury. S Afr Med J 96:969–975
6. Thomale UW, Graetz D, Vajkoczy P et al (2010) Severe traumatic brain injury in children—a single center experience regarding therapy and long-term outcome. Childs Nerv Syst 26:1563–1573
7. Yue JK, Rick JW, Deng H et al (2017) Efficacy of decompressive craniectomy in the management of intracranial pressure in severe traumatic brain injury. J Neurosurg Sci 63(4):425–440. https://doi.org/10.23736/S0390-5616.17.04133-9
8. Hawryluk GWJ, Aguilera S, Buki A, Bulger E, Citerio G et al (2019) A management algorithm for patients with intracranial pressure monitoring: the Seattle International Severe Traumatic Brain Injury Consensus Conference (SIBICC). Intensive Care Med 45(12):1783–1794. https://doi.org/10.1007/s00134-019-05805-9
9. Hutchinson PJ, Kolias AG, Timofeev IS, Corteen EA, Czosnyka M, et al; RESCUEicp Trial Collaborators (2016) Trial of decompressive craniectomy for traumatic intracranial hypertension. N Engl J Med 375(12):1119–1130. https://doi.org/10.1056/NEJMoa1605215
10. Honeybul S, Ho KM, Gillett GR (2018) Long-term outcome following decompressive craniectomy: an inconvenient truth? Curr Opin Crit Care 24:97–104
11. Jagannathan J, Okonkwo DO, Dumont AS et al (2007) Outcome following decompressive craniectomy in children with severe traumatic brain injury: a 10-year single-center experience with long-term follow up. J Neurosurg 106:268–275
12. Josan VA, Sgouros S (2006) Early decompressive craniectomy may be effective in the treatment of refractory intracranial hypertension after traumatic brain injury. Childs Nerv Syst 22:1268–1274
13. Semenova ZB, Lukianov VI, Meshcheryakov SV, Roshal LM (2018) Mean square deviation of ICP in prognosis of severe TBI outcomes in children. Acta Neurochir Suppl 126:35–37. https://doi.org/10.1007/978-3-319-65798-1_8
14. Taylor A, Butt W, Rosenfeld J et al (2001) A randomized trial of very early decompressive craniectomy in children with traumatic brain injury and sustained intracranial hypertension. Childs Nerv Syst 17(3):154–162. https://doi.org/10.1007/s003810000410
15. Mhanna MJ, Mallah WE, Verrees M et al (2015) Outcome of children with severe traumatic brain injury who are treated with decompressive craniectomy. J Neurosurg Pediatr 16:1–7
16. Rutigliano D, Egnor MR, Priebe CJ et al (2006) Decompressive craniectomy in pediatric patients with traumatic brain injury with intractable elevated intracranial pressure. J Pediatr Surg 41:83–87
17. Csykay A, Emelifeonwu JA, Fügedi L et al (2012) The importance of very early decompressive craniectomy as a prevention to avoid the sudden increase of intracranial pressure in children with severe traumatic brain swelling (retrospective case series). Childs Nerv Syst 28:441–444
18. Desgranges FP, Javouhey E, Mottolese C et al (2014) Intraoperative blood loss during decompressive craniectomy for intractable intracranial hypertension after severe traumatic brain injury in children. Childs Nerv Syst 30:1393–1398

Use of Direct Intracranial Pressure and Brain Tissue Oxygen Monitoring in Perioperative Management of Patients with Moyamoya Disease

Maya Kommer, Michael Canty, Emer Campbell, Meharpal Sangra, Anthony Amato-Watkins, Simon Young, Christopher Hawthorne, Laura Moss, Ian Piper, Martin Shaw, and Roddy O'Kane

Introduction

Moyamoya disease is characterized by chronic progressive arterial stenosis of the internal carotid arteries and proximal middle cerebral and anterior cerebral arteries. This is a result of progressive hyperplasia in smooth muscle in the arterial vessel wall. The progressive vascular stenosis precipitates development of collateral circulation from dilation of preexisting arterial perforators and formation of new ones, giving the characteristic "puff of smoke" seen on a cerebral angiogram. It may be idiopathic or secondary to treatment of other neurosurgical conditions (such as radiotherapy following tumor resection) and is responsible for 6% of pediatric cerebrovascular accidents [1]. It is also associated with other conditions such as trisomy 21 and neurofibromatosis type 1. The clinical picture is a combination of ischemic and hemorrhagic events, with the former being more common.

Medical management of moyamoya disease involves therapy with antiplatelet agents and calcium channel antagonists. There are various surgical strategies for management of moyamoya disease. These include direct revascularization, which consists of a bypass of the occluded segment, or indirect revascularization procedures, which involve laying vessels, dura, muscle, or a combination of these over the ischemic area of the brain. A recent meta-analysis of surgical outcomes of pediatric moyamoya disease found perioperative stroke risks of 4.5% with direct procedures, 9% with indirect procedures, and 6% with combined procedures [2].

Intracranial pressure (ICP) and brain tissue oxygenation ($PbtO_2$) are frequently monitored in head injury, with the goal of optimizing cerebral perfusion and oxygen delivery to tissues. We sought to determine if monitoring of ICP and $PbtO_2$ was feasible in patients with moyamoya disease. We were also interested in determining the autoregulatory status of these patients, who have abnormal cerebral vasculature.

Materials and Methods

All patients were evaluated clinically and with a digital subtraction angiogram during a separate hospital admission. Under general anesthesia with desflurane and remifentanil, an intraparenchymal Raumedic® PTO catheter was placed in the frontal lobe on the side ipsilateral to the revascularization. A radial arterial line was also inserted and zeroed at the level of the external auditory meatus. Monitoring of ICP and brain tissue oxygen was undertaken from the start of the procedure until 48 h postoperatively. The surgical procedure used in all patients was indirect pial synangiosis. After insertion of the PTO catheter, the superficial temporal artery was isolated using Doppler ultrasound and dissected free with a surrounding cuff of tissue. A large craniotomy was performed, the dura was opened widely, and a donor superficial temporal artery was placed over the exposed ischemic hemisphere along with the inverted dura. The bone flap was replaced, and the scalp was closed with absorbable sutures. All patients were managed in the pediatric intensive care unit

M. Kommer (✉) · E. Campbell · A. Amato-Watkins · S. Young
R. O'Kane
Institute of Neurological Sciences, Queen Elizabeth University Hospital, Glasgow, UK

Royal Hospital for Children, Glasgow, UK
e-mail: mayakommer@nhs.net, maya.kommer@ggc.scot.nhs.uk

M. Canty · C. Hawthorne
Institute of Neurological Sciences, Glasgow, UK

M. Sangra
Royal Hospital for Children, Glasgow, UK

L. Moss · M. Shaw
NHS Greater Glasgow Clyde, Glasgow, UK

University of Glasgow, Glasgow, UK

I. Piper
Usher Institute of Population Health and Informatics, University of Edinburgh, Edinburgh, UK

B. Depreitere et al. (eds.), *Intracranial Pressure and Neuromonitoring XVII*, Acta Neurochirurgica Supplement 131,
https://doi.org/10.1007/978-3-030-59436-7_24,

for 48 h postoperatively. A further digital subtraction angiogram was performed 6 months postoperatively to assess the success of revascularization.

Brain tissue oxygen tension was measured in millimeters of mercury. The cerebral autoregulatory status was examined across all patients, using the low-frequency autoregulatory index (LAx) [3]. ICP was plotted against the mean arterial pressure (MAP) to determine the pressure reactivity index (PRx) in each patient [4]. The cerebral perfusion pressure (CPP) was plotted against PRx to determine the optimum cerebral perfusion pressure (CPPOpt) [5]; this was the lowest point of inflection on the best-fit curve. Lower and upper limits of autoregulation were determined using the Aries methodology [6]. The patient was judged as autoregulating between the two values where the curve crossed the *x*-axis at zero.

Results

Four patients underwent seven revascularization procedures. All were in Suzuki stage 3 [7]. All patients presented with headaches and episodes of transient ischemia related to the affected hemisphere. The underlying patient characteristics are shown in Table 1. $PbtO_2$ data were available for four out of the seven operated hemispheres. For patient 1, no data were available. Patient 2 had a median $PbtO_2$ value of 55 mmHg (interquartile range (IQR) 53–57.6) at their first operation. In patient 3, the median $PbtO_2$ values were 25.2 mmHg (IQR 19.2–26.4) on the right side and 11.1 mmHg (IQR 1.5–21.1) on the left. In patient 4, the median $PbtO_2$ was 22.6 mmHg (IQR 16.2–25.8). Two of the four patients had best-fit LAx curves that crossed zero and were therefore judged to be autoregulating; these and the calculated CPPOpt values are shown in Table 2. The upper and lower limits of autoregulation in patients 2 and 3 are shown in Table 3. There were no complications of either PTO catheter insertion or craniotomy. One patient developed transient clinical ischemia on day 1 postoperatively, which responded to intravenous fluid and vasopressor infusion.

Discussion

$PbtO_2$ is frequently monitored in severe traumatic brain injury; it has been shown in a meta-analysis that combination of ICP/CPP therapy with $PbtO_2$ therapy increases the chances of a favorable outcome [8]. Our small series shows that monitoring of brain tissue oxygenation is feasible in the perioperative period in patients with moyamoya disease. It has previously been shown that cerebral blood flow is reduced in patients with moyamoya disease, using the ^{133}Xe inhalation method [9]. This, presumably, is a result of progressive luminal stenosis of the large intracranial arteries and occurs even in asymptomatic patients with moyamoya disease. As flow is reduced, the oxygen delivery to the tissues is impaired and, in theory, this should lead to lower $PbtO_2$ values. We found

Table 1 Patient characteristics

Patient number	Age (years)	Etiology	Hemisphere	Suzuki stage	Clinical symptoms
1	19	Allagile syndrome	Left	3B	Headache
			Right	3B	Ischemia
2	8	Unilateral moyamoya disease	Left	3A	Headache
			Left	3A	Ischemia
3	13	Possible chromosome 2 abnormality	Right	3B	Headache
			Left	3B	Ischemia
4	13	Unilateral, postradiotherapy	Left	3	Headache, Ischemia

Table 2 Autoregulatory status and optimal cerebral perfusion pressure (CPPOpt)

Patient number	Side	Autoregulation	CPPOpt (mmHg)
1	Left	No	
	Right	No	
2	Left	Yes	58
	Left	Yes	73
3	Right	Yes	78
	Left	Yes	60
4	Left	No	

Table 3 Limits of autoregulation

Patient number	Side	Limits (mmHg)		
		Lower	Upper	Range
2	Left	53	63	10
	Left	52	93	41
3	Right	75	98	23
	Left	46	75	29

that the majority of patients began the procedure with a low $PbtO_2$ value and that this increased during the procedure and the postoperative period. One patient had a normal $PbtO_2$ value; his follow-up angiogram showed poor revascularization. He had ongoing clinical episodes of ischemia and underwent a further revascularization procedure on the same hemisphere. Perhaps a low preoperative $PbtO_2$ value is a prerequisite for successful revascularization; study of more cases is required to determine if this is the case.

Cerebral autoregulation has been much studied within the fields of neurosurgery and neurocritical care, especially in the context of head injury. The classical model of autoregulation states that cerebral blood flow is maintained over a wide range of physiological MAP values, in accordance with Lassen's curve [10]. Autoregulation relies on the ability of the cerebral vasculature to constrict and dilate. The progressive arterial stenosis caused by moyamoya disease presumably results in reduced ability of the system to autoregulate. It is well known that these patients develop clinical ischemia in response to hyperventilation resulting from reduced partial pressure of carbon dioxide and hypotension in the context of a fever or intercurrent illness [11]. We postulate that the arteries of patients with moyamoya disease are in a state of maximal vasodilation to maintain cerebral blood flow. In our series, we found that four out of the seven hemispheres (in two patients) did show evidence of autoregulation. The range over which cerebral blood flow was maintained was, however, much smaller than that predicted by Lassen's curve [10]. The lower limit of autoregulation was increased in one of the hemispheres, whereas the upper limit was reduced in all four hemispheres that did show evidence of autoregulation.

We believe that this is the first published report of use of $PbtO_2$ and intracranial pressure monitoring in perioperative management of patients with moyamoya disease. It provides an interesting insight into the cerebrovascular physiology of patients with moyamoya disease.

Conflict of Interest **The authors declare no conflict of interest.**

References

1. Nagaraja D, Verma A, Taly AB, Kumar MV, Jayakumar PN (1994) Cerebrovascular disease in children. Acta Neurol Scand 90:251–255
2. Ravindran K, Wellons JC, Dewan MC (2019) Surgical outcomes for pediatric moyamoya: a systematic review and meta-analysis. J Neurosurg Pediatr 13:1–10
3. Depreitere B, Güiza F, Van den Berghe G, Schuhmann M, Maier G, Piper I, Meyfroidt G (2014) Pressure autoregulation monitoring and cerebral perfusion pressure target recommendation in patients with severe traumatic brain injury based on minute-by-minute monitoring data. J Neurosurg 120:1451–1457
4. Czosnyka M, Smielewski P, Kirkpatrick P et al (1997) Continuous assessment of the cerebral vasomotor reactivity in head injury. Neurosurgery 4:11–19
5. Steiner LA, Czosnyka M, Piechnik SK, Smielewski P, Chatfield D, Menon DK, Pickard JD (2002) Continuous monitoring of cerebrovascular pressure reactivity allows determination of optimal cerebral perfusion pressure in patients with traumatic brain injury. Crit Care Med 30(4):733–738
6. Aries MJ, Czosnyka M, Budohoski KP, Steiner LA, Lavinio A, Kolias AG, Hutchison PJ, Brady KM, Menon DK, Pickard JD, Smielewski P (2012) Continuous determination of optimal cerebral perfusion pressure in traumatic brain injury. Crit Care Med 40(8):2456–2463
7. Suzuki J, Takaku A (1969) Cerebrovascular "moyamoya" disease: disease showing abnormal net-like vessels in base of brain. Arch Neurol 20(3):288–299
8. Nangunoori R, Maloney-Wilensky E, Stiefel M, Park S, Kofke WA, Levine JM, Yang W, Le Roux PD (2012) Brain tissue oxygen-based therapy and outcome after severe traumatic brain injury: a systematic literature review. Neurocrit Care 17(1):131–138
9. Ogawa A, Yoshimoto J, Suzuki J, Sakurai Y (1990) Cerebral blood flow in moyamoya disease. Acta Neurochir 105:30–34
10. Lassen N (1959) Cerebral blood flow and oxygen consumption in man. Physiol Rev 39(2):183–238
11. Scott RM, Smith ER (2009) Moyamoya disease and moyamoya syndrome. N Engl J Med 360(12):1226–1237

Part V

Neuromonitoring Technology

Variability of the Optic Nerve Sheath Diameter on the Basis of Sex and Age in a Cohort of Healthy Volunteers

Karthikka Chandrapatham, Danilo Cardim, Marek Czosnyka, Alessandro Bertuccio, Anna Di Noto, Francesco Corradi, Joseph Donnelly, Paolo Pelosi, Peter J. Hutchinson, and Chiara Robba

Introduction

Increased intracranial pressure (ICP) is a dangerous condition, which may be caused by many neurological and non-neurological illnesses [1] and is associated with a poor outcome [2]. Invasive assessment of ICP with devices such as intraparenchymal probes and intraventricular catheters is the gold standard but may be contraindicated in patients with coagulopathies and may lead to complications such as infections or hemorrhages [3].

To avoid such complications, many noninvasive tools to evaluate ICP have been implemented in the past [4], such as ultrasonographic measurement of the optic nerve sheath diameter (ONSD), which is a repeatable, safe, and feasible technique. The optic nerve is surrounded by a dural sheath and the subarachnoid space, which encloses the nerve and is filled with cerebrospinal fluid (CSF); thus, increases in ICP are identifiable as ONSD increases in the anterior retrobulbar compartment approximately 3 mm behind the eyeball [5, 6].

This technique has the advantage of having low intra- and interobserver variability [7]. ICP and ONSD have a linear association in conditions of intracranial hypertension [7, 8] and in a recent meta-analysis, ONSD was shown to have an area under the hierarchical summary receiver operating characteristic curve of 0.94 [4].

There are still uncertainties regarding possible variability in ONSD in the healthy population, considering different sex and age subgroups, and this could affect the cutoff values to

Karthikka Chandrapatham and Danilo Cardim contributed equally to this work.

K. Chandrapatham (✉)
Department of Surgical Sciences and Integrated Diagnostics, University of Genoa, Genoa, Italy

D. Cardim
Brain Physics Laboratory, Division of Neurosurgery, Department of Clinical Neurosciences, University of Cambridge, Cambridge, UK

Institute for Exercise and Environmental Medicine, Texas Health Presbyterian Hospital, Dallas, TX, USA

Department of Neurology and Neurotherapeutics, University of Texas Southwestern Medical Center, Dallas, TX, USA

M. Czosnyka
Brain Physics Laboratory, Division of Neurosurgery, Department of Clinical Neurosciences, University of Cambridge, Cambridge, UK

Institute of Electronic Systems, Warsaw University of Technology, Warsaw, Poland

A. Bertuccio
Department of Neurosurgery, Azienda Ospedaliera SS Antonio e Biagio e Cesare Arrigo, Alessandria, Italy

A. Di Noto
Anaesthesia and Intensive Care, San Martino Policlinico Hospital, IRCCS for Oncology, University of Genoa, Genoa, Italy

F. Corradi
University of Pisa, Florence, Italy

J. Donnelly
Brain Physics Laboratory, Division of Neurosurgery, Department of Clinical Neurosciences, University of Cambridge, Cambridge, UK

Department of Anesthesiology, University of Auckland, Auckland, New Zealand

P. Pelosi
Department of Surgical Sciences and Integrated Diagnostics, University of Genoa, Genoa, Italy

Anaesthesia and Intensive Care, San Martino Policlinico Hospital, IRCCS for Oncology, University of Genoa, Genoa, Italy

P. Hutchinson
Division of Neurosurgery, Department of Clinical Neurosciences, Addenbrooke's Hospital, University of Cambridge, Cambridge, UK

C. Robba
Brain Physics Laboratory, Division of Neurosurgery, Department of Clinical Neurosciences, University of Cambridge, Cambridge, UK

Anaesthesia and Intensive Care, San Martino Policlinico Hospital, IRCCS for Oncology, University of Genoa, Genoa, Italy

B. Depreitere et al. (eds.), *Intracranial Pressure and Neuromonitoring XVII*, Acta Neurochirurgica Supplement 131,
https://doi.org/10.1007/978-3-030-59436-7_25,

be considered in clinical conditions on the basis of age and sex differences. The aim of this study was to assess age- and sex-related ONSD differences in a cohort of healthy volunteers.

Materials and Methods

The study protocol was approved by the relevant research ethics board in Genoa, Italy (approval number REC 031R8G2015) and followed the principles of the Declaration of Helsinki.

A total of 122 healthy volunteers were prospectively recruited between 1 September 2015 and 1 January 2018 at Galliera Hospital, Genoa, Italy. We prospectively enrolled adult (>18-year-old) Italian healthy volunteers (with an American Society of Anesthesiologists (ASA) physical classification of 1–2) undergoing preanesthetic assessment for low-risk surgical interventions at Galliera Hospital.

The inclusion criteria were the absence of any cardiovascular, respiratory, neurological, or systemic pathology, and the absence of any chronic diseases and any acute illnesses in the 4 weeks preceding the evaluation. All volunteers gave their written informed consent before enrollment. Admissible patients were evaluated, their demographic data were noted, and their arterial blood pressure (ABP) was measured noninvasively.

The cohort was stratified for sex (male versus female) and divided into three different age groups (group 1: young adults aged 18–44 years; group 2: middle-aged adults aged 45–64 years; and group 3: elderly adults aged ≥65 years).

ONSD was measured 3 mm behind the eyeball after application of ultrasound gel on both eyelids of the volunteers, who were in the supine position. Two trained investigators (CR and FC), with a background of more than 30 examinations, used a 7.5-MHz linear ultrasound probe (DC-T6, Mindray Medica, Shenzhen, China) directed at around 30° in the horizontal plane and perpendicularly in the vertical plane. The final ONSD measurement was obtained as the average of the axial and longitudinal diameters for both eyes.

Statistical analyses were done using RStudio version 3.6.0 software. Continuous variables were expressed as median (interquartile range). The data were verified for normality using the Shapiro–Wilk test. Pearson or nonparametric Spearman correlation coefficients were applied to relate continuous variables. A Welch two-sample *t* test or a nonparametric Wilcoxon rank sum test was used to evaluate the differences in ONSD between the sexes. One-way analyses of variance (parametric ANOVAs and a nonparametric Kruskal–Wallis test), followed by parametric post hoc pairwise comparison tests (using a *t* test with a pooled standard deviation) or nonparametric post hoc pairwise comparison tests (using a Wilcoxon rank sum test), with Bonferroni correction for multiplicity, were applied to evaluate the differences in ONSD with regard to age groups. A multivariable linear model was used to assess whether age, sex, and arterial blood pressure were independently related to ONSD (using the following linear model structure: ONSD ~ age + sex + ABP). The level of significance was set at *P* value of <0.05.

Results

There was a positive significant correlation between ONSD and age ($R = 0.50$, $P < 0.0001$) (Fig. 1).

A significant difference was found in ONSD between males and females (4.2 (interquartile range (IQR) 3.9–4.6) versus 4.1 (IQR 3.3–4.2) mm, $P = 0.01$) (Table 1). When the entire population was considered, ONSD showed a statisti-

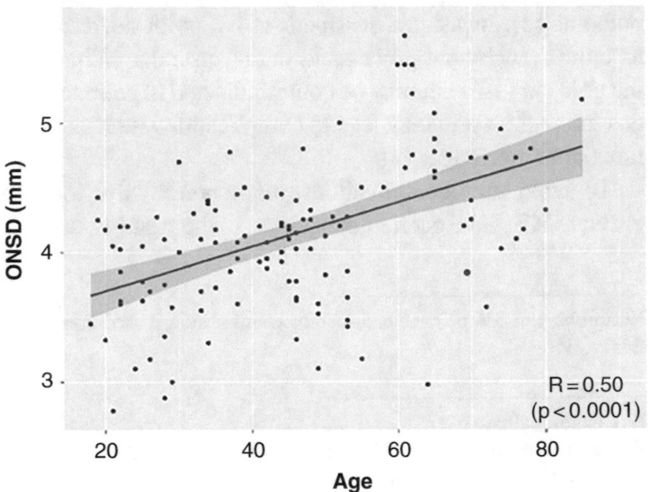

Fig. 1 Correlation between the optic nerve sheath diameter (ONSD, measured in millimeters, and age in a healthy population ($R = 0.50$, $P < 0.0001$). The *dark gray shaded areas* represent the 95% confidence intervals for the linear regressions

Table 1 Characteristics of the study cohort

	Age [years]	Optic nerve sheath diameter [mm] All volunteers	Males	Females
All volunteers	≥18	4.2 (3.8–4.4)	4.2 (3.9–4.6)	4.1 (3.6–4.2)
Age group				
Group 1	18–44	4.0 (3.7–4.2)	4.1 (3.8–4.4)	4.0 (3.6–4.2)
Group 2	45–64	4.2 (3.6–4.5)	4.3 (4.2–4.8)	3.8 (3.6–4.2)
Group 3	≥65	4.7 (4.2–4.8)	4.8 (4.5–4.9)	4.6 (4.2–4.27)

The values are expressed as median (interquartile range)

cally significant difference between age groups 1 and 3 (4.0 (IQR 3.7–4.2) versus 4.7 (IQR 4.2–4.8) mm, $P < 0.0001$) and between groups 2 and 3 (4.2 (IQR 3.6–4.5) versus 4.7 (IQR 4.8–4.2) mm, $P = 0.01$).

The multivariable linear model analysis revealed that age and sex were independently related to ONSD ($P < 0.0001$ and $P = 0.005$, respectively).

Discussion

We found significant differences between age groups and sexes in the whole cohort, and males had significantly higher ONSD values than females [9–12]. ONSD increased with age (Fig. 1), and elderly individuals had higher ONSD values than younger volunteers.

Many studies have tried to evaluate the normal ONSD thresholds in healthy populations. They have collectively proposed that ONSD remains relatively constant throughout adulthood [9, 10, 12, 13]. Conversely, our findings suggest that ONSD increases with age. This finding could be attributable to variations in cerebrospinal fluid circulation as a result of aging [14], resulting in an increased CSF volume in the space surrounding the optic nerve, which would increase ONSD.

A Korean study [15] evaluated a cohort of 585 healthy young adults (aged 18–30 years) and found that ONSD was significantly correlated with sex, height, and eyeball transverse diameter (ETD) in a simple linear regression analysis, but on multiple linear regression analysis, only ETD was independently associated with ONSD.

Goeres et al. studied 120 healthy adults and found that the mean ONSD varied between males and females but did not vary with age, weight, or height [16]. In another study, Anas showed no significant correlation of ONSD with age, sex, height, weight, or measurement side [17].

Other studies have proposed that ethnicity should be considered when ONSD thresholds are evaluated for increased ICP. For instance, a Chinese study [18] reported that the upper ONSD limit was lower than the thresholds seen in previous studies in Caucasian and African samples, and that underweight women had the lowest ONSD values. These findings highlight the importance of taking into account sex, the body mass index, and ethnicity.

This study had the following limitations. First, the ultrasound examinations were performed by two different operators, and we did not take into account interobserver variability as a potential confounder, but the operators were experienced and had a comparable level of training. Second, ethnic differences in ONSD values could have been relevant; our population was prevalently Caucasian. Further studies in different and larger cohorts are required to define this potential confounding factor.

Conclusion

ONSD increases with age and is significantly greater in males than in females in the healthy population. Larger studies in brain-injured patients are needed to further evaluate differences attributable to sex and age.

Conflict of Interest **The authors declare that they have no conflict of interest.**

References

1. Dunn LT (2002) Raised intracranial pressure. J Neurol Neurosurg Psychiatry 73(Suppl 1):i23–i27
2. Balestreri M, Czosnyka M, Hutchinson P, Steiner LA, Hiler M, Smielewski P et al (2006) Impact of intracranial pressure and cerebral perfusion pressure on severe disability and mortality after head injury. Neurocrit Care 4(1):8–13
3. Kristiansson H, Nissborg E, Bartek J, Andresen M, Reinstrup P, Romner B (2013) Measuring elevated intracranial pressure through noninvasive methods. J Neurosurg Anesthesiol 25(4):372–385
4. Robba C, Santori G, Czosnyka M, Corradi F, Bragazzi N, Padayachy L et al (2018) Optic nerve sheath diameter measured sonographically as non-invasive estimator of intracranial pressure: a systematic review and meta-analysis. Intensive Care Med 44(8):1284–1294
5. Moretti R, Pizzi B, Cassini F, Vivaldi N (2009) Reliability of optic nerve ultrasound for the evaluation of patients with spontaneous intracranial hemorrhage. Neurocrit Care 11(3):406–410
6. Geeraerts T, Menon DK, Benhamou D (2009) Measurement of optic nerve sheath diameter for the assessment of risk of raised intracranial pressure. Eur Neurol Rev 4(1):50
7. Robba C, Cardim D, Tajsic T, Pietersen J, Bulman M, Donnelly J et al (2017) Ultrasound non-invasive measurement of intracranial pressure in neurointensive care: a prospective observational study. PLoS Med 14(7):e1002356
8. Geeraerts T, Launey Y, Martin L, Pottecher J, Vigué B, Duranteau J et al (2007) Ultrasonography of the optic nerve sheath may be useful for detecting raised intracranial pressure after severe brain injury. Intensive Care Med 33(10):1704–1711
9. Amini A, Kariman H, Arhami Dolatabadi A, Hatamabadi HR, Derakhshanfar H, Mansouri B et al (2013) Use of the sonographic diameter of optic nerve sheath to estimate intracranial pressure. Am J Emerg Med 31(1):236–239
10. Maude RR, Amir Hossain M, Hassan MU, Osbourne S, Sayeed KLA, Karim MR et al (2013) Transorbital sonographic evaluation of normal optic nerve sheath diameter in healthy volunteers in Bangladesh. PLoS One 8(12):e81013
11. Chen H, Ding G-S, Zhao Y-C, Yu R-G, Zhou J-X (2015) Ultrasound measurement of optic nerve diameter and optic nerve sheath diameter in healthy Chinese adults. BMC Neurol 15(1):106
12. Moretti R, Pizzi B (2011) Ultrasonography of the optic nerve in neurocritically ill patients. Acta Anaesthesiol Scand 55(6):644–652
13. Bäuerle J, Lochner P, Kaps M, Nedelmann M (2012) Intra- and interobsever reliability of sonographic assessment of the optic nerve sheath diameter in healthy adults. J Neuroimaging 22(1):42–45
14. Lochner P, Cantello R, Brigo F, Coppo L, Nardone R, Tezzon F et al (2014) Transorbital sonography in acute optic neuritis: a case–control study. AJNR Am J Neuroradiol 35(12):2371–2375

15. Kim DH, Jun JS, Kim R (2017) Ultrasonographic measurement of the optic nerve sheath diameter and its association with eyeball transverse diameter in 585 healthy volunteers. Sci Rep 7:15906
16. Goeres P, Zeiler FA, Unger B, Karakitsos D, Gillman LM (2016) Ultrasound assessment of optic nerve sheath diameter in healthy volunteers. J Crit Care 31(1):168–171
17. Anas I (2014) Transorbital sonographic measurement of normal optic sheath nerve diameter in Nigerian adult population. Malays J Med Sci 21(5):24–29
18. Wang L, Feng L, Yao Y, Deng F, Wang Y, Feng J et al (2016) Ultrasonographic evaluation of optic nerve sheath diameter among healthy Chinese adults. Ultrasound Med Biol 42(3):683–688

A Noninvasive Method for Monitoring Intracranial Pressure During Postural Changes

Michele L. Pierro, Nikole M. Shooshan, Saukhyda Deshmukh, and Gordon B. Hirschman

Introduction

There is currently no gold standard for noninvasive assessment of intracranial pressure (ICP) and diagnosis of intracranial hypertension. Although advanced neuroimaging techniques have recently contributed to better understanding of the pathophysiology associated with different degrees of severity of TBI, limited accessibility of the imaging equipment, long examination times, and the need for diagnostic imaging expertise limit the clinical utility of such technologies in austere or everyday environments.

Traumatic brain injury (TBI) is a complex and heterogeneous disorder, which can result in a large spectrum of associated injury severity. The brain is a soft organ with delicate structures held within a fixed volume. Damage to small structures within the brain causes local swelling, and cerebral blood flow and systemic blood pressure may not necessarily decrease with brain swelling [1, 2]. This elevated ICP can in itself cause more damage, leading to a negative spiral that ends in dire health sequelae, including brain cell death and permanent brain injury or death [3, 4].

Because of the practical limitations imposed by invasive measurements of ICP and the TBI population, in this study we used body position to affect blood and fluid distribution [5] in healthy volunteers. ICP depends on the volume of cerebral blood and cerebrospinal fluid (CSF), the vascular component of which is influenced by systemic blood pressure, modified by cerebral autoregulation and venous outflow resistance [6], while the CSF component is described by Davson's equation [7] as a balance between CSF formation, CSF outflow resistance, and venous pressure in the sagittal sinus. Thus, given intact cerebral autoregulation [5] and systemic blood pressure regulation, as should be the case in healthy volunteers, positional changes in ICP are dominated by venous pressure [5], which correlates with gravitational stress (hydrostatic pressure).

Pulse wave velocity (PWV) analysis has previously been employed for effectiveness assessment of the state of the systemic vasculature—for example, calculation of vessel elasticity, impedance and reflection coefficients [8], and arterial stiffness [9]. These works have been based on the underlying principle (as presented by the Moens–Korteweg equation) that describes PWV as a function of basic properties of the vascular route, such as the internal radius and wall thickness of the vessel [8]. Different authors [10] have previously applied the PWV approach to analysis of the intracranial hemodynamic system. Specifically, the PWV was calculated in the peripheral circulation by measurement of time delays in cerebral blood flow velocity (as measured by transcranial Doppler ultrasound) obtained simultaneously from the cervical carotid artery and the ipsilateral middle cerebral artery [10].

In this study, we proposed assessment of pulse onset latency (or the pulse transit time (PTT)) as the time interval between optical signals measured at three reference locations (an earlobe, a fingertip, and a supraorbital artery) and an optical signal measuring cerebral blood volume oscillations, and we assessed the correlation between measured PTT changes and ICP variations modulated by postural changes without the need for additional electrocardiographic measurements.

Materials and Methods

Tilt Table Study

The tilt table protocol was approved by the New England Independent Review Board (approval number NEIRB 120170179), and all subjects provided written informed consent for participation. The study was conducted at Vivonics, Inc. (Bedford, MA, USA).

M. L. Pierro (✉) · N. M. Shooshan · S. Deshmukh · G. B. Hirschman
Vivonics, Inc., Bedford, MA, USA
e-mail: mpierro@vivonics.com

B. Depreitere et al. (eds.), *Intracranial Pressure and Neuromonitoring XVII*, Acta Neurochirurgica Supplement 131,
https://doi.org/10.1007/978-3-030-59436-7_26,

Ten healthy human subjects were recruited for participation in this research. The subjects were over the age of 18 years and did not have an intracranial shunt, concussion symptoms, a musculoskeletal condition contraindicating use of an inversion table, previous brain surgery, a cardiovascular disorder, a headache, or an allergy to medical tape. Female subjects were asked to report whether there was a chance of pregnancy and were excluded if the answer was yes.

Measurements were performed by having the subject lie on the inversion table, strapped in at their ankles. The blood pressure (the mean arterial pressure (MAP)), oxygen saturation (SaO_2), heart rate (HR), stroke volume (SV), cardiac output (CO), and total peripheral resistance (TPR) were calculated by use of a noninvasive continuous blood pressure monitor (Nova, Finapres Medical Systems, Enschede, the Netherlands) attached to the subject by means of a volume clamp finger cuff, brachial cuff, and pulse oxygen sensor. The subject was additionally connected to the IPASS (Intracranial Pressure Assessment and Screening System) optical sensors: a forehead sensor (1) collected data on superficial blood volume oscillations from the supraorbital artery; a cerebral sensor (2) allowed measurement of spontaneous hemodynamic oscillations from the outer surface of the brain and measured cerebral blood oscillations; and an earlobe sensor (3) and index finger sensor (4) collected data on reference blood volume oscillations. The wavelength implemented by the IPASS is 850 nm to maximize sensitivity to oxygenated hemoglobin concentration oscillations as induced by cardiac activity (~1 Hz). Raw data were postprocessed by a custom Matlab script that allowed isolation of blood volume oscillations (~1 Hz) of interest by performing a third-order polynomial detrending and band-pass filtering procedure (~0.7–10 Hz) before extrapolating instantaneous phase values by utilizing the Hilbert transform [11]. The Hilbert transform calculated the instantaneous phase of each of the optical signals measured at the four locations, and the PTT was calculated by translating the phase difference (Δϕ $\Delta\varnothing$) between each pair of signals (cranial oscillations with respect to reference signal oscillations) and converted into a time difference by use of the formula:

$$\text{PTT} = \Delta\varnothing / 2\pi f.$$

where *f* is the main frequency component associated with the filtered signal (~1 Hz).

The Nova continuous monitoring data were collected from the subject's left side and the IPASS sensor data were collected from the subject's right side. The subjects were tilted at various angles for 90 s at each angle. The angle progression was as follows: +45°, −30°, +45°, −15°, +45°, 0°, +45°, +15°, +45°, +30°, and + 45°.

From the change in hydrostatic pressure at a given tilt angle (α), the corresponding change in ICP was estimated as:

$$\text{ICP}(\alpha) = \text{ICP}(0^\circ) - \rho \times g \times h \times \sin(\alpha)$$

where ρ is the blood density, g is the gravitational acceleration, h is the distance from below the heart (at the bottom of the sternum) to the nasion, and ICP(0°) is a previously measured value of the average ICP in subjects lying at zero degrees [ICP(0°)~11 mmHg] [5]. A *t* test was used to detect statistically significant differences ($P < 0.05$) in the PTT values between the head-up (0°, +15°, +30°, and +45°) and head-down (−30° and −15°) positions.

Results

Compared with the head-up position (+45°), the head-down and supine positions (−30°, −15°, and 0°) changed the central cardiovascular variables significantly. The data reported in Fig. 1, corresponding to an individual subject, show the heart rate (HR), stroke volume (SV), cardiac output (CO), total peripheral resistance (TPR), and mean arterial pressure (MAP) as continuously measured signals throughout the entire length of the experimental protocol. Elevating the head (from −30° to +45°) increased HR from 47 ± 6.0 to 63 ± 2.0 beats/min, MAP from 50.0 ± 3.5 to 79 ± 4.2 mmHg, and TPR from 1.4 ± 0.2 to 2.1 ± 0.3 mmHg · min · mL^{-1}. A head-down tilt and supine position increased SV from 54 ± 13 mL at 45° to 87 ± 15 mL at −30° and increased CO from 3.3 ± 0.8 L/min at 45° (P <0.05) to 4.1 ± 1.1 L/min at −30°. An increase in HR and TPR in a head-up position occurred consistently in order to maintain CO within a physiological range. Figure 1f shows the averaged pulse arrival delays between the superficial and cerebral ($PTT_{S\text{-}C}$) hemodynamic oscillations (as measured on the subject's forehead) and the cerebral and finger ($PTT_{C\text{-}F}$) oscillations, against the tilt table angles. A supine position and positive tilt table angles corresponded to low ICP values (<11 mmHg), while negative tilt table angles corresponded to increased ICP values (>11 mmHg) due to hydrostatic pressure changes. Both the calculated $PTT_{S\text{-}C}$ and $PTT_{C\text{-}F}$ changed according to the changes in hydrostatic pressure, which corresponded to ICP variations. Specifically, negative tilt table angles (−15° and −30°), which increased ICP, translated into higher PTT values (>70 ms in this specific subject) (Fig. 1), while a supine position and positive angles (0°, 15°, 30°, and 45°) resulted in lower PTT values in agreement with lower ICP values. Finally, in comparison of angle-related variations in the cardiovascular variables with respect to the PTT values ($PTT_{S\text{-}C}$ and $PTT_{C\text{-}F}$), it was noticeable that the cardiovascular variables fluctuated following any postural change (positive and

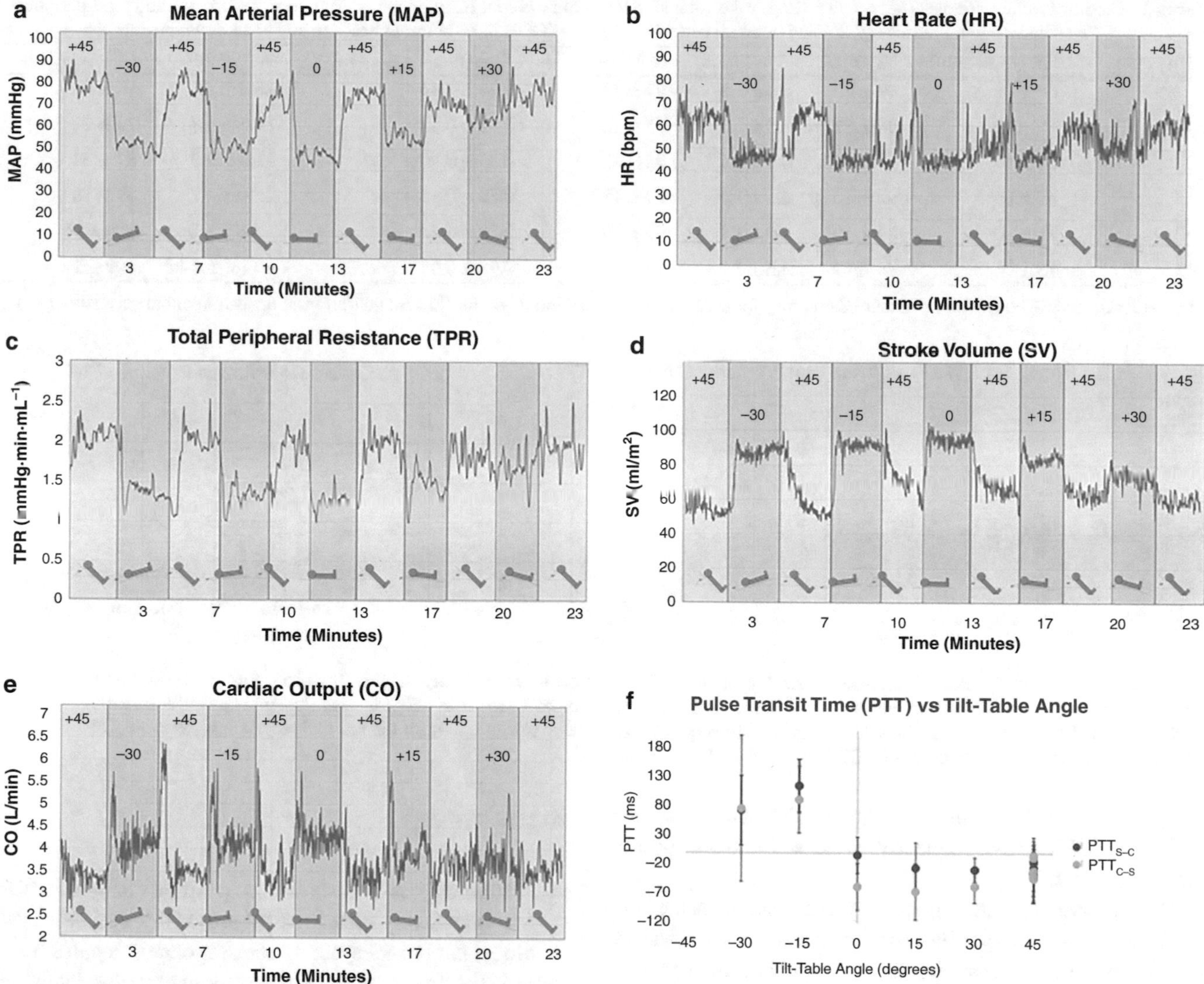

Fig. 1 Real-time measurements of cardiovascular variables: (**a**) mean arterial pressure (MAP), (**b**) heart rate (HR), (**c**) total peripheral resistance (TPR), (**d**) stroke volume (SV), and (**e**) cardiac output (CO) in an individual subject in response to our head-up and head-down tilt protocol: +45°, −30°, +45°, −15°, +45°, 0°, +45°, +15°, +45°, +30°, and +45°. (**f**) Pulse arrival delays (mean ± standard deviation) between superficial and cerebral ($PTT_{S\text{-}C}$) hemodynamic oscillations (as measured on the subject's forehead) and the cerebral and finger ($PTT_{C\text{-}F}$) oscillations in an individual subject in response to our head-up and head-down tilt protocol: +45°, −30°, +45°, −15°, +45°, 0°, +45°, +15°, and +45°

negative tilt table angles), while the PTT values changed significantly only with movement from a head-up position to a head-down position (and vice versa), but no intermediate fluctuations (for example, between different positive angles) were observed. This trend of increases and decreases across physiological signals at the various positive and negative angles was observed across all of the subjects, consistent with ICP changes.

Table 1 lists the continuously measured (in real-time) cardiovascular variables in response to the head-up and head-down tilts in only seven volunteers because of a technical problem associated with the blood pressure monitor herein used to continuously measure MAP and the other cardiovascular variables. These technical problems were not associated with any of the optical measurements performed by the IPASS. ICP values were estimated in all ten subjects, since they were independently calculated from the cardiac variables. The averaged values reported in Table 1 are consistent with the individual cardiovascular variable trends identified in the subject shown in Fig. 1. Tilting up increased HR from 68 ± 13 beats/min at −30° to 76 ± 12 beats/min at 45°, while it reduced SV from 89 ± 22 mL at −30° to 74 ± 19 mL at 45° ($P < 0.05$). CO increased from 5.6 ± 1.7 L/min at 45° to 6.0 ± 1.5 L/min at −30° during the tilt-up maneuver (from

Table 1 Cardiovascular variables (heart rate (HR), stroke volume (SV), cardiac output (CO), mean arterial pressure (MAP), and total peripheral resistance (TPR)), intracranial pressure (ICP), and cerebral perfusion pressure (CPP) in response to head-up and head-down postural changes

Tilt angle (°)	HR (beats/min)	SV (mL)	CO (L/min)	MAP (mmHg)	TPR (mmHg · min · mL^{-1})	ICP (mmHg)	CPP (mmHg)
−30	68 ± 13	89 ± 22	6.0 ± 1.5	97 ± 23	0.92 ± 0.42	26.8 ± 1.5	70 ± 23
−15	65 ± 10	96 ± 22	6.3 ± 1.7	95 ± 22	0.88 ± 0.42	19.2 ± 0.8	76 ± 22
0	64 ± 10	100 ± 22	6.4 ± 1.7	92 ± 22	0.84 ± 0.39	11.0 ± 0.0	81 ± 22
15	66 ± 10	92 ± 20	6.1 ± 1.7	92 ± 18	0.86 ± 0.42	2.8 ± 0.8	89 ± 18
30	71 ± 10	84 ± 19	6.0 ± 1.7	95 ± 15	0.89 ± 0.45	−4.8 ± 1.5	100 ± 14
45	76 ± 12	74 ± 19	5.6 ± 1.7	98 ± 12	0.98 ± 0.54	−11.4 ± 2.1	109 ± 12

The values are averaged (mean ± standard deviation) for each respective postural angle for 90 s (the duration of measurement at each tilt angle)

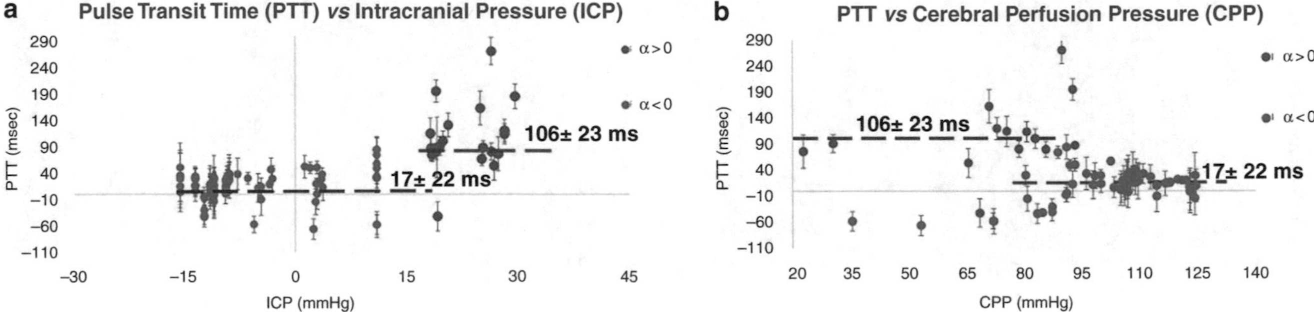

Fig. 2 Mean (± standard deviation (SD)) pulse transit time (PTT) between cerebral and finger oscillations (**a**) versus intracranial pressure (ICP) estimated from hydrostatic pressure changes in 10 subjects and (**b**) versus cerebral perfusion pressure (CPP) in 7 subjects. PTT was calculated at positive angles (0°, +15°, +30°, and +45°) and at negative angles (−15° and −30°). *Red and purple dashed lines* are the average value (mean ± SD) for the *red and purple dots* respectively

45° to −30°). As expected, the head-down maneuver increased ICP and consequently decreased cerebral perfusion pressure (CPP).

We observed that the optical signal measured at the fingertip was consistently robust in all of the subjects across the positive and negative angles, while the other reference signals degraded at negative angles, thus making PTT calculation unreliable. Figure 2 shows the plots of $PTT_{C\text{-}F}$ versus ICP and versus CPP (CPP = MAP − ICP) for all data points collected from all subjects at the different tilt table angles.

Figure 2a shows $PTT_{C\text{-}F}$ versus ICP at positive angles ($\alpha > 0$) and negative angles ($\alpha < 0$). This plot shows the increase in $PTT_{C\text{-}F}$ values from 17 ± 22 to 106 ± 23 ms ($P < 0.01$) as the subjects experienced a positional change from head-up to head-down. This postural change from positive ($\alpha > 0$) to negative ($\alpha < 0$) tilt table angles consistently correlated with increased ICP values (for negative angles: $\alpha < 0$) herein estimated from the equivalent hydrostatic pressure changes. Figure 2b compares $PTT_{C\text{-}F}$ and estimated CPP values at positive and negative angles. In this case, too, we observed significant increases in $PTT_{C\text{-}F}$ values at negative angles compared with positive angles, which also translated into lower CPP values. One subject's CPP values were found to be lower (<50 mmHg) than those in the other subjects, likely because of relatively low MAP at the beginning of the protocol (~50–60 mmHg).

Discussion

These results suggest that short-term postural changes in ICP can be noninvasively measured by use of our optical-based technology, the IPASS system, to extrapolate the pulse transit time as the time interval between peripheral blood volume oscillations (at the fingertip) and cerebral blood volume oscillations ($PTT_{C\text{-}F}$). During a head-down tilt, the measured increase in $PTT_{C\text{-}F}$ was greater than the decrease caused by a head-up tilt. These results were consistent with data reported by Petersen et al. [5], who observed that during a head-down tilt, the increase in invasively measured ICP was greater than the decrease observed during a head-up tilt. In fact, Petersen et al. [5] reported that postural changes from −20° to +20° resulted in a change in ICP from ~20 to ~0 mmHg, while postural changes at angles greater than 20° did not result in any significant ICP reduction (~0 mmHg). Petersen et al. [5] concluded that this finding was the result of formation of a smaller hydrostatic gradient at positive tilt angles, possibly caused by collapse of major neck veins in order to protect the brain from being exposed to a large negative pressure when upright. Our findings consistently showed a $PTT_{C\text{-}F}$ surge when subjects experienced a change from a head-up position ($\alpha \geq 0°$) to a head-down position ($\alpha \leq -15°$), corresponding to a $PTT_{C\text{-}F}$ change from 17 ± 22 to 106 ± 23 ms (Fig. 2).

These results highlight the value of the PPT-based method as a valid noninvasive technique for monitoring ICP.

Additionally, this work has the merit of showing that our cerebral measurements were not strongly influenced by systemic parameters such as MAP and the other cardiovascular variables. Indeed, the real-time monitoring of the cardiovascular variables (HR, MAP, TPR, SV, and CO) showed the influence of postural changes on each single cardiovascular variable at all tilt table angles independently of the estimated ICP. As opposed to that, our PTT measurements presented a significant change only in correspondence to ICP values estimated to be greater than 10 mmHg (with no significate changes across positive angles), thus indicating no correlation between PTT and cardiovascular parameters.

The ICP values reported in this work were mathematically estimated by the height of a hydrostatic fluid column calculated at each angle, which led to negative ICP estimations, as shown in Figs. 1 and 2. While we are aware that according to Petersen et al. [5], major neck veins should collapse, preventing negative ICP values, the main contribution of this work is to present a noninvasive method to monitor ICP changes and investigate PTT behavior for increased (or approaching the physiological limit: ~20 mmHg) ICP values.

Future work will be focused on estimating any extracerebral contribution to our cerebral blood volume measurements and investigating the possibility of noninvasively measuring the absolute ICP on the basis of the herein presented PTT-based method to assess relative ICP changes. The latter will require a clinical study, allowing us to establish a correlation between invasively measured—and thus accurate—ICP and IPASS PTT readings.

Acknowledgments This material is based on work supported by the US Army and by the Marine Corps System Command (MARCORSYSCOM) under contract numbers W81XWH-17-C-0006 and M67854-15-C-6528. Any opinions, findings, and conclusions or recommendations expressed in this material are those of the author(s) and do not necessarily reflect the views of the US Army or the Marine Corps System Command (MARCORSYSCOM).

Conflict of Interest **The coauthor Gordon B. Hirschman is the president and chief executive officer of Vivonics, Inc. In addition to being a salaried employee of Vivonics, Mr. Hirschman is the majority shareholder in Vivionics and the sole member of the Vivonics board of directors. Vivonics is funded by public government grants and contracts to carry out the work of researching and developing the IPASS device. As a shareholder of Vivonics, Mr. Hirschman has a financial interest in the commercial success of IPASS.**

References

1. Bouma GJ et al (1992) Ultra-early evaluation of regional cerebral blood flow in severely head-injured patients using xenon-enhanced computerized tomography. J Neurosurg 77(3):360–368
2. Kety SS, Schmidt CF (1948) The effects of altered arterial tensions of carbon dioxide and oxygen on cerebral blood flow and cerebral oxygen consumption of normal young men. J Clin Invest 27(4):484
3. Miller JD et al (1972) Concepts of cerebral perfusion pressure and vascular compression during intracranial hypertension. Prog Brain Res 35:411–432
4. Miller JD et al (1977) Significance of intracranial hypertension in severe head injury. J Neurosurg 47(4):503–516
5. Petersen LG et al (2016) Postural influence on intracranial and cerebral perfusion pressure in ambulatory neurosurgical patients. Am J Phys Regul Integr Comp Phys 310(1):R100–R104
6. Czosnyka M et al (1999) Vascular components of cerebrospinal fluid compensation. J Neurosurg 90(4):752–759
7. Davson H et al (1973) The mechanism of drainage of the cerebrospinal fluid. Brain 96(2):329–336
8. Asgari S et al (2011) An extended model of intracranial latency facilitates non-invasive detection of cerebrovascular changes. J Neurosci Methods 197(1):171–179
9. Chang HK et al (2006) Arterial stiffness in Behcet's disease: increased regional pulse wave velocity values. Ann Rheum Dis 65(3):415–416
10. Giller CA, Aaslid R (1994) Estimates of pulse wave velocity and measurement of pulse transit time in the human cerebral circulation. Ultrasound Med Biol 20(2):101–105
11. Pierro ML et al (2012) Phase-amplitude investigation of spontaneous low-frequency oscillations of cerebral hemodynamics with near-infrared spectroscopy: a sleep study in human subjects. NeuroImage 63(3):1571–1584
12. Mihalik JP et al (2017) Evaluating the "threshold theory": can head impact indicators help? Med Sci Sports Exerc 49(2):247–253

Arterial and Venous Cerebral Blood Flow Velocities in Healthy Volunteers

Karthikka Chandrapatham, Danilo Cardim, Francesco Corradi, Mypinder Sekhon, Donald Griesdale, Marek Czosnyka, and Chiara Robba

Introduction

Transcranial Doppler ultrasound (TCD) is a noninvasive, radiation-free technique through which brain hemodynamics can be evaluated with good temporal and spatial resolution [1]. It is feasible, repeatable, and applicable at the bedside [2].

The most widespread assessments are based on basic parameters derived from study of TCD waveforms, such as evaluations of systolic, diastolic, and mean cerebral blood flow velocities (FVs, FVd, and FVm, respectively) and pulsatility and resistance indices. More refined assessments may be done by advanced TCD measurements such as assessments of cerebral blood flow autoregulation, critical closing pressure, wall tension, arterial compliance, the cerebrovascular time constant, noninvasive cerebral perfusion pressure, noninvasive intracranial pressure (ICP) and assessment of cerebrovascular reactivity [1, 3, 4].

The cerebral venous compartment itself can be studied through venous TCD (vTCD), which is still underdeveloped and is mostly applied for diagnosis of stroke, dural sinus thrombosis, and head trauma [5].

In neurocritical care, vTCD has recently gained more attention because of the positive correlation between the peak venous blood flow velocity in the straight sinus (FVVs) and ICP. (In the abbreviation "FVVs," "*s*" stands for "systolic," given the resemblance of this peak blood flow velocity to an arterial systolic peak). This correlation was first described by Schoser et al. in 1999 [6] and then reconfirmed by a recent study, which demonstrated the significance of FVVs and the optic nerve sheath diameter as indirect markers of ICP [2]. However, there are still concerns regarding

Karthikka Chandrapatham and Danilo Cardim contributed equally to this work.

K. Chandrapatham (✉)
Department of Surgical Sciences and Integrated Diagnostics, University of Genoa, Genoa, Italy

D. Cardim
Brain Physics Laboratory, Division of Neurosurgery, Department of Clinical Neurosciences, University of Cambridge, Cambridge, UK

Institute for Exercise and Environmental Medicine, Texas Health Presbyterian Hospital, Dallas, TX, USA

Department of Neurology and Neurotherapeutics, University of Texas Southwestern Medical Center, Dallas, TX, USA

F. Corradi
University of Pisa, Florence, Italy

M. Sekhon
Division of Critical Care Medicine, Department of Medicine, Vancouver General Hospital, University of British Columbia, Vancouver, BC, Canada

D. Griesdale
Division of Critical Care Medicine, Department of Medicine, Vancouver General Hospital, University of British Columbia, Vancouver, BC, Canada

Department of Anaesthesiology, Pharmacology and Therapeutics, Vancouver General Hospital, University of British Columbia, Vancouver, BC, Canada

Centre for Clinical Epidemiology and Evaluation, Vancouver Coastal Health Research Institute, University of British Columbia, Vancouver, BC, Canada

M. Czosnyka
Brain Physics Laboratory, Division of Neurosurgery, Department of Clinical Neurosciences, University of Cambridge, Cambridge, UK

Institute of Electronic Systems, Warsaw University of Technology, Warsaw, Poland

C. Robba
Brain Physics Laboratory, Division of Neurosurgery, Department of Clinical Neurosciences, University of Cambridge, Cambridge, UK

Anaesthesia and Intensive Care, San Martino Policlinico Hospital, IRCCS for Oncology, University of Genoa, Genoa, Italy

B. Depreitere et al. (eds.), *Intracranial Pressure and Neuromonitoring XVII*, Acta Neurochirurgica Supplement 131, https://doi.org/10.1007/978-3-030-59436-7_27,

the impacts of age and sex on normative values of arterial and venous TCD blood flow velocities in healthy populations.

The aim of this prospective observational study was to evaluate any differences in TCD-derived arterial and venous cerebral blood flow velocities assessed in the middle cerebral arteries (MCAs) and the straight sinus (SS) in a cohort of healthy volunteers of different sexes and different ages.

Materials and Methods

The study protocol was approved by the relevant research ethics board in Genoa, Italy (approval number REC 031R8G2015) and followed the principles of the Declaration of Helsinki.

A total of 134 healthy volunteers were prospectively screened between 1 September 2015 and 1 January 2018 at Galliera Hospital, Genoa, Italy. We prospectively enrolled adult (>18-year-old) Italian healthy volunteers (with an American Society of Anesthesiologists (ASA) physical classification of 1–2) undergoing preanesthetic assessment for low-risk surgical interventions at Galliera Hospital.

The inclusion criteria were the absence of any cardiovascular, respiratory, neurological, or systemic pathology, and the absence of any chronic diseases and any acute illnesses in the 4 weeks preceding the evaluation. All volunteers gave their written informed consent before enrollment. The exclusion criteria comprised a history of head injury, pregnancy, and inadequate insonation windows (temporal and occipital (or transforaminal) windows) for detection of the MCAs and SS. Noninvasive mean arterial blood pressure (ABP), heart rate, and demographic data were collected.

Two operators with experience of performing more than 30 examinations collected the TCD measurements. Arterial TCD was performed bilaterally on the MCAs through the temporal windows at a depth of 45–65 mm, using a handheld 2-MHz probe (DC-T6, Mindray Medica, Shenzhen, China). The bilateral systolic, diastolic, and mean cerebral blood flow velocities (FVs, FVd, and FVm, respectively) were averaged to obtain the final values of these parameters.

Venous TCD was performed on the SS through the occipital window at a depth of 50–80 mm [2]. A brief Valsalva maneuver was performed to verify the venous origin of the flow [6].

The cohort was stratified for sex (male versus female) and divided into three different age groups (group 1: young adults aged 18–44 years; group 2: middle-aged adults aged 45–64 years; and group 3: elderly adults aged ≥65 years) (Fig. 1).

Statistical analyses were performed using RStudio version 3.6.0 software. Continuous variables were expressed as median (interquartile range (IQR)). The data were verified for normality using the Shapiro–Wilk test. Pearson or nonparametric Spearman correlation coefficients (R values) were used to relate continuous variables to age. A Welch two-sample t test or a nonparametric Wilcoxon rank sum test was used to evaluate the differences in flow velocities between the sexes. One-way analyses of variance (parametric ANOVAs and a nonparametric Kruskal–Wallis test) and then parametric analysis (using a t test with a pooled standard deviation) or a nonparametric analysis (using a Wilcoxon rank sum test), followed by post hoc pairwise comparison tests, with Bonferroni correction for multiplicity, were applied to evaluate the differences in blood flow velocities with regard to age groups. Multivariable linear models were used to assess whether age, sex, and ABP were independently related to cerebral blood flow velocities. The level of significance was set at P value <0.05.

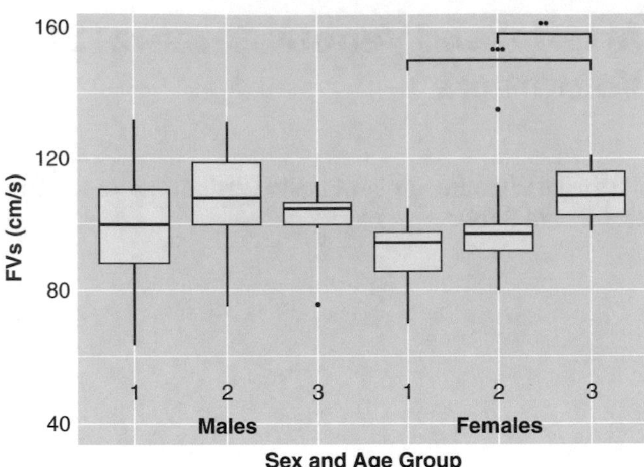

Fig. 1 Differences in systolic cerebral blood flow velocity (FVs) between males and females in group 1 (aged 18–44 years), group 2 (aged 45–64 years), and group 3 (aged ≥65 years)

Results

A total of 122 healthy volunteers were included in the analysis. The remaining 12 cases were excluded because they had inadequate occipital windows.

Considering the entire population, without distinction for age and sex subgroups, the cerebral blood flow velocities in the arterial compartment were significantly correlated with age (FVs: $R = 0.27$, $P = 0.003$; FVd: $R = 0.28$, $P = 0.002$; and FVm: $R = 0.32$, $P = 0.0004$). With regard to the venous compartment, FVVs values were significantly correlated with age ($R = 0.22$, $P = 0.01$). Males had significantly higher FVs values (104.5 (IQR 95.0–111.0) versus 96.50 (IQR 90.00–101.00) cm/s, $P = 0.01$) and FVm values (68.33 (IQR 59.92–72.83) versus 61.84 (IQR 55.50–67.83) cm/s, $P = 0.02$) than

Table 1 Variables in the whole population of healthy volunteers and in different age subgroups

	Total, $N = 122$	Age group		
		Group 1: 18–44 years, $n = 60$	Group 2: 45–64 years, $n = 41$	Group 3: ≥65 years, $n = 21$
FVs [cm/s]	100.00 (90.50–108.00)	95.00 (87.75–103.50)	100.00 (94.00–110.00)	106.00 (100.00–112.00)
FVd [cm/s]	44.00 (40.00–54.00)	45.00 (40.00–68.33)	45.00 (40.00–55.00)	54.00 (44.00–58.00)
FVm [cm/s]	64.17 (58.08–71.33)	61.00 (54.92–68.33)	65.33 (59.67–65.60)	72.00 (62.00–73.33)
FVVs [cm/s]	23.00 (16.25–32.00)	20.0 (16.00–28.00)	25.00 (20.00–38.00)	32.00 (19.00–48.00)
Age [years]	45.00 (32.25–57.25)	31.00 (24.75–38.00)	50.00 (46.00–55.00)	72.00 (67.00–76.00)

The values are expressed as median (interquartile range)
FVd diastolic cerebral blood flow velocity, *FVm* mean cerebral blood flow velocity, *FVs* systolic cerebral blood flow velocity, *FVVs* peak cerebral venous blood flow velocity

females. No differences between males and females with regard to FVd ($P = 0.12$) and FVVs ($P = 0.91$) were found.

The multivariable linear model, which included the effects of age, sex, and ABP on cerebral blood flow velocities, showed that age and sex were independently related to FVs ($P = 0.001$ and $P = 0.005$, respectively) and FVm ($P = 0.001$ and $P = 0.02$, respectively), while FVd and FVVs were related only to age ($P = 0.009$ and $P = 0.04$, respectively) (Table 1).

Discussion

Our results showed a significant difference in arterial FVs and FVm between males and females, and increasing flow velocities with age, particularly among females. Cerebral blood flow velocities in both arterial and venous compartments were significantly influenced by age, and some measurements were also influenced by sex, highlighting that these variables can affect cerebrovascular physiology [7–10].

It is important to consider any differences between different groups in order to better define blood flow velocity thresholds. Previous studies have described a decrease in arterial cerebral blood flow with aging [11] and higher flow velocities in women [7–10], proposing that there are sex- and age-related differences in brain hemodynamics. Our results contrasted with those findings, and we hypothesized that the increase in cerebral blood flow velocity across age groups in healthy volunteers may be related to the hormonal variations that women experience during the lifespan [12]. The large reduction in cerebrovascular reactivity that occurs in women after menopause could be linked to the reduction in estrogen levels. Estrogens have vasodilatory effects on endothelium through stimulation of vascular β-adrenergic receptors, which induce nitric oxide production [13]. A reduction in estrogen levels could lead to increased risks of hypertension and cerebrovascular disease [14, 15], suggesting that hormonal alterations may explain the differences in cerebral blood flow velocities between premenopausal and postmenopausal women [13].

Despite the importance of the venous compartment, which has greater compliance than the arterial one and plays a key role in the pathophysiological processes associated with intracranial hypertension, vTCD is still a poorly implemented technique.

Valdueza et al. previously studied normal flow velocities in the basal cerebral veins in both a healthy population and brain-injured patients, finding a significant decrease in FVVs in the male population aged over 40 years and unaltered FVVs in females of different ages [5]. Baumgartner et al. scanned the straight sinus in healthy volunteers aged between 20 and 59 years, and reported that the SS detection rate was lower in the older population and was challenging in deep veins in all age groups [16]. Other studies have employed venous TCD for evaluation of dural sinus thrombosis [17, 18] and cerebral autoregulation [19]. Schoser et al. performed vTCD in 30 healthy volunteers and 25 patients with elevated ICP, and found a strong correlation between ICP and FVVs. They demonstrated that in the condition of normal ICP levels, venous cerebral blood flow was comparable to control values in their data and in other studies, while increased ICP induced a shift in venous blood flow from the bridging veins toward the larger sinuses, suggesting that the maximal venous cerebral blood flow velocities in the basal veins of Rosenthal and SS were linearly related to ICP [6]. Similarly, Robba et al. demonstrated that FVVs measured in the straight sinus was a robust predictor of ICP in patients with a traumatic brain injury, whereas other arterial TCD-derived parameters did not correlate with invasive ICP [2].

We propose that TCD assessment of both arterial and venous compartments could be useful to better understand cerebral hemodynamics and the mechanisms that can buffer the rise in ICP.

This study had the following limitations. The venous sinuses tend to have anatomical variations [6], and we did not measure interobserver variability between the two operators who performed the TCD examinations. However, the operators were experienced and underwent the same training program to minimize variability between measurements.

Conclusion

Our results indicated that there are age- and sex-related differences in arterial and venous cerebral blood flow velocities. More studies in larger cohorts are needed to confirm our results and further evaluate the differences in cerebral blood flow circulation with regard to sex and the aging process. Venous TCD could advance our understanding of the compensatory mechanisms that occur in conditions of brain injury.

Conflict of Interest **The authors declare that they have no conflict of interest.**

References

1. Robba C, Cardim D, Sekhon M, Budohoski K, Czosnyka M (2018) Transcranial Doppler: a stethoscope for the brain-neurocritical care use. J Neurosci Res 96(4):720–730
2. Robba C, Cardim D, Tajsic T, Pietersen J, Bulman M, Donnelly J et al (2017) Ultrasound non-invasive measurement of intracranial pressure in neurointensive care: a prospective observational study. PLoS Med 14(7):e1002356
3. Zweifel C, Czosnyka M, Carrera E, de Riva N, Pickard JD, Smielewski P (2012) Reliability of the blood flow velocity pulsatility index for assessment of intracranial and cerebral perfusion pressures in head-injured patients. Neurosurgery 71(4):853–861
4. Robba C, Goffi A, Geeraerts T, Cardim D, Via G, Czosnyka M et al (2019) Brain ultrasonography: methodology, basic and advanced principles and clinical applications: a narrative review. Intensive Care Med 45(7):913–927
5. Valdueza JM, Schultz M, Harms L, Einhäupl KM (1995) Venous transcranial Doppler ultrasound monitoring in acute dural sinus thrombosis: report of two cases. Stroke 26(7):1196–1199
6. Schoser BGH, Riemenschneider N, Hansen HC (1999) The impact of raised intracranial pressure on cerebral venous hemodynamics: a prospective venous transcranial Doppler ultrasonography study. J Neurosurg 91(5):744–749
7. Grolimund P, Seiler RW (1988) Age dependence of the flow velocity in the basal cerebral arteries—a transcranial Doppler ultrasound study. Ultrasound Med Biol 14(3):191–198
8. Vriens EM, Kraaier V, Musbach M, Wieneke GH, van Huffelen AC (1989) Transcranial pulsed Doppler measurements of blood velocity in the middle cerebral artery: reference values at rest and during hyperventilation in healthy volunteers in relation to age and sex. Ultrasound Med Biol 15(1):1–8
9. Tegeler CH, Crutchfield K, Katsnelson M, Kim J, Tang R, Passmore Griffin L et al (2013) Transcranial Doppler velocities in a large, healthy population. J Neuroimaging 23(3):466–472
10. Krejza J, Mariak Z, Walecki J, Szydlik P, Lewko J, Ustymowicz A (1999) Transcranial color Doppler sonography of basal cerebral arteries in 182 healthy subjects: age and sex variability and normal reference values for blood flow parameters. AJR Am J Roentgenol 172(1):213–218
11. Tomoto T, Riley J, Turner M, Zhang R, Tarumi T (2019) Cerebral vasomotor reactivity during hypo- and hypercapnia across the adult lifespan. J Cereb Blood Flow Metab 40(3):600–610
12. Smulyan H, Asmar RG, Rudnicki A, London GM, Safar ME (2001) Comparative effects of aging in men and women on the properties of the arterial tree. J Am Coll Cardiol 37(5):1374–1380
13. Hart EC, Joyner MJ, Wallin BG, Charkoudian N (2012) Sex, ageing and resting blood pressure: gaining insights from the integrated balance of neural and haemodynamic factors. J Physiol 590(9):2069–2079
14. Merz AA, Cheng S (2016) Sex differences in cardiovascular ageing. Heart 102(11):825–831
15. Matteis M, Troisi E, Monaldo BC, Caltagirone C, Silvestrini M (1998) Age and sex differences in cerebral hemodynamics. Stroke 29(5):963–967
16. Baumgartner RW, Nirkko AC, Müri RM, Gönner F (1997) Transoccipital power-based color-coded duplex sonography of cerebral sinuses and veins. Stroke 28(7):1319–1323
17. Canhão P, Batista P, Ferro JM (1998) Venous transcranial Doppler in acute dural sinus thrombosis. J Neurol 245(5):276–279
18. Ries S, Steinke W, Neff KW, Hennerici M (1997) Echocontrast-enhanced transcranial color-coded sonography for the diagnosis of transverse sinus venous thrombosis. Stroke 28(4):696–700
19. Aaslid R, Newell DW, Stooss R, Sorteberg W, Lindegaard KF (1991) Assessment of cerebral autoregulation dynamics from simultaneous arterial and venous transcranial Doppler recordings in humans. Stroke 22(9):1148–1154

Comparison of Waveforms Between Noninvasive and Invasive Monitoring of Intracranial Pressure

Inês Gomes, Juliana Shibaki, Bruno Padua, Felipe Silva, Thauan Gonçalves, Deusdedit L. Spavieri-Junior, Gustavo Frigieri, Sérgio Mascarenhas, and Celeste Dias

Introduction

Intracranial pressure (ICP), which is usually measured in millimeters of mercury (mmHg), is an important invasive monitoring parameter in management of patients with acute brain injury and compromised brain compliance in an intensive care unit (ICU) setting. Likewise, there are a large number of minor neurological conditions that can benefit from continuous or occasional ICP monitoring as a diagnostic aid, as in cases of hydrocephalus, improper operation of ventriculoperitoneal valves, or intracranial hypertension caused by central nervous system infections [1].

The Monro–Kellie hypothesis states that the cranial compartment (comprising three main elements: the brain, the cerebrospinal fluid, and the blood) is an inelastic structure that maintains the same constant volume, even throughout pathological changes. Therefore, an increase in the volume of one of those elements will inevitably lead to a decrease in one or both of the others [1].

In an ICU context, ICP is monitored by an invasive sensor (with a pressure transducer) inserted into the intraventricular or intraparenchymal spaces. Although this is an extremely accurate method, it is complex and expensive, as it carries higher risks of infection and bleeding, and it can be performed only in a restricted number of hospitals that have a trained and specialized neurosurgical team available [1].

Taking into consideration the disadvantages mentioned above, the need to monitor ICP in patients whose medical condition does not justify a high-risk, continuous, and invasive procedure such as neurosurgical insertion of an internal sensor has prompted efforts to develop a noninvasive method of ICP monitoring.

In this study, we compared the waveforms of standard invasive ICP and noninvasive ICP (nICP) monitoring methods. The noninvasive values were obtained by a strain gauge mechanism (a mechanical extensometer) applied over the scalp in the temporal window (the parietal region lateral to the sagittal suture).

Our goal was to corroborate the similarities between the two ICP waveforms (invasive and noninvasive), as well as the radial arterial blood pressure (ABP), in order to validate the noninvasive method as an alternative to invasive measurements in situations where the waveform can give enough clinical information.

We also compared nICP with arterial ABP waveforms to verify the possible influence of the peripheral circulation on the nICP signal, which is one of the possible limitations of the present method.

Methods

Subjects

Fifteen patients were screened for the study. After application of the patient selection criteria, ten of them were included in the study: three with a traumatic brain injury, three with a subarachnoid hemorrhage, three with an intracranial hemorrhage, and one who had suffered an ischemic stroke.

Nine of the ten patients were male. The mean age was 58.4 ± 10.4 years, the initial Glasgow Coma Scale (GCS) score was 9 ± 4, the mean Simplified Acute Physiology Score (SAPS II) was 45.6, and the mean length of stay (LOS) in the ICU was 44 ± 45 days.

I. Gomes (✉) · C. Dias
Faculty of Medicine, University of Porto, Al. Prof. Hernâni Monteiro, Porto, Portugal
e-mail: fmup@med.up.pt

J. Shibaki · B. Padua · F. Silva · T. Gonçalves · D. L. Spavieri-Junior
G. Frigieri · S. Mascarenhas
Braincare Health Technologies, São Carlos, Brazil
e-mail: deusdedit.spavieri@brain4.care

B. Depreitere et al. (eds.), *Intracranial Pressure and Neuromonitoring XVII*, Acta Neurochirurgica Supplement 131,
https://doi.org/10.1007/978-3-030-59436-7_28,

Experimental Protocol

A strain gauge mechanism was first applied over the left or right side of the skull, in the parietal region, avoiding the temporal arteries. The system then recorded up to 30 min of waveforms (nICP, ICP, and ABP), using ICM+ software. After a minimum recording time of 30 min on the left side, the mechanism was switched over to the right side of the skull and the recording process was repeated. The times at which the recording started and ended on the right or left side were noted, as was other relevant information such as times when the patient was moved for cleaning or physiotherapy, or was turned by the nursing or medical team, which produced artifacts in the recording.

Inclusion Criteria

The study included only patients who were at least 18 years old, with an acute brain injury. Patients who had undergone decompressive craniectomy or who had an intraventricular drain were excluded.

Data Acquisition and Data Processing

The data were continuously recorded as raw data with ICM+ software. The signal preprocessing pipeline was composed of several steps: the continuously recorded physiological signals (ABP, ICP, and nICP) were initially parsed and sliced into data chunks, each 1 min in duration, and stored on a MongoDB database (MongoDB Inc., New York, NY, USA) for further analysis; the segmented signals were then decomposed to extract their pulsatile components, using spline interpolation [2]; a low-pass finite impulse response (FIR) filter with a cutoff frequency of 15 Hz was then applied to the resulting signal to eliminate high-frequency noise; pulse identification was done via the phase of the Hilbert transform [3, 4]; in sequence, the pulses obtained for each signal were aligned with the maximum slope of the pulse, and the mean pulses per minute were calculated using a nonparametric bootstrap method with a 95% confidence interval [5].

From the mean pulses obtained from the data preprocessing pipeline, we calculated the following parameters of the ICP and nICP pulses: the time to peak, the ratio between the "tidal wave" (P2) and the "percussion wave" (P1), and the Isomap [6] projections K1 and K2. The time to peak was defined as the difference between the maximal slope of the pulse and the time in which the pulse reached its maximum. The ratio between P2 and P1 waves was identified using the corresponding ABP pulse as an auxiliary signal. The Isomap dimensionality reduction method was used to summarize the pulse waveform into two dimensions (K1 and K2), preserving the similarity between the pulses in the original space. The amplitude and length of the pulses were normalized before application of the Isomap (Fig. 1).

All signal processing and analysis were performed using custom programs written in Python, using the libraries numpy [7], scipy [8], scikit-learn [9], and matplotlib [10].

Statistical Analysis

Comparisons between ICP and nICP parameters were evaluated using linear (Pearson) and nonlinear (normalized mutual information) correlations [11]. The mutual information was calculated on the basis of the respective parameters' joint histograms, using histogram bin size extrapolation as the bias correction method [12].

Results

After application of criteria for signal preprocessing to detect good-quality waveforms (signals recorded in ICM+ software that had continuous and simultaneous ABP, ICP, and nICP pulses) and slicing of those pulses into 1-min data chunks, a total of 1504 min of monitoring were studied.

Primarily, a linear correlation analysis was done to evaluate the correlation of the obtained data with ICP versus nICP signals. The calculated Pearson's coefficient showed a weak linear association in all of the ICP/nICP parameters (Table 1).

In light of these preliminary weak linear results, and to further investigate whether there was a statistical dependence between the ICP/nICP parameters, a nonlinear correlation method—normalized mutual information—was used. Normalized mutual information ranges between 0 (no statistical dependence) and 1 (maximal statistical dependence between variables). We also used a nonlinear dimensionality reduction technique—Isomap [6] projection of the pulses into a bidimensional space (K1 and K2)—to compare the entire waveform shape of the invasive and noninvasive ICP signals (Fig. 2). This last statistical analysis showed a strong nonlinear association in the K1, K2, and P2/P1 ratio variables. An exception was found in the time-to-peak variable, where the nonlinear association remained weak (Table 1, Fig. 2).

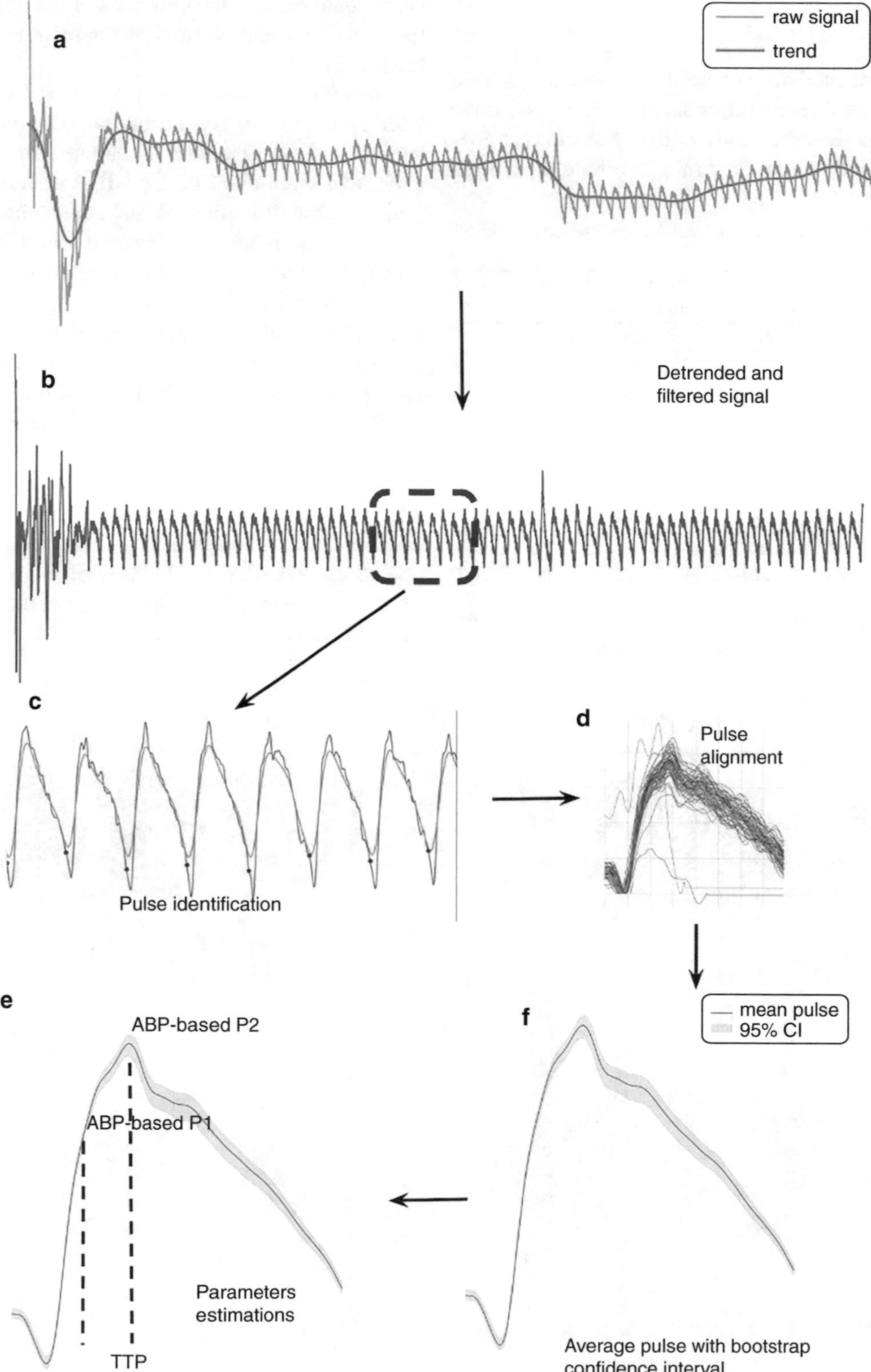

Fig. 1 Intracranial pressure and noninvasive intracranial pressure monitoring signal-processing pipeline. (**a**) Raw data and the respective spline interpolation curve. (**b**) Detrended signal. (**c**) Pulse identification based on the Hilbert transform. The *red dots* show the starts of the pulses. (**d**) Pulse alignment using, as a reference, the maximal slope before the pulse maximum. (**e**) Average pulse with bootstrap confidence interval (CI) ($a = 0.05$, $N = 1000$). (**f**) Parameter estimation. In the case of the tidal wave/percussion wave (P2/P1) ratio, we use the respective arterial blood pressure (ABP) waveform (not shown) to identify the peaks. Time to peak (TTP)

Discussion

Although the two methods we used for comparison have very different measurement approaches (one being invasive and the other over the skull), both waveforms are generated by blood inflow into the brain and therefore should share some resemblance, at least in the dominant parameters that define and summarize the main waveform characteristics [13, 14].

Therefore, we compared the ICP and nICP waveforms with the radial artery blood pressure waveform in an attempt to quantify and eliminate the interference of peripheral circulation in the nICP waveform parameters (one possible limitation of this approach). Such a limitation could be minimized if the noninvasive sensor positioning was optimized, expressly away from major vessels in the parietal region (approximating its pattern to the direct ICP waveform). Another limitation of our work was that as yet, the method developed by our team does not yield pressure values calibrated in millimeters of mercury (mmHg). Because of this, it would be interesting to evaluate and compare the waveform morphology between groups of patients with different diagnoses (when we have a larger number of patients). In that way, we could assess whether there is a waveform pattern specific to one condition or another that could provide relevant information about the state and pathophysiology of the patient without using the direct mmHg value [1].

Table 1 The studied Pearson correlation and normalized mutual information parameters

ICP/nICP parameters	Pearson	Normalized mutual information
K1	0.33 [0.27, 0.38]	0.65 [0.41, 0.91]
K2	0.22 [0.16, 0.28]	0.81 [0.62, 0.97]
Tp	0.30 [0.26, 0.36]	0.25 [0.10, 0.37]
P2/P1	0.40 [0.35, 0.46]	0.65 [0.53, 0.85]

The values displayed in square brackets are, in fact, the lower and upper confidence limits

ICP intracranial pressure, *nICP* noninvasive intracranial pressure, *P2/P1* tidal wave/percussion wave ratio, *Tp* time to peak

Parameters K1 and K2
(Based on 10 patients, 1504 minutes)

- Wilcoxon p < 0.01 (ICP < nICP)
- Pearson correlation = 0.33 **[0.27; 0.38]**
- Mutual information = 0.65 **[0.41, 0.91]**

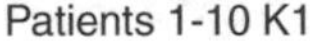

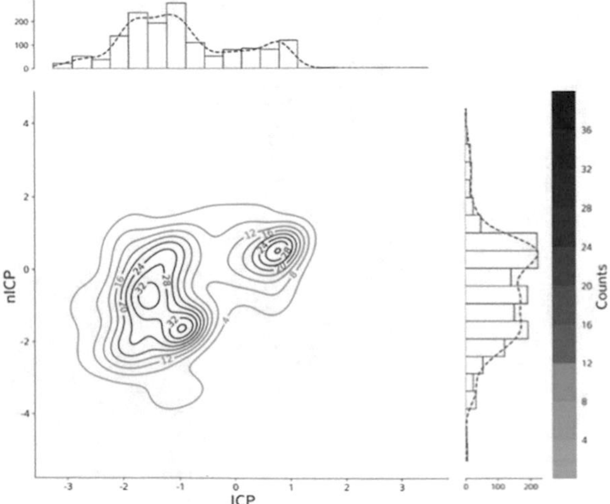

- Wilcoxon p < 0.01 (ICP < nICP)
- Pearson correlation = 0.22 **[0.16; 0.28]**
- Mutual information = 0.81 **[0.62, 0.97]**

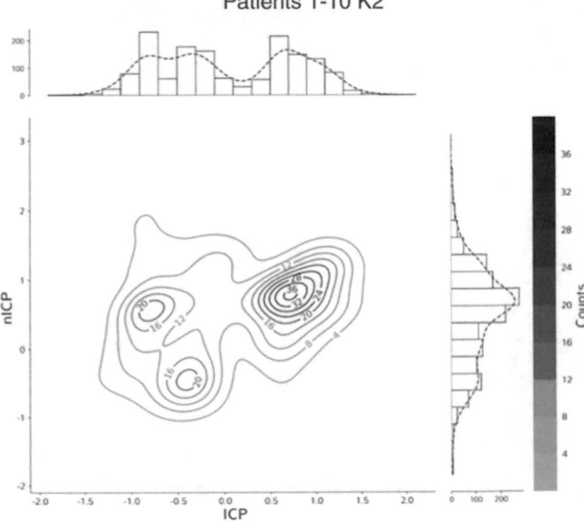

Fig. 2 Joint histograms of intracranial pressure (ICP) and noninvasive ICP monitoring (nICP) parameters. *Top left:* Time to peak (Tp). *Top right:* Tidal wave/percussion wave (P2/P1) ratio. *Bottom left:* Isomap K1. *Bottom right:* Isomap K2. Each section of the figure contains three panels: the main panel in which the joint density function approximation is shown and two adjacent panels in which the marginal histograms for the parameters can be observed. In each main panel, *dark lines* represent a higher concentration of points, as the color bar indicates. The values shown in *square brackets* are the lower and upper confidence limits. The densities were approximated by using a kernel density estimation method with optimized bandwidth selection

Parameters Time to peak and Ratio P1/P2
(Based on 10 patients, 1504 minutes)

- Wilcoxon p < 0.01 (ICP < nICP)
- Pearson correlation = 0.30 **[0.26; 0.36]**
- Mutual information = 0.25 **[0.1, 0.37]**

Patients 1-10 Time to peak

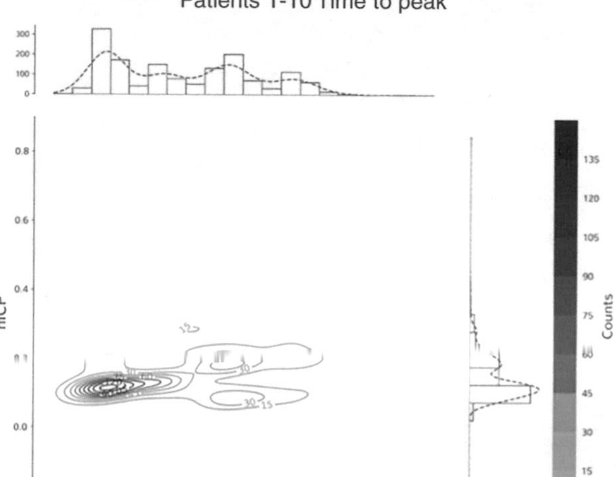

- Wilcoxon p < 0.01 (ICP < nICP)
- Pearson correlation = 0.40 **[0.35; 0.46]**
- Mutual information = 0.65 **[0.53, 0.85]**

Patients 1-10 P2/P1

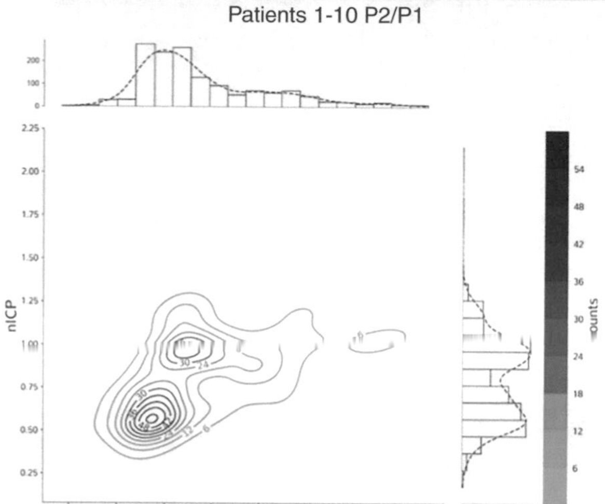

Fig. 2 (continued)

Conclusion

Although the compared waveform parameters of ICP and nICP showed strong nonlinear coupling in all but one parameter, the results presented in this work are preliminary. Therefore, mutual information analysis of a larger patient sample with a longer monitoring time would be helpful to build refined models and to improve the understanding of the waveform relationships [1].

Thus, we intend to proceed to a demographic analysis of the P2/P1 ratio and the normalized time to peak. Given the importance of ICP waveform analysis in management of the clinical state of patients with an acute brain injury, and the similarities given by the strong nonlinear correlation between the invasive and noninvasive parameters, we believe that the noninvasive method could be used for monitoring relative changes in ICP, despite the absence of absolute values in mmHg.

Conflict of Interest **Juliana Shibaki, Bruno Padua, Felipe Silva, Thauan Gonçalves, Deusdedit Spavieri-Junior, Gustavo Frigieri, and Sérgio Mascarenhas have received financial support from Braincare Health Technologies. Inês Gomes and Celeste Dias have no commercial relationship with the company.**

References

1. Kawoos U, McCarron RM, Auker CR, Chavko M (2015) Advances in intracranial pressure monitoring and its significance in managing traumatic brain injury. Int J Mol Sci 16(12):28979–28997. https://doi.org/10.3390/ijms161226146
2. Hastie T, Tibshirani R, Friedman J (2013) The elements of statistical learning: data mining, inference, and prediction. Springer, New York
3. Benitez D, Gaydecki PA, Zaidi A, Fitzpatrick AP (2001) The use of the Hilbert transform in ECG signal analysis. Comput Biol Med 31:399–406
4. Mitrou N, Laurin A, Dick T, Inskip J (2017) A peak detection method for identifying phase in physiological signals. Biomed Signal Process Control 31:452–462. https://doi.org/10.1016/j.bspc.2016.07.001
5. Zoubir AM, Boashash B (1998) The bootstrap and its application in signal processing. IEEE Signal Process Mag 15:56–76. https://doi.org/10.1109/79.647043
6. Tenenbaum JB (2000) A global geometric framework for nonlinear dimensionality reduction. Science 290:2319–2323. https://doi.org/10.1126/science.290.5500.2319
7. Oliphant TE (2015) Guide to NumPy, 2nd edn. Continuum, Austin
8. Oliphant TE (2007) Python for scientific computing. Comput Sci Eng 9:10–20. https://doi.org/10.1109/mcse.2007.58
9. Garreta R, Moncecchi G (2013) Learning scikit-learn: machine learning in Python. Packt, Birmingham
10. Hunter JD (2007) Matplotlib: a 2D graphics environment. Comput Sci Eng 9(3):90–95. https://doi.org/10.1109/mcse.2007.55

11. Vu T, Mishra A, Konapala G (2018) Information entropy suggests stronger nonlinear associations between hydro-meteorological variables and ENSO. Entropy 20(1):38
12. Strong SP, Koberle R, Van Steveninck RRDR, Bialek W (1998) Entropy and information in neural spike trains. Phys Rev Lett 80(1):197
13. Frigieri G, Andrade RAP, Dias C, Spavieri DL Jr, Brunelli R, Cardim DA, Wang CC, Verzola RMM, Mascarenhas S (2018) Analysis of a non-invasive intracranial pressure monitoring method in patients with traumatic brain injury. Acta Neurochir Suppl 126:107–110
14. Vilela GH, Cabella B, Mascarenhas S et al (2016) Validation of a new minimally invasive intracranial pressure monitoring method by direct comparison with an invasive technique. Acta Neurochir Suppl 122:97–100

Part VI

Cerebrovascular Autoregulation in Acute Brain Injury and Cardiac Surgery

An Update on the COGiTATE Phase II Study: Feasibility and Safety of Targeting an Optimal Cerebral Perfusion Pressure as a Patient-Tailored Therapy in Severe Traumatic Brain Injury

Jeanette Tas, Erta Beqiri, C. R. van Kaam, Ari Ercole, Gert Bellen, D. Bruyninckx, Manuel Cabeleira, Marek Czosnyka, Bart Depreitere, Joseph Donnelly, Marta Fedriga, Peter J. Hutchinson, D. Menon, Geert Meyfroidt, Annalisa Liberti, J. G. Outtrim, C. Robba, C. W. E. Hoedemaekers, Peter Smielewski, and Marcel J. Aries

Introduction

A raised intracranial pressure (ICP) and a reduced cerebral perfusion pressure (CPP) are long-established and important causes of secondary brain injury and are associated with worsened clinical outcomes after traumatic brain injury (TBI) [1]. Monitoring and management of ICP/CPP has become a cornerstone of severe TBI management. The 2016 Brain Trauma Foundation (BTF) guidelines recommend keeping ICP at <22 mmHg and CPP strictly between 60 and 70 mmHg [2]. Whether a fixed therapeutic CPP target range is suitable for all individual TBI patients is the subject of scientific debate. Potentially, individualizing therapies and tailoring medical treatment to dynamic pathophysiology could offer a precision medicine approach with advantages over the current 'one size fits all' strategy. The authors of the recently published SIBICC [Seattle International Severe Traumatic Brain Injury Consensus Conference] algorithm have presented expert recommendations for treatment of adult patients with ICP management [3]. In addition to formalizing what is already known, the SIBCC consensus includes new content. The authors recommend a mean arterial pressure (MAP) challenge to assess the state of cerebral autoregulation (CA). If MAP augmentation results in a reduction in ICP (confirming some degree of working CA), an increase in MAP can be used as a method to reduce ICP in an individual patient. This concept is not completely new;

J. Tas (✉) · A. Liberti · M. J. Aries
Department of Intensive Care Medicine, University of Maastricht, Maastricht University Medical Centre, Maastricht, The Netherlands
e-mail: Jeanette.tas@mumc.nl

E. Beqiri
Brain Physics Laboratory, Division of Neurosurgery, Department of Clinical Neurosciences, University of Cambridge, Cambridge, UK

Department of Physiology and Transplantation, University of Milan, Milan, Italy

C. R. van Kaam · C. W. E. Hoedemaekers
Department of Intensive Care Medicine, Radboud University Medical Centre, Nijmegen, The Netherlands

A. Ercole · D. Menon · J. G. Outtrim
University Division of Anaesthesia, University of Cambridge, Addenbrooke's Hospital, Cambridge, UK

G. Bellen · D. Bruyninckx · B. Depreitere
Department of Neurosciences, Catholic University Leuven, University Hospital Leuven, Leuven, Belgium

M. Cabeleira · M. Czosnyka · J. Donnelly · P. Smielewski
Brain Physics Laboratory, Division of Neurosurgery, Department of Clinical Neurosciences, University of Cambridge, Cambridge, UK

M. Fedriga
Brain Physics Laboratory, Division of Neurosurgery, Department of Clinical Neurosciences, University of Cambridge, Cambridge, UK

Department of Anaesthesia, Critical Care and Emergency, Spedali Civili University Hospital, Brescia, Italy

P. J. Hutchinson
Department of Clinical Neurosciences, Cambridge University, Cambridge, UK

G. Meyfroidt
Department of Cellular and Molecular Medicine, Catholic University Leuven, University Hospital, Leuven, Belgium

C. Robba
Department of Anaesthesia and Intensive Care, Policlinico San Martino, IRCCS for Oncology and Neuroscience, Genoa, Italy

B. Depreitere et al. (eds.), *Intracranial Pressure and Neuromonitoring XVII*, Acta Neurochirurgica Supplement 131,
https://doi.org/10.1007/978-3-030-59436-7_29,

it was previously proposed some decades ago, with very mixed results. In an editorial accompanying the publication of the SIBICC algorithm, Smith and Maas consider the 'one size fits all' and escalating 'staircase' approaches to ICP/CPP management undesirable and strongly support future development of recommendations for targeted individual approaches [4]. Autoregulation-guided CPP treatment could be one of the more personalized approaches to ICP management based on current understanding of the underlying pathophysiology of TBI. In healthy individuals, CA maintains constant and adequate cerebral blood flow (CBF), thereby protecting the brain from both ischaemia and hyperperfusion in the face of inevitable changes in CPP [5]. However, after TBI, CA can frequently be impaired, and this impairment is statistically related to poor outcomes [1]. This chapter describes the progress of the first randomized trial in four European centres of cerebral autoregulation-orientated management of TBI patients, with results expected to be presented early 2021.

Methods

The CPPopt Concept and COGiTATE

Czosnyka et al. first proposed use of a moving correlation coefficient (the pressure reactivity index (PRx)) between slow changes in MAP and ICP as a surrogate method for continuous bedside estimation of global CA. This concept has attracted interest in the last decade, with the observation that PRx and CPP often exhibit a U-shaped relationship over time, with a minimum PRx value occurring at a CPP value at which cerebrovascular pressure reactivity is best preserved (or least impaired) [6, 7]. These observations provide the rationale for the hypothesis that targeting a CPP value such that global CA is best could be a potential strategy for individualizing CPP targets. Indeed, deviations from this 'optimal' CPP (CPPopt) value have been associated with worse outcomes in retrospective studies [7]. However, this concept has never been studied prospectively.

In this chapter, we describe the current status of the COGiTATE [CPPopt Guided Therapy: Assessment of Target Effectiveness] study (www.cppopt.org) [8]. This is a prospective, multicentre, non-blinded, randomized, controlled trial in patients with severe TBI. Unconscious adult patients with severe TBI with an indication for ICP monitoring are recruited in the first 24 h of admission to the intensive care unit (ICU) and randomized into one of two treatment arms: the control group (with a CPP target of 60–70 mmHg in accordance with the BTF guidelines) and the intervention group (with an 'optimal' CPP target (CPPopt) based on the CA status). The duration of the intervention is maximum 5 days. Other therapies (such as measures to control ICP) are unaltered from local protocols. In this study, ICP and arterial blood pressure (ABP) are monitored as per normal clinical practice in the ICU: ICP is recorded by a parenchymal ICP probe, and ABP is monitored by invasive arterial cannulation in the radial or femoral artery and zeroed at the level of the foramen of Monro. The data are collected at a frequency ≥100 Hz (waveform resolution) and processed by means of ICM+® software (Cambridge Enterprise, Cambridge, UK; http://icmplus.neurosurg.cam.ac.uk) at the bedside. Compliance with the protocol is assessed at 4-hourly CPP treatment reviews. The 4-h interval is a pragmatic choice [9]. To facilitate the compliance assessment, a custom module has been implemented in the ICM+ software, with a system of alert and review forms designed specifically for this trial. At the review time points, a CPP target is suggested by the software, according to the randomisation group. The treating clinicians may deviate from the suggested target but must provide their proposed target and clinical rationale for deviation in a structured short questionnaire presented by the software. CPPopt is calculated using a multi-window weighted approach, inspired by Depreitere et al. [10], which was subsequently implemented in the ICM+ software and investigated in a retrospective TBI data set by Liu et al. [11]. The algorithm has been further adapted by Beqiri et al. [8] to make it more suitable for prospective bedside use. The primary end points are (1) feasibility: the percentage of monitored time with measured CPP within a range of 5 mmHg above or below the dynamic CPP target; and (2) safety: the daily (intracranial hypertension) therapy intensity level (TIL) score [12]. The secondary end points are markers that suggest differences in organ dysfunction. The study is powered to accomplish a relative increase of 20% in monitored time with CPP close to the individual CPP target. The study is not designed to assess differences in clinical outcomes. Our protocol does not allow us to perform and report any interim analysis; in this report, we provide a qualitative description of our study experiences.

Results

Three tertiary centres have been involved since the start of the study: Maastricht University Medical Centre (coordinating centre, Maastricht, the Netherlands), Cambridge University Hospitals NHS Foundation Trust (Cambridge, UK), and Catholic University Hospitals Leuven (Leuven, Belgium). The first patient was randomized in February 2018. In March 2019, a fourth study centre was added: Radboud University Medical Centre (Nijmegen, the

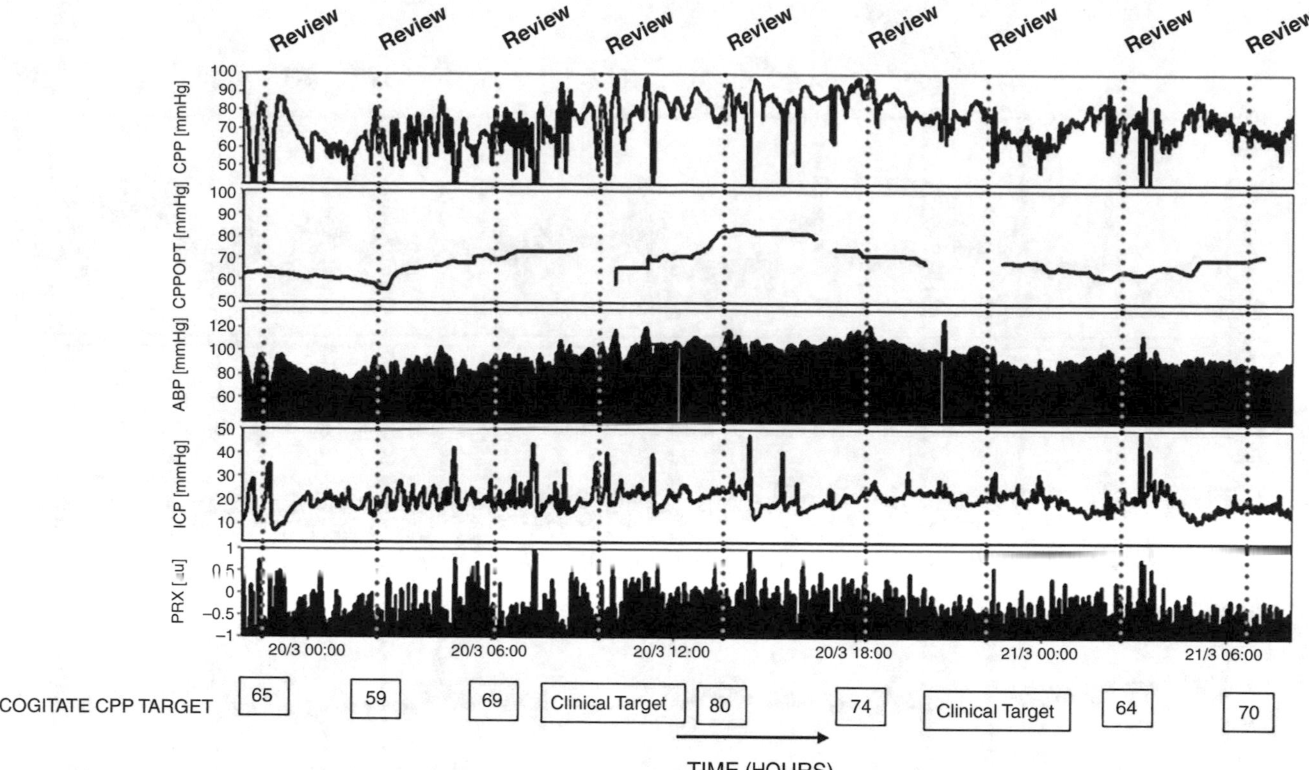

Fig. 1 Example of a (retrospective) 1.5-day recording from a patient randomized into the intervention group of the COGiTATE [CPPopt Guided Therapy: Assessment of Target Effectiveness] study. Six times daily, a CPP review is requested at the *dotted vertical line* time stamps. Physiological trends that are available to the clinical team for the cerebral perfusion pressure (CPP) target reviews are the CPP, 'optimal' CPP (CPPopt), arterial blood pressure (ABP), intracranial pressure (ICP) and pressure reactivity index (PRx). The CPP targets suggested during the reviews are displayed at the bottom of the figure. Adherence to a 'clinical' target is suggested by the software when (1) no CPPopt value can be computed or (2) the CPPopt value is out of range (<50 mmHg or >100 mmHg). Small gaps are present in the CPPopt *trend line*. The first gap can be explained by the algorithm criteria, as at least 4 h of data recording are needed before the first CPPopt value can be computed

Netherlands). Figures 1 and 2 provide examples of recordings from two randomized patients. The first example (Fig. 1) shows a recording from a patient who was randomized into the intervention group. Besides data on basic monitoring variables, data on trends in CPPopt and PRx are available to the treating clinicians. The patient in the second example (Fig. 2) was randomized into the control group, with a target CPP of 60–70 mmHg. On the overview screen, time trends in CPP, ABP and ICP are displayed. CA information is hidden from the treating clinicians. The study enrolment rate is 2.4 patients per month (Fig. 3). As of October 2019, 51 patients were randomized (85% of the intended total). At the same randomization rate, we expect enrolment to be finished around February 2020.

Discussion

In this chapter, we provide an update of the phase II COGiTATE study in severe TBI patients with ICP monitoring. This prospective evaluation of the feasibility, safety and physiological implications of autoregulation-guided management is providing evidence that will be useful in the design of a phase III outcome study. Several homeostatic processes contribute to the adequate delivery of oxygen- and nutrient-rich arterial blood to the brain to match metabolic demands. These processes operate at distinct frequencies to precisely regulate CBF. There is a long-standing belief that the lower limit of cerebral autoregulation (LLA) is 50 mmHg and that the upper limit of autoregulation (ULA) is 150 mmHg, based on a seminal report published by Lassen in 1964 [13]. However, the acceptance of these limits of autoregulation as a 'simple' guiding principle for haemodynamic management has been challenged by many studies [14]. The data support the notion that the upper and lower limits should be defined individually and cannot be determined accurately on the basis of population data. Many clinical methods of CA monitoring involve assessment of cerebrovascular reactivity (PRx) to continuously evaluate the correlation between spontaneously occurring slow-wave changes in MAP and ICP. In this way, they avoid the need to lower or raise ABP significantly in order to assess the limits of autoregulation, especially in patients who have compro-

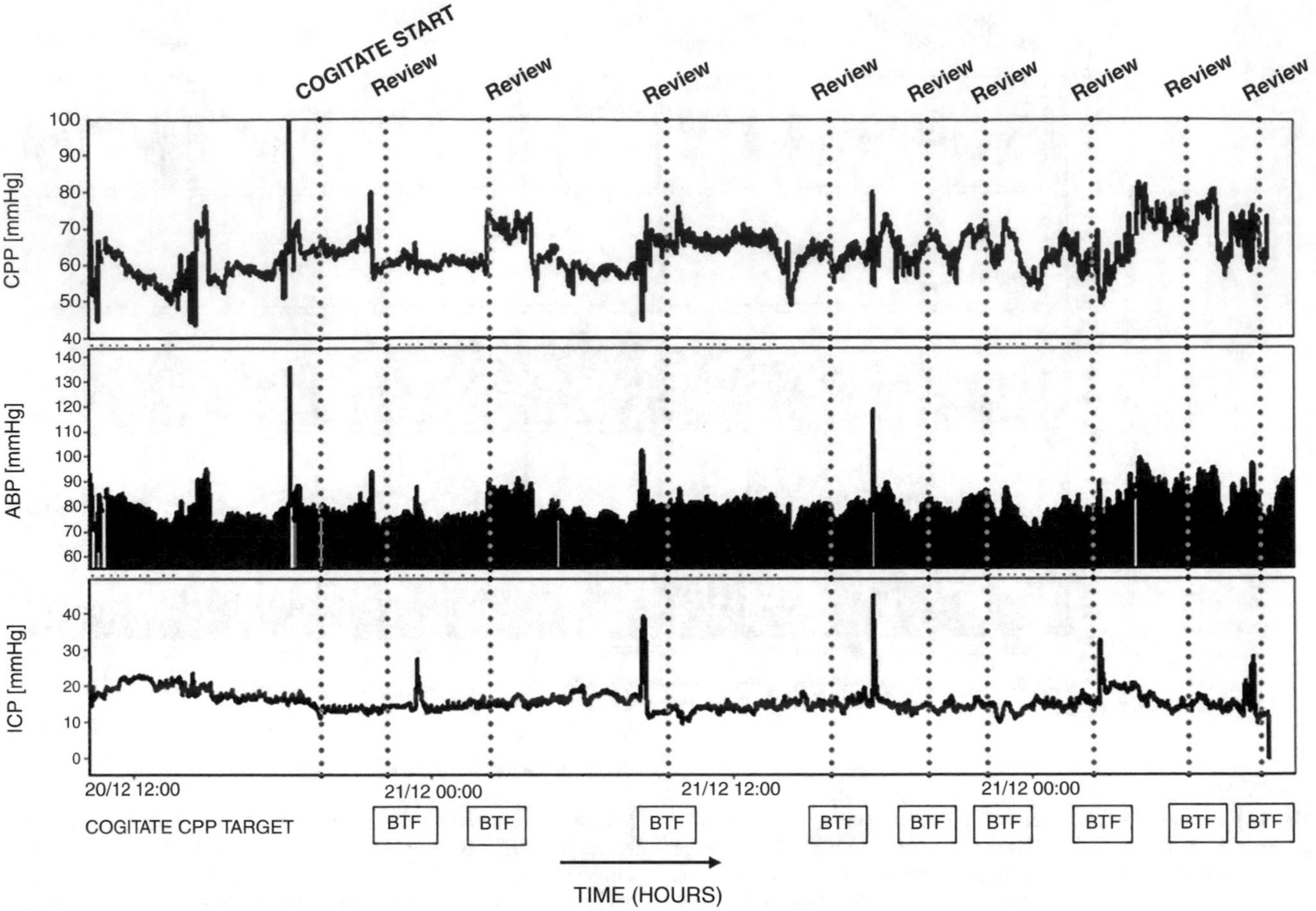

Fig. 2 Example of a 1.5-day recording from a patient randomized into the control group of the COGiTATE [CPPopt Guided Therapy: Assessment of Target Effectiveness] study. Six times daily, a review is filled in, shown by the *dotted vertical lines*. *Trend lines* for cerebral perfusion pressure (CPP), arterial blood pressure (ABP) and intracranial pressure (ICP) are shown. The CPP targets suggested during the reviews are displayed at the bottom of the figure. In the control group, the suggested targets are those recommended by the Brain Trauma Foundation (BTF) guidelines (60–70 mmHg) [2]

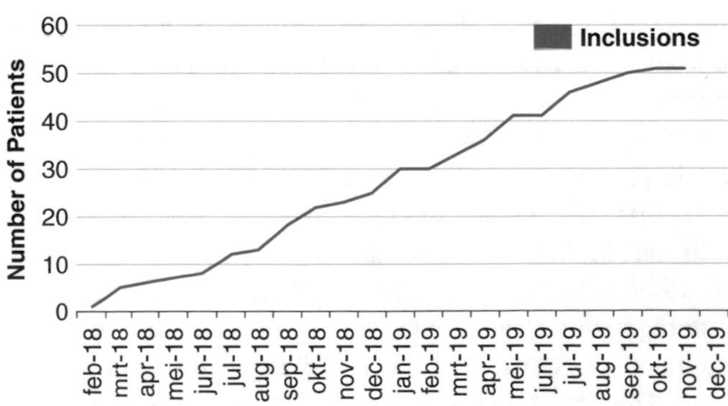

Fig. 3 The total number of study inclusions over time are presented in *blue*. The first enrolment occurred on 16 February 2018. The fourth study centre (Nijmegen, the Netherlands) started enrolling patients in March 2019. The study aims to enrol a total of 60 patients. An actual update of study inclusions can be found on www.cppopt.org. The first study results are expected early 2021

mised organ perfusion or brain swelling. The CPPopt concept relies on this latter methodology, with the compromise that often only parts of the autoregulation curve are available. However, with long-term and continuous monitoring—which is currently limited to invasive and robust monitoring signals such as ICP—the CPP value at which autoregulation is best preserved (CPPopt) can be identified.

At the moment, the benefit of autoregulation-guided perfusion therapy is being tested in different patient groups. To evaluate the importance of autoregulation-guided therapy to patient outcome after cardiac surgery, a recent prospective, randomized, single-blinded study was completed. This study assessed use of a MAP target greater than the LLA (using transcranial Doppler ultrasound measurements) during cardiopulmonary bypass versus usual institutional care in which MAP targets were chosen empirically [15]. In a subset of 199 patients (in whom postoperative delirium testing was performed), the odds of delirium were reduced by 45% in the group whose MAP targets were determined by CA monitoring (odds ratio 0.55, 95% confidence interval 0.31–0.97, P = 0.04). Petersen et al. conducted a single-centre, prospective (observational) cohort study of patients undergoing endovascular therapy (ET) after a large-vessel occlusion ischaemic stroke [16]. Autoregulatory function was measured continuously for 24 h following thrombectomy by interrogating changes in tissue oxygenation (measured by near-infrared spectroscopy) in response to changes in MAP, using time correlation analysis (TOx). The data showed that exceeding individualized thresholds of CA was associated with haemorrhagic transformation and worse functional outcomes even after adjustment for prognostic covariates.

Conclusion

ICU clinicians now have a potential tool for individualizing an 'optimal' CPP target based on continuous cerebral blood volume (autoregulation) monitoring. This intervention protocol is currently being tested in the COGiTATE feasibility and safety study, which is close to reporting its first results. Current (retrospective) data point to the limitations of using a fixed CPP range for a heterogenic TBI population because the individual's LLA or ULA may or may not be within this arbitrary range.

Acknowledgments M.J. Aries has received a clinical grant from the European Society of Intensive Care Medicine to support the COGiTATE study.

Conflict of Interest **M. Czosnyka and P. Smielewski have a financial interest in ICM+ software.**

References

1. Balestreri M, Czosnyka M, Hutchinson P, Steiner LA, Hiler M, Smielewski P, Pickard JD (2006) Impact of intracranial pressure and cerebral perfusion pressure on severe disability and mortality after head injury. Neurocrit Care 4(1):8–13. https://doi.org/10.1385/NCC:4:1:008
2. Carney N, Totten AM, O'Reilly C et al (2017) Guidelines for the management of severe traumatic brain injury, fourth edition. Neurosurgery 80(1):6–15
3. Hawryluk GWJ, Aguilera S, Buki A et al (2019) A management algorithm for patients with intracranial pressure monitoring: the Seattle International Severe Traumatic Brain Injury Consensus Conference (SIBICC). Intensive Care Med 45:1783–1794. https://doi.org/10.1007/s00134-019-05805-9
4. Smith M, Maas AIR (2019) An algorithm for patients with intracranial pressure monitoring: filling the gap between evidence and practice. Intensive Care Med 45(12):1819–1821. https://doi.org/10.1007/s00134-019-05818-4
5. Donnelly J, Aries MJ, Czosnyka M (2014) Further understanding of cerebral autoregulation at the bedside: possible implications for future therapy. Expert Rev Neurother 15(2):169–185
6. Aries MJH, Czosnyka M, Budohoski KP et al (2012) Continuous determination of optimal cerebral perfusion pressure in traumatic brain injury. Crit Care Med 40(8):2456–2463
7. Steiner LA, Czosnyka M, Piechnik SK (2002) Continuous monitoring of cerebrovascular pressure reactivity allows determination of optimal cerebral perfusion pressure in patients with traumatic brain injury. Crit Care 30(4):733–738
8. Beqiri E, Smielewski P, Robba C, Czosnyka M, Cabeleira MT, Tas J, Donnelly J, Outtrim JG, Hutchinson P, Menon D, Meyfroidt G, Depreitere B, Aries MJ, Ercole A (2019) Feasibility of individualised severe traumatic brain injury management using an automated assessment of optimal cerebral perfusion pressure: the COGiTATE phase II study protocol. BMJ Open 9(9):e030727. https://doi.org/10.1136/bmjopen-2019-030727
9. Aries MJH, Wesselink R, Elting JWJ, Donnelly J, Czosnyka M, Ercole A, Maurits NM, Smielewski P (2016) Enhanced visualization of optimal cerebral perfusion pressure over time to support clinical decision making. Crit Care Med 44(10):e996–e999
10. Depreitere B, Güiza F, van den Berghe G, Schuhmann MU, Maier G, Piper I, Meyfroidt G (2014) Pressure autoregulation monitoring and cerebral perfusion pressure target recommendation in patients with severe traumatic brain injury based on minute-by-minute monitoring data. J Neurosurg 120(6):1451–1457
11. Liu X, Maurits NM, Aries MJH et al (2017) Monitoring of optimal cerebral perfusion pressure in traumatic brain injured patients using a multi-window weighting algorithm. J Neurotrauma 34(22):3081–3088
12. Zuercher P, Groen JL, Aries MJH, Steyerberg EW, Maas AIR, Ercole A, Menon DK (2016) Reliability and validity of the therapy intensity level scale: analysis of clinimetric properties of a novel approach to assess management of intracranial pressure in traumatic brain injury. J Neurotrauma 33(19):1768–1774
13. Lassen NA (1964) Autoregulation of cerebral blood flow. Circ Res 15(Suppl):201–204
14. Brady KM, Hudson A, Hood R, DeCaria B, Lewis C, Hogue CW (2020) Personalizing the definition of hypotension to protect the brain. Anesthesiology 132(1):170–179. https://doi.org/10.1097/ALN.0000000000003005
15. Brown CH, Neufeld KJ, Tian J et al (2019) Effect of targeting mean arterial pressure during cardiopulmonary bypass by monitoring cerebral autoregulation on postsurgical delirium among older patients: a nested randomized clinical trial. JAMA Surg 154(9):819–826. https://doi.org/10.1001/jamasurg.2019.1163
16. Petersen NH, Silverman A, Wang A, Strander S, Kodali S, Matouk C, Sheth KN (2019) Association of personalized blood pressure targets with hemorrhagic transformation and functional outcome after endovascular stroke therapy. JAMA Neurol 76(10):1256–1258. https://doi.org/10.1001/jamaneurol.2019.2120

Quick Assessment of the Lower Limit of Autoregulation by Use of Transcranial Doppler Ultrasound During Cardiac Surgery

Laurent Gergelé, Younes Khadraoui, Romain Manet, and Olivier Desebbe

Introduction

Setting the mean arterial pressure (MAP) during cardiopulmonary bypass (CPB) in cardiac surgery remains a real challenge. A recent trial tested two levels of MAP (70–80 versus 40–50 mmHg) to prevent cerebral injury [1] but did not find any differences between the two treatment groups and concluded that MAP had to be individualized for each patient. This concept was largely explained in a recent review [2]. Both hypotension and hypertension during cardiac surgery are detrimental to cardiac surgical patients. Blood pressure management based on a personalized target is promising in further improving neurological outcomes after cardiac surgery [2]. The remaining question is how to identify this target in an individual patient. Currently, the best tool to determine this target is probably cerebral autoregulation monitoring, as was concluded in a recent randomized trial [3].

The cerebral autoregulation status can be measured by the mean velocity index (Mx), which is a moving Pearson correlation coefficient between paired MAP and cerebral blood flow velocity values. It is able to give the autoregulation status on a continuous basis. Other indices have been developed for use during cardiac surgery, such as the cerebral oximetry index (COx), using near-infrared spectroscopy (NIRS) technology [2, 4]. Overall, Mx is considered the best noninvasive tool to assess autoregulation in the operating room [5], and it was evaluated in a recent randomized trial where its use to set MAP during CPB decreased postoperative delirium.

Currently, in a large majority of publications, Mx is calculated as a continuous, moving Pearson's correlation coefficient between MAP and transcranial Doppler ultrasound (TCD) mean velocity (MV). Consecutive, paired, 10-s averaged values over a 300-s duration are used for each calculation, incorporating 30 data points to display an Mx value. When autoregulation is intact, there is no correlation between cerebral blood flow (CBF) and MAP, and the Mx value approaches 0. When autoregulation is impaired, the Mx value approaches 1. The length of the average window is seldom discussed in the literature. However, Mx was first developed in neurointensive care with small and slow variations in MAP and very long data recordings (lasting for several days). In the cardiac surgery field, there are bigger and faster MAP variations. Therefore, the aim of this study was to test a new setting of Mx calculation with shorter average periods. We kept the same sample with 30 data points being used to calculate Mx, but we decreased the average period from 10 to 2 s. Our hypothesis was that in cardiac surgery, the arterial pressure modification amplitude and its consequences for CBF would be better assessed with these more rapid settings.

Materials and Methods

In patients under general anaesthesia, after induction, TCD (Waki-Atys®) monitoring of the middle cerebral arteries was performed using a smart automatic robotic probe. Digitized arterial blood pressure and TCD signals were processed using OptiMAP software. OptiMAP was developed to monitor autoregulation and was installed in the TCD device (Fig. 1).

The clinicians did not use the OptiMAP software and autoregulation data to optimize haemodynamic status during

L. Gergelé (✉)
Department of Intensive Care, Ramsay Santé, Hôpital Privé de la Loire, Saint Etienne, France

Y. Khadraoui
Independent Data Scientist, Sophia Antipolis, France

R. Manet
Department of Neurosurgery B, Hôpital P. Wertheimer, Hospices Civiles de Lyon, Lyon, France

O. Desebbe
Department of Anaesthesiology and Intensive Care, Ramsay Santé, Sauvegarde Clinic, Lyon, France

B. Depreitere et al. (eds.), *Intracranial Pressure and Neuromonitoring XVII*, Acta Neurochirurgica Supplement 131,
https://doi.org/10.1007/978-3-030-59436-7_30,

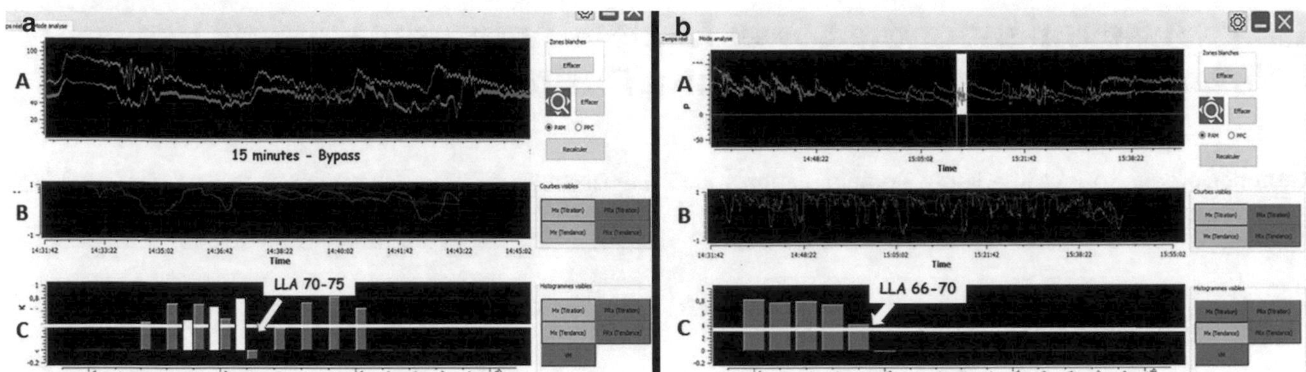

Fig. 1 Two screenshots from OptiMAP software (the post-treatment analysis screen) during cardiac surgery in the same patient. *Left panel:* Quick assessment of the lower limit of autoregulation (LLA) with Mx_{2s} (*grey bars*) and Mx_{10s} (*white bars*) during 15 min of recording. *Right panel:* LLA assessment with Mx_{10s} (*grey bars*) during the whole recording. The *top graphs* (**A**) show the mean arterial pressure (MAP) and mean velocity trends during the whole procedure; the *middle graphs* (**B**) show the Mx_{2s} and Mx_{10s} trends; and the *bottom graphs* (**C**) show the Mx values versus MAP clustered in 5-mmHg intervals, with the Mx value 0.35 shown in each graph by a *horizontal white line*

the surgery. They had access only to the absolute values of MV and other traditional markers (the systolic velocity, diastolic velocity, pulsatility index and their trends). MAP management was at the discretion of the clinicians, who could change the goals on the basis of the monitoring data.

We compared two methods of Mx calculation offline to assess the lower limit of autoregulation (LLA): Mx_{10s}, with long averaging windows of 10 s [2, 3, 5], and Mx_{2s}, with short averaging windows of 2 s. Mx_{10s} requires a minimum recording of 5 min of data to calculate the first value, and this value is refreshed every 10 s. With Mx_{2s}, the first value is available after 1 min, and this is refreshed every 2 s. Mx_{2s} and Mx_{10s} were used during a short 15-min recording to assess LLA. As described in the literature, Mx_{10s} was used as the gold standard to determine LLA on the overall recording during the surgery. Autoregulation was considered lost (defining the LLA) when Mx increased to >0.35.

Demographic and general data on the patient were collected (age, sex, and data on the timing of different aspects of the surgery), as well as haemodynamic data. The recordings were post-analysed by one investigator not involved in patient care. After the artefacts were cleaned up, the whole monitoring was analysed with Mx_{10s} and the 15-min sample was analysed with Mx_{2s} and Mx_{10s}. The Mx values were plotted as a function of MAP in 5-mmHg bins with the number of MAP values used to construct each bin (Fig. 1).

Results

Five patients (three men and two women) were enrolled in our preliminary pilot study. All results are expressed as mean ± standard deviation. The age of the patients was 71 ± 6 years. The surgery lasted for 138 ± 32 min and CBP lasted for 72 ± 33 min. MAP and MV on TCD were recorded continuously for 117 ± 24 min. MAP was very labile, varying between 33 ± 10 and 92 ± 10 mmHg throughout the entire CPB recording. During the 15-min recording, MAP was also very labile, varying from 40 ± 6.3 to 90 ± 5.5 mmHg.

During a period of 15 min with huge and rapid variations in MAP, LLA could not be calculated with Mx_{10s} in any patient (the Mx value was never under 0.35), whereas LLA was able to be calculated with Mx_{2s} in all patients.

The LLA value calculated from the whole CPB recording with Mx_{10s} was similar to that calculated using Mx_{2s} in 15 min (70 ± 2.5 versus 73 ± 3.5 mmHg).

During the whole recording, the MV value below LLA was lower than the MV value above LLA (33 ± 9 versus 40 ± 11 cm/s, $P = 0.004$). The MV value at LLA (38 ± 10 cm/s) did not differ from that at higher MAP values (40 ± 11 cm/s), pleading also for a correct LLA assessment detection with the Mx_{10s}.

In our cohort, the MAP value remained under LLA for 48 ± 12% of the recording period.

Discussion

These data show that during acute variations in MAP (from 40 ± 6.3 to 90 ± 5.5 mmHg during a 15-min recording), Mx_{2s} can rapidly provide a minimal acceptable MAP value to preserve CBF, whereas Mx_{10s} is unable to help clinicians in this way. In the area of patient-centred care, use of Mx as a tool to personalize MAP in each patient is promising.

Rapid cerebral autoregulation assessment at the start of the procedure may lead the clinician to consider LLA as a possible MAP target. Decreasing the average window exposes this marker to an increase in artefact noise on the signal; thus, it is less efficient for longer trends, such as those observed in the intensive care unit. However, in this specific setting of haemodynamic instability, Mx_{2s} can analyse cerebral autoregulation, unlike Mx_{10s}. Furthermore, despite its short period of analysis, the LLA value observed with Mx_{2s} was also comparable to that observed with Mx_{10s} during the whole recording period.

Our study had several limitations. First, we chose as a definition of autoregulation an Mx value lower than 0.35. The Mx cut-off value indicating loss of autoregulation (and thus providing the LLA) is not clearly known and has been described as being between 0.25 and 0.5 [6]; a recent prospective intervention study chose a value of 0.4 [3]. In that study, the authors suggested that individualizing MAP during CPB on the basis of cerebral autoregulation monitoring could be effective in reducing the incidence of postoperative delirium. They used LLA as the minimal tolerable MAP value during CPB. They assessed LLA during the first part of the surgery (before CPB was started). During CPB, the patient's MAP was targeted to be greater than the LLA value. In the control group, the MAP targets were determined according to institutional practice. The LLA value was determined prior to CPB on the basis of the highest MAP value at which Mx increased from <0.4 to ≥ 0.4. When Mx did not cross 0.4 clearly, LLA was defined as the blood pressure with the lowest Mx value (the MAP value with the best autoregulation). This methodological detail is very relevant. Indeed, like those authors, we experienced some difficulties in assessing LLA quickly in the first part of the procedure with the classic Mx as was described by Czosnyka et al. [5] more than 10 years ago.

The main limitation of our study was definitely the small number of patients. It was only a preliminary pilot study to provide a proof of concept. Further studies are planned to test this concept in a larger cohort.

Finally, a technical limit of Doppler measurement is the recording of surgical artefacts. Indeed, we observed that the surgeon's electrosurgical knife generated noise during the first part of the procedure. These artefacts interfere with use of TCD and compromise use of Mx in the pre-CPB period. To avoid this problem, it would be interesting to develop an automatic 'signal cleaner' at some stage.

These difficulties in recording a good signal in the operating room provide a strong argument for developing quicker LLA assessment techniques that could be used before the surgery is started. With this new specific setting of Mx and LLA calculation within a shorter period (15 min), we have proposed a new tool to help clinicians use autoregulation monitoring. With a MAP value below the LLA value 50% of the time in this observational study, traditional management of MAP may not be aggressive enough to avoid ischaemic consequences for the brain.

Conclusion

Cardiac surgery is characterized by acute haemodynamic variations. Use of a shorter Mx sampling window (2 s versus 10 s) allows accurate LLA detection within 15 min. Such rapid and sophisticated detection could assist clinicians with better MAP target management during CPB. Further studies should be performed to validate these initial findings.

Conflict of Interest **The authors have no conflicts of interest.**

References

1. Vedel AG, Holmgaard F, Rasmussen LS, Langkilde A, Paulson OB, Lange T, Thomsen C, Olsen PS, Ravn HB, Nilsson JC (2018) High-target versus low-target blood pressure management during cardiopulmonary bypass to prevent cerebral injury in cardiac surgery patients: a randomized controlled trial. Circulation 137(17):1770–1780
2. Liu Y, Chen K, Mei W (2019) Neurological complications after cardiac surgery: anesthetic considerations based on outcome evidence. Curr Opin Anaesthesiol 32(5):563–567
3. Brown CH, Neufeld KJ, Tian J et al (2019) Effect of targeting mean arterial pressure during cardiopulmonary bypass by monitoring cerebral autoregulation on postsurgical delirium among older patients: a nested randomized clinical trial. JAMA Surg 154(9):819–826. https://doi.org/10.1001/jamasurg.2019.1163
4. Ono M, Zheng Y, Joshi B, Sigl JC, Hogue CW (2013) Validation of a stand-alone near-infrared spectroscopy system for monitoring cerebral autoregulation during cardiac surgery. Anesth Analg 116(1):198–204
5. Caldas JR, Haunton VJ, Panerai RB, Hajjar LA, Robinson TG (2018) Cerebral autoregulation in cardiopulmonary bypass surgery: a systematic review. Interact Cardiovasc Thorac Surg 26(3):494–503
6. Joshi B, Ono M, Brown C, Brady K, Easley RB, Yenokyan G, Gottesman RF, Hogue CW (2012) Predicting the limits of cerebral autoregulation during cardiopulmonary bypass. Anesth Analg 114(3):503–510

Influence of Patient Demographics on Optimal Cerebral Perfusion Pressure Following Traumatic Brain Injury

Jennifer Young, Laura Moss, Martin Shaw, Elizabeth Cahya, Maya Kommer, and Christopher Hawthorne

Introduction

Despite recent advances in neurocritical care, severe traumatic brain injury (TBI) is still associated with a high mortality rate, and the majority of survivors experience some degree of ongoing disability [1]. One of the primary goals of the neurological intensive care unit (ICU) is to achieve adequate cerebral perfusion pressure (CPP) (the difference between the mean arterial pressure and intracranial pressure). Current Brain Trauma Foundation guidelines recommend aiming for 60–70 mmHg in adults [2]. Recently, attempts have been made to move away from the "one-size-fits-all" approach towards cerebral autoregulation-based management to improve patient outcomes.

Novel management strategies for patients with severe TBI involve the continuous bedside calculation and targeting of the CPP where cerebral autoregulation (CA) is optimal (CPPopt). CA is the maintenance of constant cerebral blood flow (CBF) despite changes in CPP [3]. Cerebral autoregulatory mechanisms are only active within a certain CPP range and are frequently disturbed during TBI. If CA is impaired, changes in CPP result in changes in CBF, causing further brain tissue injury [3, 4]. Since it is apparent that different patients have different CPPopts, patient outcomes may also be improved through individualised targeting of mean arterial pressure (MAP) in the pre-ICU period where intracranial pressure (ICP) is presumed elevated but CPPopt cannot be calculated [5, 6].

Several demographic and clinical characteristics are established predictors of prognosis in TBI [7, 8]. To date, the relationship between these characteristics and CPPopt has not been directly quantified. Quantifiable relationships, if they exist, would have potential for use in the prediction of CPPopt in the pre-ICU setting. Additionally, they may have significant implications for future guidelines recommending CPP targets in ICUs. Therefore, the aim of this study was to define the relationship between calculated CPPopt and clinical characteristics.

Materials and Methods

This retrospective analysis included data from TBI patients admitted to the neurological ICU at the Institute of Neurological Sciences, Glasgow, with CPPopt values calculated by applying the DATACAR-LAx method to continuous recordings of ICP and MAP [9]. The patient data had been collected as part of the Connecting Healthcare and Research Through A Data Analysis Provisioning Technology (CHART-ADAPT) project. Linear mixed effects (LME) analysis was performed using an unadjusted-adjusted approach. Variables of interest were treated as fixed effects in order to quantify their relationship with CPPopt. The random effect of study ID was included to allow the intercept to vary per patient, accounting for the correlation between repeated observations of CPPopt in each individual. Unadjusted models were created for each variable: time from initiation of ICP monitoring,

J. Young (✉) · E. Cahya
School of Medicine, Dentistry and & Nursing, University of Glasgow, Glasgow, UK
e-mail: 2174305y@student.gla.ac.uk; 2118477c@student.gla.ac.uk

L. Moss · M. Shaw
School of Medicine, Dentistry and & Nursing, University of Glasgow, Glasgow, UK

Department of Clinical Physics and Bioengineering, Institute of Neurological Sciences, Queen Elizabeth University Hospital, Glasgow, UK
e-mail: laura.moss@glasgow.ac.uk; martin.shaw@nhs.net

M. Kommer
Institute of Neurological Sciences, Royal Hospital for Children, Glasgow, UK
e-mail: mayakommer@nhs.net

C. Hawthorne
Department of Neuroanaesthesia, Institute of Neurological Sciences, Queen Elizabeth University Hospital, Glasgow, UK
e-mail: cwhawthorne@doctors.org.uk

B. Depreitere et al. (eds.), *Intracranial Pressure and Neuromonitoring XVII*, Acta Neurochirurgica Supplement 131,
https://doi.org/10.1007/978-3-030-59436-7_31,

age at admission to ICU, gender, features of the computed tomography (CT) brain scan (the presence of extradural haematoma, acute subdural haematoma, contusions, diffuse axonal injury (DAI), traumatic subarachnoid haemorrhage, midline shift and non-evacuated haematoma), multiple trauma, pre-intubation Glasgow Coma Score (GCS) and pre-intubation pupil response to light. Variables were selected for inclusion in an adjusted model at a significance level of $p < 0.10$. A second adjusted model including all variables of interest was also assessed. The level for statistical significance of covariates in adjusted models was $p < 0.05$. Only patients with data for all required variables were included in model synthesis, so no missing data were included in the final analysis. Model accuracy for predicting CPPopt was assessed by calculating the RMSE. The most effective model for predicting CPPopt was that with the lowest RMSE. Data analysis was conducted using the R statistical computing environment (version 3.5.3) [10].

Results

Characteristics of the 36 patients included in the analysis are shown in Table 1. The median age was 44.5 years (interquartile range (IQR) = 33.5–54.3 years). The majority of patients were male (83.3% male, 16.7% female). A fall was the most common mechanism by which TBI occurred (55.6%). The median CPPopt was 66.0 mmHg (IQR = 59.3–75.1 mmHg). The median total monitoring time across which ICP data were recorded in an individual patient was 2515.0 min (IQR = 1005.4–3959.9 min). The results of the unadjusted analysis are shown in Table 2. Time from initiation of ICP monitoring, age at admission to ICU and the presence of DAI reached the significance threshold for inclusion in the adjusted model. In this model, time and DAI were significant covariates (Table 3); CPPopt increases as time from initiation of ICP monitoring increases (estimate = 0.00292, $p < 0.001$), and the presence of DAI is associated with a lower CPPopt (estimate = −35.5, $p < 0.001$). Age at admission to ICU has a negative relationship with CPPopt but was not statistically significant (estimate = −0.267, $p = 0.0750$). The random effect of study ID on the intercept had a standard deviation of 10.7 mmHg. The RMSE was 8.11 mmHg. The fit of this model to the original CPPopt data is shown in Fig. 1. Figure 2 shows examples of the fit of the model to CPPopt data from individual patients included in the study. The second adjusted model contained all variables of interest. Statistically significant covariates were time from initiation of ICP monitoring, the presence of DAI and the presence of non-evacuated haematoma. According to this model, CPPopt increases as time from initiation of ICP monitoring

Table 1 Characteristics of patients included in analysis

Characteristic (n)[a]	Patients included in analysis
Age, years (36)—median (IQR)	44.5 (33.5–54.3)
Gender (36)—no. (%)	
Male	30 (83.3)
Female	6 (16.7)
Mechanism of injury (36)—no. (%)	
Fall	20 (55.6)
MVC pedestrian	5 (13.9)
MVC car	4 (11.1)
MVC motorcycle	1 (2.8)
Assault	2 (5.6)
Seizure	1 (2.8)
Sport	1 (2.8)
Unknown	2 (5.6)
Features of CT brain scan (35)—no. (%)	
EDH	7 (20.0)
ASDH	23 (65.7)
Contusions	31 (88.6)
DAI	2 (5.7)
Traumatic SAH	28 (80.0)
Midline shift	21 (60.0)
Non-evacuated haematoma	34 (97.1)
Multiple trauma (35)—no. (%)[b]	6 (17.1)
Pre-intubation GCS—median (IQR)	
Eye opening (34)	1 (1–2)
Motor response (35)	4 (2–5)
Verbal response (33)	2 (1–2)
Total (33)	7 (6–8)
Pre-intubation pupil response to light (34)—no. (%)	
Both reactive	26 (76.5)
One reactive	4 (11.8)
None reactive	4 (11.8)
Total monitoring time per patient, minutes (36)—median (IQR)	2515.0 (1005.4–3959.9)

IQR interquartile range, *MVC* motor vehicle collision, *CT* computed tomography, *EDH* extradural haematoma, *ASDH* acute subdural haematoma, *DAI* diffuse axonal injury, *SAH* subarachnoid haemorrhage, *GCS* Glasgow Coma Scale

[a]Due to missing values, total number of patients with data for each characteristic varies

[b]Multiple trauma was defined as the presence of at least one extracranial injury requiring medical treatment

[c]The Glasgow Coma Scale is used to communicate the level of consciousness of patients. Eye opening is scored from 1 to 4, motor response is scored from 1 to 6, and verbal response is scored from 1 to 5 [11]

Table 2 Unadjusted linear mixed effects analysis of relationship between demographic and clinical characteristics and optimal cerebral perfusion pressure

Variable	Estimate (SE)[a]	p-value[b]	Standard deviation of the random intercept (mmHg)
Time from initiation of ICP monitoring (min)	0.00263 (1.73×10^{-5})	<0.001	13.4
Age at admission to ICU (years)	−0.267 (0.136)	0.0576	12.9
Gender male	−4.69 (6.03)	0.442	13.5
EDH yes	−3.60 (5.78)	0.537	13.7
ASDH yes	4.30 (4.84)	0.380	13.6
Contusions yes	−8.83 (7.14)	0.225	13.4
DAI yes	−33.8 (8.09)	<0.001	11.1
Traumatic SAH yes	−7.34 (5.67)	0.204	13.4
Midline shift yes	2.15 (4.73)	0.653	13.7
Non-evacuated haematoma yes	−0.724 (13.9)	0.959	13.7
Multiple trauma yes	−0.5246 (6.17)	0.933	13.7
GCS eye opening	−1.49 (2.21)	0.505	13.9
GCS motor response	1.61 (1.47)	0.280	13.5
GCS verbal response	0.786 (2.13)	0.715	14.1
GCS total	0.454 (0.856)	0.600	14.1
Number of pupils responsive to light[c]			
One	5.22 (7.22)	0.475	13.4
None	−11.6 (7.23)	0.119	

Results presented to 3 significant figures
Equation = CPPopt ~ variable + (1 | study ID). Variables were treated as fixed effects. The random effect of study ID on the intercept was assessed, with the intercept being allowed to vary randomly according to patient. *CPPopt* optimal cerebral perfusion pressure, *ICP* intracranial pressure, *ICU* intensive care unit, *EDH* extradural haematoma, *ASDH* acute subdural haematoma, *DAI* diffuse axonal injury, *GCS* Glasgow Coma Scale
[a]Estimate of coefficient with standard error (SE)
[b]Significance level $p < 0.10$ for determining variables to include in adjusted model to reduce risk of bias and overfitting of final model
[c]Reference category was both pupils responsive to light

increases (estimate = 0.00295, $p < 0.001$), the presence of DAI is associated with a lower CPPopt (estimate = −67.5, $p < 0.001$), and the presence of non-evacuated haematoma is associated with a higher CPPopt (estimate = 62.3, $p = 0.00208$). The other covariates were not statistically significant. The random effect of study ID on the intercept had a standard deviation of 8.20 mmHg. The RMSE was 8.09 mmHg.

Table 3 Adjusted linear mixed model of optimal cerebral perfusion pressure

Variable	Estimate (SE)[a]	p-value[b]
Fixed effects		
Intercept	72.1 (5.42)	<0.001
Time from initiation of ICP monitoring (minutes)	0.00292 (1.96×10^{-5})	<0.001
Age at admission to ICU (years)	−0.211 (0.114)	0.0750
DAI yes	−35.5 (7.81)	<0.001
Random effects		
Intercept	10.7[c]	–

Results presented to 3 significant figures
Equation = CPPopt to time from initiation of ICP monitoring + age at admission to ICU + DAI + (1 | study ID). Time, age and DAI were treated as fixed effects. The random effect of study ID on the intercept was assessed, allowing the intercept to vary randomly according to patient. *CPPopt* optimal cerebral perfusion pressure, *ICP* intracranial pressure, *ICU* intensive care unit, *DAI* diffuse axonal injury
[a]Estimate of coefficient with standard error (SE)
[b]Significance level $p < 0.05$
[c]Standard deviation of random intercept

Discussion

To date, the relationship between CPPopt and clinical variables has not been directly quantified or translated into a predictive model. In this exploratory study, the relationship between CPPopt and several patient demographic and clinical characteristics was defined by LME analysis. Two LME models were produced to predict CPPopt from demographic and clinical data.

LME analysis revealed a negative relationship between age and CPPopt, which failed to reach statistical significance but was included in an adjusted model (Fig. 1). While the estimate was of small magnitude, the model indicates that an age difference of 24 years is required to cause a 5 mmHg lower CPPopt, which, over prolonged periods, is associated with increased mortality in TBI [12, 13]. Current evidence supports the hypothesis that increasing age is associated with higher CPPopt [14–16]. The contradictory finding of this study may be explained by the fact that age did not statistically significantly contribute to the model, indicating that there is a need to perform similar analyses on larger TBI cohorts to elucidate the true relationship.

It is known that CPPopt exhibits inter-individual as well as intra-individual variation over time [17]. In this study, time was highly significant in both linear models. A patient would require an ICU stay of 28.5 h to exhibit a 5 mmHg increase in CPPopt. The median duration of monitoring time for patients included in this study exceeded 28.5 h, highlighting that time has a clinically significant impact on CPPopt. However, it was clear that the positive relationship modelled did not fit the time trend exhibited by every patient (Fig. 2).

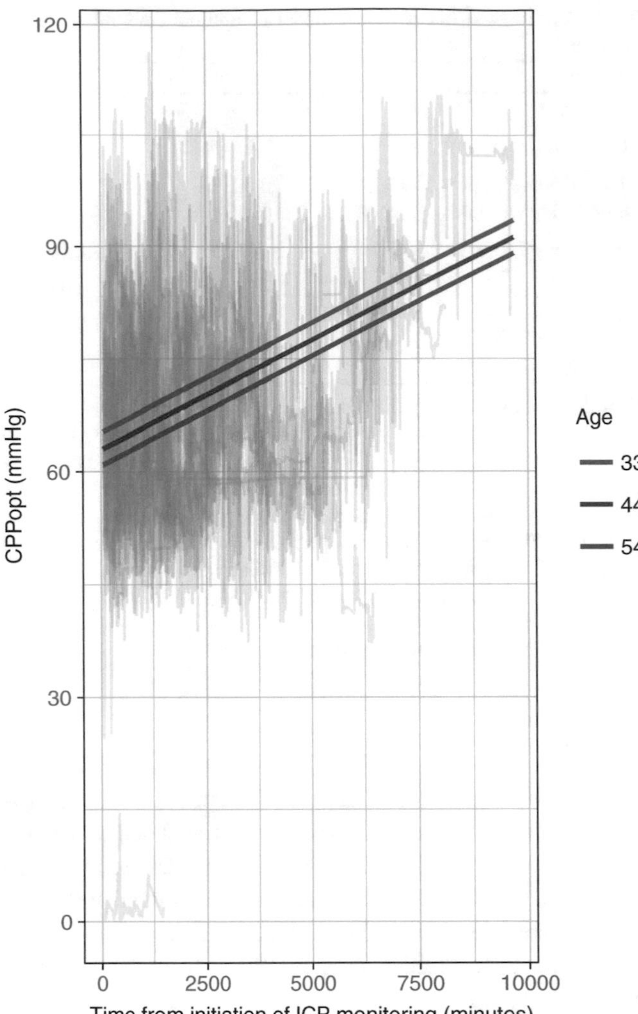

Fig. 1 Comparison of predicted optimal cerebral perfusion pressure for patients of different ages. Straight lines represent optimal cerebral perfusion pressure (CPPopt) predicted by linear mixed model with equation CPPopt to time from initiation of ICP monitoring + age at admission to ICU + DAI + (1 | study ID), for the "average" patient of age 33 (blue), 44 (red) and 54 (dark grey) years. Characteristics of the "average" patient were taken as most common observation within each variable. Light grey lines represent original data used for model synthesis, showing the trend in actual CPPopt for every patient included in the study

Overall, the results of this study emphasise the importance of continuously calculating CPPopt across a patient's entire period of ICP monitoring, rather than performing a single initial calculation.

The only CT characteristic to significantly affect CPPopt in the first adjusted model was DAI. Its presence was associated with a substantial reduction in the predicted CPPopt. However, the estimate of effect was very imprecise as only two patients in the study had DAI on CT.

The existence of a model to predict CPPopt would dramatically improve MAP targeting in patients with severe TBI prior to commencement of ICP monitoring. The RMSE for both models synthesised in this project was 8.1 mmHg, meaning that the predicted CPPopt could deviate from the true value by as much as this. Differences between CPP and CPPopt of this magnitude are known to affect patient outcomes [12, 13]. Consequently, at present, neither model adequately predicts CPPopt for application in scenarios where the ICP is not measured.

TBI is associated with very poor patient outcomes [1]. Targeting CPPopt in TBI patients may reduce the rate of unfavourable outcome, as deviation of CPP from CPPopt is associated with higher mortality and disability [9, 13, 18, 19]. The results of this study emphasise that CPPopt is a dynamic measurement which is influenced by many patient and clinical factors. Complex interactions of these variables are too patient-specific, making it difficult to accommodate a clinically useful predictive model. This supports the utility of investigating CPPopt-guided therapy as a replacement for the universal 60–70 mmHg target.

One of the strengths of this study was that, despite including data from only 36 patients, 79,375 observations of CPPopt were included in the analysis. The large number of observations mitigated the risk of model overfitting. The LME approach was well suited for making inferences regarding the relationship between single variables and CPPopt. Furthermore, this form of analysis allowed collinearity in repeated observations from each patient to be accounted for.

The principal limitation of this study was the small sample size. It is impossible to exclude the possibility that the true effect of some predictors was not elucidated owing to the small subgroup size. However, small sample sizes are characteristic of exploratory analyses such as this. The results warrant further investigation of modelling CPPopt using demographic and clinical characteristics in larger TBI cohorts. The LME approach is less suited to predictive modelling because it assumes the relationships between predictors and the outcome variable are linear. Non-linear methods may provide models which predict CPPopt more accurately, taking account of non-linear relationships, and are another avenue for future studies to explore.

Conclusions

Time from initiation of ICP monitoring, age at admission to ICU and the presence of DAI may be important predictors of CPPopt. Predictive models require further development before they can be used in calculating CPPopt when ICP is not monitored. The results of this study support the continuation of research into the feasibility and utility of CPPopt-guided therapy in TBI.

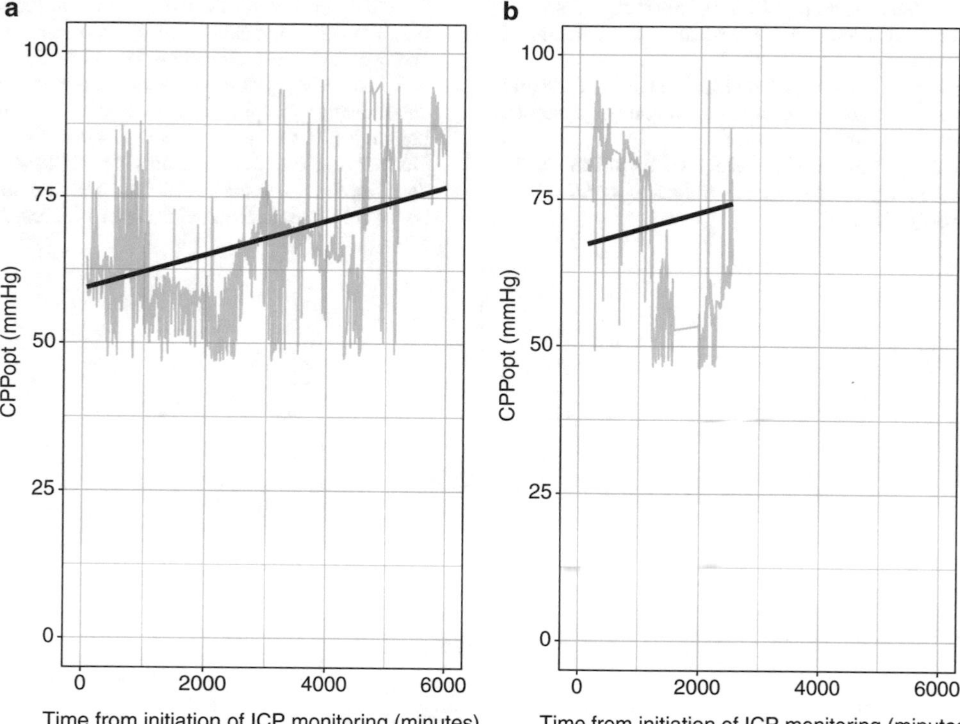

Fig. 2 Comparison of optimal cerebral perfusion pressure predictions by a linear mixed model to the trend of actual optimal cerebral perfusion pressure for individual patients. Black straight lines represent CPPopt predictions by the linear mixed model with equation CPPopt to time from initiation of ICP monitoring + age at admission to ICU + DAI + (1 | study ID). Grey lines are actual CPPopt for that individual. (**a**) The model is a good fit for this patient's data. (**b**) The model is not a good fit for this patient's data

Acknowledgements This work was financially supported by the Neuroanaesthesia and Critical Care Society of Great Britain and Ireland (NACCSGBI) through the John Snow Anaesthesia Intercalated Award.

Conflict of Interest **We declare that we have no conflict of interest.**

References

1. Rosenfeld JV, Maas AI, Bragge P, Morganti-Kossman C, Manley GT, Gruen RL (2012) Early management of severe traumatic brain injury. Lancet 380(9847):1088–1098
2. Carney N, Totten AM, O'Reilly C et al (2017) Guidelines for the management of severe traumatic brain injury, 4th edition. Neurosurgery 80(1):6–15
3. Lassen NA (1959) Cerebral blood flow and oxygen consumption in man. Physiol Rev 39(2):183–238
4. Payne S (2016) Cerebral autoregulation: control of blood flow in the brain. Springer
5. Howells T, Elf K, Jones PA et al (2005) Pressure reactivity as a guide in the treatment of cerebral perfusion pressure in patients with brain trauma. J Neurosurg 102(2):311–317
6. Jaeger M, Dengl M, Meixensberger J, Schuhmann MU (2010) Effects of cerebrovascular pressure reactivity-guided optimization of cerebral perfusion pressure on brain tissue oxygenation after traumatic brain injury. Crit Care Med 38(5):1343–1347
7. MRC CRASH Trial Collaborators (2008) Predicting outcome after traumatic brain injury: practical prognostic models based on large cohort of international patients. BMJ 336(7641):425–429
8. Steyerberg EW, Mushkudiani N, Perel P et al (2008) Predicting outcome after traumatic brain injury: development and international validation of prognostic scores based on admission characteristics. PLoS Med 5(8):e165
9. Depreitere B, Guiza F, Van den Berghe G et al (2014) Pressure autoregulation monitoring and cerebral perfusion pressure target recommendation in patients with severe traumatic brain injury based on minute-by-minute monitoring data. J Neurosurg 120(6):1451–1457
10. R Core Team (2018) R: A language and environment for statistical computing. R Foundation for Statistical Computing, Vienna, Austria. Available from: https://www.R-project.org/
11. Teasdale G. The Glasgow Structured Approach to Assessment of the Glasgow Coma Scale. Glasgow Coma Scale. Website by: Royal College of Physicians and Surgeons of Glasgow. Available from: https://www.glasgowcomascale.org/ [Accessed 15th March 2019]
12. Petkus V, Krakauskaite S, Preiksaitis A, Rocka S, Chomskis R, Ragauskas A (2016) Association between the outcome of traumatic brain injury patients and cerebrovascular autoregulation, cerebral perfusion pressure, age, and injury grades. Medicina 52(1):46–53
13. Petkus V, Preiksaitis A, Krakauskaite S et al (2017) Benefit on optimal cerebral perfusion pressure targeted treatment for traumatic brain injury patients. J Crit Care 41:49–55

14. Czosnyka M, Balestreri M, Steiner L et al (2005) Age, intracranial pressure, autoregulation, and outcome after brain trauma. J Neurosurg 102(3):450–454
15. Howells T, Smielewski P, Donnelly J et al (2018) Optimal cerebral perfusion pressure in centers with different treatment protocols. Crit Care Med 46(3):e235–e241
16. Sorrentino E, Diedler J, Kasprowicz M et al (2012) Critical thresholds for cerebrovascular reactivity after traumatic brain injury. Neurocrit Care 16(2):258–266
17. Smielewski P, Lavinio A, Timofeev I et al (2008) ICM+, a flexible platform for investigations of cerebrospinal dynamics in clinical practice. Acta Neurochir Suppl 102:145–151
18. Aries MJ, Czosnyka M, Budohoski KP et al (2012) Continuous determination of optimal cerebral perfusion pressure in traumatic brain injury. Crit Care Med 40(8):2456–2463
19. Donnelly J, Czosnyka M, Adams H et al (2018) Pressure reactivity-based optimal cerebral perfusion pressure in a traumatic brain injury cohort. Acta Neurochir Suppl 126:209–212

Secondary Cerebral Ischemia at Traumatic Brain Injury Is More Closely Related to Cerebrovascular Reactivity Impairment than to Intracranial Hypertension

Michael Dobrzeniecki, Alex Trofimov, Dmitry Martynov, Darya Agarkova, Ksenia Trofimova, Zhanna B. Semenova, and Denis E. Bragin

Introduction

Increased intracranial pressure (ICP) is one of the main causes of morbidity and mortality in a broad spectrum of pathologies, such as traumatic brain injury (TBI), nontraumatic intracerebral hemorrhage, hydrocephalus, brain tumors, and others [1]. Current guidelines recommend maintaining ICP below 21 mmHg [2, 3]. The oligemia is linked to hypoxic edema and cytotoxic cellular engorgement. The hyperemia is associated with high cerebral blood flow (CBF) and, when associated with vascular barrier impairment, may trigger interstitial edema. The development of intracranial hypertension may be linked to an excess or a lack of cerebral blood flow (CBF) and the formation of the ischemia or hyperemia. These conditions should be recognized to provide suitable treatment for ICP control [4].

Cerebral autoregulation (CA) is the mechanism responsible for maintaining a relatively constant CBF over a wide range of blood pressure which protects the brain from oligemia or hyperemia [5].

Under certain conditions, the range of CA is severely compromised, increasing the risk of cerebral edema [4, 6].

Many researchers have tried to determine the relationship between CA and ICP in the development of poor outcomes, but the significance of the cerebral ischemia formation still poorly understood [7–10].

M. Dobrzeniecki · A. Trofimov (✉) · D. Martynov · D. Agarkova
K. Trofimova
Department of Neurosurgery, Privolzhsky Research Medical University, Nizhny Novgorod, Russia

Z. B. Semenova
Department of Neurosurgery, Children's Clinical and Research Institute of Emergency Surgery and Trauma, Moscow, Russia

D. E. Bragin
Lovelace Biomedical Research Institute, Albuquerque, NM, USA

Department of Neurosurgery, University of New Mexico School of Medicine, 1 University of New Mexico, Albuquerque, NM, USA
e-mail: dbragin@salud.unm.edu

It should be noted that a compromised CA has also been shown in patients with normal ICP. It is believed that impaired CA and increased ICP can persist simultaneously and result from a breakthrough of the blood-brain barrier, disturbances to vasomotion, and subsequent brain swelling [11]. Thus, impaired CA may be a factor that triggers increases in ICP and vice versa. However, no consensus has been reached on the relationship between damaged CA and ICP in the development of secondary cerebral ischemia (SCI).

The purpose of our study was to investigate the relationship between intracranial hypertension and cerebrovascular reactivity (CVR), as quantified by the pressure reactivity index (PRx), in the development of SCI after traumatic brain injury (TBI).

Material and Methods

This nonrandomized single-center retrospective study complies with the Declaration of Helsinki, and the protocol was approved by the local ethics committee. All patients gave informed consent to participate in the study.

We included patients who had the following features: severe TBI within 6 h after a head injury with a Glasgow Coma Score (GCS) of less than 8, SCI at follow-up perfusion computed tomography (PCT), monitoring of ICP and mean arterial pressure (MAP) for at least 24 h, admission GCS and Injury Severity Score (ISS) data available. Exclusion criteria were as follows: (1) younger than 16 years, (2) GCS < 4, and (3) ISS > 60. The neuromonitoring of cerebral modalities was conducted as a part of standard patient care and archived in a database of neurophysiological monitoring. ICP exceeding 15 mmHg was treated using head elevation (15°–25°), sedation, external ventricular drainage, and mannitol. ICP was monitored continuously. Intraparenchymal (Codman MicroSensors ICP, Codman & Shurtleff, Raynham, MA,

B. Depreitere et al. (eds.), *Intracranial Pressure and Neuromonitoring XVII*, Acta Neurochirurgica Supplement 131,
https://doi.org/10.1007/978-3-030-59436-7_32,

USA) or intraventricular probes (LiquoGuard, Möller Medical GmbH & Co. K) were inserted at the bedside in the ICU or in the operating room into the frontal or parietal lobe. The intraparenchymal probes were placed in white matter on the side of the maximal lesions.

Physiological parameters were recorded continuously using a bedside monitor. In addition, these physiological variables, ICP, and cerebral compliance were recorded every 5 s on the ICU flowsheet. Dynamic PRx was estimated from the measured parameters as the moving Pearson correlation of 30 consecutive MAP and ICP, updated every minute.

Each patient was managed according to a published TBI guideline. Ventilator management was tailored to maintain PaO_2 at more than 100 mmHg and $PaCO_2$ between 30 and 35 mmHg. Albumin and crystalloid boluses and norepinephrine were used to maintain systolic blood pressure at more than 100 mmHg and central venous pressure at approximately 80 mm H_2O.

All patients were subjected to dynamic PCT by tomograph Philips Ingenuity CT (Philips Medical Systems, Cleveland, OH, USA). PCT was performed 1–2 days after TBI. We acquired noncontrast CT and postcontrast series in axial mode from the skull base to the vertex (16-cm z-axis coverage) using the following imaging parameters: 120 kV peak tube voltage, 320 mA tube current, slice thickness 5 mm, 32 cm scan field of view, 256 × 256 matrix. We acquired PCT images at the level of the basal ganglia and the third ventricle above the orbits. PCT data were transferred to a Philips Core workstation (Philips Medical Systems, Cleveland, OH, USA) and analyzed by a standardized method to create perfusion maps of mean transit time (MTT), cerebral blood flow (CBF), and cerebral blood volume (CBV). We used deconvolution software. SCI core and penumbra were established using the appropriate MTT and CBV thresholds, which are MTT > 145% of the contralateral side values and CBV > 2.0 mL/100 g for the penumbra volume and MTT > 145% of the contralateral side values and CBV < 2.0 mL/100 g for the SCI core volume [12].

Data are expressed as the mean ± standard deviation. To specify the degree of impact of changes in ICP and CVR on the SCI progression in TBI patients, logistic regression was performed. Significant p-values were < 0.05. All analyses were performed using the software package Statistica 7.0 (Statsoft, Inc., USA).

Results

In total, 89 patients with severe TBI admitted to the Nizhniy Novgorod Regional Hospital with ICP monitoring were studied. The mean age was 36.3 ± 4.8 years (range 19–45 years). There were 77 men and 12 women. The mean age was 36.3 ± 4.8 years, 53 men and 36 women. The median GCS was 6.2 ± 0.7. The median ISS score at admission was 38.2 ± 12.5.

During the described period, the mean cerebral perfusion pressure (CPP) was 81.5 ± 12.5 mmHg. The mean ICP was 19.98 ± 5.3 mmHg (minimum 11.7; maximum 51.7). The mean dynamic PRx was 0.23 ± 0.14.

The deterioration of CVR in combination with the severity of ICP has a significant impact on the increase in the prevalence rate of SCI. The post hoc comparison of the prevalence rate of SCI to different degrees of ICP and changes in CVR revealed significant differences. Thus, the increasing prevalence of SCI occurs because of both intracranial hypertension and the impairment of CVR. Logistic regression analysis for a model of the SCI dependence on intracranial hypertension and the CVR was performed. The results are shown in Table 1 and Fig. 1.

The results of the logistic regression analysis showed that the CVR was the most significant factor affecting SCI development in TBI. In particular, the probability of SCI development exceeded 50% even with an ICP level of 5 mmHg at impaired CVR. Moreover, at the upper normal values of ICP (21 mmHg) and CVR (iPRx 0.3), the probability of the development of SCI in TBI reached 75%.

Discussion

Despite numerous studies, the role of autoregulation and intracranial hypertension in the development of cerebral ischemia at TBI remains unclear.

Table 1 The logistic regression model for predicting SCI in 89 patients with severe TBI

	Const B0	iPRx	ICP
Estimate	−6.390327	14.23774	0.07451441
Standart error	2.021378	4.434144	0.06425401
t	−3.161371	3.210933	1.159685
p-level	0.00235866	0.00203311	0.2502931
−95%CL	−10.42501	5.387152	−0.053737
+95%CL	−2.355639	23.08833	0.202765
Wald χ^2	9.994267	10.31009	1.34486
p-level	0.00157174	0.00132435	0.246185
odds ratio (unit ch)	0.001677	1,525,358	1.07736
−95%CL	0.00002968	21.858	0.947681
+95%CL	0.0948329	1.064469	1.224786
odds ratio (range)		126.5745	5.15165
−95%CL		6.244066	0.306598
+95%CL		256.5813	86.56113

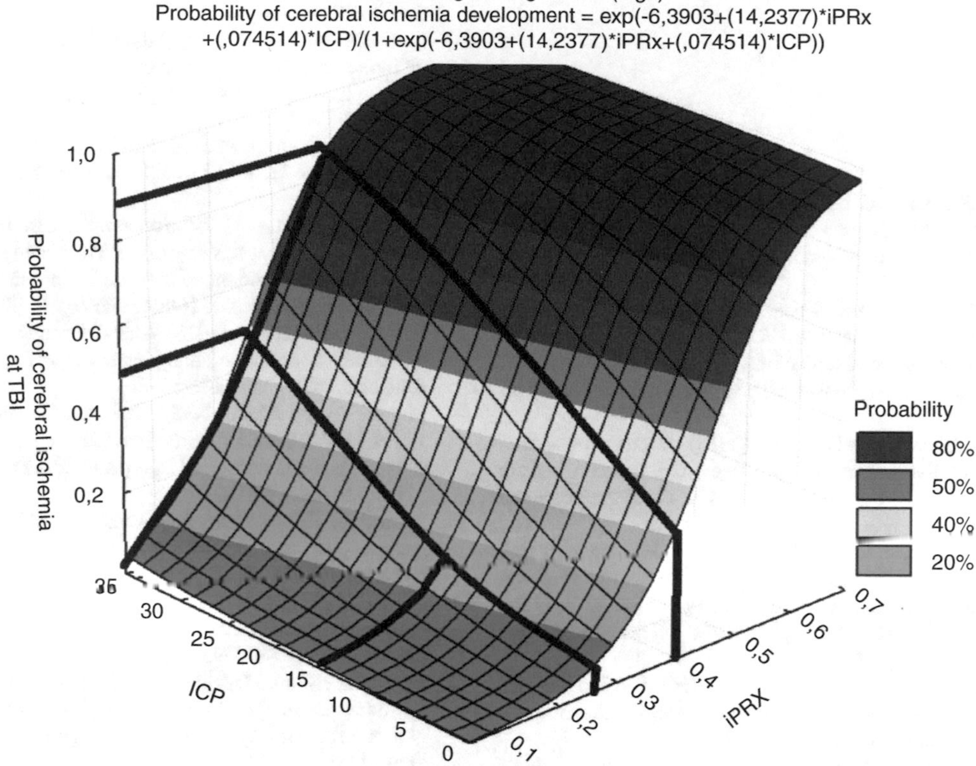

Fig. 1 Results of logistic regression analysis: probability surface of SCI development

S. Klein and B. Depreitere found a correlation between impaired autoregulation and episodes of elevated ICP; the correlation was not ideal, suggesting that autoregulation was not impaired in all episodes of elevated ICP [13]. However, in regression analysis, they showed that autoregulation disorders equally correlated only with outcomes but not SCI development.

In the normal state of CA and increased ICP, a tendency toward decreased CBF was described in just one study [10]. Meanwhile, the reverse situation is described in a large number of works [7, 14–17].

It is assumed that one of the reasons for the development of SCI at the impairment of CA may be the uncoupling of cerebral metabolism and cerebral microcirculation [18].

It has been shown that cerebral metabolic crises can play a key role in CA damage and SCI development, causing cerebral hyperemia and leading to the development of interstitial edema and intracranial hypertension [7]. Some studies have shown a persistent metabolic crisis is associated with a high lactate/pyruvate ratio, with high glutamate and low glucose levels, which was accompanied by a disruption of CA and intracranial hypertension, sometimes even despite decompressive craniectomy [19].

According to Ho et al., in all patients with signs of cerebral metabolic crisis and poor prognosis, $PtbO_2$ levels remained normal, which excluded hypoxia as the cause of malignant intracranial hypertension and increased mitochondrial dysfunction [20].

Metabolic crisis and inflammation in brain injury are also associated with a violation of CA, regardless of the level of ICP, which confirms our data [4]. On the other hand, a decrease in cerebrovascular reactivity associated with a continuing metabolic crisis may be a factor causing intracranial hypertension. However, some authors argue that intracranial hypertension itself is an independent cause of the impairment of CA [21]. Further studies are needed to clarify the proposed mechanisms of the development of SCI. The small sample size of studied patients was a limitation of our work.

Conclusions

The development of SCI in severe TBI is more dependent on CVR impairment and, to a lesser extent, on ICP level. The treatment for severe TBI patients with SCI progression should not be aimed only at intracranial hypertension correction but also at CVR recovery. The findings of this study should be validated with larger cohorts.

Acknowledgments DB was supported by NIH R01NS112808-01. AT was supported by a Grant-in-Aid for Exploratory Research from the Privolzhsky Research Medical University.

Conflict of Interest **The authors declare that they have no conflict of interest.**

References

1. Oliveira ML, Kairalla AC, Fonoff ET, Martinez RC, Teixeira MJ, Bor-Seng-Shu E (2014) Cerebral microdialysis in traumatic brain injury and subarachnoid hemorrhage: state of the art. Neurocrit Care 21:152–162
2. Hutchinson PJ, Kolias AG, Tajsic T et al (2019) Consensus statement from the International Consensus Meeting on the Role of Decompressive Craniectomy in the Management of Traumatic Brain Injury: consensus statement. Acta Neurochir 161(7):1261–1274
3. Chesnut RM, Bleck TP, Citerio G (2015) A consensus-based interpretation of the benchmark evidence from South American trials: treatment of intracranial pressure trial. J Neurotrauma 32(22):1722–1724
4. Oliveira ML, de Azevedo DS, de Azevedo MK, Nogueira RC, Teixeira MJ, Bor-Seng-Shu E (2015) Encephalic hemodynamic phases in subarachnoid hemorrhage: how to improve the protective effect in patient prognoses. Neural Regen Res 10:748–752
5. Salinet AS, Panerai RB, Robinson TG (2014) The longitudinal evolution of cerebral blood flow regulation after acute ischaemic stroke. Cerebrovasc Dis Extra 4:186–197
6. Czosnyka M (2019) In a search of pressure, which optimizes autoregulation of cerebral blood flow. Crit Care Med 47(10):1472–1473
7. Bouma GJ, Muizelaar JP, Bandoh K, Marmarou A (1992) Blood pressure and intracranial pressure-volume dynamics in severe head injury: relationship with cerebral blood flow. J Neurosurg 77:15–19
8. Lee JH, Kelly DF, Oertel M, MacArthur DL, Gleen TC, Vespa P et al (2001) Carbon dioxide reactivity, pressure autoregulation, and metabolic suppression reactivity after head injury: a transcranial Doppler study. J Neurosurg 95:222–232
9. Ter Minassian A, Dube L, Guilleux AM, Wehrmann N, Ursino M, Beydon L (2002) Changes in intracranial pressure and cerebral autoregulation in patients with severe traumatic brain injury. Crit Care Med 30:1616–1622
10. Donnelly J, Czosnyka M, Adams H (2019) Twenty-five years of intracranial pressure monitoring after severe traumatic brain injury: a retrospective, single-center analysis. Neurosurgery 85(1):E75–E82
11. Clément T, Rodriguez-Grande B, Badaut J (2020) Aquaporins in brain edema. J Neurosci Res 98(1):9–18. https://doi.org/10.1002/jnr.24354
12. Nannoni S, Cereda CW, Sirimarco G, Lambrou D, Strambo D, Eskandari A, Dunet V, Wintermark M, Michel P (2019) Collaterals are a major determinant of the core but not the penumbra volume in acute ischemic stroke. Neuroradiology 61(9):971–978
13. Klein S, Depreitere B (2018) What determines outcome in patients that suffer raised intracranial pressure after traumatic brain injury? Acta Neurochir Suppl 126:51–54
14. Munar F, Ferrer AM, de Nadal M, Poca MA, Pedraza S, Sahuquillo J et al (2001) Cerebral hemodynamic effects of 7.2% hypertonic saline in patients with head injury and raised intracranial pressure. J Neurotrauma 17:41–51
15. Voldby B, Enevoldsen EM, Jensen FT (1985) Cerebrovascular reactivity in patients with ruptured intracranial aneurysms. J Neurosurg 62:59–67
16. Lima-Oliveira M, Salinet A, Nogueira RC (2018) Intracranial hypertension and cerebral autoregulation: a systematic review and meta-analysis. World Neurosurg 113:110–124
17. Bragin DE, Statom G, Nemoto EM (2016) Dynamic cerebrovascular and intracranial pressure reactivity assessment of impaired cerebral autoregulation in intracranial hypertension. Acta Neurochir Suppl 122:255–260
18. Bor-Seng-Shu E, Oliveira ML, Teixeira MJ (2010) Traumatic brain injury and metabolism. J Neurosurg 112:1351–1353
19. Ho CL, Wang CM, Lee KK, Ng I, Ang BT (2008) Cerebral oxygenation, vascular reactivity, and neurochemistry following decompressive craniectomy for severe traumatic brain injury. J Neurosurg 108:943–949
20. Dias C, Silva MJ, Pereira E, Silva S, Cerejo A, Smielewski P et al (2014) Post-traumatic multimodal brain monitoring: response to hypertonic saline. J Neurotrauma 31:1872–1880
21. Miller JD, Stanek AE, Langfitt TW (1973) Cerebral blood flow regulation during experimental brain compression. J Neurosurg 39:186–196

Usability of Noninvasive Counterparts of Traditional Autoregulation Indices in Traumatic Brain Injury

Andras Czigler, Leanne A. Calviello, Frederick A. Zeiler, Peter Toth, Peter Smielewski, and Marek Czosnyka

Introduction

The pressure reactivity index (PRx) is one of the commonly used parameters to describe autoregulation in traumatic brain injury (TBI). It quantifies the changes in vascular smooth muscle tone that occur as a result of variations in transmural pressure. It is calculated as the moving linear correlation coefficient between mean arterial blood pressure (ABP) and intracranial pressure (ICP) [1].

In certain cases (i.e. after craniectomy), PRx might falsely indicate good autoregulation due to the increased compliance of the intracranial space and the altered status of ICP. In these situations, the correlation of ABP and the pulse amplitude of ICP (AMP) could be a better descriptor of cerebrovascular reactivity. This index is called the pressure-amplitude index (PAx) [2].

Since ICP is needed to calculate both PRx and PAx, both indices are considered to be invasively quantified markers of cerebral autoregulation. PRx and PAx are applicable for this purpose because a change in cerebral arterial blood volume (CaBV) results in a corresponding change in ICP. Therefore, PRx and PAx are indirect descriptors of the relationship between the mean arterial blood pressure (ABP) and the instantaneous blood volume inside the cranial space. However, with the help of the transcranial Doppler ultrasound (TCD) technique, it is possible to approximate CaBV noninvasively solely from cerebral blood flow velocities. The disadvantage of this method is that because of the unknown cross-sectional area of the insonated blood vessels, the direct calculation of blood volume is not possible. In this brief study, we aimed to investigate whether noninvasive estimation of relative CaBV with different models could be used to describe the cerebrovascular reactivity of TBI patients.

Materials and Methods

TBI patients received both continuous invasive (ABP and ICP) monitoring and daily noninvasive monitoring with TCD over the duration of admission to the Neurosciences Critical Care Unit (NCCU) at Addenbrooke's Hospital, Cambridge, United Kingdom. Data registered prospectively as a part of standard care were retrospectively reviewed with ICM+ soft-

A. Czigler (✉)
Brain Physics Laboratory, Division of Neurosurgery, Department of Clinical Neurosciences, University of Cambridge, Cambridge, UK

Department of Neurosurgery and Szentagothai Research Center, University of Pecs, Medical School, Pecs, Hungary

Institute for Translational Medicine, University of Pecs, Medical School, Pecs, Hungary

L. A. Calviello · P. Smielewski · M. Czosnyka
Brain Physics Laboratory, Division of Neurosurgery, Department of Clinical Neurosciences, University of Cambridge, Cambridge, UK
e-mail: ps10011@cam.ac.uk; mc141@medschl.cam.ac.uk

F. A. Zeiler
Division of Anaesthesia, Addenbrooke's Hospital, University of Cambridge, Cambridge, UK

Department of Surgery, Rady Faculty of Health Sciences, University of Manitoba, Winnipeg, Canada

Department of Human Anatomy and Cell Science, Rady Faculty of Health Sciences, University of Manitoba, Winnipeg, Canada

Biomedical Engineering, Faculty of Engineering, University of Manitoba, Winnipeg, Canada
e-mail: frederick.zeiler@umanitoba.ca

P. Toth
Department of Neurosurgery and Szentagothai Research Center, University of Pecs, Medical School, Pecs, Hungary

Institute for Translational Medicine, University of Pecs, Medical School, Pecs, Hungary

Reynolds Oklahoma Center on Aging, Donald W. Reynolds Department of Geriatric Medicine, University of Oklahoma Health Sciences Center, Oklahoma City, OK, USA

B. Depreitere et al. (eds.), *Intracranial Pressure and Neuromonitoring XVII*, Acta Neurochirurgica Supplement 131,
https://doi.org/10.1007/978-3-030-59436-7_33,

ware (Cambridge Enterprise, Cambridge, United Kingdom; http://www.neurosurg.cam.ac.uk/icmplus). The database was fully anonymized, no data on patient identifiers were available, and therefore no additional ethical approval or formal patient or proxy consent was needed. PRx and PAx were calculated as the correlation coefficients between 30 samples of 10-s averages of ABP and ICP (or the amplitude of ICP in the case of PAx).

The change in CaBV at any given time is determined by the volume of inflow and the volume of outflow from the cranial space. With TCD, only the velocity of the blood inflow is monitored. Based on the assumption made about the nature of outflow, two different methods can be used to model changes in CaBV [3]:

1. $\Delta C_{\mathrm{a}}\mathrm{BV}_{\mathrm{CFF}}(t)=\int_{t_0}^{t}\left(\mathrm{CBF}_{\mathrm{a}}(s)-\mathrm{meanCBFa}\right)\mathrm{d}s$
2. $\Delta C_{\mathrm{a}}\mathrm{BV}_{\mathrm{PFF}}(t)=\int_{t_0}^{t}\left(\mathrm{CBF}_{\mathrm{a}}(s)-\dfrac{\mathrm{ABP}(s)}{\mathrm{CVR}}\right)\mathrm{d}s$

where: *s*—the arbitrary time variable of integration, $\mathrm{CBF_a}$—cerebral blood flow, ABP—arterial blood pressure, and CVR—cerebrovascular resistance (CVR = meanABP/meanCBFa).

In a continuous flow forward (CFF) model, a non-pulsatile blood outflow is considered. The pulsatile inflow is equilibrated by a continuous outflow through the dural sinuses. Over a longer period, the outflow is considered to be equal to the inflow, so it can be calculated by averaging the inflow over several cardiac cycles (in this study, we used 5-min intervals).

The second equation presumes that the outflow—similarly to the inflow—is also pulsatile, becoming the pulsatile flow forward (PFF) model. The idea behind this theory is that the outflow is affected by the vasomotor tone of the regulating arterioles and the pulsatile ABP and can be determined by the ratio between ABP and cerebrovascular resistance.

With TCD monitoring, the cross-sectional area of the middle cerebral artery is unknown, and the CBF cannot be precisely calculated. In these equations, CBF can be replaced with CBFV, so the relative changes in CaBV can be estimated (Fig. 1).

The noninvasive counterparts of PRx (nPRx) and PAx (nPAx) were derived similarly, but with help of the estimated cerebral volumes. nPRx is calculated with CaBV instead of ICP, and nPAx with the pulse amplitude of CaBV instead of AMP. Both nPRx and nPAx were calculated using both the CFF and PFF models.

Results

Discussion

With TCD it is possible to derive noninvasive indices – nPRx and nPAx – of cerebrovascular reactivity by estimating the relative changes in CaBV. These indices can be calculated similarly to PRx and PAx if ICP is changed to CaBV. Figure 2 demonstrates that a change in CaBV is reflected in a corresponding change in ICP – which is the rationale of the usability of PRx [1]—but this could also explain the similarities between the invasive and noninvasive indices shown in Fig. 3. This analogous behavior opens up possibilities for the use of these noninvasive cerebrovascular reactivity indices: they may become clinically useful in the subacute phase of neuro-intensive care because they can provide further infor-

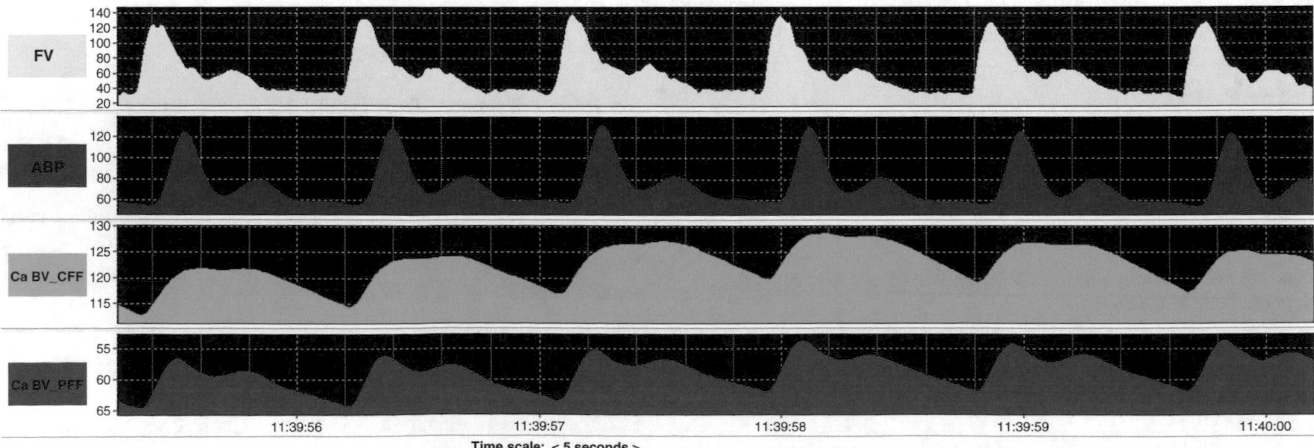

Fig. 1 Waveforms of flow velocity, arterial blood pressure and changes in CaBV, calculated both with the continuous flow forward and the pulsatile flow forward models. The pulsatile nature of CaBV with both methods is visible, but more prominent peaks appear with the PFF model

mation about autoregulation even after the removal of invasive ICP monitors. With other noninvasive techniques (continuous ABP monitoring via finger-cuff), cerebrovascular reactivity can be described without the necessity for invasive measurements, a PRx-like index can be quantified on a long-term follow-up and can be compared to PRx derived from early clinical care. In less severe cases of TBI, if invasive parameters are not available, noninvasive optimal cerebral perfusion pressure (nCPPopt) instead of traditionally invasive optimal cerebral perfusion pressure (CPPopt) could be determined and used to guide treatment.

The usability of either nPRx or nPAx is limited because these indices depend on continuous TCD monitoring technology. However, these techniques develop quickly, so further studies aimed at the investigation of nPRx and nPAx would be useful, which would enable clinicians to utilize the previously mentioned advantages immediately after the necessary improvements are made.

Acknowledgement Marek Czosnyka is supported by National Institute of Health Research, Cambridge Biomedical Research Centre.

Conflict of Interest **ICM+ is a software licensed by Cambridge Enterprise Ltd. (https://icmplus.neurosurg.cam.ac.uk). PS and MC have a financial interest in a fraction of licensing fees.**

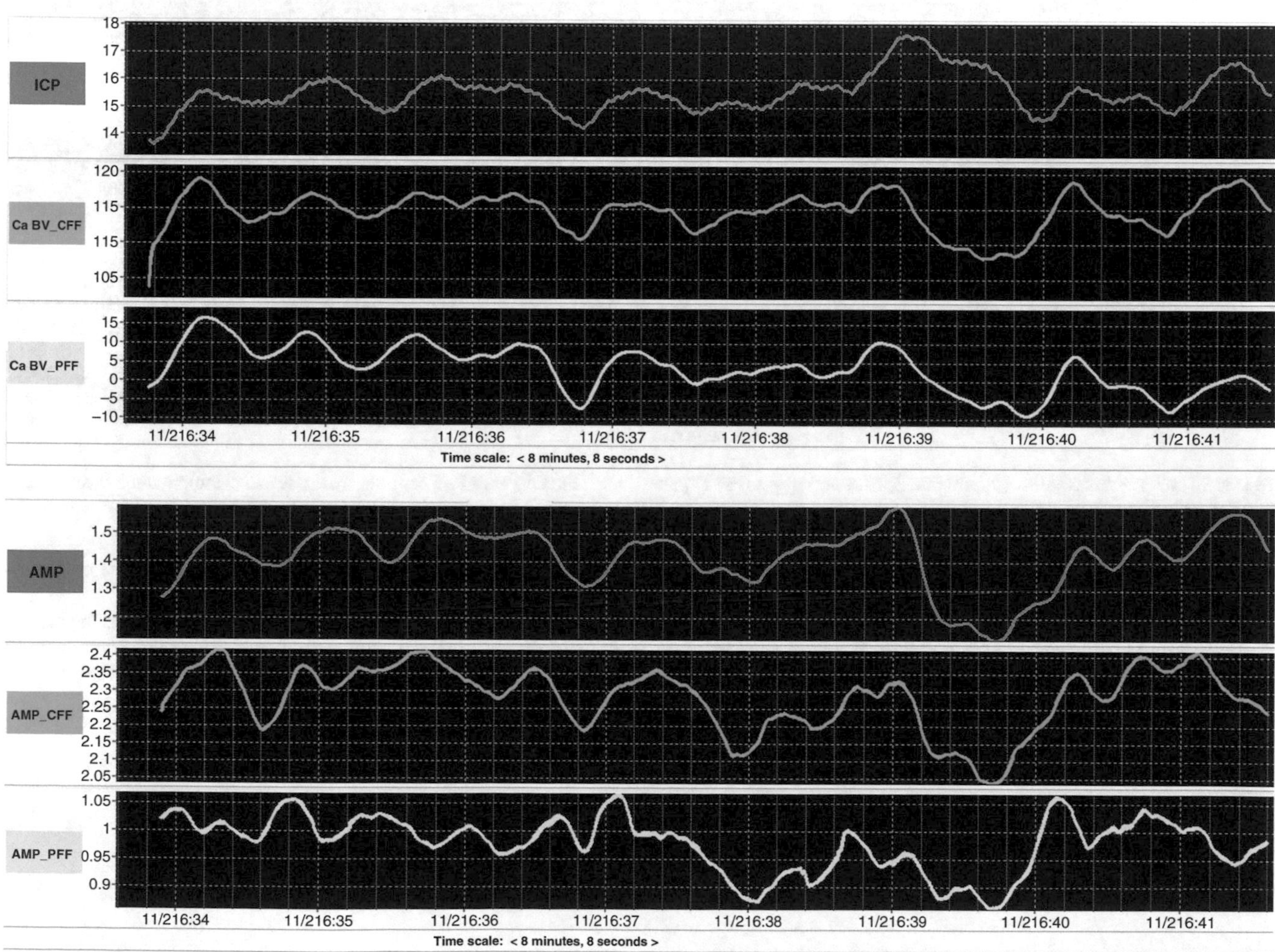

Fig. 2 A representative example of good coherence between slow waves in ICP and CaBV (upper panel) and between slow waves of AMP and pulse amplitude of CaBV (lower panel). Both the CFF and PFF models were used for the calculations

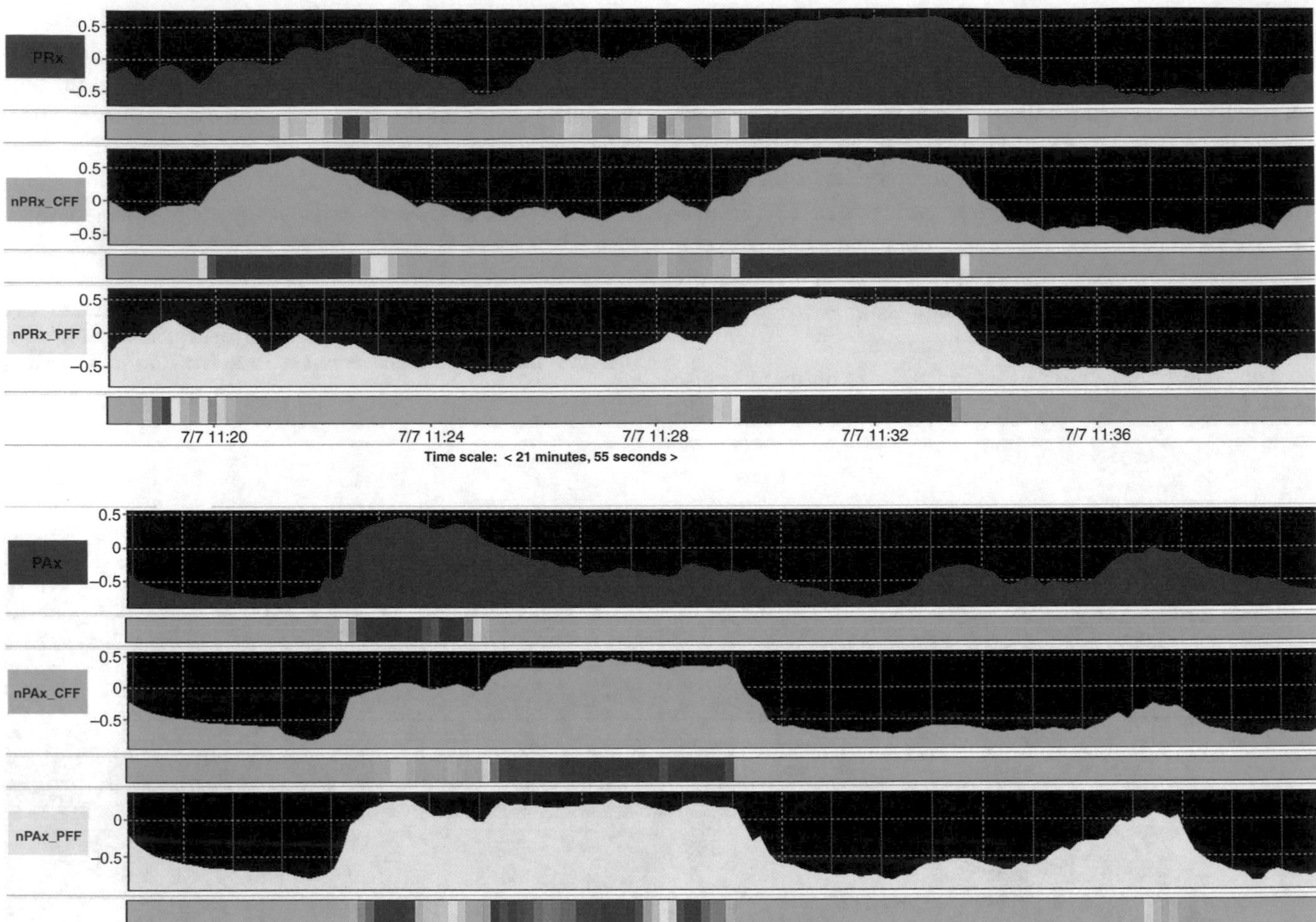

Fig. 3 Signals of PRx, nPRx (upper panel), PAx and nPAx (lower panel). Both the CFF and PFF models were used to calculate noninvasive autoregulation indices

References

1. Czosnyka M, Smielewski P, Kirkpatrick P, Laing RJ, Menon D, Pickard JD (1997) Continuous assessment of the cerebral vasomotor reactivity in head injury. Neurosurgery 41(1):11–19
2. Aries MJH, Czosnyka M, Budohoski KP, Kolias AG, Radolovich DK, Lavinio A, Pickard JD, Smielewski P (2012) Continuous monitoring of cerebrovascular reactivity using pulse waveform of intracranial pressure. Neurocrit Care 17(1):67–76
3. Uryga A, Kasprowicz M, Calviello L, Diehl RR, Kaczmarska K, Czosnyka M (2019) Assessment of cerebral hemodynamic parameters using pulsatile versus non-pulsatile cerebral blood outflow models. J Clin Monit Comput 33(1):85–94

Patient's Clinical Presentation and CPPopt Availability: Any Association?

Annalisa Liberti, Erta Beqiri, Ari Ercole, Manuel Cabeleira, Jeanette Tas, Frederick A. Zeiler, Marek Czosnyka, Peter Smielewski, Marcel J. Aries, and CENTER-TBI High Resolution Substudy Participants and Investigators

Introduction

Cerebral autoregulation (CA) is defined as the ability of the cerebrovascular system to maintain adequate cerebral blood flow (CBF) despite fluctuations in cerebral perfusion pressure (CPP) [1]. In patients with severe traumatic brain injury (TBI), CA is often impaired and related to worse outcomes. Over the years, the new concept of personalized therapy based on a patient's autoregulation has been introduced. Autoregulation-based individualized management of CPP promises to be a successful strategy, and it has already been proven from retrospective analysis that it might be related to outcome [2]. One of the methods created to estimate CA continuously at the bedside is the pressure reactivity index (PRx) [3]. PRx is calculated as the moving Pearson correlation between the slow waves of intracranial pressure (ICP) and mean arterial pressure (MAP) and it has proven to be able to detect the lower limit of autoregulation in animal models [4]. Several retrospective observations have shown correlations between average PRx and worse outcome when PRx values are above 0.2–0.3 [5–7]. In 2002, the CPPopt concept was introduced by plotting the values of PRx against CPP over the whole monitoring period for TBI patients [8]. The PRx/CPP relationship showed a U-shaped curve, with its nadir corresponding to the CPP at which PRx is the lowest and therefore the pressure reactivity is best preserved (CPPopt). Recent developments have made it possible to assess CPPopt automatically in individual patients and display it continuously at the bedside in real time (Fig. 1) [2, 9]. CPPopt guided therapy might therefore improve

Senior authors P. Smielewski and M. J. Aries contributed equally to this work.

CENTER-TBI High Resolution Sub-Study Participants and Investigators

A. Liberti (✉)
Department of Intensive Care, University Maastricht, Maastricht University Medical Center, Maastricht, The Netherlands

Department of Physiology and Transplantation, Milan University, Milan, Italy

E. Beqiri
Department of Physiology and Transplantation, Milan University, Milan, Italy

Brain Physics Laboratory, Division of Neurosurgery, Department of Clinical Neurosciences, University of Cambridge, Cambridge, UK

A. Ercole
Division of Anesthesia, University of Cambridge, Cambridge, UK
e-mail: ae105@cam.ac.uk

M. Cabeleira · M. Czosnyka · P. Smielewski
Brain Physics Laboratory, Division of Neurosurgery, Department of Clinical Neurosciences, University of Cambridge, Cambridge, UK
e-mail: mc916@cam.ac.uk; mc141@medschl.cam.ac.uk; ps10011@cam.ac.uk

J. Tas · M. J. Aries
Department of Intensive Care, University Maastricht, Maastricht University Medical Center, Maastricht, The Netherlands
e-mail: Jeanette.tas@mumc.nl; marcel.aries@mumc.nl

F. A. Zeiler
Division of Anesthesia, University of Cambridge, Cambridge, UK

Department of Surgery, Rady Faculty of Health Sciences, University of Manitoba, Winnipeg, Canada

Department of Anatomy and Cell Science, Rady Faculty of Health Sciences, University of Manitoba, Winnipeg, Canada

Biomedical Engineering, Faculty of Engineering, University of Manitoba, Winnipeg, Canada

Centre on Aging, University of Manitoba, Winnipeg, Canada
e-mail: frederick.zeiler@umanitoba.ca

B. Depreitere et al. (eds.), *Intracranial Pressure and Neuromonitoring XVII*, Acta Neurochirurgica Supplement 131,
https://doi.org/10.1007/978-3-030-59436-7_34,

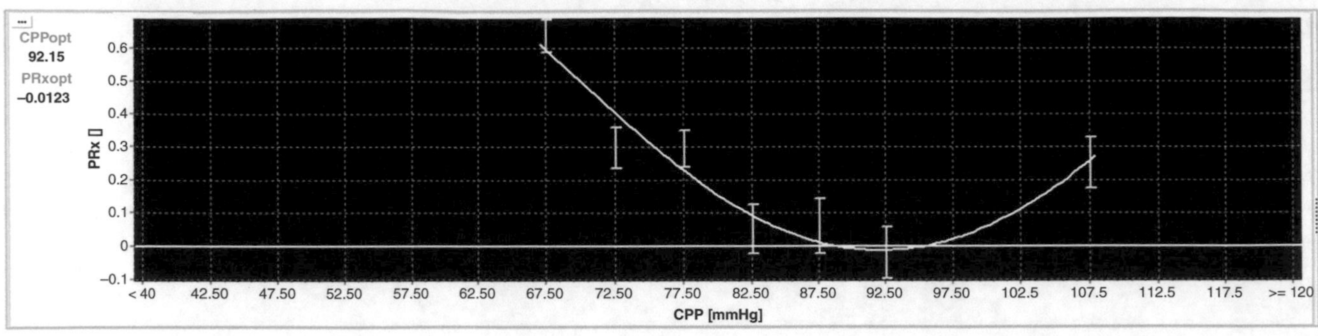

Fig. 1 The CPP-PRx error bar over a certain period in a single patient with a fitted U-shaped curve (for more information about CPPopt and the fitting process, visit the website www.cppopt.org). In this example, the CPPopt would be around 92 mmHg

autoregulation, and its feasibility, safety, and effectiveness are currently being tested in a randomized controlled trial in four European centers (CPPOpt Guided Therapy: Assessment of Target Effectiveness, COGiTATE, www.cppopt.org) [10].

In the traditional CPPopt calculations based on a 4-h moving window, the yield was shown to be 50–60% of the total CPP monitored time [2]. With the weighted multiwindow approaches, the CPPopt availability improved to 94 ± 2.1% (mean ± SD) [9]. The importance of achieving high yield is crucial for the management of TBI patients in the light of future trials because it is important to know whether there are particular categories that are not likely to benefit from this approach, because CPPopt might not be readily available most of the time (Fig. 2a, b). This prompted our research question to investigate the relationship between demographic, clinical, and admission factors and the average CPPopt yield.

Material and Methods

This retrospective analysis was performed using ICP and ABP waveforms from the high-resolution cohort of the Collaborative European NeuroTrauma Effectiveness Research in TBI (CENTER-TBI) study. Patients in this cohort were not treated taking PRx or CPPopt information into account. The total cohort contained 271 TBI patients. After the exclusion of 41 patients who received ICP monitoring by an external ventricular drainage system with noisy or unreliable signals (due to continuous or intermittent Cerebrospinal fluid (CSF) drainage), 230 patients were left for analysis. CPPopt was calculated with ICM+ software (https://icmplus.neurosurg.cam.ac.uk) using a weighted multiwindow approach with the calculation criteria used in the COGiTATE study [10]. Several admission variables were selected: sex, age, hypoxia and hypotension at the trauma scene, Marshall computed tomography (CT) score, admission Glasgow Coma Scale (GCS), injury severity score (ISS), therapeutic intensity level (TIL) for the first 24 h, pupil reactivity, and decompressive craniectomy (DC) (Tables 1 and 2). The admission variables hypoxia, hypotension, and pupils were dichotomized into present or absent. Pupil reactivity was scored as bilateral reactive, bilateral unreactive, or unilateral unreactive. Pupils were then reclassified as a binary into normal if both pupils were reactive and pathological when one or both pupils were not reactive to light. The GCS at admission was divided into two groups, above and below 8, as an estimate of initial head trauma severity (mild/moderate if GCS > 8 and severe if GCS ≤ 8). CPPopt yield was considered as the percentage of monitored time (%) with CPPopt available given the presence of CPP. The TIL score was considered as an estimate of intracranial hypertension severity and the need for intensive treatment [11]. The aim of TIL is to produce a quantitative estimate of the interventions by assigning numerical scores to each TIL intervention and summing these. The maximum score is 38. DC was investigated as a contributing factor because there are worries that the pressure-volume characteristics necessary for reliable PRx calculations are violated [12]. In this cohort of patients, DC refers to both primary and secondary craniectomy. Statistical analysis was done with R Studio software (version 3.5.1). Nonparametric tests were used after testing the distribution of the variables through a Shapiro-Wilk test. Linear regression models were used comparing the CPPopt yield (%) to continuous variables (age, ISS, and 24-h TIL score for the first day). Mann-Whitney U and Kruskal-Wallis tests were used to compare CPPopt yield (%) for categorical and ordinal variables. A *p*-value <0.05 was considered for statistical significance.

Results

The patient characteristics are listed in Tables 1 and 2. The median CPPopt yield was 80.7% (interquartile range (IQR) 70.9–87.4) for the whole ICP/CPP monitoring period, suggesting the availability of CPPopt values during most of the

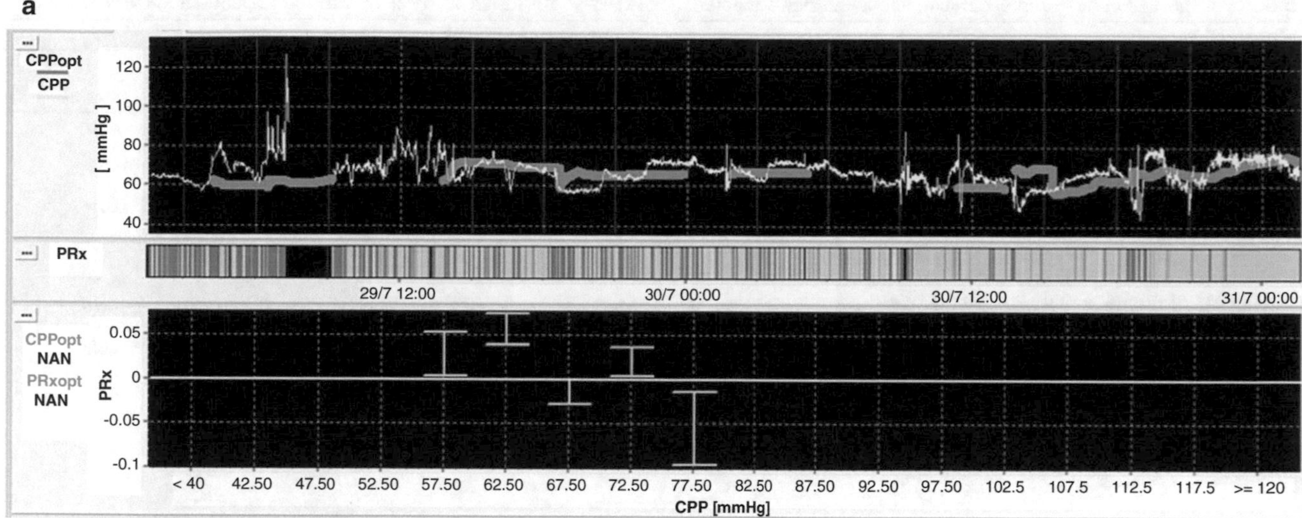

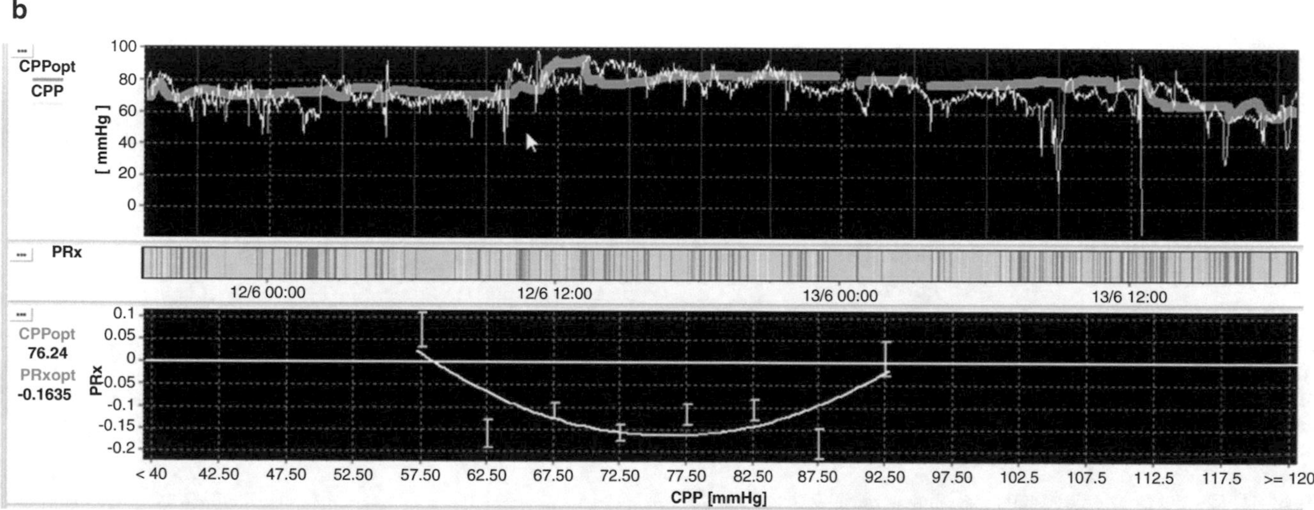

Fig. 2 Examples of CPPopt time trends generated by continuous automated algorithm: CPPopt (thick line), CPP (thin line), PRx risk bar (with bold values indicating impaired autoregulation). PRx and CPP are selected for plotting the error bar chart. (**a**) An example when the (multiwindow and weighted) CPPopt time trend has several gaps limiting its use for CPP individualized management. Of note, the PRx/CPP relationship chart over this selected monitored period does not in fact form a proper U-shaped curve. (**b**) In this example, the CPPopt value is almost always available. Of note, the PRx/CPP plot over the selected period in this example shows a U-shaped curve

recording period. All variables had a nonparametric distribution, showing the heterogeneity of the TBI population in this multicenter cohort. In the cohort analyzed, the median 24-h TIL score for the first day was 6 (IQR 4–9), and the median ISS score was 34 (IQR 25–43). No statistical relationship between any of the considered variables and CPPopt yield was found (Table 3).

Discussion

None of the admission demographic variables correlated with the CPPopt yield over the whole monitored period in a multicenter cohort of TBI patients. The importance of the CPPopt guided therapy concept lies in the fact that it might improve CA and, therefore, could improve the clinical outcome in TBI patients [13]. An important prerequisite of the application of the CPPopt concept at the bedside is the continuous availability of the automatically generated values of CPPopt, so that they could be used as clinical CPP targets. The first observation by Steiner et al. in 2002 about the CPPopt concept considered the total monitored time period identifying a single CPPopt value for all the patients and thus not ready for clinical use at the bedside [8]. Over the years the CPPopt algorithm and the bedside software interface have been modified using initially a 4-h moving single window [2] and later with a weighted multiwindow algorithm approach to improve the yield and stability of the CPPopt target [9, 10]. Weersink et al. investigated the relationship

Table 1 Categorical demographic, clinical, and admission variables

Categorical variable	*N* (%)
Gender	Male 178 (77.4)
	Female 51 (22.2)
	NA 1 (0.4)
Hypoxia at trauma scene	Yes 16 (6.9)
	No 213 (92.6)
	NA 1 (0.4)
Hypotension at trauma scene	Yes 7 (3)
	No 222 (96.9)
Marshall CT score	I 7 (3)
	II 71 (30)
	III 13 (5.7)
	IV 3 (1.3)
	V 6 (2.6)
	VI 71 (30)
	NA 59 (25.7)
Pupil reactivity	Bilateral reactive 159 (69.1)
	Unilateral reactive 19 (8.2)
	Both unreactive 39 (17)
	NA 13 (5.7)
Decompressive craniectomy[a]	Yes 48 (20.1)
	No 180 (78.3)
	NA 2 (0.9)

NA Not available
[a]These variables consist of primary and secondary decompressive craniectomies

Table 2 Continuous demographic and clinical variables

Variable	Median (IQR)
Age, years	49 (30–63)
Intracranial pressure (first 24 h), mmHg	11.9 (8.6–15.9)
Cerebral perfusion pressure (whole recorded period), mmHg	71.4 (64.9–77.9)
"Optimal" cerebral perfusion pressure (whole recorded period), mmHg	72.0 (65.4–77.4)
Admission Glasgow Coma Score	6 (3–15)
24-h therapeutic intensity level (TIL) of first day	6 (4–9)
Injury severity score (ISS)	34 (25–43)

between the absence of a CPPopt curve and physiological and therapy variables in a two-center study [14]. Conditions related to the absence of a CPPopt curve were a high amount of sedative drugs, administration of high-dose vasopressors, using neuromuscular blockers, low variance in slow ABP waves, and status after DC. The absolute ICP values were also associated with an absence of CPPopt. CPPopt appeared

Table 3 Univariate analysis of selected variables and CPPopt yield

Continuous Variables			
Variable	CPPopt yield correlation coefficient (*r*)		*p*-value
Age, years	−0.09		0.16
ISS	0.03		0.64
24-h TIL (day 1)	0.03		0.59
Categorical variables			
Variable	CPPopt yield % (Median (IQR))		*p*-value
Sex	Male	80.6 (71.3–88.3)	0.48[a]
	Female	81.1 (69.9–85.9)	
Hypoxia	Present	76.6 (56.4–83.8)	0.14[a]
	Absent	81.1 (71.9–87.6)	
Hypotension	Present	86.2 (81.7–88.4)	0.16[a]
	Absent	80.7 (70.5–87.3)	
Marshall CT score	I	83.3 (75.5–87.3)	0.99[b]
	II	81.3 (72–87.8)	
	III	79.2 (74.5–86.1)	
	IV	78.7 (75.6–83.9)	
	V	59 (52.1–68.6)	
	VI	78.4 (71.6–86.7)	
Admission GCS	GCS ≤ 8	80.9 (71.6–87)	0.85[a]
	GCS > 8	81.9 (66.8–87.6)	

Table 3 (continued)

Continuous Variables				
Variable	CPPopt yield correlation coefficient (*r*)			*p*-value
Pupil Reactivity	Normal	Bilateral reactive	77.1 (63.8–85.6)	0.97[a]–0.33[b,c]
	Pathological	Unilateral reactive	83 (70.9–87.7)	
		Unreactive	81.6 (72–88)	
Decompressive craniectomy	Present		80.8 (71.6–86.3)	0.99[a]
	Absent		80.7 (70.5–87.6)	

[a]Mann-Whitney *U* test used
[b]Kruskal Wallis test used
[c]We dichotomized pupil reactivity in "normal" (both pupils reactive) or "pathological" (unilateral or bilateral unreactive) using a Mann-Whitney *U* test. A further analysis tested three categories (bilateral reactive/unilateral reactive/bilateral not reactive) through a Kruskal-Wallis test

more frequently in periods with higher ICP levels, perhaps owing to fact that a stronger association is present between slow fluctuations in ABP and ICP in the steep part of pressure-volume curves, thereby producing possibly more robust pressure reactivity values [3]. The multiwindow approach increased the yield considerably (reaching values above 90%) [9]. This algorithm was adapted to prospective bedside use within the COGiTATE study, introducing safety and stability measures that decreased the yield from the original multiwindow algorithm [10]. However, the retrospective analysis performed in this multicenter database showed that a high overall CPPopt yield was found (>80% of monitored time) with the algorithm suggested for prospective use by the COGiTATE study. Moreover, the yield was neither negatively influenced by admission criteria including demographic variables like sex and age or clinical variables like hypoxia and hypotension at the trauma scene, Marshall CT score, admission GCS, pupil reactivity, and DC. Furthermore, the 24-h ISS and TIL scores—as an estimate of (head) trauma severity—were not related to CPPopt yield.

Conclusions

This retrospective analysis showed no association between CPPopt yield and demographic, clinical, and management characteristics.

Acknowledgements The data used here were collected as part of a study supported by the European Union seventh Framework Programme (Grant 602150), Collaborative European NeuroTrauma Effectiveness Research in Traumatic Brain Injury (Center-TBI).

CENTER-TBI High-Resolution (HR ICU) Substudy Participants and Investigators: Audny Anke, Ronny Beer, BoMichael Bellander, Andras Buki, Marco Carbonara, Arturo Chieregato, Giuseppe Citerio, Endre Czeiter, Bart Depreitere, Shirin Frisvold, Raimund Helbok, Stefan Jankowski, Danile Kondziella, Lars-Owe Koskinen, Ana Kowark, David K. Menon, Geert Meyfroidt, Kirsten Moeller, David Nelson, Anna Piippo-Karjalainen, Andreea Radoi, Arminas Ragauskas, Rahul Raj, Jonathan Rhodes, Saulius Rocka, Rolf Rossaint, Juan Sahuquillo, Oliver Sakowitz, Nino Stocchetti, Nina Sundström, Riikka Takala, Tomas Tamosuitis, Olli Tenovuo, Peter Vajkoczy, Alessia Vargiolu, Rimantas Vilcinis, Stefan Wolf, Alexander Younsi.

Disclosure **Authors MC and PS have a financial interest in part of the licensing fees for ICM+ software.**
MC is supported by NIHR, Biomedical Research Centre, Cambridge, UK.

References

1. Lassen NA (1968) Autoregulation of cerebral blood flow. Circ Res 15(Suppl):201–204
2. Aries MJH et al (2012) Continuous determination of optimal cerebral perfusion pressure in traumatic brain injury. Crit Care Med 40(8):2456–2463
3. Czosnyka M et al (1997) Continuous assessment of the cerebral vasomotor reactivity in head injury. Neurosurgery 41(1):11–19
4. Brady KM, Lee JK, Kibler KK, Easley RB, Koehler RC, Shaffner DH (2008) Continuous measurement of autoregulation by spontaneous fluctuations in cerebral perfusion pressure: comparison of 3 methods. Stroke 39:2531–2537
5. Lavinio A et al (2008) Cerebrovascular reactivity and autonomic drive following traumatic brain injury. Acta Neurochir Suppl 102:3–7. https://doi.org/10.1007/978-3-211-85578-2_1
6. Petkus V, Krakauskait S, Preiksaitis A et al (2016) Association between the outcome of traumatic brain injury patients and cerebrovascular autoregulation, cerebral perfusion pressure, age, and injury grades. Medicina (Lithuania) 52(1):46–53
7. Sorrentino E, Diedler J, Kasprowicz M, Budohoski KP, Haubrich C, Smielewski P, Outtrim JG, Manktelow A, Hutchinson PJ, Pickard JD, Menon DK, Czosnyka M (2012) Critical thresholds for cerebrovascular reactivity after traumatic brain injury. Neurocrit Care 16(2):258–266
8. Steiner LA, Czosnyka M, Piechnik SK, et al. (2002) Continuous monitoring of cerebrovascular pressure reactivity allows determination of optimal cerebral perfusion pressure in patients with traumatic brain injury. Critical Care, 30(4):733–738
9. Liu X et al (2017) Monitoring of optimal cerebral perfusion pressure in traumatic brain injured patients using a multi-window weighting algorithm. J Neurotrauma 34:3081–3088
10. Beqiri E, Smielewski P, Robba C et al (2019) Feasibility of individualised severe traumatic brain injury management using an automated assessment of optimal cerebral perfusion pressure: the COGiTATE phase II study protocol. BMJ Open 9:e030727. https://doi.org/10.1136/bmjopen-2019-030727

11. Maset AL, Marmarou A, Ward JD, Choi S, Lutz HA, Brooks D, Moulton RJ, DeSalles A, Muizelaar JP, Turner H (1987) Pressure-volume index in head injury. J Neurosurg 67:832–840
12. Timofeev et al. (2008) "Effect of decompressive craniectomy on intracranial pressure and cerebrospinal compensation following traumatic brain injury"J Neurosurg; 108(1):66–73
13. Dias C et al (2015) Optimal cerebral perfusion pressure management at bedside: a single-center pilot study. NCC 23:92–102
14. Weersink C.S.A et al. (2015) Clinical and physiological events that contribute to the success rate of finding "Optimal" cerebral perfusion pressure in Severe Brain Trauma Patients Crit Care Med; 43(9):1952–63

Optimal Cerebral Perfusion Pressure Based on Intracranial Pressure-Derived Indices of Cerebrovascular Reactivity: Which One Is Better for Outcome Prediction in Moderate/Severe Traumatic Brain Injury?

Alexander Lilja-Cyron, Frederick A. Zeiler, Erta Beqiri, Manuel Cabeleira, Peter Smielewski, and Marek Czosnyka

Introduction

Intracranial pressure (ICP) is a key component of multimodal monitoring in neurocritical care [1]. ICP-derived indices of cerebrovascular reactivity (and, indirectly, autoregulation of cerebral blood flow) have been developed as measures to improve understanding of brain status from available neuromonitoring variables. These indices are moving correlation coefficients between slow-wave vasogenic fluctuations in ICP (or ICP pulse wave amplitude, AMP) and mean arterial blood pressure (MAP) or cerebral perfusion pressure (CPP) [2–4]. If cerebrovascular autoregulation is intact, the vascular bed reacts to an increase in arterial blood pressure (ABP) with a vasoconstriction causing a decrease in ICP [2]. Thus, theoretically, an intact cerebrovascular reactivity corresponds to a negative value of these indices (i.e., a negative correlation coefficient), whereas a positive value corresponds to a passive transmission of ABP to ICP (i.e., a positive correlation coefficient).

The pressure reactivity index (PRx), i.e., the correlation coefficient between ICP and MAP, is the most extensively studied measure of cerebrovascular reactivity [5–7]. In retrospective clinical studies, PRx is an independent predictor of outcome in patients with traumatic brain injury (TBI) [8]. Plotted against CPP, a theoretical "optimal" CPP (CPPopt) can be derived from the lowest point of this U-shaped curve [9], and deviation of the actual CPP from this CPPopt is associated with outcomes following TBI: CPP below CPPopt is associated with increased mortality, while CPP above CPPopt is associated with increased rate of severe disability [10]. Therapeutic targeting of CPPopt is now being tested in patients with TBI in an ongoing randomized clinical feasibility study (COGiTATE, ClinicalTrials.gov identifier: NCT02982122). Additional ICP-derived indices of cerebral autoregulation are PAx (correlation coefficient between AMP and MAP) and RAC (correlation coefficient between AMP and CPP) [11, 12].

The objective of this study is to compare the association between CPPopt calculated from different ICP-derived

A. Lilja-Cyron (✉)
Brain Physics Laboratory, Division of Neurosurgery, Department of Clinical Neurosciences, Addenbrooke's Hospital, University of Cambridge, Cambridge, UK

Department of Neurosurgery, Rigshospitalet, Copenhagen, Denmark

F. A. Zeiler
Division of Anaesthesia, Addenbrooke's Hospital, University of Cambridge, Cambridge, UK

Rady Faculty of Health Sciences, Department of Surgery, University of Manitoba, Winnipeg, Canada

Clinician Investigator Program, Rady Faculty of Health Sciences, University of Manitoba, Winnipeg, Canada
e-mail: Frederick.Zeiler@umanitoba.ca

E. Beqiri
Brain Physics Laboratory, Division of Neurosurgery, Department of Clinical Neurosciences, Addenbrooke's Hospital, University of Cambridge, Cambridge, UK

Department of Pathophysiology and Transplantation, University of Milan, Milano, Italy

M. Cabeleira · P. Smielewski
Brain Physics Laboratory, Division of Neurosurgery, Department of Clinical Neurosciences, Addenbrooke's Hospital, University of Cambridge, Cambridge, UK
e-mail: mc916@cam.ac.uk; ps10011@cam.ac.uk

M. Czosnyka
Brain Physics Laboratory, Division of Neurosurgery, Department of Clinical Neurosciences, Addenbrooke's Hospital, University of Cambridge, Cambridge, UK

Institute of Electronic Systems, Warsaw University of Technology, Warsaw, Poland
e-mail: mc141@medschl.cam.ac.uk

B. Depreitere et al. (eds.), *Intracranial Pressure and Neuromonitoring XVII*, Acta Neurochirurgica Supplement 131,
https://doi.org/10.1007/978-3-030-59436-7_35,

indices of cerebrovascular reactivity (PRx, PAx, and RAC) and clinical outcomes in patients with moderate to severe TBI with a special focus on time spent with CPP below CPPopt and "dose" of cerebral hypoperfusion, i.e., integrating both time and severity of CPP below CPPopt.

Methods

Patient Demographics

This retrospective study includes 200 patients admitted to the neurocritical care unit of Addenbrooke's Hospital with moderate to severe TBI between 2003 and 2015. Patients were randomly sampled from our database based on functional outcome at 6 months measured on the Glasgow Outcome Scale (GOS) [13], i.e., we identified a sample population including 100 patients who were dead (GOS 1) at 6 months and 100 patients who had good recovery (GOS 4–5). We chose to study cerebral hypoperfusion (CPP below CPPopt) in particular because this was previously associated with increased mortality, whereas cerebral hyperperfusion (CPP above CPPopt) was associated with severe disability [10]. This methodology was chosen in order to maximize outcome prediction capabilities using the different indices and thresholds. Additional patient demographic data obtained from the database were age, sex, and admission Glasgow Coma Score (GCS). Continuous recording of ABP and ICP was performed as part of a local monitoring protocol and treatment in the Neurosciences Critical Care Unit (NCCU) at Addenbrooke's Hospital. The treatment protocol was a CPP/ICP-oriented algorithm with target CPP above 60 mmHg and ICP below 20 mmHg [14]. All data were fully anonymized, and no attempt was made to re-access clinical records for additional information.

Data Acquisition

ABP was monitored invasively through an arterial line (radial or femoral) using a standard pressure monitoring kit (Baxter Healthcare, CardioVascular Group, Irvine, CA) and was zeroed at the level of the right atrium. ICP was monitored using an intraparenchymal strain-gauge probe (Codman ICP MicroSensor, Codman & Shurtleff, Raynham, MA) inserted into the frontal cortex. All signals were sampled at 50 Hz or higher and recorded using ICM+ software (Cambridge Enterprise, Cambridge, UK, http://www.neurosurg.cam.ac.uk/icmplus, version 8.4) digitally directly from GE Solar monitors. ICM+ was later used for the retrospective analysis. Signal artifacts (e.g., caused by tracheal suctioning or arterial line flushing) were visually identified in each patient recording and removed manually. Data were recorded and analyzed anonymously as part of a standard audit approved by the Neurocritical Care Users Group Committee.

Signal Processing

Postacquisition signal processing of ICP and ABP recordings was performed using the ICM+ software (referenced earlier). CPP was calculated as CPP = MAP – ICP, and AMP was calculated as the fundamental Fourier amplitude of the ICP pulse wave in a 10-second window. Ten-second moving averages (updated every 10 s to avoid data overlap) were calculated for all recorded signals: ICP, ABP (producing MAP), AMP, and CPP. Averages over 10 s were used to suppress the influence of the pulse and respiratory waves on the recorded signals, focusing on slow-wave vasogenic fluctuations in signals associated with cerebrovascular reactivity. Time-dependent values for PRx, PAx, RAC, and, based on these, CPPopt were calculated for all patients as described in the following sections. Finally, data for further statistical analyses were provided in the form of patient-specific minute-by-minute time series, including all variables of interest. These were exported from ICM+ into comma-separated value (CSV) files, and these were collapsed into one continuous data sheet (compiled from all patients). In this dataset and using SAS (described in what follows), time spent with CPP below CPPopt and dose of CPP below CPPopt (the area between the actual CPP curve and the CPPopt curve with the unit mmHg*hour) was calculated for each patient.

Calculation of Indices of Cerebrovascular Reactivity (PRx, PAx, and RAC)

The ICP-derived indices of autoregulation were calculated in ICM+ every minute as the moving Pearson correlation coefficient between ICP and MAP (for PRx), AMP and MAP (for PAx), or AMP and CPP (for RAC), using 30 consecutive 10-s windows (5 min of data, i.e., 80% overlap of data).

Calculation of CPPopt

For each of the three indices, we calculated CPPopt using the multiwindow weighting algorithm recently published by Liu et al. [15]. In short, this approach uses varying window length ranging from 2 to 8 h with 10-min increments instead of the fixed 4-h window used in previous investigations. Hence, using this optimization algorithm 36 CPP-PRx plots are generated for each time point, and these plots are weighted based on three rules: (1) a longer window duration receives a lower weight (i.e., recent data are weighted higher); (2) a smaller curve fit error receives a higher weight (using full fit error); and (3) a nonparabolic curve receives a lower weight. Finally, a CPPopt value is computed as the weighted average of the 36 available CPP values.

Statistical Analysis

Baseline demographics for the entire cohort and separated by outcome group are presented as absolute values, percentages, and median values/interquartile range (IQR), as appropriate. Neuromonitoring data are presented as mean and standard deviation. Statistical analysis was carried out using SAS 9.3 (SAS Institute, Cary, NC, USA). For all tests described in what follows, *P*-values lower than 0.05 were considered statistically significant. Differences in baseline variables between outcome groups (GOS 1 = dead vs. GOS 4–5 = good recovery) were tested using a chi-squared test for categorical variables and Wilcoxon signed-rank test for numerical variables. Univariate binary logistic regression analysis was performed for the predictor variables obtained (time/dose of CPP below CPPopt) based on CPPopt estimation using the three ICP-derived indices of cerebrovascular reactivity (PRx, PAx, and RAC). The binary outcome was good recovery (GOS 4–5) vs. death (GOS 1) at 6-month follow-up. Multivariate binary logistic regression analyses (with the same outcome and predictor variables) were performed, which included baseline demographic variables: age, sex, and admission GCS. Additionally, we performed receiver operating curve (ROC) analyses using area under the curve (AUC). Comparison of the AUCs from multivariate models including the different predictor variables was conducted using Delong's test.

Results

Patient Characteristics

In total, we included 200 patients with moderate to severe TBI. Median age was 38 years (IQR 23–56 years), and 80.5% of the included patients were male. Baseline characteristics for patients in the two outcome groups are displayed in Table 1. There was no significant difference between patients with good recovery (GOS 4-5) and those who died (GOS 1) in connection with sex (77 vs. 85%, $P = 0.28$), length of the multimodal monitoring period (135.7 vs. 137.3 h, $P = 0.27$), and MAP (93.9 vs. 95 mmHg). Patients with good recovery were younger (29.5 vs. 40.0 years, $P < 0.001$), had higher admission GCS (8 vs. 6, $P < 0.002$), had lower ICP (14.4 vs. 19.3 mmHg, $P < 0.001$), and had higher CPP (79.5 vs. 76.4 mmHg, $P < 0.001$).

Table 1 Baseline demographics and calculated intracranial pressure–derived indices of cerebrovascular reactivity

	All patients	Dead (GOS 1)	Good recovery (GOS 4–5)	P
No.	200	100	100	
Age (years)	38 [23–56]	47 [30–60]	29.5 [20–45]	<0.001*
Sex (F/M)	39/161	16/84	23/77	0.28
Admission GCS	3 [7–9]	6 [3–8]	8 [5–11]	<0.002*
Duration of monitoring (hours)	137.3 [68–216]	137.3 [69.4–212]	135.7 [68–222]	0.27
ICP (mmHg)	16.8 (8.4)	19.3 (10.4)	14.4 (4.9)	<0.001*
MAP (mmHg)	94.4 (8.2)	95.0 (8.9)	93.9 (7.5)	0.37
CPP (mmHg)	77.9 (9.6)	76.4 (11.6)	79.5 (6.7)	<0.001*
PRx	0.089 (0.185)	0.165 (0.203)	0.014 (0.129)	<0.001*
PAx	−0.007 (0.067)	0.007 (0.074)	−0.021 (0.056)	0.002*
RAC	−0.062 (0.068)	−0.045 (0.075)	−0.078 (0.056)	<0.001*

Numerical variables presented as either median [IQR] or mean (SD). *CPP* cerebral perfusion pressure, *GCS* Glasgow Coma Score, *GOS* Glasgow Outcome Scale, *ICP* intracranial pressure, *MAP* mean arterial pressure, *PAx* pulse-amplitude index, *PRx* pressure reactivity index, *RAC* correlation coefficient between intracranial pulse wave amplitude and CPP

[*] *P*-value < 0.05

Table 2 Optimal cerebral perfusion pressure (CPPopt) calculated from intracranial pressure (ICP)-derived indices of cerebrovascular reactivity

	All patients	Dead (GOS 1)	Good recovery (GOS 4–5)	*P*
Calculated CPPopt value: (mmHg)				
– PRx	77.4 (7.7)	77.5 (8.0)	77.2 (7.4)	0.532
– PAx	78.5 (8.6)	77.9 (9.1)	79.1 (8.0)	0.646
– RAC	77.1 (8.6)	77.0 (8.7)	77.2 (8.5)	0.970
Monitoring time with valid CPPopt curve (%)				
– PRx	92.9 [81.2–97.2]	92.7 [74.7–97.5]	96.8 [93.0–99.9]	0.129
– PAx	86.7 [73.1–93.0]	83.9 [68.7–91.6]	93.2 [87.9–100.0]	0.071
– RAC	84.6 [72.4–91.3]	84.9 [70.8–91.5]	91.0 [84.2–99.9]	0.869
Difference between observed CPP and calculated CPPopt: (mmHg)				
– PRx	0.8 (6.1)	−1.2 (6.9)	2.7 (4.4)	<0.001*
– PAx	−0.2 (5.0)	−1.4 (5.5)	1.0 (4.1)	0.001*
– RAC	0.8 (5.9)	−0.9 (6.3)	2.5 (5.0)	<0.001*

Numerical variables presented as either median [IQR] or mean (SD). *CPP* cerebral perfusion pressure, *CPPopt* optimal cerebral perfusion pressure, *PAx* pulse-amplitude index, *PRx* pressure reactivity index, *RAC* correlation coefficient between intracranial pulse wave amplitude and CPP
**P*-value < 0.05

Indices of Autoregulation and CPPopt

Patients with good recovery had lower values of all autoregulatory indices compared to patients who died (Table 1): PRx (0.014 vs. 0.165, $P < 0.001$), PAx (−0.021 vs. 0.007, $P = 0.002$), and RAC (−0.078 vs. −0.045, $P < 0.001$). Based on these indices, it was possible to obtain a CPPopt curve in 92.9% (PRx), 86.7% (PAx), and 84.6% (RAC) of the total monitoring period with equal length of monitoring in the two outcome groups (Table 2). Overall, there was no difference between the calculated CPPopt values in the patients with good recovery vs. those who died, but in the latter group, observed CPP was lower than calculated CPPopt (using any of the three indices of cerebrovascular reactivity) and significantly lower than in patients with good recovery (Table 2).

Time/Dose of CPP Below CPPopt

Using the different indices of cerebrovascular reactivity to calculate CPPopt, overall time spent with CPP below CPPopt ranged from 46.7% (using PRx) to 50.3% (using PAx), and the difference between observed CPP and calculated CPPopt was positive (i.e., CPP was above CPPopt) for patients with good recovery and negative for patients who died (Table 2). For all indices, patients with good recovery spent less time with CPP below CPPopt (all $P \leq 0.001$) (Table 3). Doses of CPP below CPPopt ranged from 504 mmHg*hour (using RAC) to 617 mmHg*hour (PAx) and was only significantly lower in patients with good recovery when the CPPopt calculation was based on PRx (479 vs. 689 mmHg*hour) and RAC (442 vs. 567 mmHg*hour) (Table 3).

Table 3 Time/dose spent with cerebral perfusion pressure (CPP) below optimal CPP (CPPopt)

	All patients	Dead (GOS 1)	Good recovery (GOS 4–5)	*P*
Monitoring time with CPP below CPPopt (%)				
– PRx	46.7	52.1	41.3	<0.001*
– PAx	50.3	53.8	47.0	0.001*
– RAC	47.4	52.3	42.7	<0.001*
*Dose of CPP below CPPopt (mmHg*hour)*				
– PRx	583.6	689.4	478.9	0.009*
– PAx	617.1	660.4	574.7	0.13
– RAC	504.0	567.0	441.7	0.016*

PAx pulse-amplitude index, *PRx* pressure reactivity index, *RAC* correlation coefficient between intracranial pulse wave amplitude and CPP
**P*-value < 0.05

Outcome Prediction Using Time/Dose of CPP Below CPPopt

In the univariate logistic regression analyses, the percentage of monitoring time spent with CPP below CPPopt (calculated from all indices) was significantly associated with outcome (death vs. good recovery) (Table 4), with ROC AUCs ranging from 0.635 (PAx) to 0.693 (RAC). Using dose of cerebral hypotension (CPP below CPPopt), only calculations from PRx were associated with outcome (Table 4), with ROC AUCs of 0.823 (time) and 0.802 (dose).

In the multivariate analysis, the baseline model, which included age, sex, and admission GCS, had an AUC of 0.762 ($P < 0.0001$), with only age and sex being independently associated with outcome (data not shown). When adding time/dose of CPP below CPPopt, all multivariate models predicted the dichotomous outcome measure, but additional value of the prediction was only significantly added by the PRx-based calculations of time spent with CPP below CPPopt and dose of CPP below CPPopt (Table 4).

Table 4 Outcome prediction (good recovery vs. death) at 6-month follow-up based on time spent with cerebral perfusion pressure (CPP) below optimal cerebral perfusion pressure (CPPopt)

	Univariate		Multivariate			
	AUC	*P*	AUC	*P*	AUC[a]	*P*
Baseline model (age, sex, and GCS)	–	–	0.762	<0.0001*	–	–
Monitoring time with CPP below CPPopt						
– PRx	0.670	0.0002*	0.823	<0.0001*	0.0607	0.017*
– PAx	0.635	0.0012*	0.782	<0.0001*	0.0194	0.20
– RAC	0.693	<0.0001*	0.803	<0.0001*	0.0402	0.072
Dose of CPP below CPPopt						
– PRx	0.609	0.020*	0.802	<0.0001*	0.0393	0.031*
– PAx	0.566	0.33	0.771	<0.0001*	0.0086	0.28
– RAC	0.600	0.071	0.775	<0.0001*	0.0125	0.29

In multivariate logistic regression analysis, baseline variables were age, sex, and admission GCS. AUC for the baseline model was 0.762 ($P < 0.0001$). *AUC* area under the receiver operating curve (ROC), *PAx* pulse-amplitude index, *PRx* pressure reactivity index, *RAC* correlation of pulse wave amplitude and cerebral perfusion pressure

[a]AUC added to baseline multivariate model (age, sex, and admission GCS) by the variable

**P*-value < 0.05

Discussion

We designed this study to investigate the effect of cerebral hypotension on outcome following moderate/severe TBI. Cerebral hypotension was defined as CPP below CPPopt calculated using three ICP-derived indices of cerebrovascular reactivity (PRx, PAx, and RAC). These indices all have their theoretical advantages in different patient populations, but we wanted to test their performance in a mixed population of patients with moderate to severe TBI. Our study has three main findings. First, using an optimized ICM+ profile, we were able to obtain a valid CPPopt curve in 85-93% of the total monitoring period (highest for PRx, lowest for RAC), supporting the potential use of these indices in a clinical setting. Second, there was no difference between calculated CPPopt (using either of the indices) in patients with good recovery compared to those who died. Third, time spent with CPP below CPPopt was significantly associated with outcome, but in our multivariate logistic regression model, additional information was only added to the prediction by time/dose of CPP below CPPopt when using the PRx-based calculations.

Stability of the CPPopt curve is a prerequisite for widespread clinical use of real-time assessment of cerebrovascular reactivity, and this was previously a limitation of technology, e.g., a valid CPPopt curve was only present 55% of the monitoring period in the initial publication documenting an association between CPPopt and clinical outcome [10]. Liu et al. were able to obtain a mean yield of 94% of the total monitoring period studied using an optimized ICM+ profile for CPPopt calculation, and in the present investigation we confirm this finding through documentation of a CPPopt curve in 93% of the monitoring period (using PRx). It is worth emphasizing that even though the difference did not reach statistical significance, a trend was observed toward a higher yield in patients with good recovery compared to those who died, especially for the PAx-based calculations. In future studies, this should be considered when evaluating and optimizing the algorithm because there might be a higher prevalence of disturbed cerebrovascular reactivity (requiring tight blood pressure control) in patients with more severe injuries. The current multiwindow approach uses a weighting algorithm assigning higher priority to recent calculation windows, ensuring stability of the estimation without compromising relevancy at the specific CPPopt calculation time point. Thus, the multiwindow approach has an equally strong association with patient outcome compared to the single-window approach [16].

The average observed CPP in the entire study population was 77.9 mmHg (using MAP calibrated to the right atrium of the heart), which corresponds to the aggressive CPP oriented treatment protocol employed in the NCCU at Addenbrooke's Hospital [14]. Average CPPopt was 77.1–78.5 mmHg (calculated using RAC and PRx, respectively), with no difference between patients with good recovery and those who died for any of the indices. However, patients with good recovery had observed CPP above calculated CPPopt, whereas patients who died had CPP below CPPopt. This supports the use of CPPopt across clinical settings and the previous finding that CPP below CPPopt is associated with increased mortality [10]. Because we wanted to test the three indices in a mixed population of TBI patients, we did not, for example, exclude patients with terminal intracranial hypertension or those treated with decompressive craniectomy, even though both these situations theoretically might influence the relationship between the physiological parameters that we study through these indices.

The main objective of this study was to investigate the effect of cerebral hypotension on outcome following moderate/severe TBI. Cerebral hypotension was defined as CPP below CPPopt, which was calculated by different ICP-derived indices of autoregulation. In the present investigation, the time/dose of CPP below CPPopt only had predictive value (i.e., adding predictive power to the baseline model including age, sex, and admission GCS) in relation to the dichotomous outcome chosen (good recovery vs. death) when calculated using PRx. Thus, the information important for outcome prediction in the calculations using

PAx and RAC somehow is contained within the baseline model already. The calculation of PRx, and thus CPPopt estimation based on PRx, relies on the assumption that changes in cerebrovascular resistance are reflected in cerebral blood volume (CBV) and that changes in CBV are reflected in ICP. This assumption is satisfied when intracranial compliance is low (ICP is high) but may be challenged at low ICP values or in increased compliance settings (e.g., in patients after decompressive craniectomy). The pulse-amplitude index (PAx) is the correlation coefficient between MAP and AMP and is thought to address this issue: when autoregulation is intact, a decrease in ABP causes a compensatory vasodilatation, resulting in an increased CBV promoting a stronger transmission of the pulse wave to ICP, i.e., a stronger relationship between MAP and AMP [17]. In a study of 327 patients with TBI, PAx was in fact superior to PRx in predicting dichotomized 12-month outcome (dead vs. alive) in the subgroup of 120 patients with ICP < 15mmHg [18]. Interestingly, in the same study, PAx performed equally well as PRx in predicting outcome in the subgroup of patients with ICP > 15 mmHg and, thus, has the potential to be applied in a broader clinical setting than PRx. In our study population, however, average ICP was 17 mmHg, which might explain the superiority of outcome prediction in the PRx-based calculations.

There are some limitations to the findings described here that deserve mention. This preliminary investigation represents a retrospective analysis of prospectively gathered clinical and multimodal neuromonitoring data and, thus, is limited by the information collected at the time. Data on, e.g., pupillary status and surgical procedures would have strengthened the study, but such data were not available. Furthermore, patients with moderate/severe TBI are subjected to a wide range of therapeutic interventions, and the retrospective observational design inflicts risks of selection and information biases as well as a risk of misclassification of outcome. However, choosing to include patients who either died or had good recovery minimizes this concern, although the GOS is a crude measure of functional outcome. In contrast, choosing this patient population limits the direct clinical applicability since indices found to be inferior in our study might be stronger in predicting outcome in patients with, e.g., moderate/severe disability. Finally, this study's design and the current status of CPPopt research in general do not exclude the possibility that deranged indices of cerebrovascular reactivity are merely indicators of more severe brain damage and that therapeutic interventions targeting these measures do not improve outcome.

In conclusion, we find PRx-based calculations of time/dose of cerebral hypotension (CPP below CPPopt) to predict outcome better than similar calculations using PAx and RAC in a mixed cohort of patients with moderate to severe TBI.

Conflict of Interest **No conflict of interest regarding the data presented in the present paper. Of note, MC and PS have a financial interest in part of the licensing fees for ICM+ software (Cambridge Enterprise Ltd., UK).**

References

1. Carney N, Totten AM, O'Reilly C et al (2017) Guidelines for the management of severe traumatic brain injury, 4th edition. Neurosurgery 80(1):6–15
2. Czosnyka M, Smielewski P, Kirkpatrick P, Laing RJ, Menon D, Pickard JD (1997) Continuous assessment of the cerebral vasomotor reactivity in head injury. Neurosurgery 41(1):11–19
3. Fraser CD III, Brady KM, Rhee CJ, Blaine Easley R, Kibler K, Smielewski P, Czosnyka M, Kaczka DW, Andropoulos DB, Rusin C (2013) The frequency response of cerebral autoregulation. J Appl Physiol 115:52–56
4. Howells T, Johnson U, McKelvey T, Enblad P (2014) An optimal frequency range for assessing the pressure reactivity index in patients with traumatic brain injury. J Clin Monit Comput 29(1):97–105
5. Needham E, McFadyen C, Newcombe V, Synnot AJ, Czosnyka M, Menon D (2017) Cerebral perfusion pressure targets individualized to pressure-reactivity index in moderate to severe traumatic brain injury: a systematic review. J Neurotrauma 34(5):963–970
6. Rivera-Lara L, Zorrilla-Vaca A, Geocadin R, Ziai W, Healy R, Thompson R, Smielewski P, Czosnyka M, Hogue CW (2017) Predictors of outcome with cerebral autoregulation monitoring: a systematic review and meta-analysis. Crit Care Med 45(4):695–704
7. Zeiler FA, Donnelly J, Calviello L, Smielewski P, Menon DK, Czosnyka M, Smieleweski P, Menon DK, Czosnyka M (2017) Pressure autoregulation measurement techniques in adult traumatic brain injury, Part II: A scoping review of continuous methods. J Neurotrauma 34(23):5086
8. Sorrentino E, Diedler J, Kasprowicz M et al (2012) Critical thresholds for cerebrovascular reactivity after traumatic brain injury. Neurocrit Care 16(2):258–266
9. Steiner LA, Czosnyka M, Piechnik SK (2002) Continuous monitoring of cerebrovascular pressure reactivity allows determination of optimal cerebral perfusion pressure in patients with traumatic brain injury. Crit Care 30(4):733–738
10. Aries MJH, Czosnyka M, Budohoski KP et al (2012) Continuous determination of optimal cerebral perfusion pressure in traumatic brain injury*. Crit Care Med 40(8):2456–2463
11. Zeiler FA, Donnelly J, Menon DK, Smielewski P, Hutchinson PJA, Czosnyka M (2018) A description of a new continuous physiological index in traumatic brain injury using the correlation between pulse amplitude of intracranial pressure and cerebral perfusion pressure. J Neurotrauma 35(7):963–997
12. Zeiler FA, Donnelly J, Smieleweski P, Menon D, Hutchinson PJ, Czosnyka M (2018) Critical thresholds of ICP derived continuous cerebrovascular reactivity indices for outcome prediction in non-craniectomized TBI patients: PRx, PAx and RAC. J Neurotrauma 160:1315–1324
13. Jennett B, Bond M (1975) Assessment of outcome after severe brain damage: a practical scale. Lancet 305(7905):480–484
14. Patel HC, Menon DK, Tebbs S, Hawker R, Hutchinson PJ, Kirkpatrick PJ (2002) Specialist neurocritical care and outcome from head injury. Intensive Care Med 28:547–553
15. Optimal Cerebral Perfusion Pressure (CPPopt) research website. http://cppopt.org/. Accessed 20 Aug 2018

16. Liu X, Maurits NM, Aries MJH et al (2017) Monitoring of optimal cerebral perfusion pressure in traumatic brain injured patients using a multi-window weighting algorithm. J Neurotrauma 2017:5003
17. Radolovich DK, Aries MJH, Castellani G, Corona A, Lavinio A, Smielewski P, Pickard JD, Czosnyka M (2011) Pulsatile intracranial pressure and cerebral autoregulation after traumatic brain injury. Neurocrit Care 15(3):379–386
18. Aries MJH, Czosnyka M, Budohoski KP, Kolias AG, Radolovich DK, Lavinio A, Pickard JD, Smielewski P (2012) Continuous monitoring of cerebrovascular reactivity using pulse waveform of intracranial pressure. Neurocrit Care 17(1):67–76

Optimal Cerebral Perfusion Pressure Assessed with a Multi-Window Weighted Approach Adapted for Prospective Use: A Validation Study

Erta Beqiri, Ari Ercole, Marcel J. Aries, Manuel Cabeleira, Andras Czigler, Annalisa Liberti, Jeanette Tas, Joseph Donnelly, Xiuyun Liu, Marta Fedriga, Ka Hing Chu, Frederick A. Zeiler, Marek Czosnyka, and Peter Smielewski

Introduction

Cerebrovascular pressure reactivity index (PRx)-cerebral perfusion pressure (CPP) relationships over a given time period can be used to detect an optimal value of CPP at which PRx shows the best autoregulation (CPPopt). Algorithms for continuous automated assessment of CPPopt in traumatic brain injury (TBI) patients reached the desired high yield using the multi-window approach (CPPopt_MA, published by Liu et al. (2017) [1]). However, the calculations were tested on retrospective datasets, in which artefacts were removed manually and CPP was scarcely managed according to CPPopt. Moreover, CPPopt 'false positive' values can be generated from non-physiological variations of intracranial pressure (ICP) and arterial blood pressure (ABP) [2]. Therefore, the algorithm was fine-tuned to improve its robustness and making it more suitable for prospective bedside application (currently used in the COGiTATE trial—www.cppopt.org [3]). The aim of this study was to validate the CPPopt revised algorithm in a large single-centre retrospective cohort of TBI patients by testing its relationship with outcome and comparing it with the current Brain Trauma Foundation (BTF) guidelines [4].

E. Beqiri (✉)
Brain Physics Laboratory, Division of Neurosurgery, Department of Clinical Neurosciences, University of Cambridge, Cambridge, UK

Department of Physiology and Transplantation, Milan University, Milano, Italy

A. Ercole
Division of Anaesthesia, Department of Medicine, Addenbrooke's Hospital, University of Cambridge, Cambridge, UK
e-mail: ae105@cam.ac.uk

M. J. Aries · J. Tas
Department of Intensive Care, Maastricht UMC, HX Maastricht, The Netherlands
e-mail: marcel.aries@mumc.nl; jeanette.tas@mumc.nl

M. Cabeleira · J. Donnelly · K. H. Chu · M. Czosnyka · P. Smielewski
Brain Physics Laboratory, Division of Neurosurgery, Department of Clinical Neurosciences, University of Cambridge, Cambridge, UK
e-mail: mc916@cam.ac.uk; khc42@cam.ac.uk; mc141@medschl.cam.ac.uk; ps10011@cam.ac.uk

A. Czigler
Brain Physics Laboratory, Division of Neurosurgery, Department of Clinical Neurosciences, University of Cambridge, Cambridge, UK

Department of Neurosurgery and Szentagothai Research Center, University of Pecs, Medical School, Pecs, Hungary

A. Liberti
Department of Physiology and Transplantation, Milan University, Milano, Italy

Department of Intensive Care, Maastricht UMC, HX Maastricht, The Netherlands

X. Liu
Department of Anesthesiology and Critical Care Medicine, School of Medicine, Johns Hopkins University, Baltimore, MD, USA

M. Fedriga
Brain Physics Laboratory, Division of Neurosurgery, Department of Clinical Neurosciences, University of Cambridge, Cambridge, UK

Department of Anesthesia, Critical care and Emergency, Spedali Civili University Hospital, Brescia, Italy

F. A. Zeiler
Division of Anaesthesia, Department of Medicine, Addenbrooke's Hospital, University of Cambridge, Cambridge, UK

Department of Surgery, Rady Faculty of Health Sciences, University of Manitoba, Winnipeg, MB, Canada

Department of Anatomy and Cell Science, Rady Faculty of Health Sciences, University of Manitoba, Winnipeg, MB, Canada

Biomedical Engineering, Faculty of Engineering, University of Manitoba, Winnipeg, MB, Canada
e-mail: Frederick.Zeiler@umanitoba.ca

B. Depreitere et al. (eds.), *Intracranial Pressure and Neuromonitoring XVII*, Acta Neurochirurgica Supplement 131,
https://doi.org/10.1007/978-3-030-59436-7_36,

Materials and Methods

We performed a retrospective analysis of ICP and ABP waveforms and Glasgow Outcome Score (GOS) using 6-month data of TBI patients requiring ICP monitoring admitted in Addenbrooke's Hospital Neuro Critical Care Unit from 1996 to 2018. Patients who underwent craniectomy were excluded. ICP and ABP waveforms were processed with ICM+ software (https://icmplus.neurosurg.cam.ac.uk). For each patient, only the first 5 days from the date of injury were considered. For each recording the following variables were calculated: CPPopt, CPPopt_MA, target, yield, stability, ΔCPPopt, ΔCPP60 and ΔTarget (Fig. 2), defined as in Table 1.

Details about the algorithm used to calculate CPPopt are shown in Fig. 1, and further explanations are available at the website cppopt.org. Here the main differences from the previous algorithm (CPPopt_MA) are highlighted.

First of all, the CPP values taken into account for generating the curve are filtered so that scarcely represented values given by short spikes and drops (which are common in the clinical daily environment and would have been manually removed in the retrospective analysis) but not given by the physiological trend will be disregarded. A 5-min-duration median filter is applied to CPP before the data points are divided into bins of 5 mmHg. Furthermore, the percentage of the total data count that each CPP bin must represent is increased to 3%.

Secondly, when the second-order polynomial is fitted in the PRx-CPP plots over a certain time window, the curves might appear only in their descending or ascending part, not including the nadir, referred to here as non-parabolic. These fits, by their nature, result in 'optimum' values at the extreme ends of the available CPP bins range and are usually produced by relatively short periods of transient up and down swings of CPP. Including these in the combined, weighted-average calculations often leads to sudden discontinuities in the resulting CPPopt, of magnitude more than 10 mmHg. It is unlikely that the physiology of autoregulation changes in this way. Therefore, in the new algorithm, only U-shaped parabolic curves are considered, decreasing the overall yield but increasing substantially stability of the calculation and ensuring physiological values of CPPopt.

Finally, the U-shape curves generated by the PRx-CPP plots were screened for their determination coefficient R^2_{full}, which gives a measure of the variability explained by the fitting curve compared to the total variability of the data. The 'full' subscript denotes that the calculations of R^2 are done on the complete set of bins, rather than on only the subset selected for the curve fitting process, as part of the fitting algorithm heuristics. The curves that produce values of $R^2_{full} < 0.2$ are rejected. All the remaining curves were combined using R^2_{full} as a weighting factor in the weighted average.

In the COGiTATE protocol, the clinicians would adopt new recommendations for CPP management target only at fixed review times, not adjusting it until the next such time. These were scheduled once every 4 h. In addition, the new target value would have been restricted to the clinically safe range of 50–100 mmHg and not allowed to change by more than 10 mmHg at a time. To simulate this in our retrospective analysis, we introduced a new variable called Target, which was only updated once every 4 h and truncated at that safety zone margins and with the imposed limit on change of 10 mmHg (Fig. 2).

Student's *t*-test was used to assess ΔCPPopt, ΔCPP60, and ΔTarget ability in discriminating mortality and survival. AUCs (confidence interval (CI) 95%) were calculated and compared with the DeLong test.

Table 1 Calculated variables and their brief description

Variable	Explanation
CPPopt	PRx-CPP relationship is assessed with the multi-window approach using a selected set of calculation heuristics, which were chosen based on their performance in a selected dataset and on the greatest discrimination from values generated from surrogate signals (Fig. 1)
CPPopt_MA	PRx-CPP relationship is assessed with the multi-window approach using calculation heuristics as described in [3]
Target	The CPPopt value is sampled every 4 h in order to simulate the CPP Target provided to the clinical team as per COGiTATE protocol [3], which included a clinical 'safe range' of 50–100 mmHg imposed on the Target and a limit of maximum change of ±10 mmHg from the previous Target value (Fig. 2)
Yield	Percentage of total CPP recorded time with CPPopt (or CPPopt_MA) values available
Stability	Standard deviation of difference in two consecutive values of CPPopt (or CPPopt_MA)
ΔCPPopt	Average deviation from CPPopt (ΔCPPopt = CPP − CPPopt) (Fig. 2)
ΔCPP60	Average deviation from BTF guidelines 60 mmHg (ΔCPP60 = CPP − 60) (Fig. 2)
ΔTarget	Average deviation from Target (ΔTarget = CPP − Target) (Fig. 2)

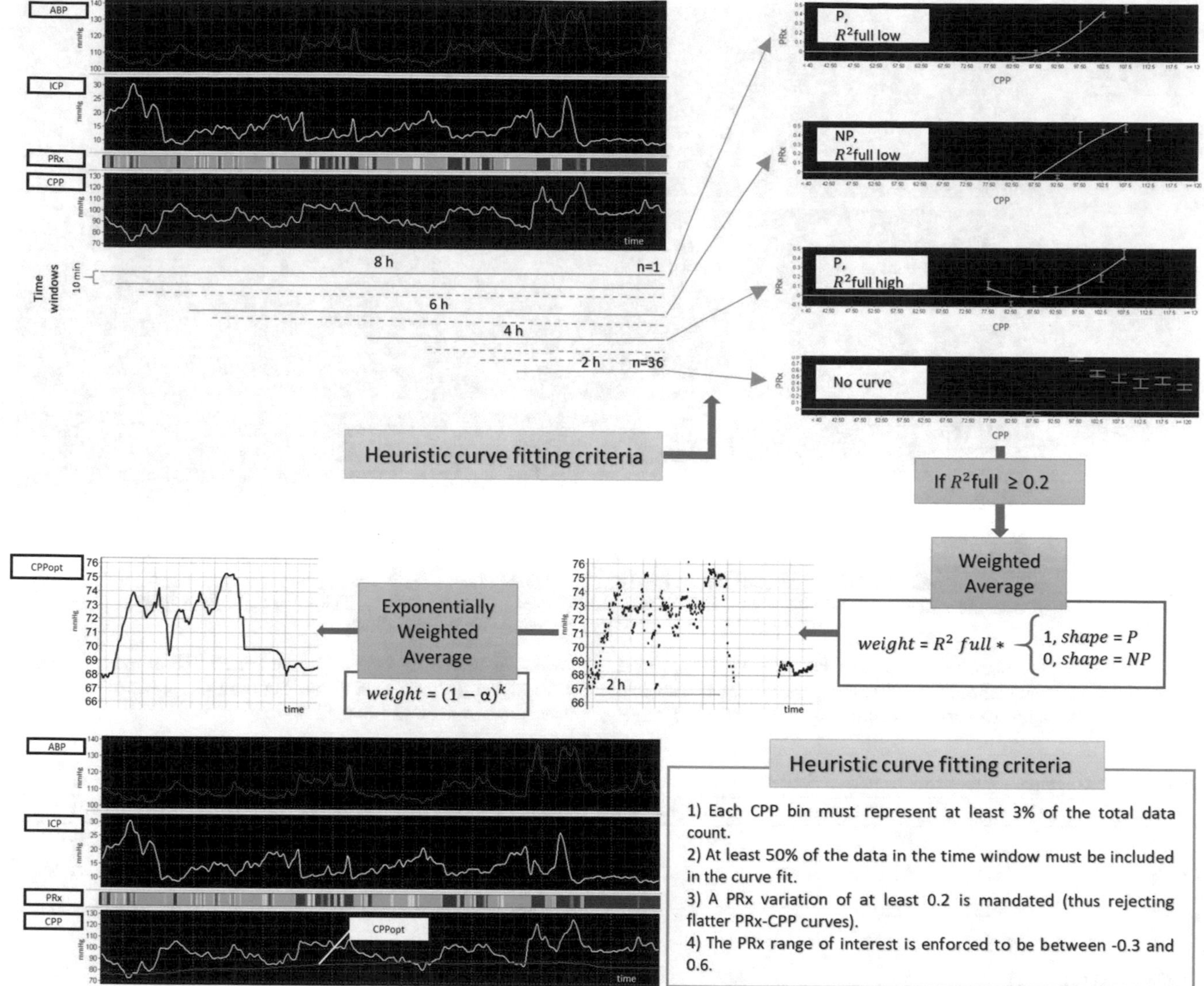

Fig. 1 CPPopt calculation. At each time point, 36 PRx-CPP (5-min median filter) plots are generated from past data windows of increasing duration ranging from 2 to 8 h, using incremental steps of 10 min. The data points are divided into groups corresponding to CPP bins of 5 mmHg length, within a CPP range of 40–120 mmHg. For each bin, mean PRx and CPP values are used to fit a second-order polynomial describing the theoretical U shape, with its nadir determining CPPopt, according to the curve fitting criteria. This process is repeated for each progressively longer data window. Only parabolic curves (P = parabolic; NP = non-parabolic) with $R^2_{\text{full}} > 0.2$ are then combined using weighted average operation. The calculations are repeated every minute and the resulting time series is finally subjected to an exponentially weighted average filter of 2 h duration forming the CPPopt time. The missing data limit of the calculation is set at 50%, so at least 4 h of data are necessary to generate the first CPPopt value

Results

The study included 813 TBI patients; 74% of the patients had a severe TBI (GCS < 9) (Table 2), and 23% were dead at GOS assessment at 6 months (Table 2). CPPopt showed a lower yield (83 % (range 75–90)) compared with CPPopt_MA (89% (range 81–93)), $p < 0.001$; however the stability was significantly increased with the new algorithm ($p < 0.001$). ΔCPPopt and ΔTarget work better in distinguishing mortality and survival outcome than ΔCPP60 ($p < 0.05$ and $p < 0.001$, Table 3).

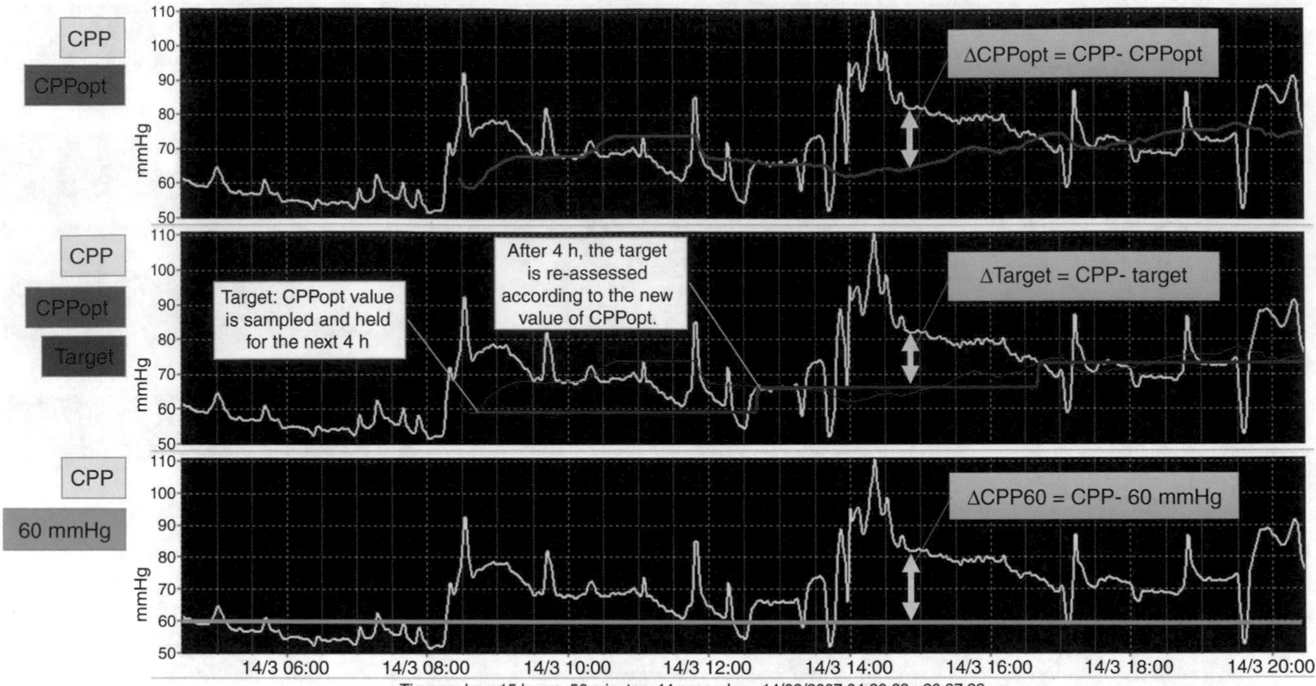

Fig. 2 CPP trend is shown along with CPPopt, the CPPopt target value, and the BTF guidelines limit (60 mmHg). The Target is assessed as CPPopt value sampled every 4 h in order to simulate the CPP target provided to the clinical team as per the COGiTATE protocol; no Target can be higher or lower than 10 mmHg from the previous one. Target values range from 50 to 100 mmHg

Table 2 Demographic and outcome characteristics

Variable		*N* (or median)	% (or IQR)
Age		38	24–89
GCS	14–15	37	5
	9–13	166	22
	1–8	569	74
GOS 6 months	D	191	23
	VS	15	2
	SD	259	32
	MD	202	25
	GR	146	18

GCS Glasgow Coma Score, *GOS* Glasgow Outcome Score, *D* dead, *VS* vegetative state, *SD* severe disability, *MD* mild disability, *GR* good recovery

Table 3 Assessment of ability to distinguish outcome groups

Variable	Dead	Alive	*P*	AUC (CI 95%)
ΔCPPopt	−1.73	1.1	<0.001	0.65 (0.60–0.70)
ΔCPP60	15.4	18	0.001	0.58 (0.53–0.63)
ΔTarget	−2	1.6	<0.001	0.66 (0.62–0.71)
DeLong test				***P***
ΔCPPopt vs. ΔCPP60				0.014
ΔTarget vs. ΔCPP60				<0.001

P-values of *t*-test (dead vs alive) and AUC values are presented for ΔCPPopt, ΔCPP60 and ΔTarget. The DeLong test shows that both ΔCPPopt and ΔTarget could offer an advantage over ΔCPP60. ΔCPPopt, ΔCPPopt = CPP − CPPopt; ΔCPP60, ΔCPP as per BTF guidelines = CPP − 60 mmHg; ΔTarget, ΔCPP Target = CPP − Target

Discussion

We validated in a large cohort of TBI patients a new algorithm, proposed for the prospective use of automated CPPopt at the bedside as part of the COGiTATE study. This CPPopt algorithm seems more stable, robust and able to distinguish between outcome groups.

A large amount of retrospective work has been done on improving the technology for the continuous assessment of CPPopt in TBI patients. With the multi-window approach inspired by Depretiere et al. [5] and implemented in ICM+ by Liu et al. (CPPopt_MA) [1], the yield was considerably improved compared with the previous 4-h-based algorithm [6]. CPPopt_MA could be available for more than 90% of the time, calculated on the whole monitored time. This rendered it clinically useful, making it possible to start thinking about the prospective application of CPPopt assessed continuously and automatically at the bedside; therefore the COGiTATE study—the first randomized control trial assessing the feasibility and safety of managing CPP according to CPPopt in TBI patients—was designed [3]. The fact that CPPopt needed to be assessed prospectively in real time at the bedside and that clinical recommendations for treating patients would be managed according to CPPopt values, raised two issues: (1) CPPopt was previously largely studied in retrospective cohorts, where waveform artefacts were cleaned both manually and automatically; (2) the individual values generated by the automatic semi-continuous algorithm would need to be reliable and, more importantly, safe enough to make it suitable for clinical use. Therefore, the algorithm was modified and implemented with heuristics chosen for their ability to discriminate between estimations performed on the original versus surrogate (randomized) signals. We checked the robustness of the calculation (low inter-point variability), avoidance of non-physiological sudden jumps in the CPPopt time trend, and the reliability of the values in reflecting the cerebral autoregulation status.

The combination of the new heuristics made the algorithm more robust and stable and suitable for bedside use, but the relationship previously found with outcome had not been re-apprised. For this reason, we validated the new algorithm against outcome and showed that the average deviation from CPPopt calculated with this algorithm, for the first 5 days from the date of injury, could distinguish mortality and survival and performed better than the current guidelines threshold. The down side of using the more restrictive criteria is that the yield of CPPopt would decrease, as our analysis showed. However, the yield here is still higher than when using the single-window approach, and at 83% it should still be clinically useful.

This validation study is still retrospective, and the dataset is composed of a large cohort of TBI patients admitted in a single centre over a large time span. The data were partially cleaned manually and partially automatically. However, the results are comparable with the previous algorithm (CPPopt_MA), and both analyses were subject to the same limitations.

Conclusion

We demonstrated that the new algorithm is not only more robust and stable but also maintains the ability of the new algortihm in discriminating outcome groups is maintained and is better than the ability of the fixed BTF guidelines. Thus, we believe it is suitable for prospective use in TBI patients in future trials.

Acknowledgement MC is supported by NIHR Cambridge Biomedical Research Centre.

The authors would also like to express their gratitude to all doctors and nursing staff of the Neuro Critical Care Unit of Addenbrooke's Hospital, Cambridge, UK, for their professional help and support in computer-bedside data monitoring conducted by the Brain Physics Laboratory team.

Conflict of Interest **PS and MC have a financial interest in a part of the ICM+ software (https://icmplus.neurosurg.cam.ac.uk) licensing fees.**

References

1. Liu X, Maurits NM, Aries MJH et al (2017) Monitoring of optimal cerebral perfusion pressure in traumatic brain injured patients using a multi-window weighting algorithm. J Neurotrauma 34(22):3081–3088
2. Cabeleira M, Czosnyka M, Liu X, Donnelly J, Smielewski P (2018) Occurrence of CPPopt values in uncorrelated ICP and ABP time series. Acta Neurochir Suppl.:143–146
3. Beqiri E, Smielewski P, Robba C et al (2019) Feasibility of individualised severe traumatic brain injury management using an automated assessment of optimal cerebral perfusion pressure: the COGiTATE phase II study protocol. BMJ Open 9(9):e030727
4. Carney N, Totten AM, Hawryluk GWJ et al (2016) Guidelines for the management of severe traumatic brain injury, 4th edn
5. Depreitere B, Güiza F, Van Den BG, Schuhmann MU, Maier G, Piper I, Meyfroidt G (2014) Pressure autoregulation monitoring and cerebral perfusion pressure target recommendation in patients with severe traumatic brain injury based on minute-by-minute monitoring data. J Neurosurg 120(120):1451–1457
6. Aries MJH, Czosnyka M, Budohoski KP et al (2012) Continuous determination of optimal cerebral perfusion pressure in traumatic brain injury*. Crit Care Med. https://doi.org/10.1097/CCM.0b013e3182514eb6

Monitoring of Cerebrovascular Reactivity in Intracerebral Hemorrhage and Its Relation with Survival

Ana V. Ferreira, Isabel Maia, and Celeste Dias

Introduction

Spontaneous intracerebral hemorrhage (ICH), also known as hemorrhagic stroke, is the second most common cerebrovascular event and carries exceptionally high morbidity and mortality [1]. Clinical presentation may range from a few symptoms to critical states with the need for intensive care, surgery, and extensive rehabilitation. This high variability is one of the main concerns when investigating ICH [2]. Mortality may affect as much as 60% of patients per year, and only 20% will have functional independence at 6 months after the event [3].

Neuromonitoring analysis for spontaneous intracerebral hemorrhage (ICH) is still scarce, especially regarding vascular reactivity patterns. Intracerebral pressure (ICP) is most frequently monitored by an intraparenchymal pressure sensor used in brain lesion patients that require mechanical ventilation for neurological assessment while sedated. Augmented ICP and impaired cerebrovascular autoregulation have been recognized as important mechanisms to contribute to secondary brain injury after brain trauma, subarachnoid, and ischemic stroke [4, 5].

There is some evidence that ICP variability and frequency above 20 mmHg is associated with mortality and poor outcome in ICH patients [6]. However, neuromonitoring data regarding ICH to guide neurocritical care are still scarce and are mainly based on transferred information from traumatic brain injury (TBI) patients [7].

PRx is an index, recorded by ICM+ software, obtained from the correlation between arterial blood pressure (ABP) and ICP. A negative correlation (up to a maximum value of 0.25) is considered normal, since, in physiological conditions, it is expected that with an increase in ABP, cerebral vasculature may be able to increase resistance to maintain a stable ICP. This is considered a preserved cerebrovascular autoregulation.

Cerebral perfusion pressure (CPP) is the driving force that leads blood into cranial vessels and is calculated by the difference between ABP and ICP (ABP-ICP). Its value may be calculated in real time at bedside and is frequently described in the literature as a value that should be maintained between 60 and 80 mmHg. However, in the last few years, tailoring CPP based on cerebrovascular autoregulation status driven by PRx has been associated, in retrospective studies, with better outcomes for TBI patients. This concept is referred to as optimal CPP (CPPopt) [8, 9].

The need for neuromonitoring research and defining its utility in neurocritical care for ICH patients has been expressed often. Considering ICH management guideline assessment of ICP and CPP is important for secondary brain injury prevention; however, information regarding cerebrovascular reactivity is still scarce and its importance for patient management and association with outcome is yet to be established [10].

Our goal was to determine the association, if any, between the presence/absence of cerebrovascular autoregulation and patient 28-day survival.

Materials and Methods

At our Neuro Critical Care Unit (NCCU), patients with intracerebral lesions that need to be sedated have placement of an ICP Codman® probe for intracranial neuromonitoring. The neuromonitoring integration data system used is ICM+ ® (Cambridge Enterprise UK). This allows us to calculate in real time and at bedside not only ICP, but also indices associated with ICP and ABP such as CPP, PRx, and optimal PRx.

A. V. Ferreira (✉)
Department of Neurosurgery, Centro Hospitalar São João, Porto, Portugal

I. Maia · C. Dias
Department of Intensive Care Medicine, Centro Hospitalar São João, Porto, Portugal

B. Depreitere et al. (eds.), *Intracranial Pressure and Neuromonitoring XVII*, Acta Neurochirurgica Supplement 131,
https://doi.org/10.1007/978-3-030-59436-7_37, © Springer Nature Switzerland AG 2021

With the availability of these data from our unit, neuromonitoring records between 2013 and 2016 of adult patients, with spontaneous supra-tentorial ICH, were retrospectively reviewed. To be considered eligible, records had to have a minimum of 24 h of good-quality signals for each patient.

Variables considered for analysis were ICP, CPP, CPPopt, and PRx, as well as ICP dose, PRx dose, and time percentage above critical value (T%abv). ICP dose and PRx dose were calculated as secondary analysis using ICM® software and correspond to the area beneath the histogram curve relating time of exposure and ICP and PRx values. Information regarding demographics, surgical drainage, external ventricular drain (EVD) placement, and 28-day mortality was recorded. A *t*-test and Kaplan-Meier curves were used for statistical analysis. Significance value was considered at 0.05. Approval for data collection was obtained from our local ethics committee.

Results

We analyzed data from 46 patients, representing a mean duration of 263 ± 173 h of signal records and a median length of stay in the intensive care unit (ICU) of 22 (interquartile range (IQR) of 13) days. The mean age was 62.6 ± 11.8 years, and 24 (52%) of the patients were male. The EVD for cerebrospinal fluid (CSF) drainage was applied in addition to an ICP probe in 50% of patients, and 32.6% were sent to surgery for ICH evacuation (Table 1). Patients who died within 28 days (37.0%) had significantly higher mean ICP, PRx, ICP dose, PRx dose, and T%abv compared to those who survived (Table 2 and Fig. 1). Although patients who died had relatively low values of mean ICP (13.73 ± 7.75 mmHg), under the critical value of 20 mmHg, they presented a mean PRx of over 0.25, indicating impaired cerebrovascular reactivity (0.30 ± 0.26). Patients with PRx over 0.25 had significantly lower survival, with a proportion of 14% survival at 28 days, as opposed to 85% of those with PRx under 0.25 ($p < 0.001$) (survival curves in Fig. 2).

Table 1 Demographics data

n	46
Male	24 (52.2%)
Age	62.6 ± 11.75
LOS ICU	22 (13)
Duration of records (h)	263 ± 172
EVD	23 (50%)
ICH drainage	15 (32.6%)
DC	4 (8.7%)
Mortality at 28th day	17 (36.9%)

Values described as mean ± standard deviation, absolute value (%), and median (IQR). *DC* decompressive craniectomy, *EVD* external ventricular drainage, *ICH* intracerebral hemorrhage, *LOS ICU* length of stay at intensive care unit

Table 2 Neuromonitoring data

	Alive (29)	Dead (17)	*p*
PRx > 0.25 (*n*)	2	12	
ICP (mmHg)	9.1 ± 3.2	13.7 ± 7.7	0.006
CPP	89.0 ± 4.9	77.5 ± 11.7	<0.001
PRx	0.026 ± 0.147	0.30 ± 0.264	0.001
ICP dose	1.24 (2.33)	8.90 (21.25)	0.001
PRx dose	1.59 ± 1.016	2.58 ± 1.449	0.002
ICP T%abv 20 mmHg (%)	1.4 (11.4)	7.53 (37.12)	<0.001
PRx T%abv 0.25 (%)	26.0 (17.8)	57.6 (40)	<0.001
CPP-CPPopt	0.67 ± 4.32	−6.57 ± 7.50	0.037

Values presented as mean ± standard deviation or median (interquartile range). *T%abv* time percentage above critical value

Discussion

Although mean ICP in ICH patients was under the critical value of 20 mmHg, the ICP dose and percentage of time above critical value was higher in patients with worse outcomes. The variability of intracranial pressure is high and the exposure of brain to higher pressure may not be well represented by mean ICP but better by ICP dose and T%abv. It is hypothesized that these measures of exposure representativity may have prognostic value in ICH patients.

Regarding cerebrovascular pressure reactivity, the mean values were higher than 0.25 in patients with worse outcomes (mortality at 28 days), as were PRx dose and T%abv.

In our cohort, patients with ICH were more exposed to autoregulation impairment than to increased ICP. When taking into account the patient's outcome, ICH patients who died in the first 28 days had worse cerebrovascular reactivity indices, namely PRx, PRx dose, and time above the critical value of 0.25. Optimal CPP was particularly challenging to identify and achieve in these patients. However, our analysis had limitations in that our cohort was retrospectively analyzed. Based on our data, we may hypothesize that treatments aimed at keeping PRx as low as possible may be associated with better outcomes for ICH patients. Besides being an individualized value, most ICH patients have been chronically exposed to elevated blood pressure (one of the main risk factors in ICH), this is why it is possible that CPP intervals considered to TBI may not be adequate for all ICH patients. Individual adjustment, through continuous evaluation of PRx, may positively influence outcomes [9].

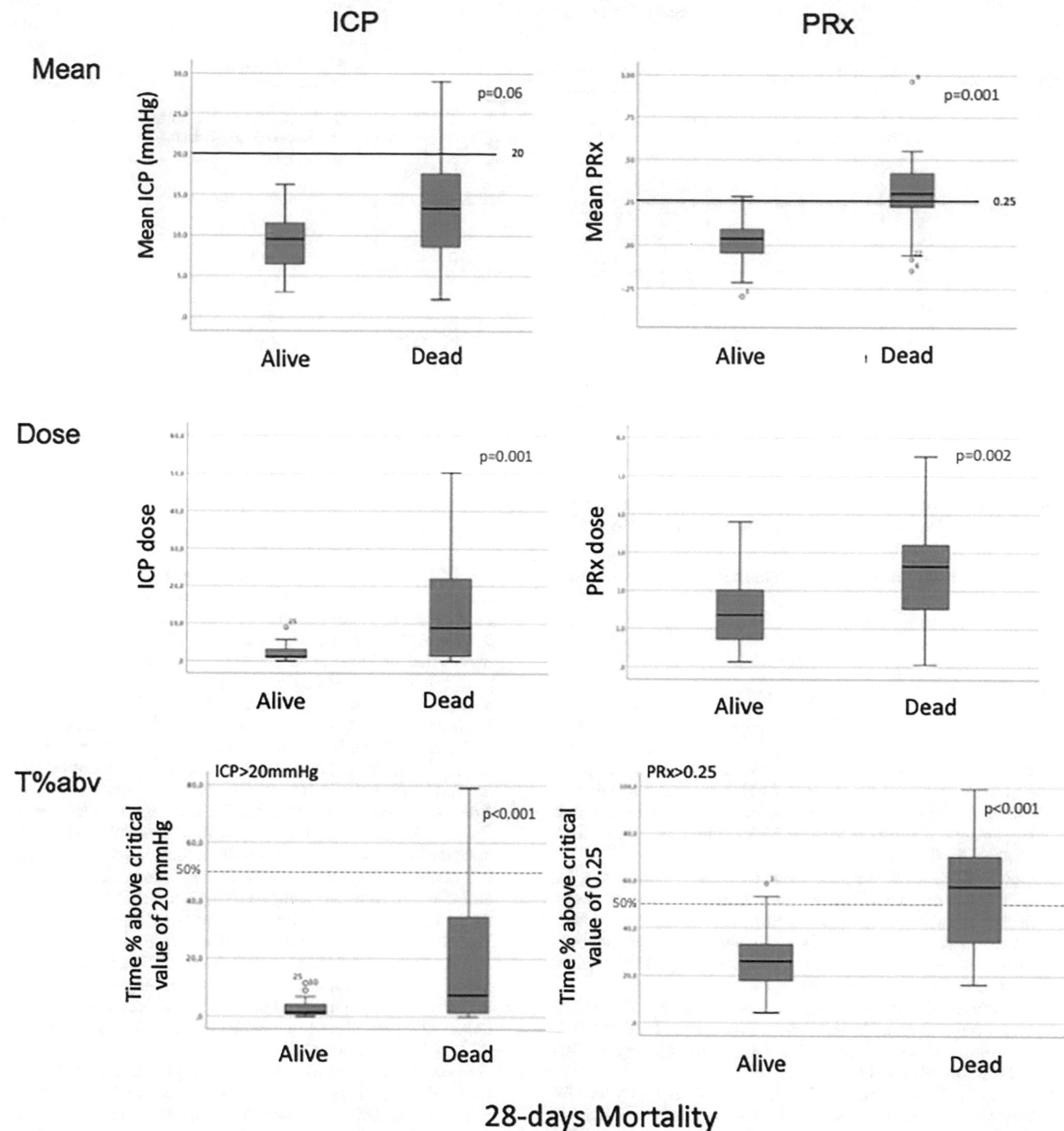

Fig. 1 Monitoring variable distribution of alive and dead patients at 28 days. *ICP* intracerebral cranial pressure, *PRx* cerebrovascular reactivity index; dose calculated by Unit*Time; *T%abv* time percentage above critical value

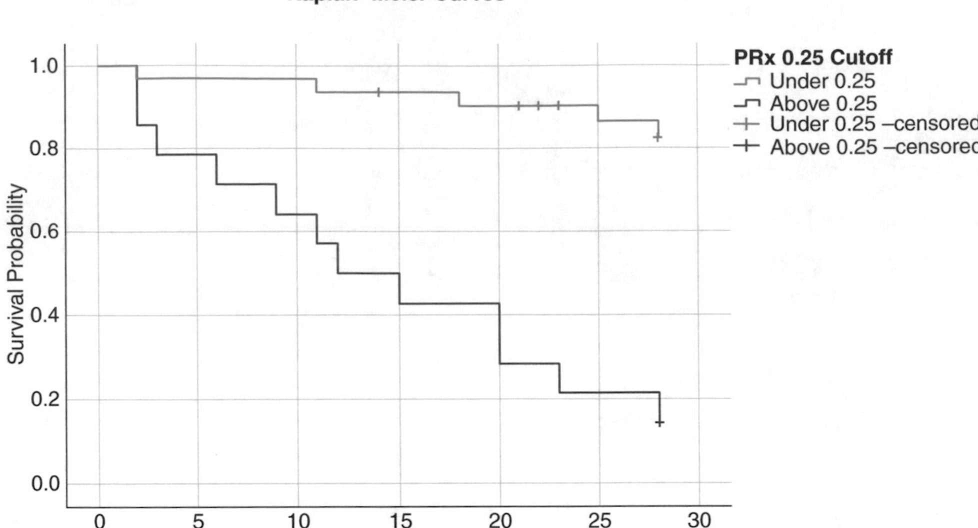

Fig. 2 Kaplan-Meier survival curves. Patients with a mean PRx < 0.25 had higher 28-day survival rates compared to those with PRx > 0.25 ($p < 0.001$). Median survival time for patients with PRx > 0.25 was 12 days

Conflict of Interest: **The authors declare that they have no conflict of interest.**

References

1. Roh D, Sun CH, Schmidt JM, Gurol E, Murthy S, Park S, Agarwal S, Connolly ES, Claassen J (2018) Primary intracerebral hemorrhage: a closer look at hypertension and cerebral amyloid angiopathy. Neurocrit Care 29:77–83. https://doi.org/10.1007/s12028-018-0514-z
2. Guo R, Blacker DJ, Wang X, Arima H, Lavados PM, Lindley RI, Chalmers J, Anderson CS, Robinson T (2017) Practice patterns for neurosurgical utilization and outcome in acute intracerebral hemorrhage: intensive blood pressure reduction in acute cerebral hemorrhage trials 1 and 2 studies. Neurosurgery 81:980–985. https://doi.org/10.1093/neuros/nyx129
3. Cordonnier C, Demchuk A, Ziai W, Anderson CS (2018) Intracerebral haemorrhage: current approaches to acute management. Lancet 392:1257–1268. https://doi.org/10.1016/s0140-6736(18)31878-6
4. Carney N, Totten AM, O'Reilly C, Ullman JS, Hawryluk GW, Bell MJ, Bratton SL, Chesnut R, Harris OA, Kissoon N, Rubiano AM, Shutter L, Tasker RC, Vavilala MS, Wilberger J, Wright DW, Ghajar J (2017) Guidelines for the management of severe traumatic brain injury, fourth edition. Neurosurgery 80:6–15. https://doi.org/10.1227/NEU.0000000000001432
5. Ko SB (2013) Multimodality monitoring in the neurointensive care unit: a special perspective for patients with stroke. J Stroke 15:99–108. https://doi.org/10.5853/jos.2013.15.2.99
6. Sykora M, Steinmacher S, Steiner T, Poli S, Diedler J (2014) Association of intracranial pressure with outcome in comatose patients with intracerebral hemorrhage. J Neurol Sci 342:141–145. https://doi.org/10.1016/j.jns.2014.05.012
7. Diedler J, Sykora M, Rupp A, Poli S, Karpel-Massler G, Sakowitz O, Steiner T (2009) Impaired cerebral vasomotor activity in spontaneous intracerebral hemorrhage. Stroke 40:815–819. https://doi.org/10.1161/STROKEAHA.108.531020
8. Aries MJ, Czosnyka M, Budohoski KP, Steiner LA, Lavinio A, Kolias AG, Hutchinson PJ, Brady KM, Menon DK, Pickard JD, Smielewski P (2012) Continuous determination of optimal cerebral perfusion pressure in traumatic brain injury. Crit Care Med 40:2456–2463. https://doi.org/10.1097/CCM.0b013e3182514eb6
9. Beqiri E, Smielewski P, Robba C, Czosnyka M, Cabeleira MT, Tas J, Donnelly J, Outtrim JG, Hutchinson P, Menon D, Meyfroidt G, Depreitere B, Aries MJ, Ercole A (2019) Feasibility of individualised severe traumatic brain injury management using an automated assessment of optimal cerebral perfusion pressure: the COGiTATE phase II study protocol. BMJ Open 9:e030727. https://doi.org/10.1136/bmjopen-2019-030727
10. Hemphill JC 3rd, Greenberg SM, Anderson CS, Becker K, Bendok BR, Cushman M, Fung GL, Goldstein JN, Macdonald RL, Mitchell PH, Scott PA, Selim MH, Woo D (2015) Guidelines for the management of spontaneous intracerebral hemorrhage: a guideline for healthcare professionals from the American Heart Association/American stroke association. Stroke 46:2032–2060. https://doi.org/10.1161/str.0000000000000069

Part VII

Neuroinformatics and Artificial Intelligence

Spectral Cerebral Blood Volume Accounting for Noninvasive Estimation of Changes in Cerebral Perfusion Pressure in Patients with Traumatic Brain Injury

Danilo Cardim, Peter Smielewski, and Marek Czosnyka

Introduction

Cerebral perfusion pressure (CPP) is one of the fundamental modalities in neurocritical care [1]. However, its accuracy in direct monitoring depends on the precision of two independent pressure transducers, for arterial blood pressure (ABP) and intracranial pressure (ICP).

ABP is usually measured with an external transducer, with input blood pressure transmitted via an indwelling arterial catheter. It is typically zeroed at the heart level, but for neurocritical care patients requiring monitoring of CPP, it should be zeroed at the level of the auditory meatus and re-zeroed following every change of body position. Because most patients receiving neurocritical care are managed with head elevation (to ease brain venous return), zeroing the ABP transducer at the heart level may produce overestimation of CPP from 10 to 20 mmHg [2]. With head elevation in sedated patients (in whom depleted baroreflex compromises cerebral haemodynamics [3]), blood flow has to overcome gravitational effects to reach the cerebral arteries, and it is assumed there is a reduction in ABP directly related to the water column between the heart and the brain (usually a reduction of 1 mmHg for each 1.35 cm) [4]. Furthermore, contemporary ICP micro-transducers are zeroed against atmospheric pressure only once during implantation. Their drift over time (usually not above 1 mmHg per day [5]) may accumulate over long monitoring periods (sometimes 2–3 weeks), adding additional considerable errors in CPP monitoring.

Therefore, direct invasive monitoring of mean CPP is more complex than it appears. Various studies have been conducted to measure CPP noninvasively (nCPP), most of them based on transcranial Doppler (TCD) monitoring of arterial cerebral blood flow velocity profiles ($CBFV_a$) in the middle cerebral artery (MCA) [6–10]. The relative accuracy for such estimation has been reported to vary from 12 to 20 mmHg [6–10].

In this study, we test the performance of a new TCD-based method for nCPP estimation (spectral nCPP or $nCPP_s$) presented elsewhere [11]. This method is based on accounting for changes in pulsatile cerebral arterial blood volume (C_aBV) applied to the analysis of a simplified hydrodynamic model of cerebral blood flow (CBF) and cerebrospinal fluid (CSF) dynamics [12–14]. The spectral feature of the method permits independence from the inaccuracy associated with zeroing the ABP transducer at the heart level and accounts

D. Cardim (✉)
Brain Physics Laboratory, Division of Neurosurgery, Department of Clinical Neurosciences, Cambridge Biomedical Campus, Addenbrooke's Hospital, University of Cambridge, Cambridge, UK

Department of Neurology and Neurotherapeutics, University of Texas Southwestern Medical Center, Dallas, TX, USA

Institute for Exercise and Environmental Medicine, Texas Health Presbyterian Hospital Dallas, Dallas, TX, USA

P. Smielewski
Brain Physics Laboratory, Division of Neurosurgery, Department of Clinical Neurosciences, Cambridge Biomedical Campus, Addenbrooke's Hospital, University of Cambridge, Cambridge, UK
e-mail: ps10011@cam.ac.uk

M. Czosnyka
Brain Physics Laboratory, Division of Neurosurgery, Department of Clinical Neurosciences, Cambridge Biomedical Campus, Addenbrooke's Hospital, University of Cambridge, Cambridge, UK

Institute of Electronic Systems, Warsaw University of Technology, Warsaw, Poland
e-mail: mc141@medschl.cam.ac.uk

B. Depreitere et al. (eds.), *Intracranial Pressure and Neuromonitoring XVII*, Acta Neurochirurgica Supplement 131,
https://doi.org/10.1007/978-3-030-59436-7_38,

for the issue of time delay between peripheral ABP and $CBFV_a$ since these parameters are calculated in the frequency domain [11].

As a primary goal, since the absolute comparison of $nCPP_s$ to direct CPP has limitations, we focused on cases where CPP is changing: (1) a rise during vasopressor-induced augmentation of ABP and (2) a decrease during spontaneous changes in ICP (plateau waves). Then we compared changes in $nCPP_s$ versus changes in direct CPP to rule out problems secondary to ABP zeroing. Secondarily, to account for a broader variety of clinical events other than specific increases or decreases in CPP, we analysed $nCPP_s$ in a population presenting wider ranges of CPP.

Material and Methods

Patients

Patients admitted to the Neurosciences Critical Care Unit at Addenbrooke's Hospital, Cambridge, UK, with severe (admission Glasgow Coma Score (GCS) < 8) or moderate (admission GCS < 12) traumatic brain injury (TBI) with secondary neurological deterioration requiring intubation and mechanical ventilation were eligible for inclusion in this study. All patients were intubated and mechanically ventilated, sedated with propofol and fentanyl, and paralysed with atracurium.

Three cohorts of patients were analysed. The first cohort consisted of 20 TBI patients with induced rise in ABP producing rises in CPP levels (median patient age was 27.5 years (interquartile range (IQR) 41–21.5)), as previously described by Steiner et al. [15]. The local research ethics committee approved the data collection for this study (2001–2002), and informed consent was obtained from the next of kin of all patients. The second and third cohorts were derived from a database of 446 adult TBI patients (median patient age was 30 years (IQR 78–18)), with simultaneous recordings of ABP, ICP and TCD collected between 1995 and 2016 during routine clinical TCD investigations of cerebral autoregulation (included in Protocol 30 REC 97/290). The second cohort consisted of a subset of patients presenting plateau waves identified as sudden and spontaneous increases in ICP (and pulse amplitude of ICP), during which CPP and mean cerebral blood flow velocity dropped with a relatively stable ABP. The third cohort consisted of 340 patients who presented wider ranges of CPP across time.

For patients monitored before 1997, the Neurocritical Care Users' Committee allowed TCD examinations for the assessment of TBI patients. Informed consent was obtained from the next of kin of all patients. Further use of the anonymised data was allowed as a part of clinical audits.

Monitoring and Data Analysis

ABP was measured directly from the radial artery calibrated at the level of the heart (Baxter Health Care Corp., CardioVascular Group). ICP was monitored continuously using a microtransducer placed in the brain parenchyma (MicroSensors ICP Transducer; Codman and Shurtleff, Inc.). CPP was calculated as the difference between the mean ABP and ICP. $CBFV_a$ was obtained bilaterally from the left and right MCAs using a TCD ultrasonography system (DWL Multidop X4, DWL Elektronische Systeme GmbH), with the probe held in place during the entire recording using a head frame. Mean $CBFV_a$ was calculated as the average between left and right $CBFV_a$. Raw signals were digitised using an analog–digital converter (DT 2814, Marlborough, California, USA) sampled at a frequency of 100 Hz and recorded with ICM+ ® (Cambridge Enterprise, https://icmplus.neurosurg.cam.ac.uk/). The recorded signals were subjected to manual artefact removal and analysed with ICM+ ®. All parameters were calculated and averaged. All calculations were performed over a 10-s-long sliding window.

Noninvasive CPP Formula

The noninvasive CPP formula was simply derived from a mathematical equation explaining the value and changes in the spectral pulsatility index [16]:

$$\mathrm{nCPP_s} = \frac{a1}{\mathrm{sPI}} \times \sqrt{\left(R_a \cdot C_a\right)^2 \cdot HR^2 \cdot \left(2\pi\right)^2 + 1} \ \ (\mathrm{mmHg})$$

where

$$\mathrm{sPI} = \frac{f1}{\mathrm{CBFV}_a}$$

sPI denotes the spectral pulsatility index; *HR* is expressed in Hz; *f1* and $a1$ are first harmonics of $CBFV_a$ and ABP signal amplitudes; C_a is cerebral arterial compliance; and R_a is cerebrovascular resistance.

Statistical Analysis

Statistical analysis was conducted with R Studio software (R version 3.6.0). We calculated the correlation coefficient in the time domain (R) between direct CPP and $nCPP_s$ for cohorts 1 and 2. Correlation coefficients in the time domain were obtained for individual patients and then averaged within cohorts 1 and 2. For cohort 3, individual recordings were treated as independent events and used for the correlation analysis. For this patient cohort, the correlation analysis was performed over CPP bins of 25 mmHg, ranging from 0 to 125 mmHg. We also calculated the Spearman correlation coefficient for mean values between CPP and $nCPP_s$ considering the difference (delta [Δ = magnitude of changes]) between the baseline and plateau phases for cohort 2 and between baseline and ABP increase for patients in cohort 1. To assess the prediction ability of the model, we calculated the area under the curve (AUC) with a receiver operating characteristic analysis (ROC). To integrate this assessment for cohorts 1 and 2, the prediction threshold chosen was determined as the median value of the absolute difference (absolute ΔCPP) between ICP plateau/ABP increase and baseline phases for direct CPP in these two cohorts together. The threshold obtained was ΔCPP ≥ 23.2 mmHg. This test permits, independently of the direction of changes in CPP, to assess whether $nCPP_s$ can predict the magnitude of these changes reliably. We also assessed the prediction ability of the method to detect low CPP (<70 mmHg) in cohort 3. The prediction capability is considered reasonable when AUC is higher than 0.7 and strong when AUC exceeds 0.8 [17].

Results

The analysis involved 16 patients from cohort 1, and 14 patients were identified in which at least one plateau wave occurred during the monitoring period in cohort 2. A total of 21 plateau waves were analysed. A wide range of CPP, from 12.61 to 123.75 mmHg, was found for the cohort encompassing the 340 TBI patients in cohort 3, for whom 879 recordings with ABP, ICP and TCD data were performed.

Figures 1 and 2 demonstrate examples of changes in ABP, ICP, $CBFV_a$, CPP and $nCPP_s$ in the patient cohorts undergoing induced ABP increase and ICP plateau waves, respectively. Table 1 presents values of the physiological variables and $nCPP_s$ estimator assessed, displayed as median (IQR).

The average correlation in the time domain between CPP and $nCPP_s$ for patients undergoing induced rises in ABP was 0.95 ± 0.07, and 0.86 ± 0.14 during ICP plateau waves. Δ correlations between mean values of CPP and $nCPP_s$ were 0.73 ($p = 0.002$) and 0.78 ($p < 0.001$) respectively for induced rises in ABP and ICP plateau wave cohorts (Fig. 3). A Fisher z-transformation did not indicate a statistically significant difference between these two Δ correlation coefficients ($z = -0.32$ ($p = 0.75$)).

The average correlation in the time domain between CPP and $nCPP_s$ for cohort 3 was 0.63 ± 0.37. nCPPs had correlation coefficients higher than 0.60 across all CPP ranges. Most of the recordings presented CPP in the 50- to 100-mmHg range ($N = 805$ recordings (91%)).

ROC analysis of the combined threshold for CPP prediction (ΔCPP ≥ 23.2 mmHg) in cohorts 1 and 2 revealed an AUC of 0.71 (95% confidence interval (CI): 0.54–0.88). The AUC for predicting low CPP below 70 mmHg was 0.82 (95% CI: 0.79–0.85).

Discussion

Our proposed spectral nCPP method estimates CPP by accounting for changes in pulsatile cerebral blood volume based on a simplified hydrodynamic model of CBF and CSF dynamics. The spectral feature of the method has some advantages: it creates partial independence from the inaccuracy associated with zeroing the ABP transducer at heart level and partially eliminates the issue of time delay between peripheral ABP and $CBFV_a$ in the MCA. In addition, $nCPP_s$ produces patient-specific CPP estimates and does not require calibration datasets.

The magnitude of changes observed in $nCPP_s$ correlated well with direct CPP considering all patient populations. In cohorts 1 and 2, this indicates that, independently of its degree of accuracy, $nCPP_s$ can reliably detect the magnitude of changes in CPP (Fig. 3). Moreover, $nCPP_s$ demonstrated reasonable AUC for the prediction of CPP changes ≥23.2 mmHg in both patient cohorts analysed jointly (AUC = 0.71). Over a wider CPP range presented by cohort 3, $nCPP_s$ demonstrated even stronger prediction ability to detect low CPP, ≤70 mmHg (AUC = 0.82).

Our method only represents a step towards an alternative to nCPP estimation since it could not produce a clear improvement in the accuracy of estimating CPP in absolute numbers at the current stage of development. However, accuracy may not be the primary performance measure in every clinical situation, and such drawbacks may be compensated for by the ability of the method to track changes and trends in ICP over time, rather than its absolute value. Despite the lack of individual calibration, $nCPP_s$ presented reliable accuracy in tracking changes in CPP across time during increases in ABP and plateau waves (Figs. 1 (cohort 1) and 2 (cohort 2)), with a slightly better performance in the former patient cohort. For instance, plateau waves are recurrent phenomena in TBI patients, affecting approximately 25% of cases and a predictor of poor outcome [18], and pharmacologically induced ABP rise is a common clinical management strategy. Therefore, the identification of these CPP changes noninvasively could represent a useful application of $nCPP_s$. In clinical practice, it could provide a better understanding of the state of a patient and guide oriented treatments in situations where CPP is drastically changing. In a previous assessment and description of this method in paediatric TBI patients [11], we obtained a similar outcome profile wherein it showed good correlation with invasively measured CPP (R = 0.67, $p < 0.0001$), as well as an acceptable ability to track CPP changes over time ($R = 0.55 \pm 0.42$). The ability of

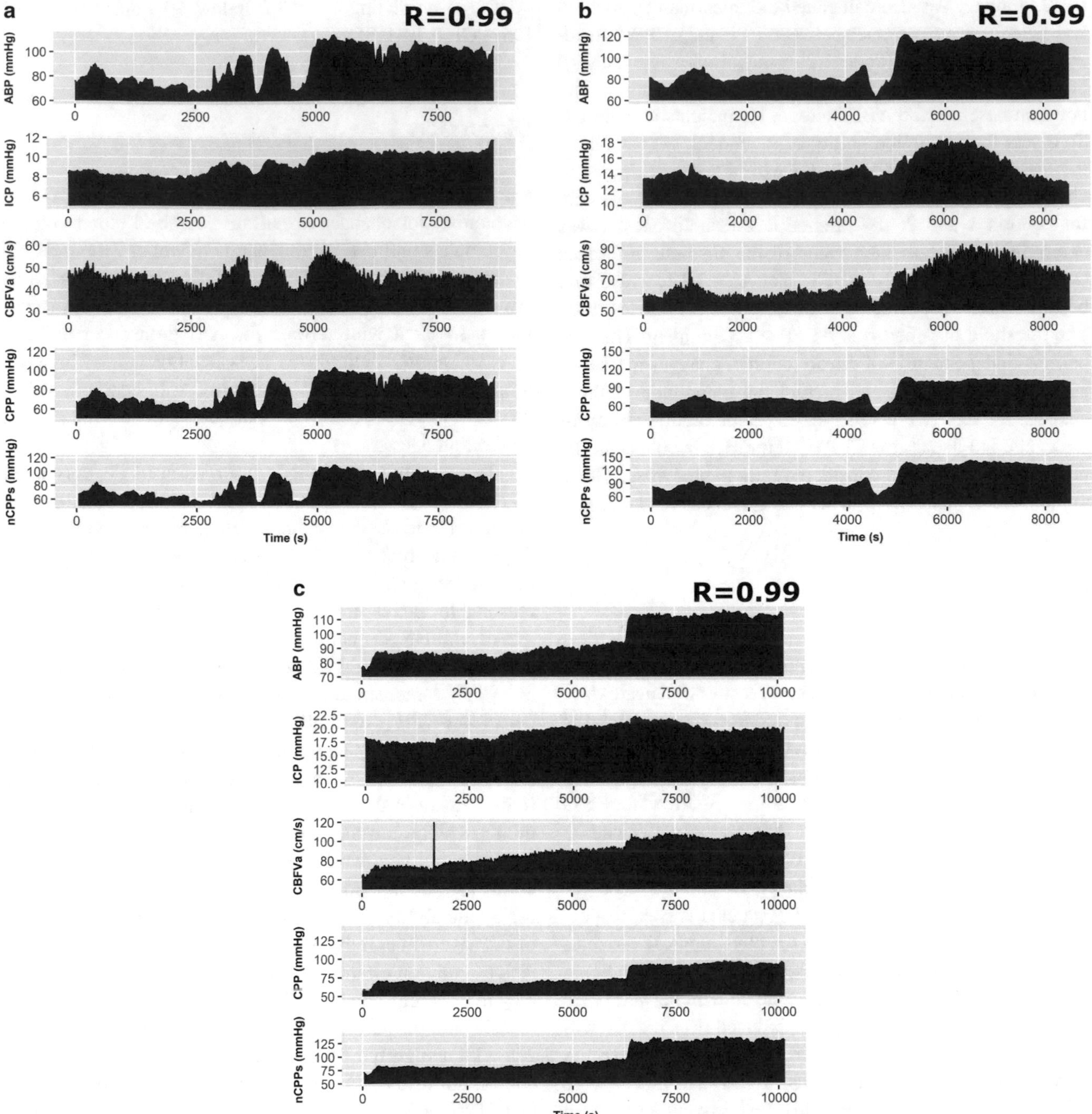

Fig. 1 Example of individual cases (**a**, **b**, **c**) showing correlation in time domain between CPP and $nCPP_s$ (R) in patients with induced rises in ABP. *ABP* arterial blood pressure, *ICP* intracranial pressure, *CPP* cerebral perfusion pressure, $nCPP_s$ noninvasive cerebral perfusion pressure according to spectral method

$nCPP_s$ to predict values of CPP below 70 mmHg was strong (AUC = 0.91 (95% CI = 0.83–0.98)). However, $nCPP_s$ overestimated CPP by 19.61 mmHg, with a wide 95% CI of ±40.4 mmHg.

Finally, the mathematical beauty of the $nCPP_s$ formula is that "nCPP = a1/sPI" was proposed as an estimator of noninvasive CPP many years ago by the 'father' of TCD ultrasonography, Dr. Rune Aaslid [19]. Our proposed formula is the result of a simple correction of his equation by including factors such as cerebrovascular compliance and resistance and heart rate.

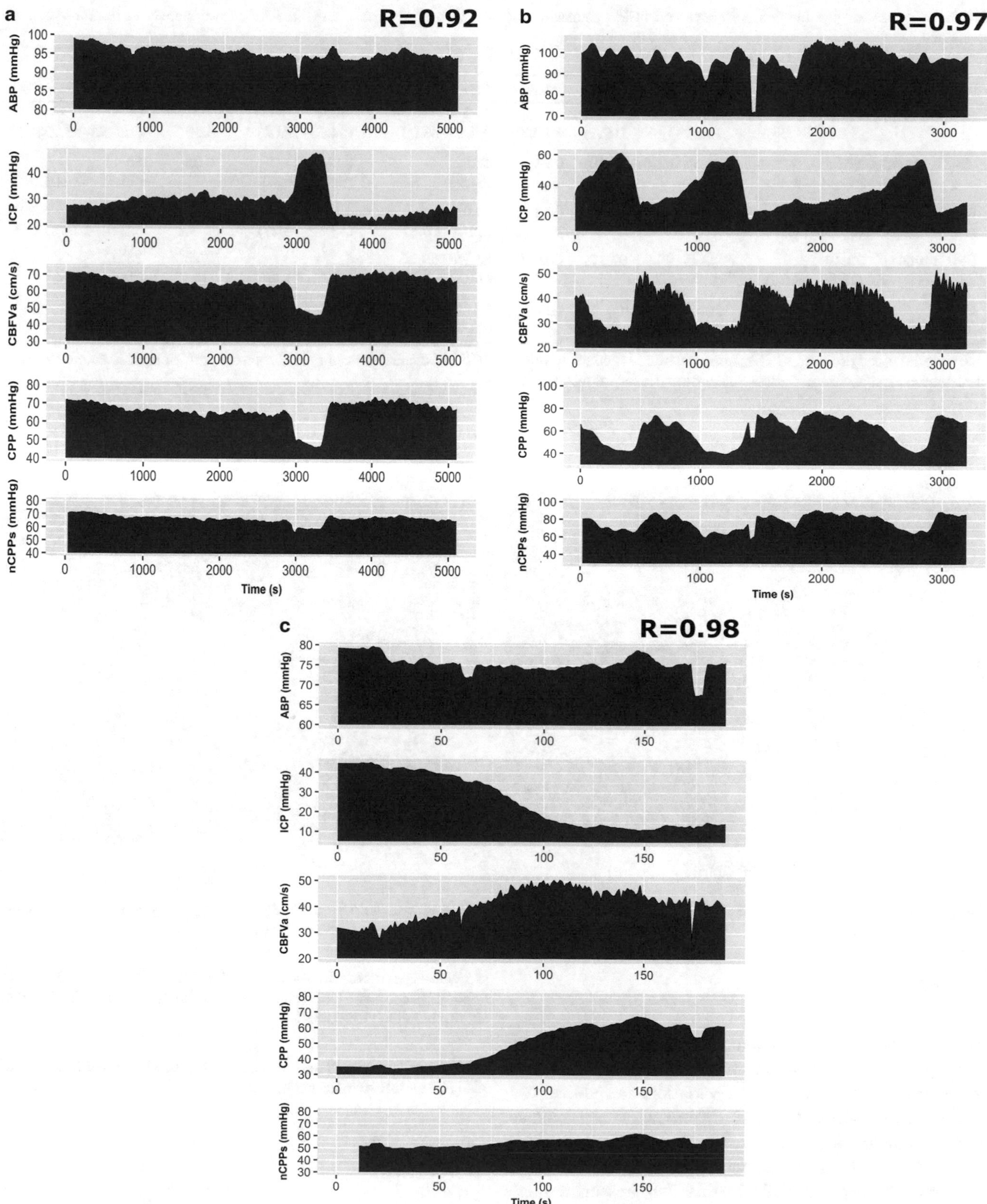

Fig. 2 Example of individual cases (**a**, **b**, **c**) showing correlation in time domain between CPP and $nCPP_s$ (R) in patients presenting ICP plateau waves. *ABP* arterial blood pressure, *ICP* intracranial pressure, *CPP* cerebral perfusion pressure, $nCPP_s$ noninvasive cerebral perfusion pressure according to the spectral method

Table 1 Values of physiological variables and $nCPP_s$ estimator assessed, displayed as median (IQR) for measurements in the three cohorts evaluated

	Cohort 1 (N = 16)			Cohort 2 (N = 14)			
Parameter	Baseline	Increase phase	p-value	Baseline	Plateau	p-value	Cohort 3 (N = 879)
ABP (mmHg)	86.92 (91.19–81.08)	110.9 (114.4–107.1)	<0.0001	91.21 (97.97–83.00)	90.77 (94.05–78.00)	0.39	91.37 (100.96–83.23)
$CBFV_a$ (cm/s)	59.03 (69.51–49.23)	72.56 (81.84–53.40)	0.22	47.51 (64.92–42.84)	35.87 (60.46–30.70)	0.05	56.41 (75.17–41.90)
ICP (mmHg)	13.93 (19.00–11.53)	15.19 (20.60–12.70)	0.33	25.08 (28.76–16.81)	48.26 (53.86–38.07)	<0.0001	17.52 (23.61–12.46)
CPP (mmHg)	73.19 (76.68–68.80)	93.25 (96.93–92.17)	<0.0001	66.35 (74.04–58.24)	41.74 (47.91–35.29)	<0.0001	74.02 (82.86–63.92)
$nCPP_s$ (mmHg)	82.73 (85.41–78.53)	109.85 (113.15–103.04)	<0.0001	72.82 (83.27–64.40)	61.97 (69.01–54.04)	<0.01	84.54 (97.03–74.75)

ABP arterial blood pressure, *$CBFV_a$* arterial cerebral blood flow velocity, *ICP* intracranial pressure, *CPP* cerebral perfusion pressure, *$nCPP_s$* noninvasive cerebral perfusion pressure according to spectral method

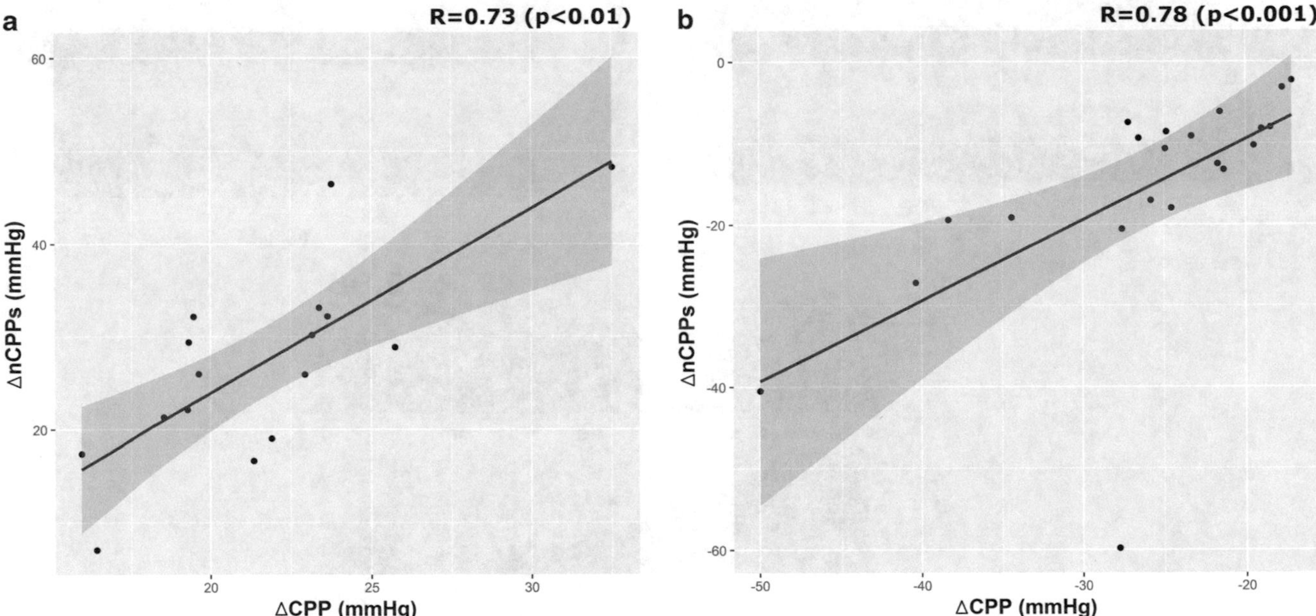

Fig. 3 Correlation plots between changes (Δ) of both CPP and $nCPP_s$ in induced rises in ABP (**a**) and plateau wave (**b**) cohorts. R represents Spearman correlation coefficient. *CPP* cerebral perfusion pressure, *$nCPP_s$* noninvasive cerebral perfusion pressure according to spectral method

Limitations

For the proposed $nCPP_s$ method, we assume that the cerebrovascular diameter is constant; however, changes in cerebrovascular resistance produced by variations in end-tidal CO_2 and partial pressure of CO_2 may disturb $nCPP_s$ and could act as a confounding factor since these parameters were unavailable [20, 21]. The presented model of the vascular input to the brain is very simplistic in that it represents a single (lumped) model of input vascular compliance and resistance. The non-linearity of vascular resistance and compliance is not considered, and the pulsatility of intracranial pressure is neglected, which may limit the accuracy of estimation. Our main intention was, however, to suggest that such a 'modelling' approach to noninvasive estimation of CPP was generally feasible.

Acknowledgements MC is supported by NIHR, Biomedical Research Centre, Cambridge UK. Project was also supported by NIHR Brain Injury MedTech Co-operative.

Conflict of Interest **PS and MC have a financial interest in a part of the ICM+ software licensing fees.**

References

1. Czosnyka M, Pickard JD (2004) Monitoring and interpretation of intracranial pressure. J Neurol Neurosurg Psychiatry 75:813–821
2. Czosnyka M, SR W RJ (2015) Calculation of cerebral perfusion pressure in the management of traumatic brain injury: joint position statement by the councils of the Neuroanaesthesia and Critical Care Society of Great Britain and Ireland (NACCS) and the Society of British Neurological Surgeons (SBNS). Br J Anaesth 115(4):487–488

3. Smith JJ, Porth CM, Erickson M (1994) Hemodynamic response to the upright posture. J Clin Pharmacol 34(5):375–386
4. Van Aken H, Miller E (2000) Deliberate hypotension. In: Miller R (ed) Anesthesia, 5th edn. Churchill Livingstone, New York, pp 1470–1490
5. Zacchetti L, Magnoni S, Di Corte F, Zanier ER, Stocchetti N (2015) Accuracy of intracranial pressure monitoring: systematic review and meta-analysis. Crit Care 19(1):420
6. Czosnyka M, Matta BF, Smielewski P, Kirkpatrick PJ, Pickard JD (1998) Cerebral perfusion pressure in head-injured patients: a noninvasive assessment using transcranial Doppler ultrasonography. J Neurosurg 88:802–808
7. Edouard AR, Vanhille E, Le Moigno S, Benhamou D, Mazoit J-X (2005) Non-invasive assessment of cerebral perfusion pressure in brain injured patients with moderate intracranial hypertension. Br J Anaesth 94(2):216–221
8. Schmidt EA, Czosnyka M, Gooskens I, Piechnik SK, Matta BF, Whitfield PC, Pickard JD (2001) Preliminary experience of the estimation of cerebral perfusion pressure using transcranial Doppler ultrasonography. J Neurol Neurosurg Psychiatry 70(2):198–204
9. Schmidt EA, Czosnyka M, Matta BF, Gooskens I, Piechnik S, Pickard JD (2000) Non-invasive cerebral perfusion pressure (nCPP): evaluation of the monitoring methodology in head injured patients. Acta Neurochir Suppl 76:451–452
10. Varsos GV, Kolias AG, Smielewski P, Brady KM, Varsos VG, Hutchinson PJ, Pickard JD, Czosnyka M (2015) A noninvasive estimation of cerebral perfusion pressure using critical closing pressure. J Neurosurg 123(3):638–648
11. Abecasis F, Cardim D, Czosnyka M, Robba C, Agrawal S (2019) Transcranial Doppler as a non-invasive method to estimate cerebral perfusion pressure in children with severe traumatic brain injury. Childs Nerv Syst. https://doi.org/10.1007/s00381-019-04273-2
12. Czosnyka M, Piechnik S, Richards HK, Kirkpatrick P, Smielewski P, Pickard JD (1997) Contribution of mathematical modelling to the interpretation of bedside tests of cerebrovascular autoregulation. J Neurol Neurosurg Psychiatry 63(6):721–731
13. Ursino M, Di Giammarco P (1991) A mathematical model of the relationship between cerebral blood volume and intracranial pressure changes: the generation of plateau waves. Ann Biomed Eng 19(1):15–42
14. Ursino M, Lodi CA (1997) A simple mathematical model of the interaction between intracranial pressure and cerebral hemodynamics. J Appl Physiol 82(4):1256–1269
15. Steiner LA, Coles JP, Johnston AJ et al (2003) Assessment of cerebrovascular autoregulation in head-injured patients. Stroke 34(10):2404–2409
16. De Riva N, Budohoski KP, Smielewski P, Kasprowicz M, Zweifel C, Steiner LA, Reinhard M, Fábregas N, Pickard JD, Czosnyka M (2012) Transcranial doppler pulsatility index: what it is and what it isn't. Neurocrit Care 17(1):58–66
17. Hosmer D, Lameshow S (1989) Applied logistic regression. John Wiley & Sons, New York
18. Castellani G, Zweifel C, Kim D-J, Carrera E, Radolovich DK, Smielewski P, Hutchinson PJ, Pickard JD, Czosnyka M (2009) Plateau waves in head injured patients requiring neurocritical care. Neurocrit Care 11:143–150
19. Aaslid R, Lundar T, Lindegaard KF, Nornes H (1986) Estimation of cerebral perfusion pressure from arterial blood pressure and transcranial Doppler recordings. In: Miller JD, Teasdale GM, Rowan JO, Galbraith SL, Mendelow AD (eds) Intracranial pressure VI. SpringerVerlag, Berlin, pp 226–229
20. Grüne F, Kazmaier S, Stolker RJ, Visser GH, Weyland A (2015) Carbon dioxide induced changes in cerebral blood flow and flow velocity: role of cerebrovascular resistance and effective cerebral perfusion pressure. J Cereb Blood Flow Metab 35(9):1470–1477
21. Verbree J, Bronzwaer A-SGT, Ghariq E, Versluis MJ, Daemen MJAP, van Buchem MA, Dahan A, van Lieshout JJ, van Osch MJP (2014) Assessment of middle cerebral artery diameter during hypocapnia and hypercapnia in humans using ultra-high-field MRI. J Appl Physiol 117(10):1084–1089

Empirical Mode Decomposition-Based Method for Artefact Removal in Raw Intracranial Pressure Signals

Isabel Martinez-Tejada, Jens E. Wilhjelm, Marianne Juhler, and Morten Andresen

Introduction

The most common way of analysing the intracranial pressure (ICP) signal in clinical practice is by visually inspecting the presence of macro patterns and waveform abnormalities. However, this approach relies on the experience of the observer, and hence the outcome might not be consistent. Automated and standardized methods of detecting wave patterns are thus desired to enable better detection of ICP deviations for diagnostic and therapeutic purposes. However, ICP signals are often contaminated by artefacts and the presence of segments of missing values. Some of these artefacts can be observed as very high and short spikes with a physiologically impossible high slope and value. These spikes can be generated by different sources, e.g. connection errors and movement of the monitoring system during data collection [1]. The presence of these spikes reduces the accuracy of pattern recognition techniques because they mask the characteristic appearance of ICP patterns.

Several methods have been used to identify the presence of spikes in ICP signals, from signal thresholding [2] to wavelet analysis. Signal thresholding fails to work if the signal-to-noise ratio (SNR) is low or if the ICP rises in an unphysiologically short time. Techniques using low-pass filtering are not appropriate in the case of the ICP signal since they are non-stationary (i.e. statistical properties change over time), as shown in the top graph of Fig. 1, where trends varying in time can be observed [3]. Alternative non-linear methods are based on wavelet transformation, whose output performance is highly influenced by the choice of a basis function [4]. These basis functions are fixed, hindering their match with the nature of the input signal at a given time. To overcome this drawback, more recent papers decompose the signal using the empirical mode decomposition (EMD) method, where the mother functions are derived from the signal, making the decomposition adaptive [4, 5].

Therefore, in this paper we propose a modified EMD method for automatic spike removal in raw ICP signals. The method is adaptive in non-linear and non-stationary signals because it involves breaking down signals into different frequency modes without leaving the time domain. It relies on the principle that some of these modes, also referred to as intrinsic mode functions (IMFs), capture the noise in signals so no a priori information on the data is required. This is important because there is no a priori knowledge of noise, so no procedures can be fixed beforehand to decrease the contribution of noise in signals.

Methods

EMD Algorithm

Huang et al. [6] presented EMD as a sifting method for adaptively decomposing non-stationary signals into a finite number of IMFs. An IMF is described as a function with two requirements: first, the number of extrema must be equal to zero-crossing or differ mostly by one and, second, the mean value of its lower and upper envelopes is zero. The EMD algorithm used for IMF extraction is briefly described for a given input ICP signal $s(t)$ as follows:

I. Martinez-Tejada (✉)
Clinic of Neurosurgery, Copenhagen University Hospital, Rigshospitalet, Denmark

Department of Health Technology, Technical University of Denmark, Lyngby, Denmark
e-mail: imate@dtu.dk

J. E. Wilhjelm
Department of Health Technology, Technical University of Denmark, Lyngby, Denmark
e-mail: jwil@dtu.dk

M. Juhler · M. Andresen
Clinic of Neurosurgery, Copenhagen University Hospital, Rigshospitalet, Denmark

B. Depreitere et al. (eds.), *Intracranial Pressure and Neuromonitoring XVII*, Acta Neurochirurgica Supplement 131,
https://doi.org/10.1007/978-3-030-59436-7_39,

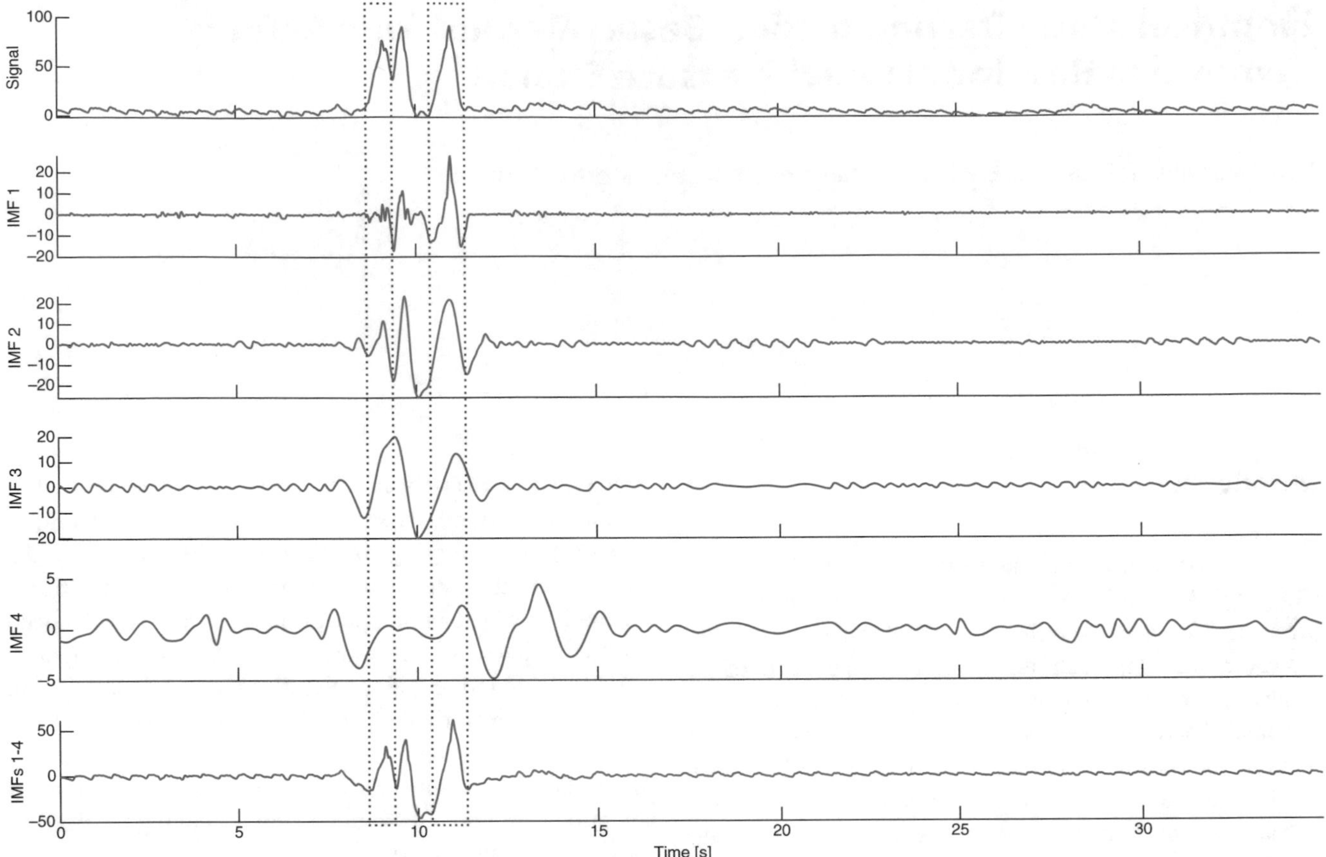

Fig. 1 Examples of peaks in ICP signals and IMF1–4

1. Find signal $x(t)$ extrema to which splines are fitted to generate both lower and upper envelopes. In the first iteration, $x(t) = s(t)$.
2. Calculate the arithmetic average of the two envelopes, $m(t)$.
3. Generate a candidate IMF $h(t)$ by subtracting the average envelope from the signal: $h(t) = x(t) - m(t)$.
4. If $h(t)$ is not an IMF according to the preceding requirements, then $x(t)$ must be replaced with $h(t)$ and steps 1–3 repeated. However, if $h(t)$ is treated as an IMF and the stopping criteria are not reached, the residue $r(t) = x(t) - h(t)$ is assigned to $x(t)$ and steps 1–3 are repeated. The stopping condition is usually a very small value to which the mean squared difference between the last two extracted successive IMFs is compared.

At the end of this iterative process, the original signal $s(t)$ can be expressed as the sum of all extracted IMFs plus the final residue. Note that the later an IMF is extracted, the lower will be its frequency content.

Proposed EMD-Based Algorithm

Spikes have a band-limited waveform, which implies that the frequency content is limited only to certain consecutive IMFs. *Band-limited* means that the frequency domain of the signal is zero beyond a certain finite frequency. The summation of the successive IMFs that contain part of a spike's dominant frequency would then help to temporally localize the spike event.

For localization and later removal of spikes from the ICP signal, we propose the following method:

1. Break down ICP signal into sixteen IMFs via EMD, as described above. Based on the physiological properties of the ICP signal as well as previous experiences by Feng et al. [7], breaking down the signal into 16 IMFs was considered the best trade-off between the signal length and computational time [8].
2. Spike detection from estimated IMFs.
3. Spike imputation in the original signal.

It must be noted that missing values are also randomly present in the ICP signal and they must be temporarily replaced with zeroes before EMD. In our monitored ICP signals, missing values are most likely due to sensor detachment during several minutes. Thus, temporal replacement by zeros during only the decomposition would not have any effect on higher frequency IMFs, which are the ones we are interested on for denoising. Instead, it will affect the low-frequency part, *i.e.* the local trend. Given the simplicity and lower computational time of this shortcoming and its ability to achieve an effective technical solution, it is preferred over the interpolation of values.

After decomposition, as visually demonstrated in Fig. 1, high amplitude oscillations in the first IMF align with the location of spikes in the ICP signal. Because the spikes have band-limited waveforms, dominant oscillations are found in various consecutive IMFs. Thus, a more effective event duration estimation is obtained when various successive IMFs are taken into account. In our case, only the location of peaks in $IMF_{1–4}$ aligns with the location of peaks in the ICP signal, so summing these four IMFs enhances spike episodes: $IMF_{1-4} = \sum_{k=1}^{4} IMF_k(t)$. It is assumed then that the oscillations that build a spike are present in these four successive IMFs at the same temporal location as the signal artefact.

To identify the peaks in the summed IMFs, an adaptive thresholding approach is proposed (Fig. 2). ICP samples outside the bounded region in $[-P_{th}, P_{th}]$ will be identified as spikes. The threshold is determined based on the noise level in the summed IMFs: $P_{th} = \widehat{\sigma}\sqrt{2 \times \log L}$, where σ is the standard deviation of the signal and L the number of samples in the summed IMF [1]. Because σ is always unknown given the presence of artefacts in the signal, it must be estimated using e.g. the median absolute deviation: $\hat{\sigma} = \frac{MAD}{0.6745}$, where $MAD = Me \mid IMF_{1-4} - Me(IMF_{1-4}) \mid$ [9]. If two identified spikes lie within a window of 0.4 s, the ICP samples between them are also treated as spike events. ICP spikes identified can either be removed or imputed with a moving average calculated over a sliding window of 10 s. An example of the results can be seen in Fig. 3.

Results

To both prove the non-stationarity of the signals and test the ability of the proposed method to detect spikes, real ICP signals are used. A total of 26 h are investigated from five different monitoring sequences. The Kwiatkowski–Phillips–Schmidt–Shin (KPSS) test for stationarity is applied to selected artefact-free segments of increasing size [10]. With a 1-s window size, ICP signals are non-stationary with p-values around 0.03 for a significance level (critical alpha) equal to 0.05. Increasing window sizes reject the null hypothesis for the stationarity of the time series with even lower p-values (i.e. values close to 0.01).

To investigate the performance of the proposed algorithm, ICP segments containing unwanted dominant spikes are examined. Segments are visually inspected by an expert using a spike template. This template is established just for visual inspection purposes and is based on the determination of two spike characteristics: a duration shorter than 0.5 s and an abrupt ICP value increase. The artefact events visually

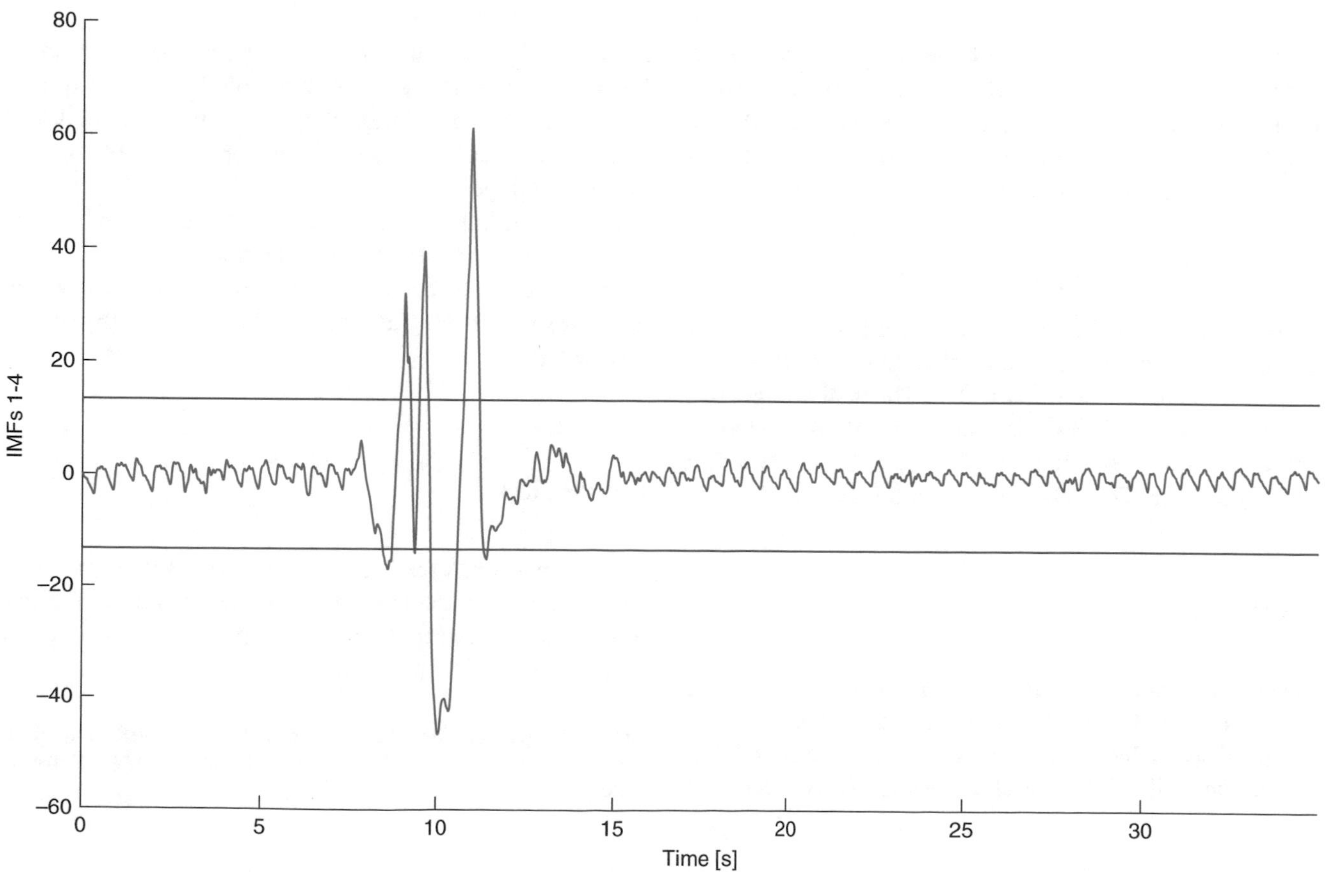

Fig. 2 ICP signals with lower and upper thresholds marked in red

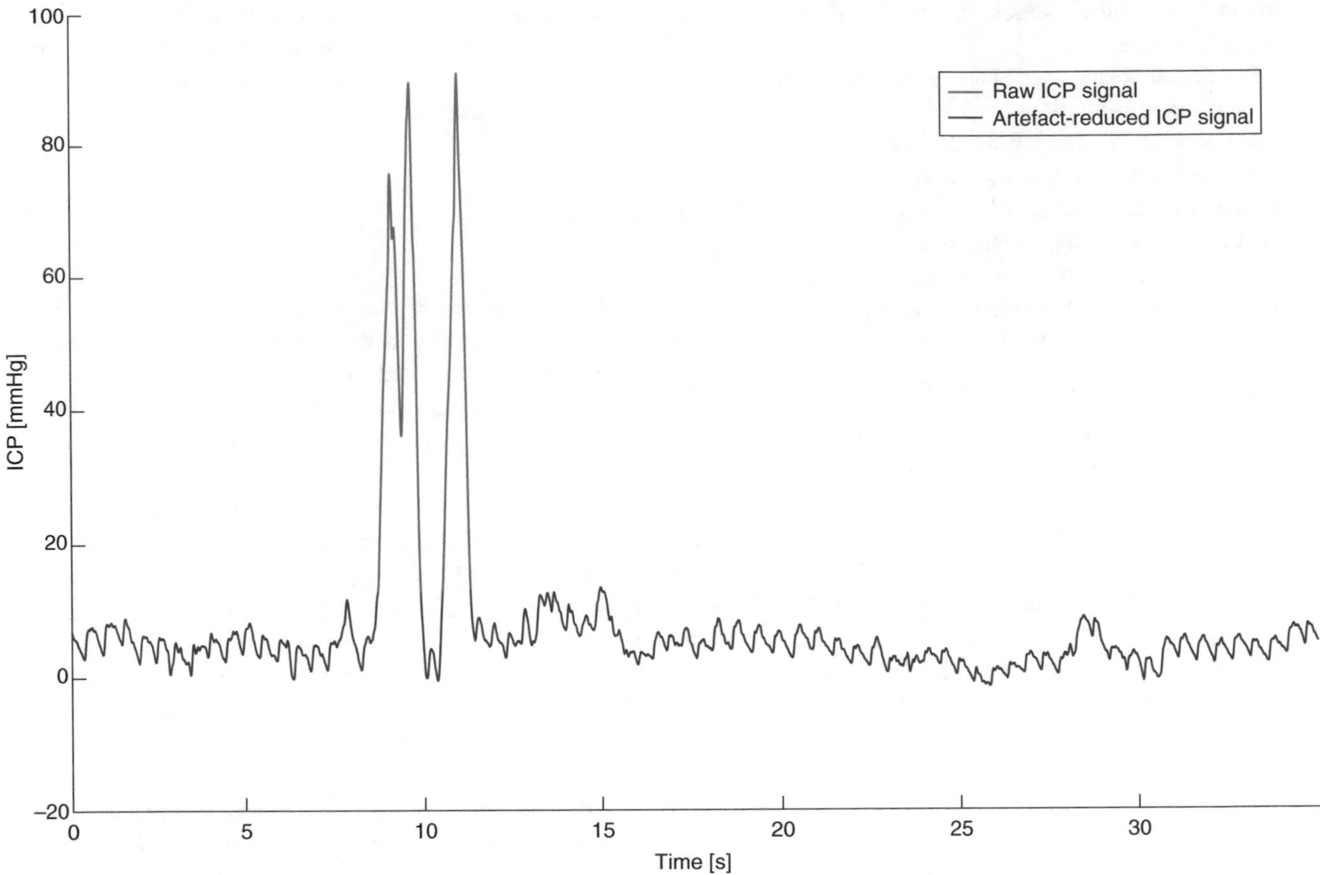

Fig. 3 Artefact-reduced ICP signal where detected spike has been removed

identified with the presence of the template are used as ground truth, and the ability of the method to identify them is then examined. The performance of the proposed method is quantified based on how well it estimates the location of the spikes using precision and recall metrics:

$$\text{precision} = \frac{\text{TP}}{\text{TP} + \text{FP}} \qquad \text{recall} = \frac{\text{TP}}{\text{TP} + \text{FN}}$$

where TP is the number of correctly identified spikes, FP is the number of spikes identified that were not spikes, and FN is the number of unidentified spikes. The goal is to get both values as close to 100% as possible. The proposed algorithm can detect spikes achieving an 84% precision and a 77% recall, given that TP = 114, FP = 21 and FN = 34.

Discussion

Results show that there are some artefact-free signal segments that are incorrectly classified as artefacts, given that the precision achieved is not 100%. The recall is lower, which shows that some artefact events are not identified. This is likely to be due to the magnitude of the episodes being smaller than the adaptive threshold P_{th} calculated. This limitation could be addressed by performing an additional spike identification iteration based on the slopes of the summed IMF peaks.

The algorithm also presents the drawback of not establishing a method to deal with the identified artefacts. We will further investigate this in our ongoing research, for which autoregressive moving average (ARMA) models [5] will be considered.

Conclusion

In this paper, a new methodology based on EMD is proposed for the removal of unphysiological spikes in clinical ICP signals, which is essential for correct patient evaluation and diagnosis in clinical practice.

Acknowledgement The authors are thankful for contributions from the Novo Nordisk Fonden Tandem Programme and Otto Mønsteds Fond.

Conflict of Interest **The authors declare that they have no conflict of interest.**

References

1. Andresen M, Juhler M, Thomsen OC (2013) Electrostatic discharges and their effect on the validity of registered values in intracranial pressure monitors. J Neurosurg 119:1119–1124
2. Obeid I, Wolf PD (2004) Evaluation of spike-detection algorithms for a brain-machine interface application. IEEE Trans Biomed Eng 51(6):905–911. https://doi.org/10.1109/TBME.2004.826683
3. Han B, Muma M, Feng M, Zoubir AM (2013) An online approach for intracranial pressure forecasting based on signal decomposition and robust statistics. In: 2013 IEEE International Conference on Acoustics, Speech and Signal Processing (ICASSP), pp. 6239–6243
4. Andrade AO, Nasuto S, Kyberd P, Sweeney-Reed CM, Van Kanijn FR (2006) EMG signal filtering based on empirical mode decomposition. Biomed Signal Process Control 1(1):44–55
5. Farashi S, Abolhassani M, Kani M (2014) An empirical mode decomposition based method for action potential detection in neural raw data. World Academy of Science, Engineering and Technology, Open Science Index 85. Int J Med Health Sci 8(1):45–49
6. Huang NE, Shen Z, Long SR, Wu MC, Shih HH, Zheng Q, Yen N, Tung C, Liu HH (1998) The empirical mode decomposition and the Hilbert spectrum for nonlinear and non-stationary time series analysis. Proc Math Phys Eng Sci 454(1971):903–995
7. Feng M, Loy LY, Zhang F, Guan C (2011) Artifact removal for intracranial pressure monitoring signals: a robust solution with signal decomposition. In: Proceedings of the annual international conference of the IEEE Engineering in Medicine and Biology Society, EMBS, vol 6090182. IEEE, pp 797–801
8. Sanchez JL, Ortigueira M, Rato R, Trujillo J (2016) An improved empirical mode decomposition for long signals. In: SIGNAL 2016: The First International Conference on advances in signal, image and video processing
9. Signal noise reduction. Proceedings of World Academy of Science, Engineering and Technology, 2, 93–96
10. Kwiatkowski D, Phillips PCB, Schmidt P, Shin Y (1992) Testing the null hypothesis of stationarity against the alternative of a unit root. J Econ 54(54):159–178. https://doi.org/10.1016/0304-4076(92)90104-Y

RAQ: A Noise-Resistant Calibration-Independent Compliance Surrogate

Andreas Spiegelberg, Matthias Krause, Juergen Meixensberger, and Vartan Kurtcuoglu

Introduction

The intracranial pressure-volume relationship contains important information for diagnosing hydrocephalus and other space-occupying pathologies. To quantify the pressure-volume relationship, the craniospinal compliance and pressure volume index (PVI) can be calculated based on volume loading [1]. However, this procedure is time-consuming and carries the risk of infection. Furthermore, the regression coefficient of the amplitude/pressure) characteristic (RAP) [2] can be calculated. However, all changes in intracranial pressure (ICP), including non-compliance-changing ones, are reflected in RAP.

The aims of this study were to design and test a parameter that (a) does not reflect artificial and noncompliance influencing changes in ICP, (b) can be calculated from the ICP time course without volume loading, and (c) is independent of calibration and zero offsets of ICP.

Furthermore, we aimed to design a MATLAB program that can calculate the parameter from overnight recordings, to test the program on synthetic ICP signals, and to retrospectively apply the new method on overnight ICP recordings of two groups of patients with different etiologies of hydrocephalus.

A. Spiegelberg (✉)
University of Zurich, The Interface Group, Institute of Physiology, Zurich, Switzerland
e-mail: andreas.spiegelberg@uzh.ch

M. Krause · J. Meixensberger
Universitaetsklinikum Leipzig AoeR, Klinik und Poliklinik für Neurochirurgie, Leipzig, Germany
e-mail: krause@kinderneurochirurgie-leipzig.de; juergen.meixensberger@medizin.uni-leipzig

V. Kurtcuoglu (✉)
University of Zurich, The Interface Group, Institute of Physiology, Zurich, Switzerland

University of Zurich, Zurich Center for Integrative Human Physiology and Neuroscience Center Zurich, Zurich, Switzerland
e-mail: vartan.kurtcuoglu@uzh.ch

Methods

The new parameter, the respiratory amplitude quotient (RAQ), quantifies the modulation of the pulse amplitude by the respiratory wave in the ICP time course. RAQ is defined as the ratio of the amplitude of the respiratory wave in the ICP signal to the amplitude of the respiration-induced wave in the course of the heartbeat-dependent pulse amplitude.

RAQ can theoretically be calculated for single respiratory cycles, fixed consecutive time windows, or select time periods.

Figure 1 shows in a time window containing several heartbeats the mean ICP (MICP) calculated beat by beat and the time courses of the pulse amplitude in the ICP signal (A_{vp}), the amplitude of the respiratory wave in the MICP signal (A_{rp}), and the amplitude of the respiratory wave in the A_{vp} signal (AA_{vp}). RAQ is then calculated as

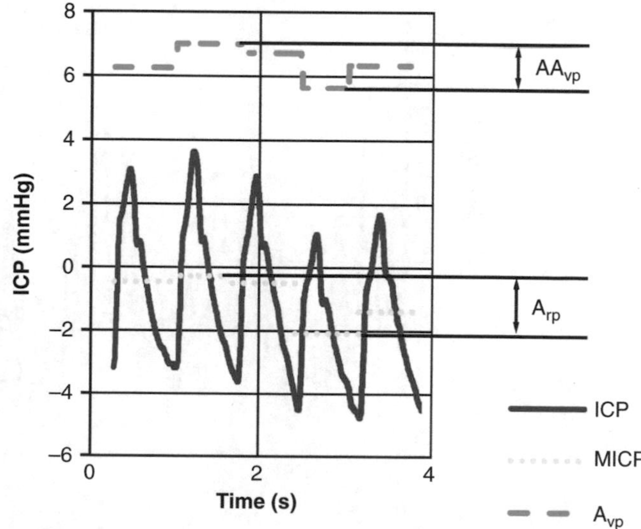

Fig. 1 Course over time of ICP, mean ICP calculated beat by beat (MICP), course of pulse amplitude in ICP signal (A_{vp}), amplitude of respiratory wave in MICP signal (A_{rp}), and amplitude of respiratory wave in A_{vp} signal (AA_{vp})

B. Depreitere et al. (eds.), *Intracranial Pressure and Neuromonitoring XVII*, Acta Neurochirurgica Supplement 131,
https://doi.org/10.1007/978-3-030-59436-7_40, © Springer Nature Switzerland AG 2021

$$\mathrm{RAQ} = A_{\mathrm{rp}} / \mathrm{AA}_{\mathrm{vp}} \quad (1)$$

We designed a MATLAB program to calculate RAQ in which the duration of the analyzed time window can be randomly selected. To calculate the pulse amplitudes, we use the automatic multiscale-based peak detection (AMPD) algorithm, which finds the systolic and diastolic points from the ICP signal in the time domain [3]. Then we calculate the half-period amplitudes (A_{vp}) and forme a time series from them. We further determine, for each half-period, the MICP and forme a time series from it. To calculate the respiratory amplitudes in both the time series of the MICP and the time series of the pulse amplitude, we apply the fast Fourier transform [4] on the corresponding time series and then select the highest amplitude within the respiratory frequency range.

We used the MATLAB program to calculate RAQ in a number of different synthesized ICP signals using time windows of 10 min duration. We then compared the results to theoretical values.

On overnight recordings of patients, we calculated the mean value of RAQ during all B-wave containing periods. The time windows for RAQ calculation were set to the duration of each individual B-wave containing period. B-waves were recognized using the method described in [5]. To compare the RAQ values between the two hydrocephalus groups, we employed the Mann-Whitney U test, because the data were not normally distributed.

Material

To test the method, we used synthetically generated ICP time series under the influence of sinusoidal volume pulse waves and sinusoidal respiratory volume waves for different pressure-volume relationships and different respiratory amplitudes. The signals were synthesized according to

$$\mathrm{ICP} = \mathrm{ICP}_0 + \mathrm{ICP}_1 \cdot e^{k \cdot V} \quad (2)$$

with V being the change in craniospinal blood volume giving rise to the pulse [6]. V is the difference between the pulsatile amount of blood supplied to the craniospinal system by the afferent vascular system and the simultaneous pulsatile blood outflow through the efferent venous system. The venous outflow is influenced by the intrathoracic pressure, which is modulated by the respiration. k is the exponential coefficient, and ICP_0 and ICP_1 are constants.

Figure 2 shows the synthesized ICP for an exponential coefficient of $k = 0.15$/mL.

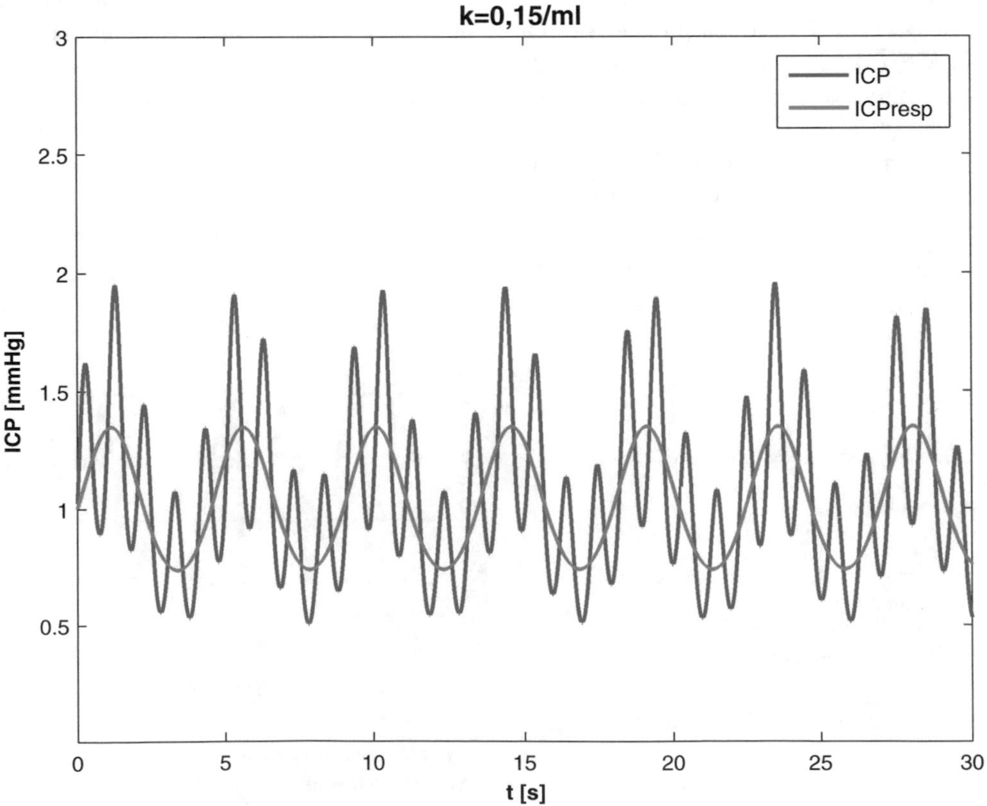

Fig. 2 Synthesized ICP for exponential coefficient $k = 0.15$

We then applied the method to overnight intraparenchymal ICP recordings of two groups of patients presenting with Hakim's triad:

- 8 aqueductal stenosis patients (AQ), morphologically diagnosed using magnetic resonance imaging (MRI)
- 20 non-normal-pressure hydrocephalus patients (NNPH), MRI morphologically diagnosed hydrocephalus patients with no positive response to external lumbar drainage or no positive response to ventriculoperitoneal shunting.

Local ethics committee approval was obtained for the study (Ethikkommission Universität Leipzig Az 014-13-28,012,013). Written informed consent was obtained from the patients before their participation in the study.

Results

The values of RAQ determined with our MATLAB program match those expected by theory. For the synthesized ICP shown in Fig. 2 with an exponential coefficient of $k = 0.15$/ml, RAQ theoretically is 1.303. Our program determined RAQ to be 1.322. Similar results were obtained for $k = 0.1$/ml and $k = 0.125$/ml with a mean error of 0.44%.

Figure 3 shows the pressure-volume relationships for three different values of k and the resulting RAQs. Table 1 shows the RAQ values for the AQ group and the NNPH group. RAQ was found to be lower in the AQ group ($p = 0.031$).

Discussion

Using spectral analysis to calculate RAQ, we ensure narrow band selectivity for the effect caused by respiration. As opposed to RAP, which reflects all changes in ICP, RAQ is not affected by events occurring in other frequency ranges,

Table 1 Mean RAQ values and standard deviations for non-NPH (comparison) and AQ (aqueductal stenosis) patient groups

	RAQ
NNPH	1.065 ± 0.195
AQ	0.872 ± 0.107

The values are significantly different ($p = 0.031$)

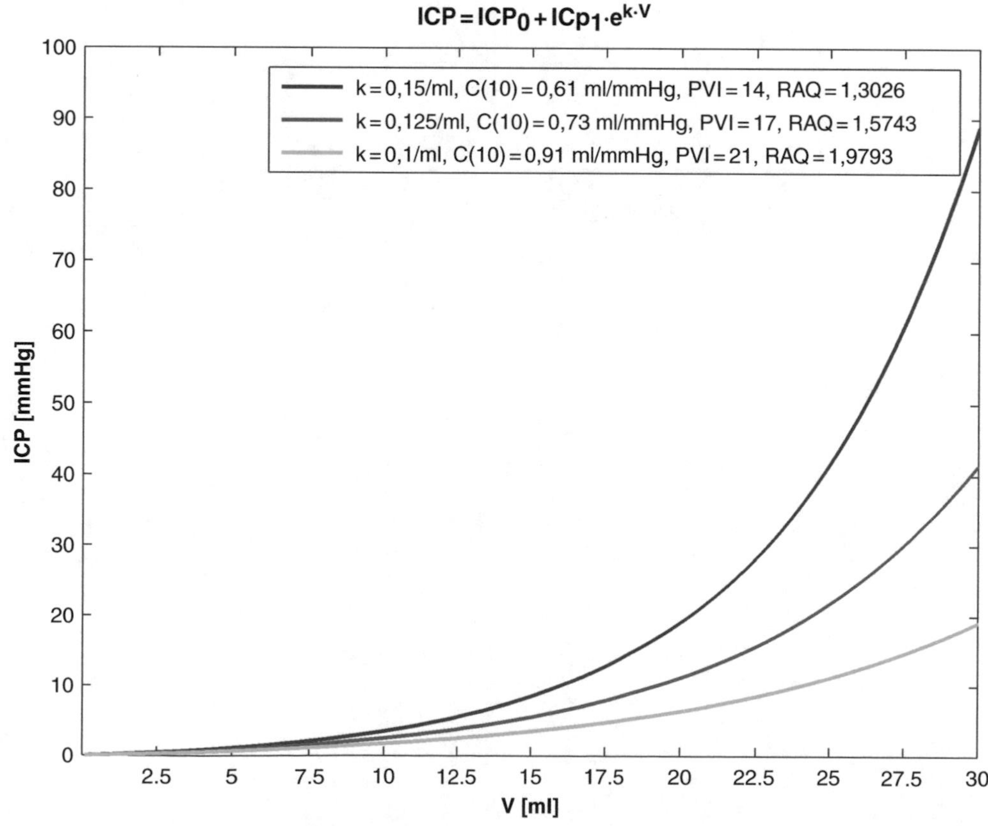

Fig. 3 Pressure-volume relationships for three different values of k and resulting RAQs. C(10) is the compliance at 10 mmHg indicated for each curve

e.g., position changes, B-waves, A-waves, and spike-like artifacts. Being a quotient of amplitudes, RAQ is independent of the calibration and zero offset of ICP signals. Consequently, RAQ can be calculated from uncalibrated signals, including noninvasively measured ICP surrogates. Furthermore, it is not influenced by zero point drifts as encountered in epidural pressure monitoring and long-term telemetric monitoring.

RAQ is constant on a given pressure volume curve and is independent of the depth of respiration.

Conclusion

RAQ is a new parameter that has distinct advantages. We found a significant difference in RAQ for the two aforementioned evaluated groups. RAQ may be beneficial for the evaluation of overnight ICP recordings for normal-pressure hydrocephalus diagnostics and diagnostics for other space-occupying pathologies.

Conflict of Interest **Vartan Kurtcuoglu and Andreas Spiegelberg are inventors, Andreas Spiegelberg and the University of Zurich are applicants for patents DE102018100697A1 and WO2018206799A1. Andreas Spiegelberg is the owner of Cephalotec, a manufacturer of devices that use RAQ. Matthias Krause and Juergen Meixensberger declare that they have no conflict of interest.**

References

1. Bergsneider M (2005) The value of supplemental prognostic tests for the preoperative assessment of idiopathic normal-pressure hydrocephalus. Neurosurgery 57:17–28
2. Price JD, Czosnyka M, Williamson M (1993) Attempts to continuously monitor autoregulation and compensatory reserve in severe head injuries. In: Intracranial pressure, vol VIII. Springer, Berlin, Heidelberg, pp 61–66
3. Scholkmann F, Boss J, Wolf M (2012) An efficient algorithm for automatic peak detection in noisy periodic and quasi-periodic signals. Algorithms 5:588–603
4. Cooley JW, Tukey JW (1965) An algorithm for the machine calculation of complex Fourier series. Math Comput 19:297–301
5. Spiegelberg A, Krause M, Meixensberger J, Seifert B, Kurtcuoglu V (2018) Significant association of slow vasogenic ICP waves with normal pressure hydrocephalus diagnosis. In: Intracranial pressure neuromonitor XVI. Springer, Cham, pp 243–246
6. Avezaat C, van Eijndhoven JHM (1984) Cerebrospinal fluid pulse pressure and craniospinal dynamics: a theoretical, clinical and experimental study

Methodological Consideration on Monitoring Refractory Intracranial Hypertension and Autonomic Nervous System Activity

Marta Fedriga, András Czigler, Nathalie Nasr, Frederick A. Zeiler, Erta Beqiri, Stefan Wolf, Shirin K. Frisvolf, Peter Smielewski, and Marek Czosnyka

Introduction

Intracranial hypertension is a consequence of the fact that the cerebrospinal system content cannot accommodate any additional volume [1, 2]. *Refractory intracranial hypertension* (RIH) constitutes a dramatic increase in ICP that runs from normal or moderately increased values to gross intracranial hypertension. It is refractory to medical or surgical treatment and leads to a patient's death by meeting brain death criteria or major brain damage [3, 4]. Detrimental sequelae of raised ICP in acute brain injury (ABI) are unclear because the pathophysiological mechanisms underlying raised ICP in ABI remain uncertain.

One of the potential factors involved in developing ICP and related to the detrimental effects of high ICP itself could be the autonomic nervous system (ANS).

Impairment of the ANS has been demonstrated to be correlated with outcomes in ABI patients [5–8], although it remains hypothetical how autonomic changes contribute intracranial hypertension sequelae.

The ANS can be assessed in patients monitored with electrocardiogram (ECG) and arterial blood pressure (ABP) through the analysis of heart rate variability (HRV) and baroreflex sensitivity. HRV can be assessed in the beat-to-beat

The authors P. Smielewsky and M. Czosnyka share joint senior authorship.

M. Fedriga (✉)
Brain Physics Laboratory, Division of Neurosurgery, Department of Clinical Neurosciences, University of Cambridge, Cambridge, UK

Department of Anesthesia, Critical Care and Emergency, Spedali Civili University Hospital, Brescia, Italy

A. Czigler
Brain Physics Laboratory, Division of Neurosurgery, Department of Clinical Neurosciences, University of Cambridge, Cambridge, UK

Department of Neurosurgery and Szentagothai Research Center, University of Pecs, Pecs, Hungary

N. Nasr
Départément de Neurologie CHU de Toulouse, Université de Toulouse III, Toulouse, France

F. A. Zeiler
Department of Surgery, Rady Faculty of Health Sciences, University of Manitoba, Winnipeg, MB, Canada

Department of Human Anatomy and Cell Science, Rady Faculty of Health Sciences, University of Manitoba, Winnipeg, MB, Canada

Biomedical Engineering, Faculty of Engineering, University of Manitoba, Winnipeg, MB, Canada

Division of Anaesthesia, Department of Medicine, University of Cambridge, Cambridge, UK

E. Beqiri
Brain Physics Laboratory, Division of Neurosurgery, Department of Clinical Neurosciences, University of Cambridge, Cambridge, UK

Department of Physiology and Transplantation, Milan University, Milan, Italy

S. Wolf
Department of Neurosurgery Charite Hospital, Berlin, Germany

S. K. Frisvolf
Department of Intensive Care, University Hospital, Tromso, Norway

P. Smielewski · M. Czosnyka
Brain Physics Laboratory, Division of Neurosurgery, Department of Clinical Neurosciences, University of Cambridge, Cambridge, UK

B. Depreitere et al. (eds.), *Intracranial Pressure and Neuromonitoring XVII*, Acta Neurochirurgica Supplement 131,
https://doi.org/10.1007/978-3-030-59436-7_41, © Springer Nature Switzerland AG 2021

interval (also called the R-R interval), which is an intrinsic characteristic of healthy cardiac functioning. Baroreflex sensitivity can be described as the response in heartbeat intervals to a change in blood pressure; it is also used as a marker of healthy ANS and is usually calculated as the slope of the regression line between ABP and R-R intervals.

Therefore, the aim of our study was to assess the feasibility of assessing changes in autonomic activity during the development of RIH using our adopted methodology.

Materials and Methods

Data Collection

The study was conducted as a retrospective analysis of a prospectively maintained database cohort (2009–2018) in which physiological monitoring data had been archived in three different hospitals: Department of Neurosurgery Charite Hospital, Berlin, Germany; Department of Intensive Care, University Hospital, Tromsø, Norway; and Neurocritical Care, Addenbrooke's University Hospital, Cambridge, UK. Monitoring was conducted using ICM+® software (Cambridge Enterprise, Ltd., Cambridge, UK, http://icmplus.neurosurg.cam.ac.uk).

ABI patients with a clinical need for ICP monitoring and computerized signal were included. The monitoring was part of standard patient care and archived in an anonymized way. All demographic/clinical data (Table 1) were extracted from hospital records and were fully anonymized, and no data on patient identifiers were available; therefore, formal patient or proxy consent and institutional ethics approval was not required.

Table 1 Patient demographics and descriptive statistics

Number of patients	24
Age mean (years)	37
ABI/TBI (num)	21
ABI/SAH (num)	3
Initial GCS (min)	3
Initial GCS (max)	14
Monitoring length hours (mean, SD)	52 ± 32
Decompressive craniectomy YES	5
NO	17
NA	2
Csf drainage with EVD	5
Death (%)	100
Withdrawal of treatment (num)	11
Brain death	4
NA	9

ABI acute brain injury, *TBI* traumatic brain injury, *SAH* subarachnoid hemorrhage, *CSF* cerebrospinal fluid, *EVD* external ventricular drain, *NA* information not available

Data Processing

Signals were acquired at a sampling frequency of at least 100 Hz. The time-average values of ICP and ABP were calculated on a 10-s calculation window.Secondary parameters reflecting autonomic activity were computed in the time and frequency domains through the continuous measurements of HRV. According to guidelines [9], we calculated the standard deviation (SD), that is, the SD of HRV in the time domain, and simultaneously calculated the power spectral density of different ranges that also had their own physiological meaning: high-frequency (HF) range within 0.15–0.4 Hz, modulated by the parasympathetic nervous system, low-frequency (LF) range within 0.04–0.15 Hz, modulated by both the sympathetic and parasympathetic nervous system, and the ratio between the two, which seems to mirror the sympathetic activity (LF/HF) [9].

The HRV in the time domain was analyzed using a 300-s time series of R-R intervals that were updated every 10 s. In the frequency domain, the Lomb-Scargle periodogram was used to calculate the spectral power of the R-R interval time series.

Baroreflex sensitivity was measured in ms/mmHg using the cross-correlation method, also referred to as the Baroindex or x-BRS [10]· which resulted in having a lower intra- and interindividual variability in the EUROBAVAR database. The x-BRS calculation algorithm was implemented in ICM+ software using a 10-s window moving along the time axis. To remove the influence of an unknown time delay of the baroreceptor response, a cross-correlation function was used to maximize the correlation coefficient, which meant that the actual total window length used in each calculation was 17 s. Valid x-BRS was returned only if the correlation coefficient was significant at $p < 0.01$.

The artifacts were manually cleaned in the raw data: in the ABP and ICP signal, the nonpulsatile chunks were removed. From the ECG, arrhythmic events and flat lines were removed, and ectopic beats were detected by the software.

Statistical Analysis

The R statistical language was used to perform the statistical analysis [R: A language and environment for statistical computing. R Foundation for Statistical Computing, Vienna, Austria. URL http://www.R-project.org/. version 3.3.3]. The nonnormal distribution of the data was established by a Shapiro-Wilk test [11].

A Wilcoxon test was used to make comparisons after variables were extracted as the mean value ±SD during the three different periods.

Results

We selected for retrospective review 24 ABI patients who had developed RIH with an initial baseline of ICP (mean value 15 mmHg ±8) followed by a rise to over 40 mmHg. Criteria for exclusion were the lack of ECG signal, frequent artifacts, lack of raw data, or absence of baseline ICP recording before hypertension evolved. Demographic/clinical data are shown in Table 1. Patients were monitored with at least ICP, ABP, and ECG.

Initial analysis showed that the profiles that formed for ICM+ worked correctly. Data processing with ICM+ revealed the detection of R complex from ECG time series, plotting the R-R interval versus time (Fig. 1).

The calculation of variables of HRV in the time domain was then performed (Fig. 2). Moreover, the decomposition of the R-R signal into its constituent frequencies was calculated and the power of the spectrum divided by a specific range of HRV was shown (Fig. 2). Baroreflex sensitivity was successfully calculated in the time domain as the Baroindex.

Consistent trends of parameters of interest were obtained during the development of RIH, and the autonomic variables could then be observed and studied in a dynamic way throughout the time trend (Fig. 3).

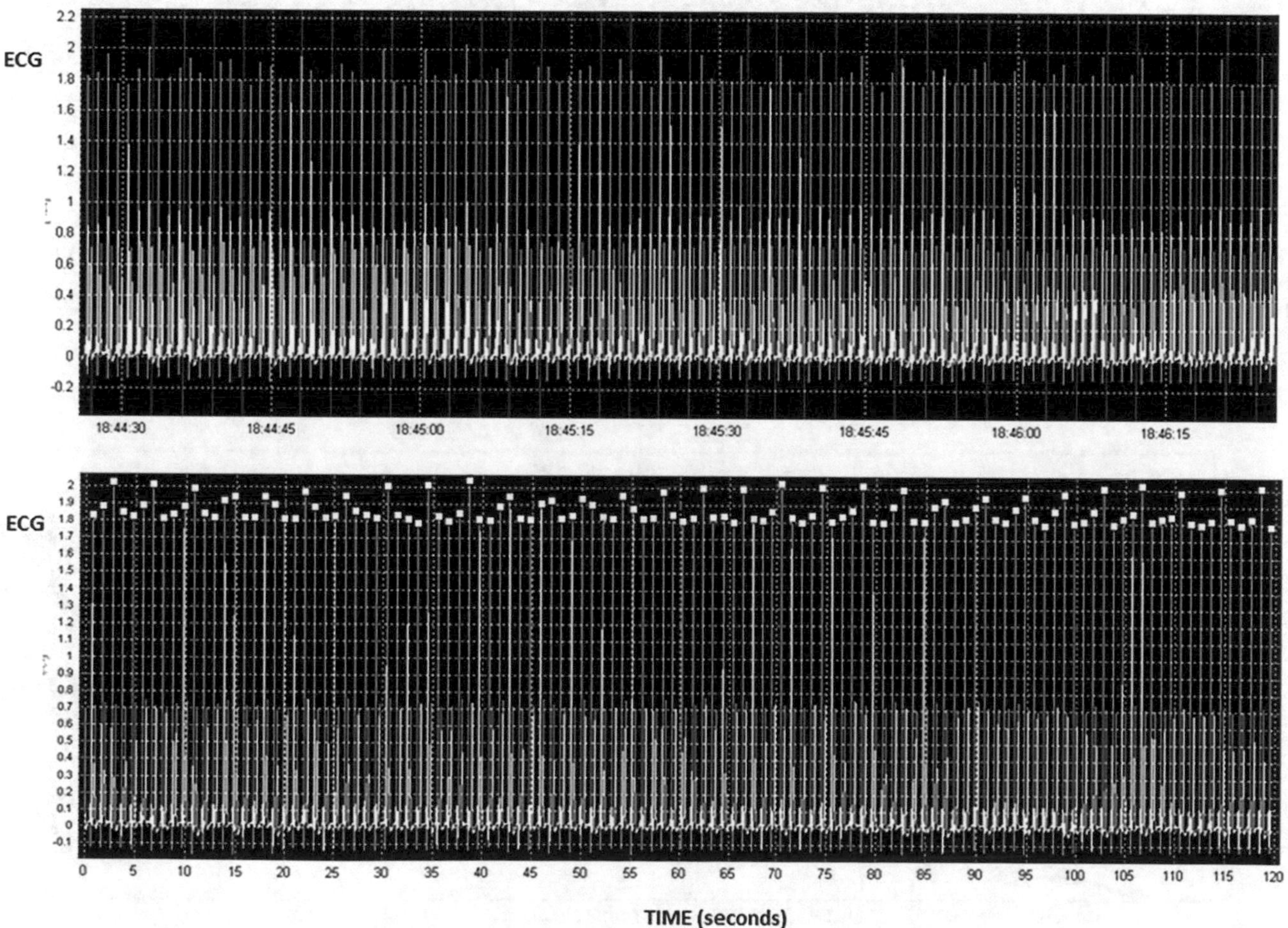

Fig. 1 Data processing with ICM+ showing detection of R complex from ECG time series, plotting of R-R interval versus time

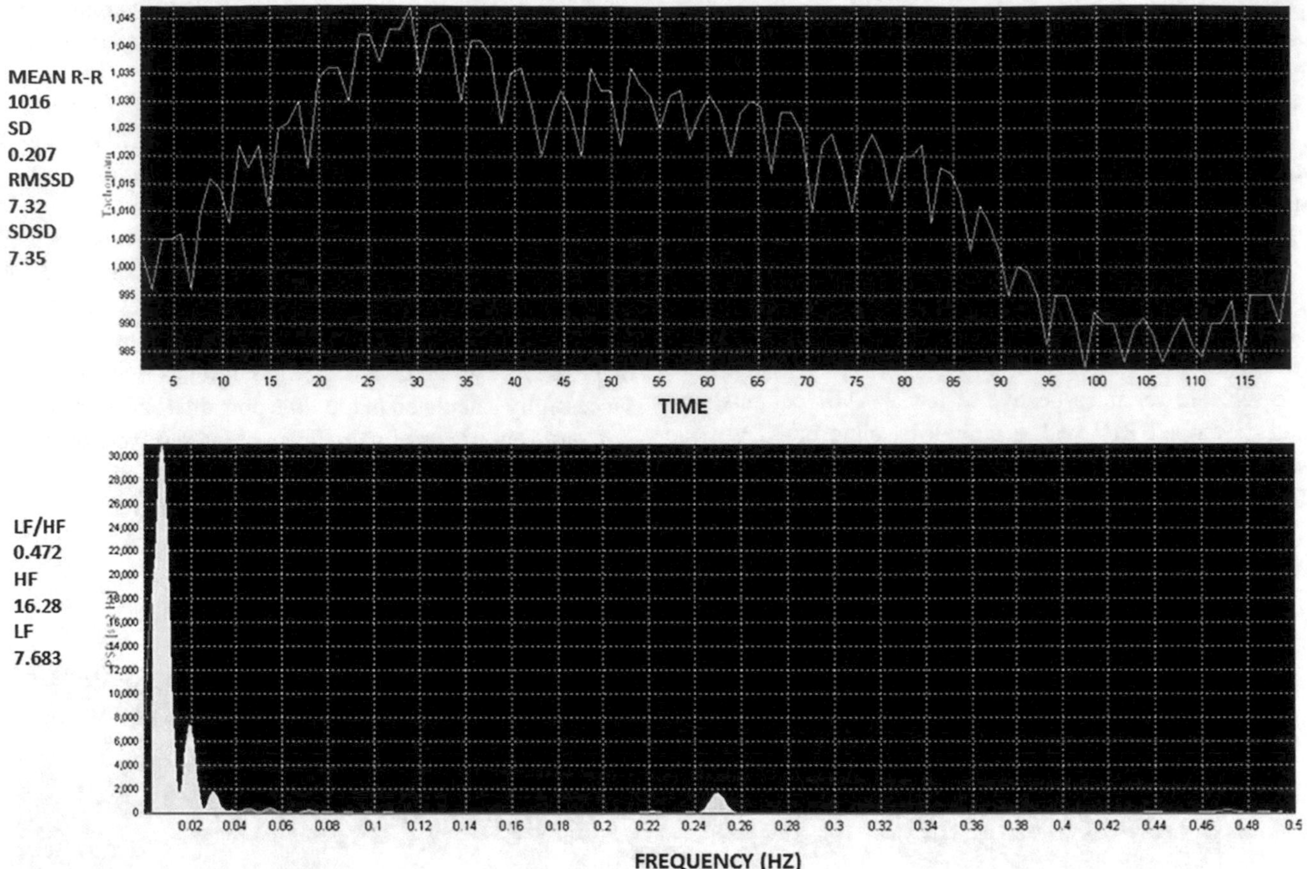

Fig. 2 Calculation of HRV variables in time domain: tachogram and automatic calculation of standard deviation (SD), standard deviation of difference between sequential beats (SDSD), and square root of mean squared difference between sequential beats (RMSSD) Decomposition of R-R signal into constituent frequencies, calculation of power spectral density divided by specific frequency range: high-frequency component (HF), low frequency (LF), low-frequency/high-frequency ratio LF/HF

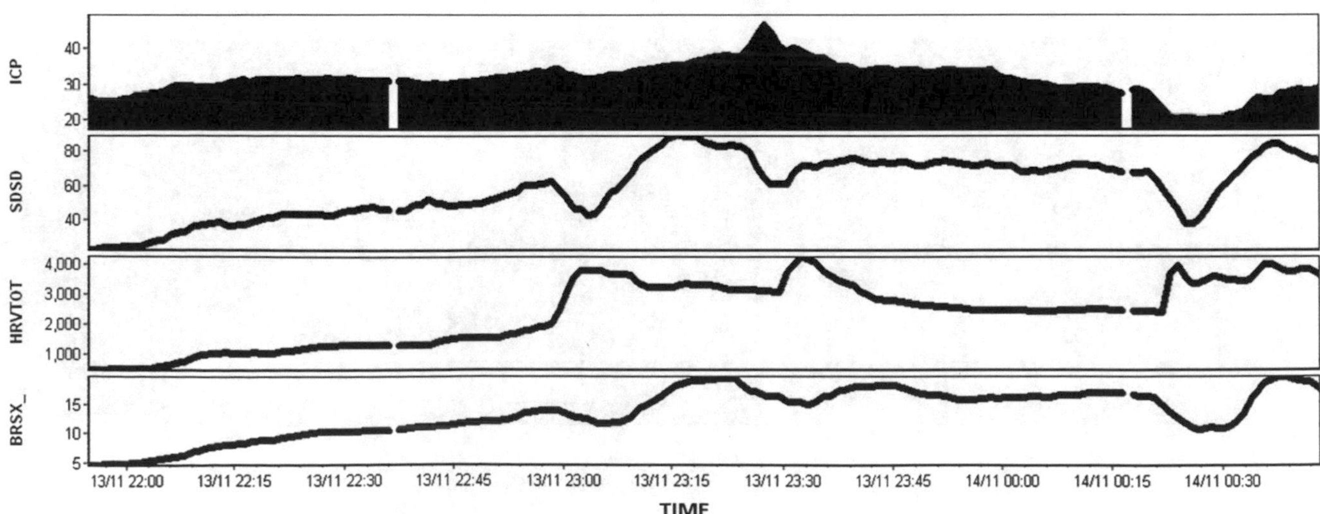

Fig. 3 Data processed with ICM+ showing trend of ICP and trend of HRV variables and baroreflex

Discussion

Our results suggest that the relationship between changes in ICP and ANS activity can be studied in retrospective time series using ICM+ methodology. Detailed results will be discussed in a separate publication. Limitations on the methodology are the effect of drugs on autonomic variables and of signal artifacts. The latter effect must be taken into account when applying the same approach to real-time data streams because in that case they cannot be eliminated manually. Automated treatment of those cases is possible but requires further investigation in this context in order to find a robust way of performing equivalent analysis on prospective data making it possible to monitor autonomic events reliably as they occur at bedside. In this way, the methodology will gain acceptance for practical application in intensive care, with the possibility of predicting RIH before it occurs.

Acknowledgments F.A. Zeiler's research program is supported by the United States National Institutes of Health (NIH) through the National Institute of Neurological Disorders andStroke (NINDS), the Canadian Institute for Health Research (CIHR), the Canadian Foundation for Innovation (CFI), the University of Manitoba Centre on Aging, the University of Manitoba VPRI Research Investment Fund (RIF), the University of Manitoba Rudy Falk Clinician-Scientist Professorship, and the Health Sciences Centre Foundation in Winnipeg.

M. Czosnyka is supported by NIHR Cambridge Biomedical Research Centre.

Conflicts of Interest **P. Smielewsky and M. Czosnyka receive part of the licensing fees for multimodal brain monitoring software ICM+, licensed by Cambridge Enterprise Ltd., University of Cambridge, UK. There are no other conflicts of interest to declare.**

References

1. Kellie G (1824) Appearance observed in the dissection of two of three individuals presumed to have perished in the storm of the 3rd and whose bodies were discovered in the vicinity of Leith on the morning of 4th November 1821 with some reflections on the pathology of the brain 1:84–122
2. Monro A (1783) Observation on the features and functions of the nervous system, illustrated with tables. Lond Med J 4: 113–135
3. Salih F, Finger T, Vajkoczy P, Wolf S (2017) Brain death after decompressive craniectomy: incidence and pathophysiological mechanisms. J Crit Care 39(2017):205–208
4. Salih F, Holtkamp M, Brandt SA, Hoffmann O, Masuhr F, Schreiber S, Weissinger F, Vajkoczy P, Wolf S (2016) Intracranial pressure and cerebral perfusion pressure in patients developing brain death. J Crit Care 34:1–6
5. Colivicchi F, Bassi A, Santini M, Caltagirone C (2005) Prognostic implications of right-sided insular damage, cardiac autonomic derangement, and arrhythmias after acute ischemic stroke. Stroke 36(8):1710–1715
6. Nasr N, Gaio R, Czosnyka M et al (2018) Baroreflex impairment after subarachnoid hemorrhage is associated with unfavorable outcome. Stroke 49(7):1632–1638
7. Sykora M, Czosnyka M, Liu X, Donnelly J, Nasr N, Diedler J, Okoroafor F, Hutchinson P, Menon D, Smielewski P (2016) Autonomic impairment in severe traumatic brain injury. Crit Care Med 44(6):1173–1181
8. Szabo J, Smielewski P, Czosnyka M, Jakubicek S, Krebs S, Siarnik P, Sykora M (2018) Heart rate variability is associated with outcome in spontaneous intracerebral hemorrhage. J Crit Care 48:85–89
9. Camm AJ, Bigger JT, Breithardt G, Cerutti S, Cohen RJCP (1996) Guidelines heart rate variability. Eur Heart J 17:354–381
10. Westerhof BE, Gisolf J, Stok WJ, Wesseling KH, Karemaker JM (2004) Time-domain cross-correlation baroreflex sensitivity. J Hypertens 22(7):1371–1380
11. Shapiro S, Wilk MB (1972) An analysis of variance test for normality. Biometrika 52:591–611

Evaluation of Software for Automated Measurement of Adherence to ICP-Monitoring Threshold Guideline

Anthony Stell, Laura Moss, Christopher Hawthorne, Roddy O'Kane, Maya Kommer, Martin Shaw, and Ian Piper

Introduction

Current methods of clinical guideline development face two formidable challenges: (1) there is often a long time-lag between the key results and incorporation into recommended best practices and (2) the measurement of adherence to those guidelines is often qualitative and difficult to standardise into measurable impact. This paper presents a validation test of a framework developed to use empirical physiological and treatment data to independently measure guideline adherence within a neurological intensive care unit (ICU).

The primary technological concept underpinning this framework is that of process models—a construct used in corporate and business domains to model time-varying processes and identify efficiencies. The process models are used to measure the adherence of clinicians to the intracranial pressure (ICP)-threshold traumatic brain injury (TBI)guideline [1] using physiological and treatment data from bedside machines in neurological ICUs. Similarly, the relevant guideline text from the Brain Trauma Foundation (BTF) is represented using Business Process and Model Notation (BPMN) so that a comparable process model can be constructed. Building on previous comparative work between process models [2], a 'distance' between the two models is then calculated and applied as a metric of guideline adherence, along with the qualitative components making up that metric.

There are several technical steps involved in this work:

1. The classification of events in physiological output known as Edinburgh University Secondary Insult Grade (EUSIG) events and compilation of an event log from this.
2. The expression of those event logs as process models.
3. The extraction of clinical guideline texts into process models.
4. The comparison of two process models using complex similarity/distance algorithms.

Together, these steps—outlined schematically in Fig. 1—form the framework through which the possibilities of quantitative, real-time guideline adherence monitoring can be explored.

This model has been developed into a web-enabled application that can readily feed back the non-adherence measurements in a clinical environment for any given cohort of patients with standard physiological and treatment output. Full technical details of the framework can be found in [3].

The work described in this manuscript attempts to validate the use of the framework against contextual information from clinical domain experts who work in neurological ICUs and would be the target users of the system in its production form.

Materials and Methods

Key technical factors that support this framework are the definition of EUSIG events and the factors that influence non-adherence to guidelines.

Figure 2 shows a schematic of a single physiological EUSIG event, with a time window for treatment overlaid, which allows treatment annotation to be associated with an event. A threshold is crossed and remains high for a specific period (the hold-down), indicating that a EUSIG event has started. The clear hold-down indicates that the EUSIG event has ended.

A. Stell (✉) · L. Moss · M. Shaw · I. Piper
Department of Clinical Physics, University of Glasgow, Queen Elizabeth University Hospital, Glasgow, UK
e-mail: a.stell.1@research.gla.ac.uk

C. Hawthorne · R. O'Kane · M. Kommer
Institute of Neurological Sciences, Queen Elizabeth University Hospital, Glasgow, UK

B. Depreitere et al. (eds.), *Intracranial Pressure and Neuromonitoring XVII*, Acta Neurochirurgica Supplement 131,
https://doi.org/10.1007/978-3-030-59436-7_42,

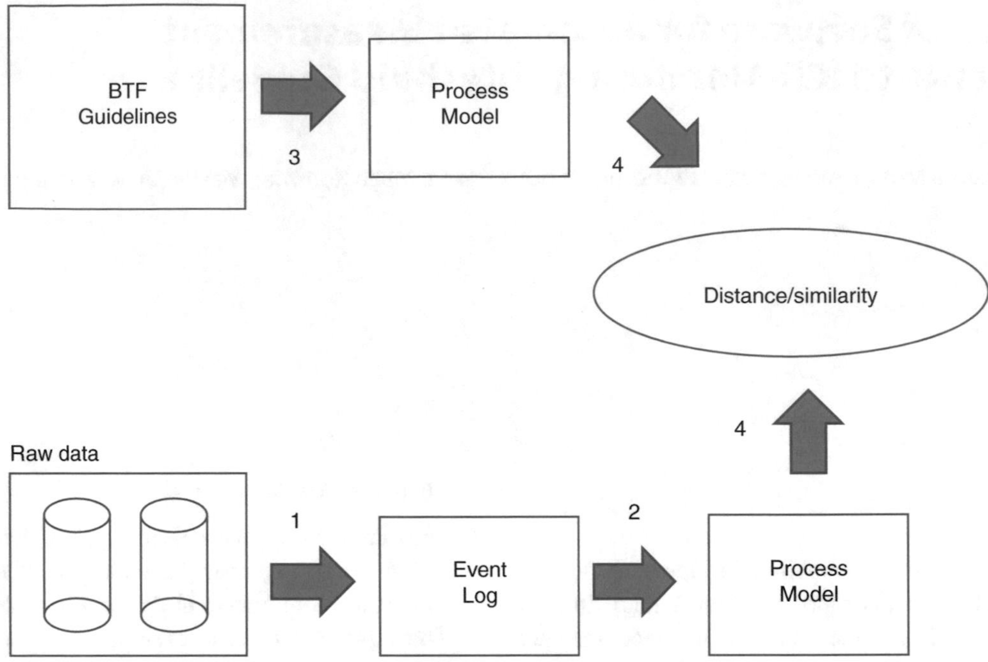

Fig. 1 Distance metric between models derived from bedside data and guidelines

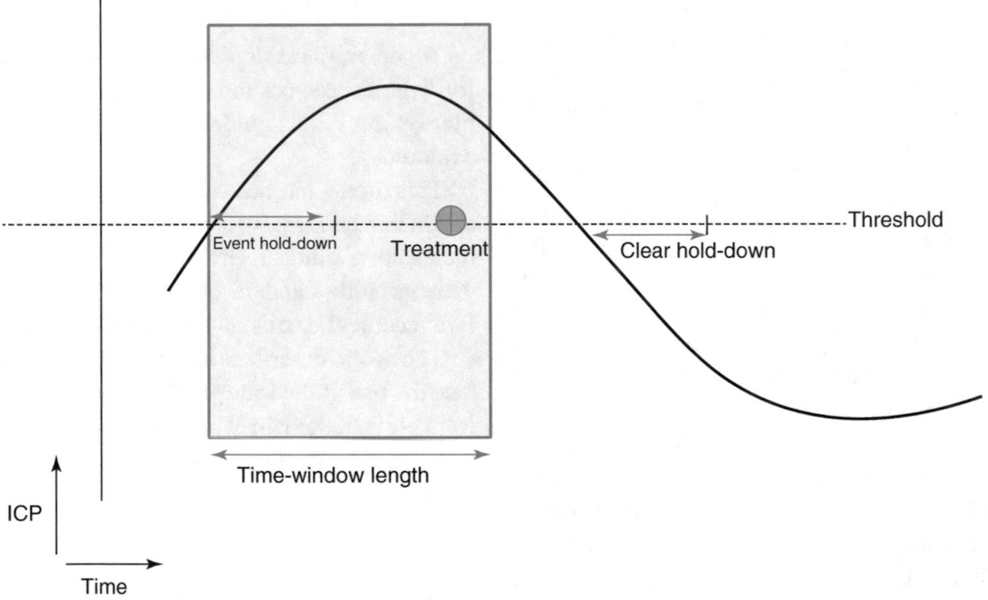

Fig. 2 EUSIG-event definition for a given time-varying physiological data stream. Time to treatment is from the start of an event to time of treatment

Table 1 shows the different factors that are considered to influence adherence to guidelines. The type indicates the drug categories (see discussion for the implications of these definitions), whilst the nature of the intervention (single or repeat) and the time taken from event to treatment are also considered. These factors are calculated using concepts of string-edit and graph-edit similarity, additional details of which can be found in [3].

A process model, similar in nature to a flowchart, is a sequence of time-varying events that, in this case, capture the overall management of patients during their stay in a neurological ICU. In this work, two process models are calculated, one derived from physiological and treatment data extracted from the bedside (i.e. the "real" situation), and the other taken from the authoritative guidelines in the space, the pressure threshold guidelines published by the BTF.

On a minute-by-minute basis, the distance between these two models is calculated, giving a quantitative metric representing how far from or near the so-called ideal state of complete adherence to the guideline, given the reality of an ever-changing ICU environment. This metric is calculated using two concepts, known as string-edit and graph-edit similarity, which are mathematical means to work out how similar two extended process models are (similar to flowcharts in nature). A suitable analogy is to consider what the minimum number of steps is, where a step is a transformation of either a node or an edge, required to turn one process model into another. The inputs to these formulae include three factors—time taken, dosage, and nature—and these are allocated weightings based on their considered importance to the clinical situation. In each minute during the stay, the numbers for these factors are put into the formula and this outputs the non-adherence number for that minute. Figure 3 shows an example.

The default state is a concept that emerged due to a general lack of annotations in the dataset. The numbers associated with this common state would always output 36.2% (though this could be recalibrated to 100% to signify complete non-adherence if desired). The clinical interpretation is simply that the patient, according to the system, requires an intervention, but none has been provided.

Table 1 Node label possibilities for the different nodes in each process model

Node	Label options
Treatment type	Ventilation, sedation, analgesia, paralysis, volume expansion, inotropes, anti-hypertensives, anti-pyretics, hypothermia, steroids, cerebral vasoconstriction, osmotic therapy, cerebrospinal fluid (CSF) drainage, head elevation, barbiturates, other
Nature of treatment	Single, repeat
Time taken	Time between event and treatment

Pilot Study Outline

A dataset collected from the Philips Intellivue Critical Care and Anaesthesia (ICCA) system was chosen for this evaluation because it is a popular bedside patient management software commonly used in ICUs in the UK [4]. Three TBI patients were selected for analysis by domain experts, with the following data characteristics:

- A prevalence of EUSIG events in ICP output
- Active management of ICP required

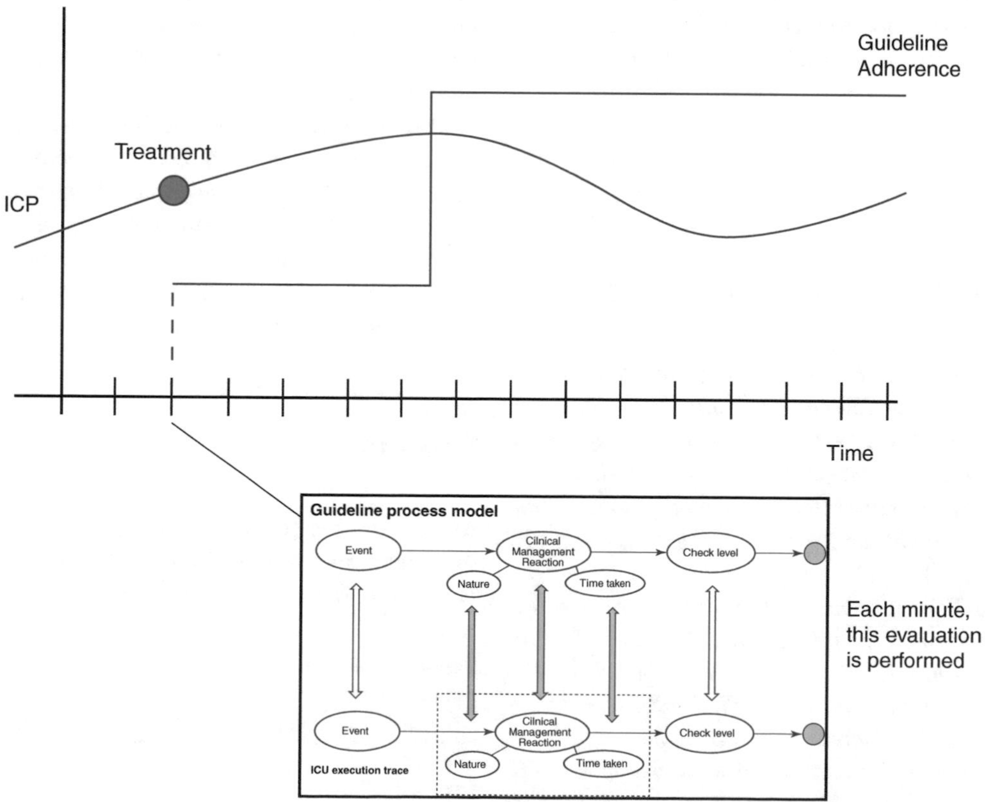

Fig. 3 Comparison of process models (inner box) in a single time point, which will then be repeatedly evaluated throughout the EUSIG event (outlined in outer box)

- Two patients (numbers 1 and 3) required non-intervention due to the nature of the ICP events
- One patient (number 2) had one large refractory event throughout the course of stay

Clinical management of the patients was carried out in accordance with a number of relevant treatment protocols and guidelines (not just BTF), which deliberately tested the ability of this system to provide useful guidance despite competing clinical priorities and possible comorbidities.

The physiological data structure of the ICP data in the ICCA dataset was millisecond wave form, down-sampled to minute-by-minute for this evaluation. This was achieved by averaging the contributing millisecond readings across the corresponding minute, which would incur some loss of precision in the recorded variation across that minute (considered acceptable at this resolution). The treatment data were primarily ventilation support and drug administration, obtained by manual inputs to, and then drawn from, the integrated ICCA system.

The results of guideline adherence output from these patients are presented in three sections:

1. An audit of overall counts of EUSIG events (where the EUSIG definition is varied by changing the threshold value) and treatment annotations;
2. Overall adherence measures for all three patients, including non-adherence instance tables, a chart of contributing reasons, and an interquartile range of instances;
3. Individual instances of non-adherence shown in a time-varying chart.

Results

The detailed clinical notes for the individual patients were as follows:[1]

- ***Patient 1***—*"Infusions of propofol, morphine, midazolam, noradrenaline; repeat CT scan on 12 July 2017—decision to stop sedation, disconnect ICP and assess; repeat CT scan performed—no surgical options; decision that, because ICP is not controlled by medical management, ICP monitor should be removed, stop sedation and assess".*
- ***Patient 2***—*"ICP consistently >20, overall upward trajectory of ICP (despite infusions of propofol 2% 400 mg/h; morphine 3 mg/h; midazolam 13 mg/h 11:00; cisatracurium 30 mg/h; thiopentone 125 mg/h 14:00; noradrenaline 0.1 mg/h 13:34—increased to 0.2 mg/h at 14:00".*
- ***Patient 3***—*"ICP > 20; associated with rise in $ETCO_2$; optimisation of ventilation by increasing pressure support (documented at 09:00 15 December 2016); decrease in CO_2 leads to decrease in ICP"* [therefore non-intervention was recommended as the ICP increase was expected to be transient].

[1]These are reproduced verbatim except the square brackets in patient 3, which were added as a separate note by one of the clinicians to provide added clarity.

Event and Treatment Counts

The number counts in Table 2 were compiled once the ICCA sample dataset had been processed into the *"treatment_profiles"* database (which supports the guideline adherence framework holding the physiological and treatment information [3]). The EUSIG definition is varied according to the threshold definition in order to obtain a variety of values.

The total EUSIG event number was **21**, and the total treatment annotation number was **1721.8.** EUSIG events were associated with treatments, which was **80%** of the most frequently used EUSIG threshold definition. This suggests that the count of annotations was high relative to the physiological output (i.e. a high proportion of EUSIG events detected was associated with a treatment annotation). This summary count of events and treatments provides an estimate of confidence to the non-adherence measurement. In this case, the level of 80% association is slightly misleading because there are few EUSIG events, against a very dense number of treatment annotations. Whilst this latter fact provides valuable information (and is unusual in a typical neuro-ICU environment), confidence the in accuracy of the association is not correspondingly high.

Patients 1 and 3 provided the most variety in terms of non-adherence states, so all four metrics are shown for patient 1 and the table and chart of instances are shown for patient 3 (distributions removed to save space). Patient 2 only had a single instance of non-adherence due to a refractory ICP event. This is considered in the discussion, but the table/chart results are not shown.

Patient 1

Most instances for patient 1 are variation due to time to treatment and a contributing factor of incorrect type (Fig. 4). However, for two instances, the dosage/nature is

Table 2 Count of individual mean ICP EUSIG events from ICCA sample dataset

Threshold value (mmHg)	Count
10	3
15	10
20	2
25	3
30	3

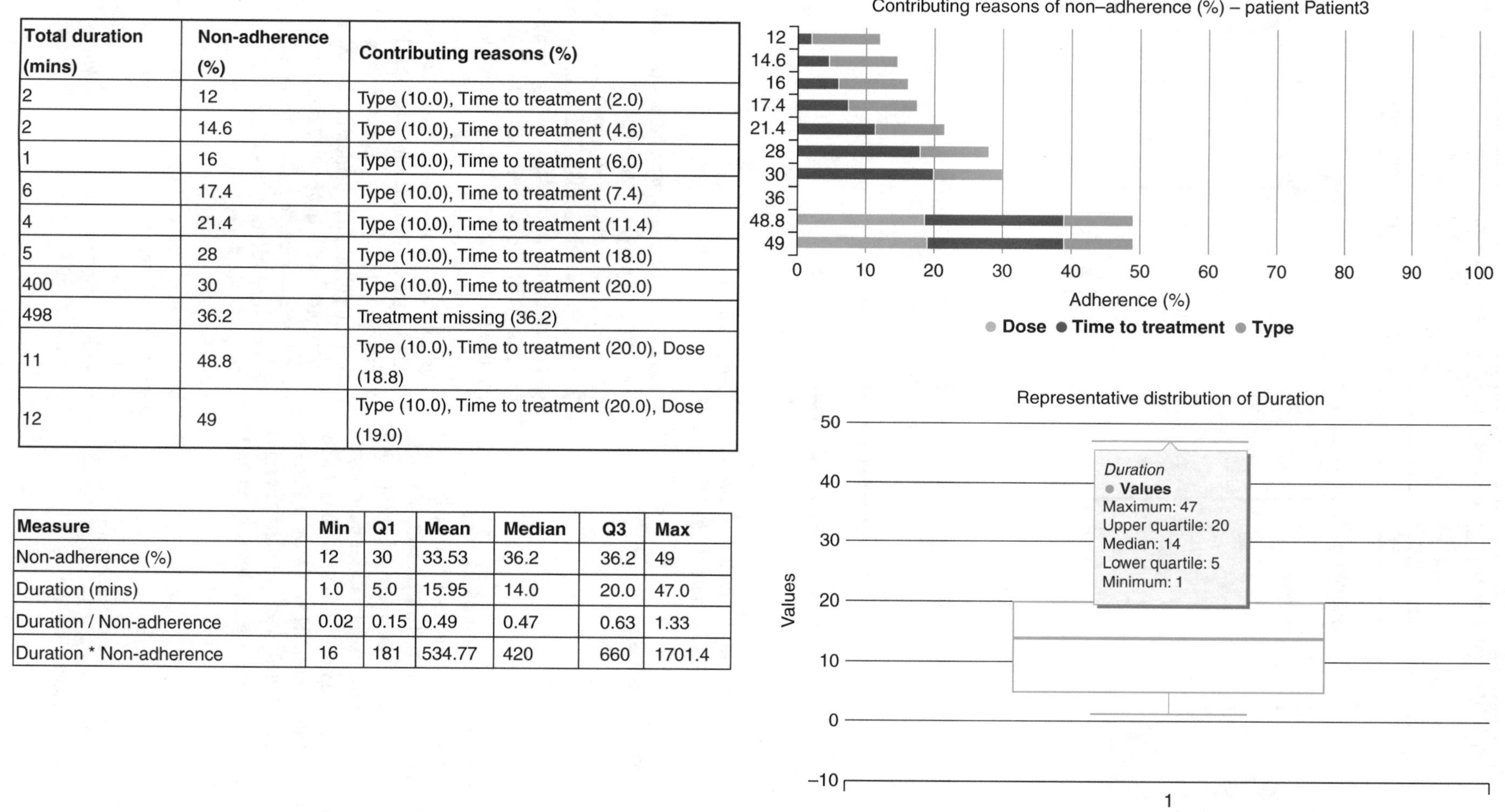

Total duration (mins)	Non-adherence (%)	Contributing reasons (%)
2	12	Type (10.0), Time to treatment (2.0)
2	14.6	Type (10.0), Time to treatment (4.6)
1	16	Type (10.0), Time to treatment (6.0)
6	17.4	Type (10.0), Time to treatment (7.4)
4	21.4	Type (10.0), Time to treatment (11.4)
5	28	Type (10.0), Time to treatment (18.0)
400	30	Type (10.0), Time to treatment (20.0)
498	36.2	Treatment missing (36.2)
11	48.8	Type (10.0), Time to treatment (20.0), Dose (18.8)
12	49	Type (10.0), Time to treatment (20.0), Dose (19.0)

Measure	Min	Q1	Mean	Median	Q3	Max
Non-adherence (%)	12	30	33.53	36.2	36.2	49
Duration (mins)	1.0	5.0	15.95	14.0	20.0	47.0
Duration / Non-adherence	0.02	0.15	0.49	0.47	0.63	1.33
Duration * Non-adherence	16	181	534.77	420	660	1701.4

Fig. 4 Top left shows instances of non-adherence for patient 1, top right shows factors contributing to those instances, bottom left shows interquartile range table (with "default state" removed), and bottom right shows corresponding boxplot for duration aspect of non-adherence

Total duration (mins)	Non-adherence (%)	Contributing reasons (%)
3	13.4	Type (10.0), Time to treatment (3.4)
4	18.6	Type (10.0), Time to treatment (8.6)
170	30	Type (10.0), Time to treatment (20.0)

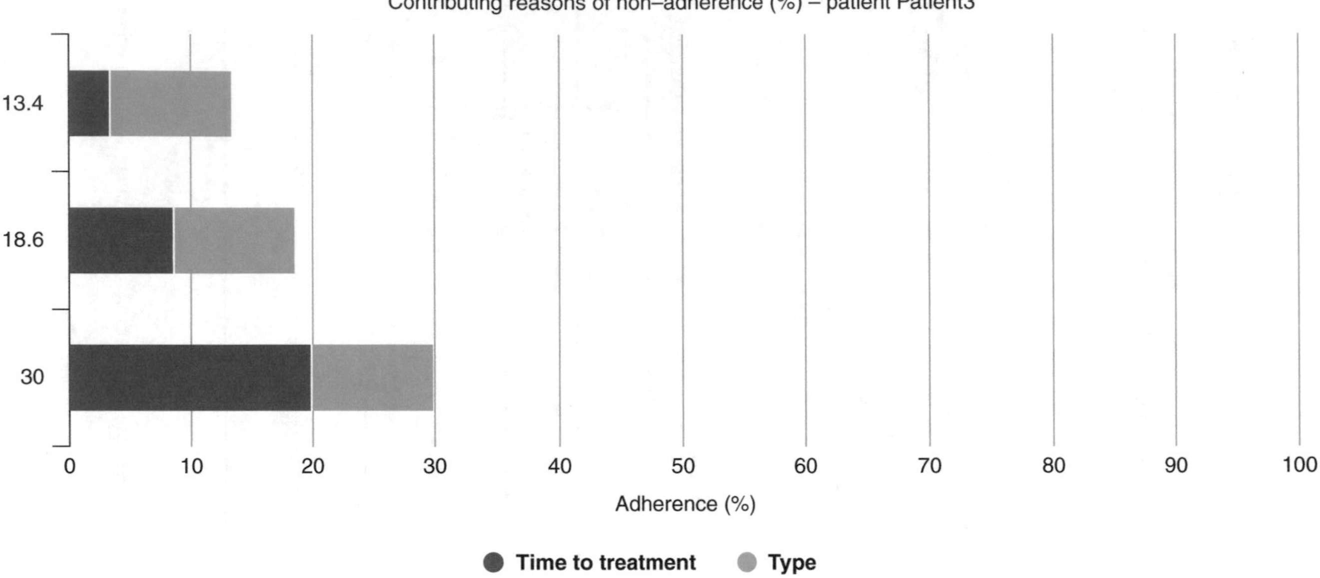

Fig. 5 Table of instances, with default state removed, and contributing reasons for patient 3

a contributing factor as well. The majority of the non-adherence duration is in the "default state"[2] (36.2%) and in a lower, but similar, value of 30%. The distribution appears to be spread evenly among all four factors.

Patient 3

Figure 5 show the instances of non-adherence for patient 3.

Two instances of individual timelines of non-adherence, for each patient, are shown in Fig. 6. This presents a minute-by-minute rendering of the non-adherence against the ICP and treatment output. The red line in the figures indicates the non-adherence and has a "stepped" character due to the nature of the distance calculation. This allows a detailed view of the non-adherence relative to an individual event or treatment annotation (e.g. when trying to identify an exact moment of non-adherence).

[2]*Default state* refers to the distance in a given dataset which occurred when there were large "gaps" due to low numbers of treatment annotations. In this case, the distance calculated was 36.2%.

Discussion

Considering the strengths of this work, this framework was developed to provide immediate, detailed and independent feedback on adherence at a level of clinical management. The vision for this application would be to fit it into audit procedures, such as weekly meetings to assess compliance or to assist with the review and further development of the guidelines themselves. The presentation styles chosen—individual view charts, interquartile range representation, aggregate information—were all carefully chosen so as to maximise the utility of the information, in a way that informs a clinician as rapidly as possible about a patient's status relative to the guideline considered. The trace of non-adherence reasons provides a qualitative detail to the overall quantitative non-adherence, so information—whilst hidden for easier viewing—can still be "unpacked" and reviewed if required.

In terms of limitations, the adherence output generated from the three patients highlighted several issues with the system. One major general issue was the categorisation of treatments. The direct drug name was listed in the treatment tables of the framework database, which can either be categorised according to the BrainIT listing (as defined in [3] or from the original BrainIT specification [5]) or individually incorpo-

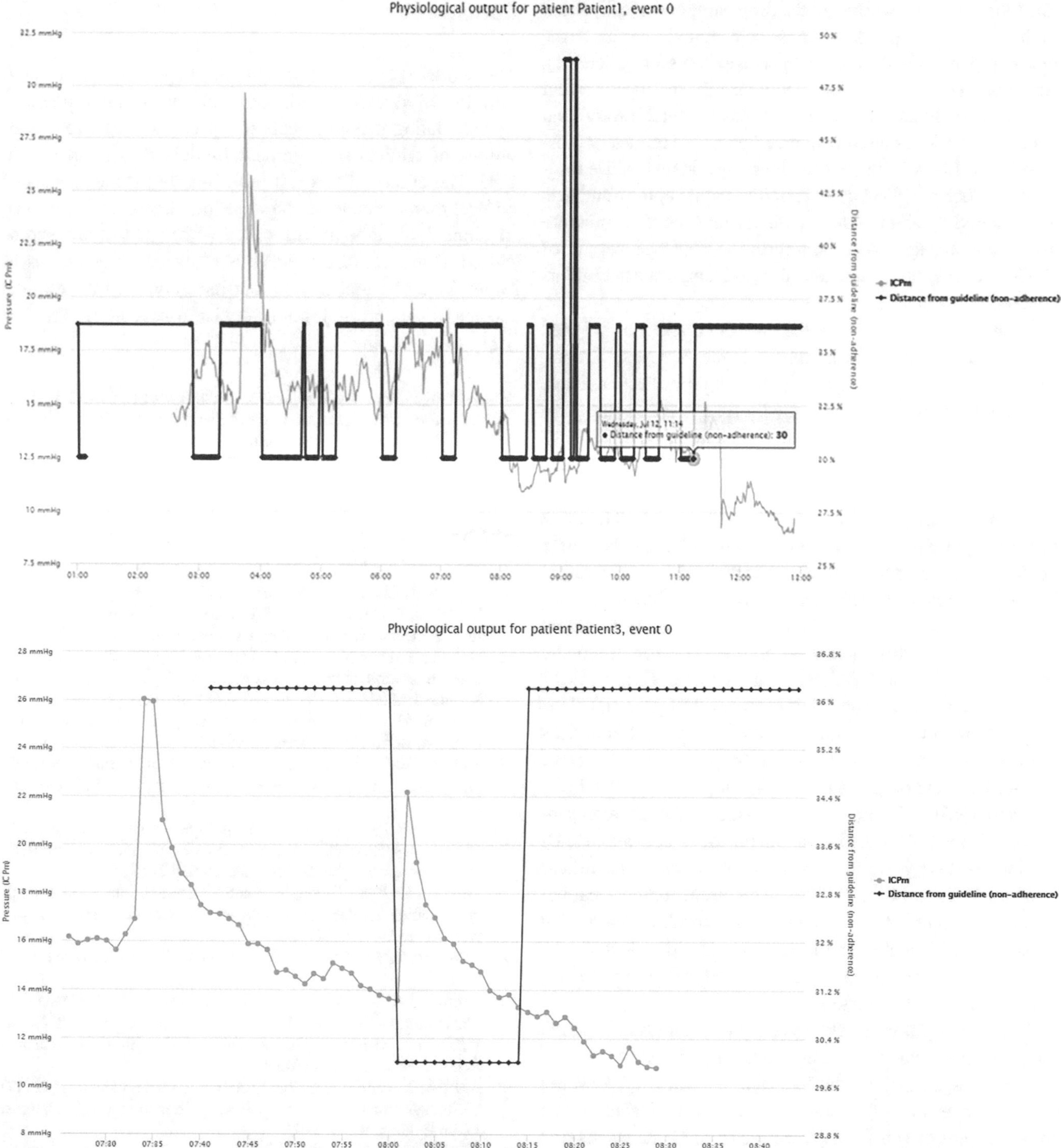

Fig. 6 Top diagram represents a timeline of event 0 ICPm—the EUSIG event definition was a threshold of 10 mmHg, a hold-down of 20 min and a time window overlaid of 15 min. The bottom diagram represents a timeline of event 0, patient 3—the EUSIG event definition was a threshold of 15 mmHg, a hold-down of 20 min and a time window overlaid of 15 min. In both diagrams, the blue line represents ICPm and the red line represents the distance from guideline (non-adherence)

rated into the framework (e.g. the drug name specifically listed in the code where pressors/fluids are captured to evaluate the type comparison in the cerebral perfusion pressure guideline). An improved categorisation would specify the measurement of adherence output more closely. From patient 2 it was found that the adherence output responded poorly to refractory pressure events (those with constant increase and no positive resolution). When a clinical context of intentional non-treatment is encountered (patient 3 had regular transient ICP pressure events that appeared to synchronise with the rise and fall of ETCO2 levels), the system also fails to incorporate this into its adherence evaluation.

In the wider TBI context, the project most closely aligned to this work in the clinical sphere is the European Union–funded CENTER-TBI project [6]. Many publications have been made by this group over the lifetime to date of the project, with a particular focus on living systematic reviews (LSRs). They cover several areas, such as the need for combining human and machine effort (suggestions for approach) [7], and recommendations for the curation and development of living guidelines [8]. However, these publications largely detail the issues and challenges experienced so far rather than outlining a full implementation of procedure.

Most instructive in the clinical space has been the recent review of the sixth International Initiative for Traumatic Brain Injury Research (InTBIr) conference in October 2017 [9] (a worldwide collaboration of major TBI projects). This reflected the progress of many of the leading TBI initiatives worldwide, with particular interest, from the point of view of this study, in the progress in data development by CENTER-TBI and TRACK-TBI [10]. In the same meeting, a representative of the BTF noted that on the development of TBI guidelines there is a lot of progress on literature identification/synthesis and evidence-based recommendations, but not on the development of protocols and algorithms that would assist technologically in the revision and development of guidelines. The framework validated in this work would be a very good fit for this vision.

In terms of future work, a variety of avenues of research and refinement can be pursued. Tasks that should be immediately addressed include the technical limitations discovered during the evaluation phases of the work, including the improvement of sensitivity to refractory EUSIG events and of the processing of multiple treatments and events in one time window. In terms of contextual application, it would be ideal to apply the framework to a subset of the CENTER-TBI dataset and to approach the BTF to demonstrate as a possible application of technological algorithms to the feedback and development of TBI guidelines.

Conclusion

The work described in this manuscript outlines a small pilot test of a guideline adherence framework that operates by calculating distances between process model representations of clinical management models in a neurological ICU. The output of this test indicates that some aspects of clinical management can be identified and correlated back to clinical opinion on the cases (through the notes provided). However, further work is required, with studies of larger patient numbers, to outline more subtle clinical nuance to support auditing or decision-making in a neurological ICU setting.

Acknowledgements We would like to acknowledge the work of the BrainIT Group investigators and participating centres in the BrainIT dataset without whom this work could not have been conducted.

References

1. Bullock R, Chesnut R, Clifton G, Ghajar J, Marion D, Narayan R, Newell D, Pitts L, Rosner M, Wilberger J (1996) Guidelines for the management of severe head injury. Eur J Emerg Med 2:109–127
2. Dijkman R, Dumas M, García-Bañuelos L (2009) Graph matching algorithms for business process model similarity search. In: Dayal U, Eder J, Koehler J, Reijers HA (eds) Business process management. BPM 2009. Lecture notes in computer science, vol 5701. Springer, Berlin, Heidelberg, pp 48–63
3. Stell A (2019) Evaluating clinical variation in traumatic brain injury data. PhD thesis, University of Glasgow. http://theses.gla.ac.uk/74263
4. ICCA (2018) https://www.usa.philips.com/healthcare/product/HCNOCTN332/intellispace-critical-care-and-anesthesia-critical-care-information-system. Accessed 10 Sep 2018
5. Piper I et al (2009) The brain monitoring with information technology (BrainIT) collaborative network: EC feasibility study results. Acta Neurochir 102:217–221
6. CENTER-TBI (2018) https://www.center-tbi.eu/. Accessed 2 Oct 2018
7. Thomas J, Noel-Storr A, Marshall I, Wallace B, McDonald S, Mavergames C, Glasziou P, Shemilt I, Synnot A, Turner T, Elliott J (2017) Living systematic reviews: 2. Combining human and machine effort. J Clin Epidemiol 91:31–37
8. Akl EA, Meerpohl J, Elliott J, Kahale L, Schunemann H (2017) Living systematic reviews: 4. Living guideline recommendations. J Clin Epidemiol 91:47–53
9. InTBIr (2017) International Initiative for Traumatic Brain Injury Research—local PDF file, shared by participants, available on request. Accessed 1 Oct 2018
10. McMahon P, Hricik A, Yue J, Puccio A, Inoue T, Lingsma H, Beers S, Gordon W, Valadka A, Manley G, Okonkwo D (2014) Symptomatology and functional outcome in mild traumatic brain injury: results from the prospective TRACK-TBI study. J Neurotrauma 31(1):26–33

Time Series Analysis and Prediction of Intracranial Pressure Using Time-Varying Dynamic Linear Models

Martin Shaw, Chris Hawthorne, Laura Moss, Maya Kommer, Roddy O'Kane, Ian Piper, and On Behalf of the BrainIT Group

Introduction

The international incidence of traumatic brain injury (TBI) is currently estimated at 69 million people per year [1]. The incidence of TBI is 30–40% of all injury-related deaths internationally and is projected to account for the greatest burden of healthy years lost to disability of any neurological disorder until 2030 [2]. Due to the long-term patient support required following a TBI, conservative estimates in the USA place the economic burden at $81 million in direct and $2.3 billion in indirect health costs [3]. This implies that any improvement upon current clinical management strategies has the potential to reduce both patient recovery times and the need for so much long-term support.

The measurement of intracranial pressure (ICP) is a key clinical tool in the assessment and management of TBI patients in a neuro-intensive care unit (neuro-ICU). Increased incidence of elevated ICP has been shown to be linked to worsening patient outcomes and higher mortality rates [4]. As such, a deeper understanding of how standard clinical therapies affect an individual patient's ongoing ICP wave form would be beneficial to the clinical decision-making process.

Current guidance and advice on the management of elevated ICP is moving from a standardised 'staircase' approach for all patients to targeted approaches on an individual level [5]. It would therefore be useful to be able to assess these therapeutic approaches in the context of each patient. To achieve this aim, a combination of time series modelling of existing patients' ICP waveforms and both factual and counterfactual simulation could be applied to newly collected data. This would enable estimation of the ICP under actual conditions, factual simulation and, under hypothetical conditions that did not apply to the patient at that time, counterfactual simulation.

Time series modelling is a branch of statistical analysis that is concerned with understanding serially generated values both for inter- and intra-related values of sets of recorded signals, not necessarily from the same source [6]. In the context of physiological monitoring it is concerned with understanding both the relationships between successive time points in a single patient's recorded vital-sign signals and the relationship between each temporaneously recorded different vital-sign signals, such as arterial blood pressure's (ABP) influence on ICP. There are a number of ways to approach analysing and modelling a set of times series vital-sign

On Behalf of the BrainIT Group

M. Shaw (✉)
Department of Clinical Physics and Bioengineering, Queen Elizabeth University Hospital, Glasgow, UK

School of Medicine, Dentistry & Nursing, University of Glasgow, Glasgow, UK

Academic Unit of Anaesthesia, Pain & Critical Care Medicine, University of Glasgow, Glasgow, UK
e-mail: martin.shaw@nhs.net

C. Hawthorne
School of Medicine, Dentistry & Nursing, University of Glasgow, Glasgow, UK

Department of Neuroanaesthesia, INS, Queen Elizabeth University Hospital, Glasgow, UK

L. Moss
Department of Clinical Physics and Bioengineering, Queen Elizabeth University Hospital, Glasgow, UK

School of Medicine, Dentistry & Nursing, University of Glasgow, Glasgow, UK

M. Kommer · R. O'Kane
Department of Neurosurgery, INS, Queen Elizabeth University Hospital, Glasgow, UK

I. Piper
Usher Institute of Population Health and Informatics, University of Edinburgh, Edinburg, UK

B. Depreitere et al. (eds.), *Intracranial Pressure and Neuromonitoring XVII*, Acta Neurochirurgica Supplement 131,
https://doi.org/10.1007/978-3-030-59436-7_43,

signals [7]; one of the most flexible, however, is using a time-varying dynamic linear model (DLM) [8].

A DLM is also known as a state-space model because it represents each observation as a distinct state that the signal, or space, equals at an instance in time. Secondly, a single DLM can represent multiple input and output signals at the same time. Finally, each state can be influenced by the states that directly precede it or are simultaneous with it. This ability to build complex relationships between the signals and their states lends itself well to modelling physiological signals that can have multiple external influences such as ICP.

Mathematically this would be represented for each state at a time point t as

$$\theta_t = G_t \theta_{t-1} + \omega_t$$

where θ_t is the underlying temporal process driving the changes in the output signals, G_t is known as the evolutional matrix that will encode the known time series effects on the input processes, and ω_t is an estimate of Gaussian noise inherent in the process. This underlying process would then generate the output signal via.

$$y_t = F_t \theta_t + \nu_t$$

where y_t is the output signal being modelled at a time point t, F_t is known as the observational matrix that will define the structure of how each signal interacts with the underlying temporal process, and finally ν_t is any measurement error associated with the output signal, as illustrated in Fig. 1.

The evolutionary matrix G_t can be created to represent a number of simultaneous time series concepts such as varying baseline signal trend using both polynomial and Fourier factors, autoregressive moving average (ARMA) effects on the estimated errors and, finally, seasonal components for cyclical effects on signals, where the time-varying aspect of a model can be accounted for with changes to both G_t and F_t as the time t increases.

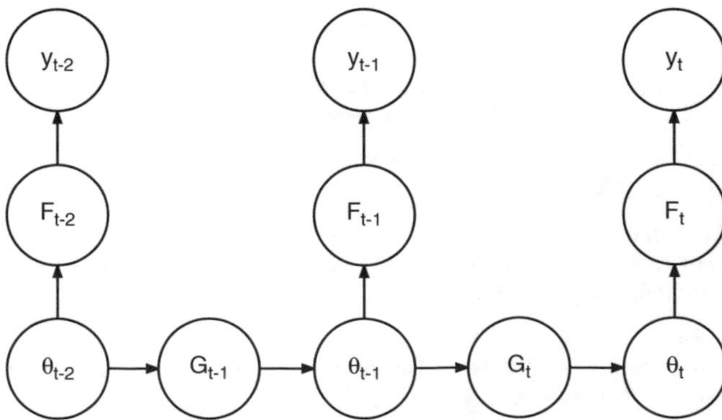

Fig. 1 Illustration of state relationships in typical dynamic linear model, where θ_t is the underlying temporal process, G_t is the evolutional matrix, y_t is the output signal being modelled at a time point t, and F_t is the observational matrix

Forecasting with Additive Switching of Seasonality, Trend and Exogenous Regressors (FASSTER) is a new time-varying DLM implementation which was recently developed [9]. It incorporates multi-DLM switching to more accurately model external influences on a time series [10]. This technique models multiple DLMs under different specified conditions and transitions between them over the course of the time series as the conditions change.

Materials and Methods

A pilot application of the FASSTER time-varying DLM implementation was conducted using R version 3.6.1 [11] on the BrainIT database, a multi-centre dataset collected from 22 European countries containing 261 patients and over 2.8 million recorded minute-by-minute data points from multiple vital-sign channels, such as ICP and ABP, with temporaneous treatment information [12]. This latter point is key to the conduct of the study due to the need for known interventional therapies, which are intended to target aspects of management for the ICP signal.

The database was subdivided into patients with at least 27 h of sequential ICP recordings, which could include missing values over that period, and those who have less than that amount. This amount was required so that 24 h could be used to train a model, 2 h as the true values when calculating any goodness-of-fit metrics, and a final hour to ensure that the tested 2-h prediction was not directly at the end of a sequence where more clinical manipulation could be encountered. This gave the study 106 patients who have the required 27 h of data, on which the FASSTER model would be applied, and 155 patients, the remaining cohort from the original 261 patients in the BrainIT database, so that modelling features could be assessed to create the evolution matrix G_t. The demographics for the complete database and for the 106-patient subgroup are shown in Table 1.

Table 1 Selected demographics of the 106 patients included in the FASSTER time series modelling

	Female (N = 26)	Male (N = 80)
Age	33.4 (17.9–54.7)	31.5 (19.0–46.0)
Initial pH	7.42 (7.33–7.47)	7.40 (7.34–7.44)
GCS: Eye	1.00 (1.00–1.33)	1 (1–2)
GCS: Motor	4 (1–5)	5 (2–5)
GCS: Verbal	1 (1–2)	1 (1–2)
Mean ICP	13 (9–17)	13 (9–18)
Mean ABP	86 (78–94)	86 (77–96)
Heart rate	86 (75–97)	80 (69–93)
Core temperature	37.4 (37.0–37.8)	37.6 (37.0–38.0)
SaO_2	99 (98–100)	99 (98–100)

There was a median (interquartile range (IQR) 2.1% (0%, 11.2%)) of values missing per ICP signal over the 106 patients; these values were included without manipulation in the analysis because DLMs can analyse data containing non-stationary processes, missing values and non-uniform sampling.

To start to create the evolution matrix G_t, a number of strategies were employed to assess the underlying structures in the time series. Firstly, Fourier analysis was performed on the 155-patient training subgroup to assess what, if any, baseline trends existed in the dataset. Then autocorrelation (ACF) and partial autocorrelation (PACF) analyses were performed to investigate the order of any ARMA errors for the ICP signal. Domain knowledge was employed to add seasonal components to the signal at 5- and 30-min intervals to account for ongoing clinical manipulation of the patients at bedside and enable ABP, age and gender to influence the general state of the ICP signal. Finally, the top three prevalent interventional therapies given to target ICP changes were chosen to enable the switching between each of these therapeutic states, and a summary of the prevalence is given in Table 2.

The constructed FASSTER model was then trained on the first 24 h of each of the 106 testing patients' ICU stays, and then the next 2 h of ICP was forecast. These time intervals were chosen, both 24 and 2 h, to ensure enough time had passed in which at least one of the three interventional therapies could have occurred. Each of these 2-h forecasts were then assessed using a median absolute error against what actually happened to the patients' ICP signal in the same period.

Table 2 Prevalence of clinical therapy states from the106 patients extracted from the BrainIT dataset

Therapy	Count (%)
Analgesia	1490 (20.5)
Sedation	1441 (19.8)
Osmotic therapy	1401 (19.3)
Paralysis	1049 (14.4)
Head elevation	509 (7.0)
Ventilation	420 (5.8)
Other therapy	409 (5.6)
Volume expansion	154 (2.1)
Barbiturate therapy	132 (1.8)
Anti-pyretics	107 (1.5)
Anti-hypertensives	66 (0.9)
CSF drainage	36 (0.5)
Hypothermia	28 (0.4)
Steroid therapy	22 (0.3)
Inotropes	10 (0.1)

Results

The analysis of the 155 training patients showed, via Fourier analysis, that there was a significant periodicity at 298 min in this dataset. Secondly, from the ACF and PACF analysis an ARMA(1,3) model was shown to be adequate in estimating more accurate errors.

The three most prevalent therapeutic categories were shown to be analgesia, n = 1490 (20.5%), osmotic therapy, n = 1441 (19.8%), and paralysis, n = 1401 (19.3%).

The accuracy assessment of the FASSTER time-varying DLM implementation shows the overall median absolute error, with 95% confidence intervals, was 2.98 (2.41–5.24) mmHg calculated using all 106 two-hour forecasts, with a representative forecast shown in Fig. 2.

Discussion

Prediction of ICP is not a new idea; however, the dichotomous task of predicting whether ICP is higher than a pre-specified target threshold has been shown to be inadequate [13]. It would therefore be better to attempt to predict the actual ICP value and assess how it changes over the period of interest.

Farhadi et al. [7] investigated time series prediction of ICP values at a 30-min horizon in children using a number of classical approaches. They highlighed the need for exogenous regressors, such as other vital-sign channels and medication delivery, to augment any single-signal analysis. These key points form the basis of why the FASSTER implementation is useful in this context. The simple autoregressive integrative moving average (ARIMA) model from that paper was assessed and found to have similar order values to this current studies ARMA assessment on the 155-patient training set, (1,1,4) and (1,3) respectively, where the first-order differencing component in the ARIMA model is accounted for elsewhere in the FASSTER model.

A median absolute error of 2.98 (2.41–5.24) mmHg is within clinically acceptable limits, and this is in line with the mean absolute errors seen by Farhadi et al. [7], though it should be noted that this current paper assessed the values over all forecast time points in the subsequent 2 h, whereas Farhadi et al. were forecasting only the next 30 min.

The median or mean absolute errors are only summaries of what the minute-to-minute errors actually are. As seen in Fig. 2, there are several points in which the variability of the true ICP signal is not replicated by the FASSTER-implemented ICP forecast. This highlights the need for more information to be included in the modelling process to improve the final fit. The current model could be simply

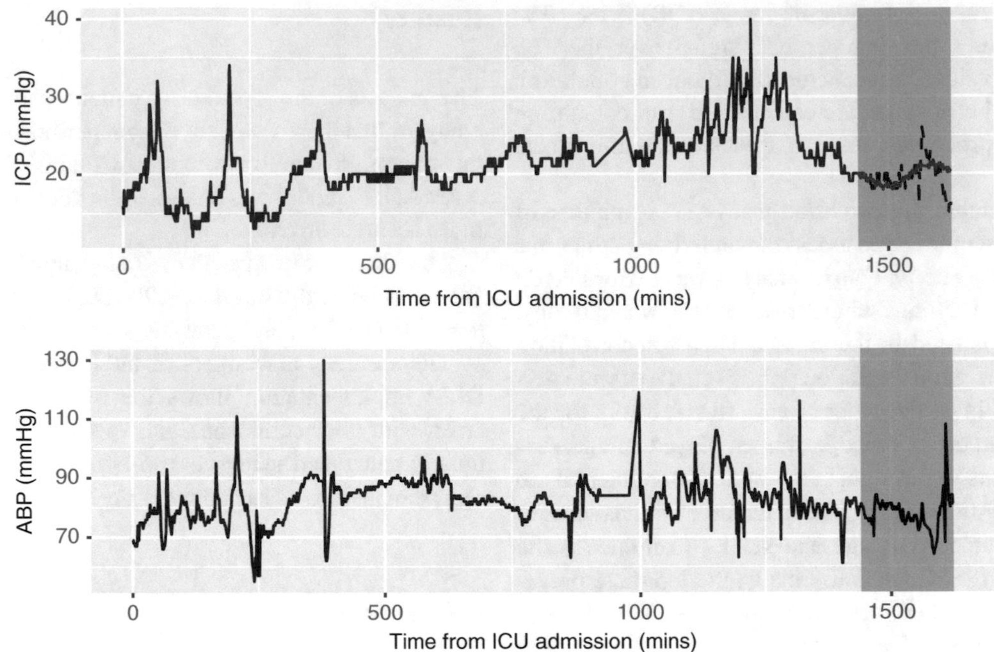

Fig. 2 Representative example forecast of mean ICP, shown in blue with red background, and the actual mean ICP, shown in black, using mean ABP as one of the exogenous regressors

extended to incorporate this new information either by adding more switchable therapeutic states or adding more exogenous regressors.

This current work only looks to forecast what actually happened to the ICP signal to enable assessment of the FASSTER implementation as a new modelling technique. However, it also has the ability to simulate counterfactual forecasts under hypothetical conditions. A counterfactual forecast can be created using any exogenous regressors that could be targeted with a clinical intervention, such as ABP, or any of the included therapeutic states, analgesia, osmotic therapy or paralysis. This hypothetical forecast can generate a possible ICP signal under the chosen combination of exogenous regressors and therapeutic states enabling exploration of possible outcomes in which different clinical interventions are applied.

Currently these counterfactual simulations are limited by the original model's ability to learn how an individual patient's ICP signal reacts to a given therapeutic state, implying that if a patient has not been in that state during the training period, of the previous 24 h, then a less accurate forecast will be generated under those unknown hypotheses. To counter this inherent limitation of the current technique, it is proposed that an average patient reaction to all therapeutic states be learned across all patients in the current dataset. These general effects could then be used as baseline exogenous input to all per-patient models to better influence a forecast's overall trend when an unknown counterfactual is encountered.

Conclusion

The FASSTER time-varying DLM implementation is a novel technique which shows some promise for forecasting with an adequate accuracy of approximately 3 mmHg. It will require further optimisation to become a usable clinical tool for both factual and counterfactual simulations of a patient's ICP signal.

Conflict of Interest **There are no known conflicts of interest from any authors associated with this work.**

References

1. Dewan MC, Abbas R, Saksham G, Baticulon RE, Ya-Ching H, Maria P et al (2018) Estimating the global incidence of traumatic brain injury. J Neurosurg 130:1080–1097
2. World Health Organization (2006) Neurological disorders: Public Health Challenges. http://www.who.int/mental_health/neurology/neurological_disorders_report_web.pdf. Accessed 26 Oct 2019
3. Humphreys I, Wood RL, Phillips CJ, Macey S (2013) The costs of traumatic brain injury: a literature review. Clinicoecon Outcomes Res 5:281–287
4. Magni F, Pozzi M, Rota M, Vargiolu A, Citerio G (2015) High-resolution intracranial pressure burden and outcome in subarachnoid hemorrhage. Stroke 46:2464–2469
5. Smith M, Maas AIR (2019) An algorithm for patients with intracranial pressure monitoring: filling the gap between evidence and practice. Intensive Care Med 45:1819–1821

6. Gooijer JGD, Hyndman RJ (2006) 25 years of time series forecasting. Int J Forecast 22:443–473
7. Farhadi A, Chern J, Hirsh D, Davis T, Jo M, Maier F et al (2018) Intracranial pressure forecasting in children using dynamic averaging of time series data. Forecasting 1:47–58
8. Petris G, Petrone S, Campagnoli P (2009) Dynamic linear models with R. Springer, Dordrecht
9. O'Hara-Wild M, Hyndman RJ. Forecasting with additive switching of seasonality, trend and exogenous regressors. https://github.com/tidyverts/fasster. Accessed 26 Oct 2019
10. Liu Z, Hauskrecht M (2017) A personalized predictive framework for multivariate clinical time series via adaptive model selection. Proc ACM Int Conf Inf Knowl Manag 2017:1169–1177
11. R Core Team (2019) R: a language and environment for statistical computing. R foundation for statistical computing, Vienna, Austria. https://www.R-project.org/
12. Piper I, Citerio G, Chambers I, Contant C, Enblad P, Fiddes H et al (2003) The BrainIT group: concept and core dataset definition. Acta Neurochir 145:615–628; discussion 628–9
13. Güiza F, Depreitere B, Piper I, Van den Berghe G, Meyfroidt G (2013) Novel methods to predict increased intracranial pressure during intensive care and long-term neurologic outcome after traumatic brain injury: development and validation in a multicenter dataset. Crit Care Med 41:554–564

Automatic Pulse Classification for Artefact Removal Using SAX Strings, a CENTER-TBI Study

Manuel Cabeleira, Marta Fedriga, and Peter Smielewski

Introduction

A patient stay in a modern intensive care unit (ICU) generates large volumes of high-resolution data that encode underlying information about the patient's physiology. This information can then be used directly at the bedside to help in patient management and lead to better outcomes. To assess this information, the data generated must be collected and subjected to further analysis.

Because of the nature of the data collection process and the continuous interventions made to these patients, the raw data collected are very often polluted with artefacts that mask the underlying physiology. In this scenario some of the artefactual data recorded originated from sensor disconnection, misplacement, recalibration routines or flushing of the signal-conducting channels. The data generated by these occurrences are completely invalid and must be eliminated before any meaningful and reliable analysis can be done. Other types of artefact are generated when the patient is subject to any kind of bedside intervention such as suctions and patient repositioning maneuvers. These types of artefacts should be dealt with in a different manner than the ones described previously because the data measured are likely correct, i.e. the patient will experience the effects of these interventions and the response measured will be true, albeit artificially induced.

It is therefore of paramount importance to devise preprocessing methods that can distinguish different types of artefacts and deal with them in an effective and systematic way. The gold standard method for identifying and marking artefacts remains the manual mark-up, but, although this technique is sensitive to different types of artefacts, it is also very time-consuming, highly dependent on the criteria, bias and experience of the investigator marking the recording and can only be applied on retrospective data.

Another commonly used technique makes use of simple heuristics like thresholding using the accepted physiological values as limits or detecting the lack of pulsatility of otherwise pulsatile modalities to detect artefactual periods. Even though these methods can be applied to real-time data processing and systematically following the same rules throughout the processing, these algorithms are often tailored to specific types of artefacts and will usually not eliminate the artefactual sections in their totality.

An ideal artefact detection technique is one that can reliably and systematically discern between different types of artefacts whilst being applicable in real-time analysis scenarios. Such an algorithm should also support the means of selecting families of artefacts to be removed from analysis depending on the phenomena being studied.

A good candidate for this task is the Symbolic Aggregate aproXimation (SAX) algorithm, which can extract information about the shape of individual pulses of periodic modalities, like arterial blood pressure (ABP) or intracranial pressure (ICP), and determine whether the pulse is artefactual. Though these signals are highly dynamic, if unperturbed, they will maintain highly stable and very well-defined shapes. On the other hand, interventions will influence the shape of the pulses, and these changes will be detected and marked as artefacts.

In this work we present the application of the SAX algorithm as an automatic artefact detection technique that can be

M. Cabeleira (✉) · P. Smielewski
Brain Physics Lab, Division of Neurosurgery, Department of Clinical Neurosciences, Addenbrooke's Hospital, University of Cambridge, Cambridge, UK

Neurosurgery Unit, Addenbrooke's Hospital, Cambridge, UK
e-mail: mc916@cam.ac.uk

M. Fedriga
Brain Physics Lab, Division of Neurosurgery, Department of Clinical Neurosciences, Addenbrooke's Hospital, University of Cambridge, Cambridge, UK

Neurosurgery Unit, Addenbrooke's Hospital, Cambridge, UK

Department of Anesthesia, Critical Care and Emergency, Spedali Civili University Hospital, Brescia, Italy

B. Depreitere et al. (eds.), *Intracranial Pressure and Neuromonitoring XVII*, Acta Neurochirurgica Supplement 131,
https://doi.org/10.1007/978-3-030-59436-7_44, © Springer Nature Switzerland AG 2021

comparatively as sensitive to different types of artefacts as the manual mark-up but can be applied in real time. Here we will also evaluate the performance of this method against the gold standard method, the manual mark-up.

Materials and Methods

The dataset used to evaluate the performance of this algorithm was composed of high-resolution ABP signals (>100 Hz sampling frequency) from the CENTER-TBI project [1]. The data were collected between January 2015 and December 2017 and comprised continuous streams of data from patients with moderate to severe traumatic brain injury from 21 centres in the European Union. The data collection software was ICM+ [2], and the files were then processed further in MATLAB [3].

The information about the shape of the pulses was obtained using the SAX algorithm [4], which converts a pulse represented in the time domain into a 'word', called a SAX string (SAXS) (Fig. 1). Similar pulses will naturally aggregate into the same or very similar SAXS. To distinguish between SAXS generated from artefactual and physiological pulses, a classifier based on a support vector machine (SVM) [5] was used.

To calculate the SAXS, the raw signal was cut into individual pulses, this was done using an algorithm published in [6]. The cut pulses were then normalized so that their mean value was 0 and standard deviation was 1, and they were also rescaled to a length of 100 data points. The length of the SAXS was chosen to be six with an alphabet of six characters, so that the number of SAXS generated would be manageable for manual classification (6^6 possible SAXS). To attribute a value to each letter of the SAXS, the pulse was cut into six equally sized chunks, and the mean value of each chunk was calculated. This mean value was then encoded by a letter by dividing the letter axis into six areas of equal size and matching the mean value to a letter (Fig. 1).

This algorithm was then applied to the raw ABP of 50 randomly chosen patients from the dataset and a dictionary composed of pairs of SAXS—a mean pulse (calculated from all pulses encoded by the same SAXS)—was created, yielding 3330 entries.

From this dictionary the 700 most commonly occurring SAXS, composing 99.75% of the total number of pulses analysed, were manually classified as physiological or artefactual and used as the training dataset for the SVM classifier.

To evaluate the performance of the technique, a new dataset composed of a balanced number of artefactual and physiological pulses was created from another eight randomly chosen patients from the CENTER-TBI dataset (Fig. 2). Each individual pulse in this new dataset was then automatically classified by the trained SVM classifier and two independent researchers. The evaluation of the two independent researchers was then compared to the results of the automatic classification.

Results

The created dictionary relating the SAXS/average pulse pairs proved to be a very effective way of generating the classified data to train the classifier. Fig. 1 shows examples of

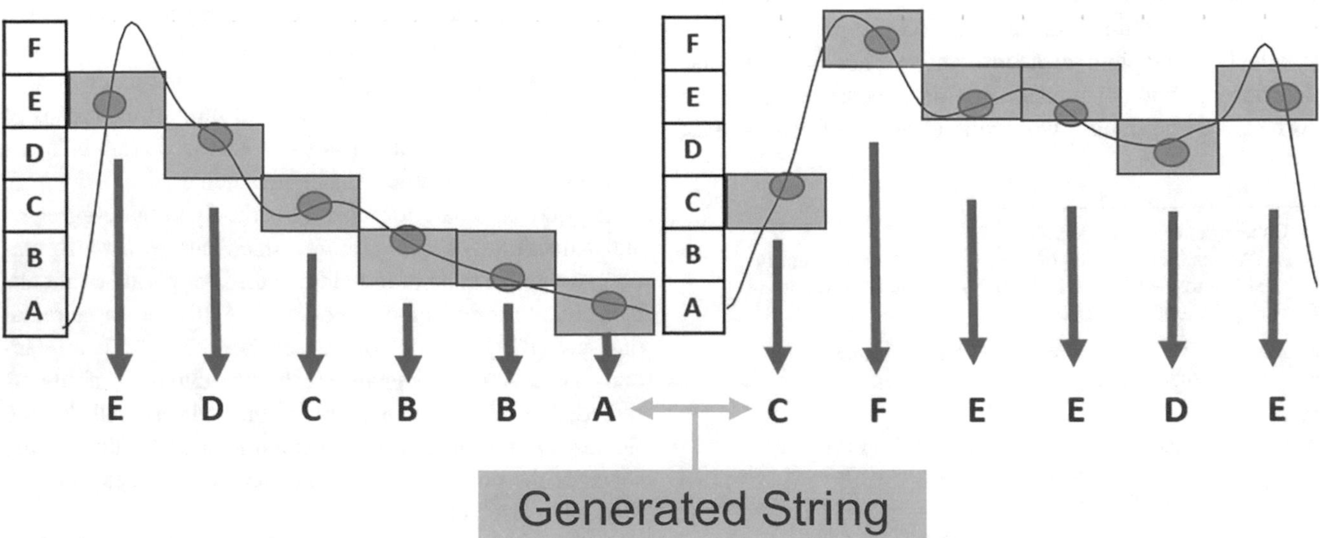

Fig. 1 Diagram depicting calculation of SAX string for individual pulse. On the *y*-axis is the SAXS generated for each pulse, on the *x*-axis the alphabet used to calculate the letters for the SAXS

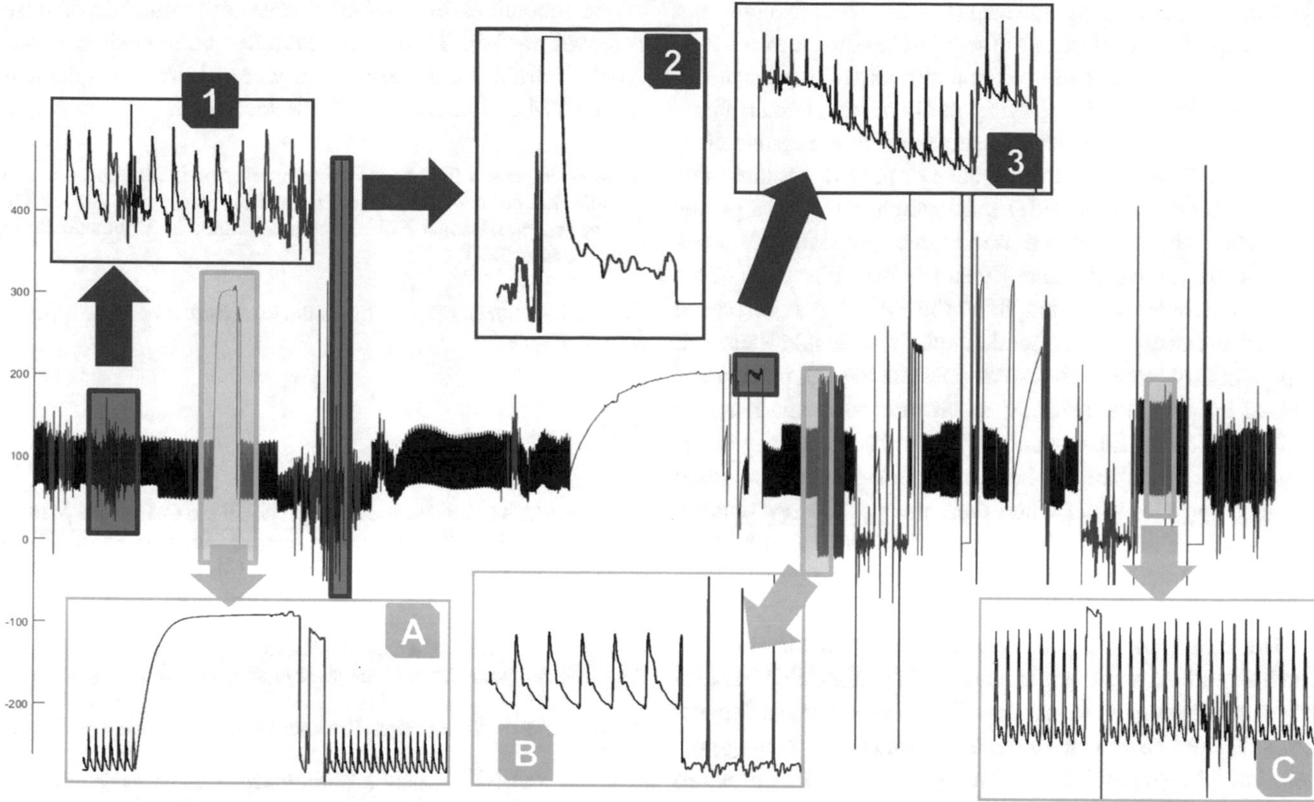

Fig. 2 The time series in the centre of the figure was used to evaluate the performance of the algorithm. *1*—Example of misclassified pulse due to presence of noise. *2*—Example of misclassified pulse due to having an acceptable SAX but with non-physiological values. *3*—Same as 2. *A*—Example of an accurately rejected line flush. *B*—Example of accurately rejected pulses from different modalities. *C*—Example of accurately rejected pulses where sensor was perturbed. In black are pulses classified as physiological, in blue are pulses classified as artefactual and in red are pulses rejected by the algorithm before classification

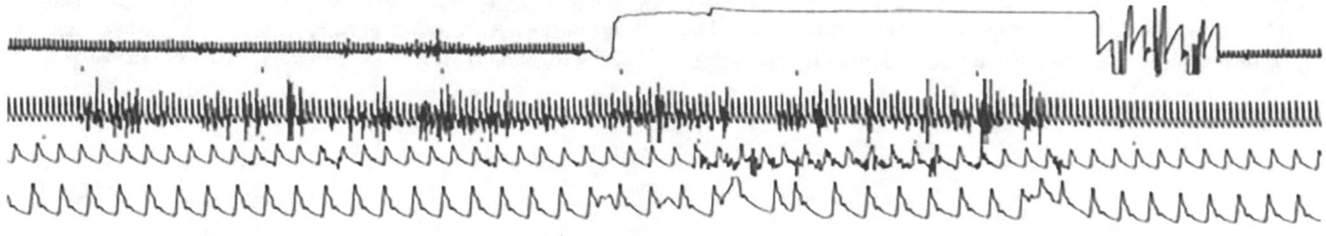

Fig. 3 Results of pulse classification; pulses in blue were accepted as physiological; those in red were rejected as artefacts

SAXS generated by a physiological pulse and an artefactual pulse. The testing dataset contained examples of the most common types of artefacts described that allowed us to evaluate the algorithm in different scenarios. Fig. 2 shows a snapshot of this dataset and the result of the pulse classification by the algorithm. Fig. 3 presents examples of the application of the algorithm to detect artefacts in some ABP time series.

Compared with the two independent researchers, the algorithm achieved a sensitivity of 97.2% and 95.4% and a specificity of 87.7% in both comparisons.

Discussion

The very high sensitivity displayed by the algorithm guarantees that the majority of physiological pulses are allowed through, with a high rejection rate of artefactual pulses verified by the specificity. This result is remarkable because the classification is based solely on information about the overall shape of the pulses, ignoring all other commonly used measures. The algorithm was also shown to be very highly sensitive to various families of artefacts, successfully eliminating line flushes, noisy signals, sensor interference and even sections of data with signal swap (Fig. 2). This technique can also be applied in real time at the bedside since it works on a pulse-by-pulse basis and is computationally inexpensive.

Despite its overall satisfying performance, certain families of pulses would lend themselves to false negative classifications. This is partially because of the low resolution of the SAXS (six letters wide) that sometimes groups pulses that would be considered noisy into physiological ones because they have the same mean value (Fig. 2(1)). This could be avoided if the length of the SAXS were increased and the alphabet used to encode them, but it would lead to an exponentially larger universe of possible SAXS, making the task of training the classifier much more difficult. Another factor generating false positives is the absence of any information other than shape; this leads to the detection of some pulses as physiological when the values of the raw data go outside of the physiological ranges (Fig. 2(2, 3)). Errors in the pulse extraction phase also lead to some otherwise true positives being classified as artefacts.

The requirement of supervised training of the classifier can also influence the performance of the algorithm because it will still be subject to the same limitations as manual markup. This can bias the classifier, and because the training process is highly repetitive and time-consuming, it is prone to erroneous and slightly inconsistent annotations.

Overall the algorithm performed highly satisfactorily, and our results serve as a proof of concept that information about pulse shape can constitute an effective tool for detecting and removing common artefacts in physiological signals that carry cardiac rhythm variability. Future iterations of this algorithm would use better performing pulse-cutting algorithms to minimize the number of pulses wrongly cut. The algorithm would also have to consider physiological ranges of the modalities in order to decrease the number of false positives further. To be able to fully distinguish between types of artefacts, the algorithm would have to implement more SVM classifiers trained to detect them.

Acknowledgments This study was supported by the European Union Seventh Framework Programme (grant 602150) for Collaborative European NeuroTrauma Effectiveness Research in Traumatic Brain Injury (Center-TBI).

Conflict of Interest **The authors declare that they have no conflict of interest.**

References

1. Maas AIR, Menon DK, Steyerberg EW, Citerio G, Lecky F, Manley GT, CENTER-TBI Participants and Investigators et al (2015) Collaborative European NeuroTrauma Effectiveness Research in Traumatic Brain Injury (CENTER-TBI): a prospective longitudinal observational study. Neurosurgery 76(1):67–80. https://doi.org/10.1227/NEU.0000000000000575
2. ICM+ software. https://icmplus.neurosurg.cam.ac.uk. Accessed 3 Nov 2019
3. MATLAB Software. https://uk.mathworks.com/. Accessed 3 Nov 2019
4. Lin J, Keogh E, Lonardi S, Chiu B (2003) A symbolic representation of time series, with implications for streaming algorithms. Proceedings of the 8th ACM SIGMOD Workshop on Research Issues in Data Mining and Knowledge Discovery, DMKD '03. https://doi.org/10.1145/882082.882086
5. Tongsimon S, Koller D (2002) Support vector machine active learning with applications to text classification. Support Vector Machine Active Learning with Applications to Text Classification. https://doi.org/10.1162/153244302760185243
6. Scholkmann F, Boss J, Wolf M (2012) An efficient algorithm for automatic peak detection in noisy periodic and quasi-periodic signals. Algorithms 5:588–603. https://doi.org/10.3390/a5040588

DeepClean: Self-Supervised Artefact Rejection for Intensive Care Waveform Data Using Deep Generative Learning

Tom Edinburgh, Peter Smielewski, Marek Czosnyka, Manuel Cabeleira, Stephen J. Eglen, and Ari Ercole

Introduction

Critically ill patients in an intensive care unit (ICU) may experience life-threatening deterioration, sometimes over minutes or even seconds. Care of these patients is therefore highly dependent on data [1], which, by necessity, may be voluminous and complex. An extreme example of this are high-frequency physiological waveforms, such as invasive arterial blood pressure (ABP), electrocardiogram and other vascular or intracranial pressures, which provide a wealth of complex, heterogeneous, yet highly structured data at optimal sampling frequencies of 100Hz or even more. Continuous monitoring of these waveforms form the basis of clinical research and care, in particular alerting clinicians to changes in the patient state in real time, and they may be further processed to derive other useful parameters, for example measures for tracking cerebral autoregulation [2] and heart-rate variability [3], which have repeatedly been shown to be determinants of physiological integrity. Further, more sophisticated metrics of these waveforms, based on non-linear dynamics [4] or information theory [5], may form novel digital biomarkers for precision care in the future (e.g. [6]).

Waveform artefacts arise from a variety of internal and external sources, such as sensor noise, patient movement and clinical intervention. Such artefacts may reduce reliability in the estimation of derived indices, confound analysis and create uncertainty in clinical decision-making. In the same manner, the handling of missing data is closely related and is often treated using simple methods, such as linear interpolation of observed data, that are biased and underestimate variability. Imputation methods that maintain some statistical properties or features of the data offer a useful alternative [7]. Artefact detection is also important for ICU alerting systems [8] and reduces the likelihood of false positive alarm incidents. A high rate of false alarms carries a significant risk because alarm fatigue often leaves clinical staff perceiving the alarms to be generally unhelpful and can therefore potentially result in delays in the appropriate clinical intervention [9].

Artefact detection has traditionally been a difficult and costly task, requiring time-consuming human annotation or thresholding based on signal-specific feature engineering [10]. Due to the complex morphologies of waveforms, annotation by experienced clinicians remains a gold standard for ICU multimodality monitoring, despite inherent biases and issues with replicability. Many standard supervised learning methods require samples that are annotated in this way in order to learn a model, though a recent study used active learning to query and propose samples for annotation in an efficient manner [11]. An alternative unsupervised approach has foundations in spectral anomaly detection [12]. These methods seek an embedding of data in an 'information bottleneck' lower-dimensional space, where the anomaly or artefact is separated from the normal data, and then form a reconstruction of the input from its lower-dimensional representation back to the original input space. Embedding in the 'bottleneck' latent space is a lossy transformation, and the aim is to capture salient features of the data whilst disregarding anomalous features. Subsequently, the reconstruction should restore the underlying 'true' behaviour, and the error in the reconstruction, compared to the input, can then be used to discriminate artefacts.

Generative modelling describes a class of models in which we want to learn a distribution $p_\theta(x)$ to approximate the true distribution of data X in a dataset. We can sample directly from this learnt distribution to generate new example data that

T. Edinburgh (✉) · S. J. Eglen
Department of Applied Mathematics and Theoretical Physics, University of Cambridge, Cambridge, UK
e-mail: te269@cam.ac.uk

P. Smielewski · M. Czosnyka · M. Cabeleira
Brain Physics, Department of Clinical Neurosciences, University of Cambridge, Cambridge, UK

A. Ercole
Division of Anaesthesia, Department of Medicine, University of Cambridge, Cambridge, UK

B. Depreitere et al. (eds.), *Intracranial Pressure and Neuromonitoring XVII*, Acta Neurochirurgica Supplement 131,
https://doi.org/10.1007/978-3-030-59436-7_45,

captures some statistical properties and features of the true distribution of the data. A subset of this are latent variable models, which condition on unobserved variables or features z, with a family of deterministic functions $f(z;\theta)$ mapping z to the data space via a decoder network, which is parameterised by θ. The aim is maximum likelihood estimation of the marginal (model evidence) $p(x) = \int p(x,z)dz = \int p_\theta(x|z)p(z)dz$ with respect to θ, but this is often intractable. Variational autoencoders (VAEs) [13] resolve this using variational Bayesian inference, reproducing this 'bottleneck' architecture (Figure 1) via coupled but distinct encoder and decoder modules, where the encoder describes a variational distribution $q_\phi(z|x)$ that approximates the true posterior $p(z|x) = p(x|z)p(z)/p(x)$. During training, it learns both to encode some information about each data point in its latent representation, $z \sim q_\phi(z|x)$, and stochastic sampling from this distribution allows the model to abstract and generate new candidate data, $x \sim p_\theta(x|z)$, that accurately reconstructs inputs from the assumed underlying random process. This enables it to discriminate artefacts despite never being explicitly exposed to any, since we assume different latent mechanisms govern the waveform behaviour of any artefacts, and so model prediction over an input containing such an artefact will have low reconstruction probability and high reconstruction error [14]. For further details, comprehensive summaries of VAEs can be found in the literature, e.g. [15–17].

In this work, we demonstrate the potential for deep generative learning, in particular VAEs, in the detection of artefacts in physiological waveforms, developing a VAE-based model and pipeline, which we name DeepClean. We investigate whether, by training DeepClean on largely clean ABP recordings as an example, regions of artefactual data can be identified in a self-supervised way without explicitly showing DeepClean any artefact exemplars. Furthermore, we aim to determine whether the DeepClean generative model can impute missing data over such regions. This work is a shortened version of a preprint we archived recently [18]; the reader is encouraged to refer to that paper for a fuller discussion.

Methods

Fully anonymous ABP data from a standard indwelling arterial line connected to a pressure transducer (Baxter Healthcare Corp. CardioVascular Group, Irvine, CA) was obtained as part of routine ICU clinical care. The data used in this study are ABP waveforms from a single anonymised adult patient monitored almost continuously throughout a stay of several days in the ICU. The signal was sampled at frequency of 125Hz using ICM+ software (Cambridge Enterprise Ltd., Cambridge, UK, http://icmplus.neurosurg.cam.ac.uk). Under UK regulations, ethical approval was not required for the reuse of anonymous data obtained as part of routine clinical practice for research.

DeepClean was trained and tested on 10s windows of preprocessed data. To learn a generative model describing 'clean' physiological waveforms, we first removed large, grossly abnormal sections by applying basic thresholding heuristics (for further detail, see [18]), to obtain largely 'clean' training data without human mark-up at a beat-to-beat level. This is a far easier task than manual mark-up of a waveform but inevitably leaves artefacts in the training set. Removing this preprocessing step does not prevent the learning of a generative model, but without it training can be more difficult and the final generative model suboptimal because such training samples will make a larger contribution to the overall loss function. Though DeepClean is self-supervised, we required a labelled test set to determine model performance against manual expert mark-up. We selected this test set randomly from the unprocessed data to avoid potential sources of selection bias, but with higher probability of selecting regions marked as abnormal in preprocessing, because we assumed waveform artefacts were rare compared to normal beats and we required a balanced test set, with a similar proportion of artefacts and valid signals (again, see [18]). The test set and preprocessing-marked regions were then removed from the dataset and the remaining data split into 10s samples, shuffled, and divided into training and vali-

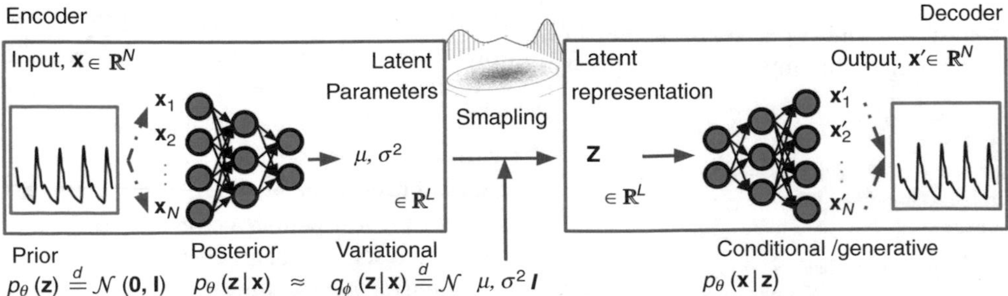

Fig. 1 A variational autoencoder learns a generative model, $p_\theta(x|z)$, and a variational approximation, $q_\phi(z|x)$, to the posterior distribution for the latent variables, $p_\theta(x|z)$, and we can generate new data by sampling from the latent and generative distributions in order. The weights of the encoder are the variational parameters, ϕ, and the weights of the decoder are the generative parameters, θ. The output of the encoder acts as a mean and standard deviation to the Gaussian variational distribution. Figure also in [18]

dation sets with a ratio of 9:1. Training, validation and test sets were then standardised by the training set mean and standard deviation. Each 10s test sample was labelled as either containing an artefact or being artefact free by expert review (TE, AE). Furthermore, for samples judged to contain an artefact, sections of the waveform *within* each 10s window were also annotated. We also assessed performance by comparison to principal component analysis (PCA), which performs a similar dimensionality reduction and reconstruction. The number of principal components is comparable to the latent dimension of a VAE, so we refer to both as the latent dimension for brevity.

We built a variational autoencoder with deep convolutional neural networks (CNNs) for both encoder and decoder modules. CNNs allow a network to learn translation-invariant local patterns, with successive layers building a spatial hierarchy of increasing scale, a sensible approach in this context where physiological signal data are quasi-periodic and highly structured. We fixed an encoder network architecture with three relatively small convolutional layers, alternated with two pooling layers to increase the receptive field, and finally two dense layers that split the network graph into separate branches for the two parameters that define the latent space. The decoder architecture mirrored this in reverse, with pooling replaced by up-sampling. Both encoder and decoder contained approximately 20,000 trainable parameters. We then trained separate models with increasing latent space dimension. For each latent dimension, we repeated training five times, presenting the model that minimised the validation loss. To train DeepClean, we used an NVidia Pascal P100 graphical processing unit (GPU), with code written in Python using the Keras library [19] with TensorFlow backend [20]. We optimised the evidence lower bound objective (ELBO) [13, 15, 17] and made typical assumptions about the distributional families of the prior, variational and conditional.

We assessed the performance of our approach in detecting whether or not a 10s sample of data contained an artefact or not via the mean squared error (MSE) between the sample and its reconstruction, with a suitable threshold. The goal of this work was to develop a 'blind' self-supervised classification procedure, and so any threshold on a metric applied to the reconstruction error must be chosen independently of the test data. Figure 2 illustrates that the MSE values are generally not independent of hyperparameter choice. Therefore, without prior knowledge of a suitable threshold, a pragmatic approach was to set a threshold based on the 90th percentile of the same metric calculated instead on the training data and their corresponding reconstructions. Note that, by decreasing the threshold on a metric, we classified more samples as artefacts, regardless of the correctness of this classification, and therefore increased the specificity at the cost of decreasing the sensitivity (Fig. 2). We assessed the model performance by comparing the DeepClean classification to our annotation, using measures widely employed in clinical settings: accuracy, sensitivity and specificity. With samples identified as artefacts, we could then use a metric on subsets of the sample (such as a sliding window approach) to identify artefacts more precisely within these samples [18].

Results

We worked with 486,984 s of ABP waveform data from a single anonymised adult patient. We marked 11,082s of 486,984s (2.28%) as grossly abnormal in preprocessing, leaving training and validation sets of 37,821 and 4728 10s samples. Training required under 10 min of computation time on average, although this increased with latent dimension. Subsequent prediction, on test data or on new data, is inexpensive and requires only milliseconds. Our annotation marked 130 test samples out of a test set of 200 as containing an artefact.

DeepClean was able to reconstruct much more accurately the waveform inputs than PCA. In particular, DeepClean was able to encode subpulse components, such as the dicrotic notch, even for minimal latent dimensions. The PCA reconstruction is particularly poor for a small number of principal components but is much better for larger latent dimensions (as seen in the training set log-MSE values in Fig. 2). DeepClean significantly outperformed the baseline PCA in sample-wide artefact detection in model sensitivity (Table 1), using our training set–defined threshold. Whilst we give a heuristic for identifying this threshold, DeepClean also had a significantly higher receiver operating characteristic area under the curve (ROC AUC) than PCA. There is in general a clear distinction between the log-MSE of artefacts and valid data for the DeepClean reconstruction since DeepClean is able to distinguish samples similar to and unlike those belonging to the underlying generative process of the waveform from the training set data. In contrast, the range of log-MSE values for PCA reconstructions were similar for both training set and test set artefacts, so the latter could not be easily identified in this way. In both cases, the non-artefact test samples followed a distribution similar to that of the training data, so the specificity was generally close to the training set 90th-percentile threshold. Because PCA reconstructions have a higher error than DeepClean unless the number of principal components is very large, the threshold was different for each method, and so an identical reconstruction may be identified differently by DeepClean and PCA. In particular, a poor DeepClean reconstruction of a sample containing an artefact may be identified as such when an identical reconstruction from PCA may not.

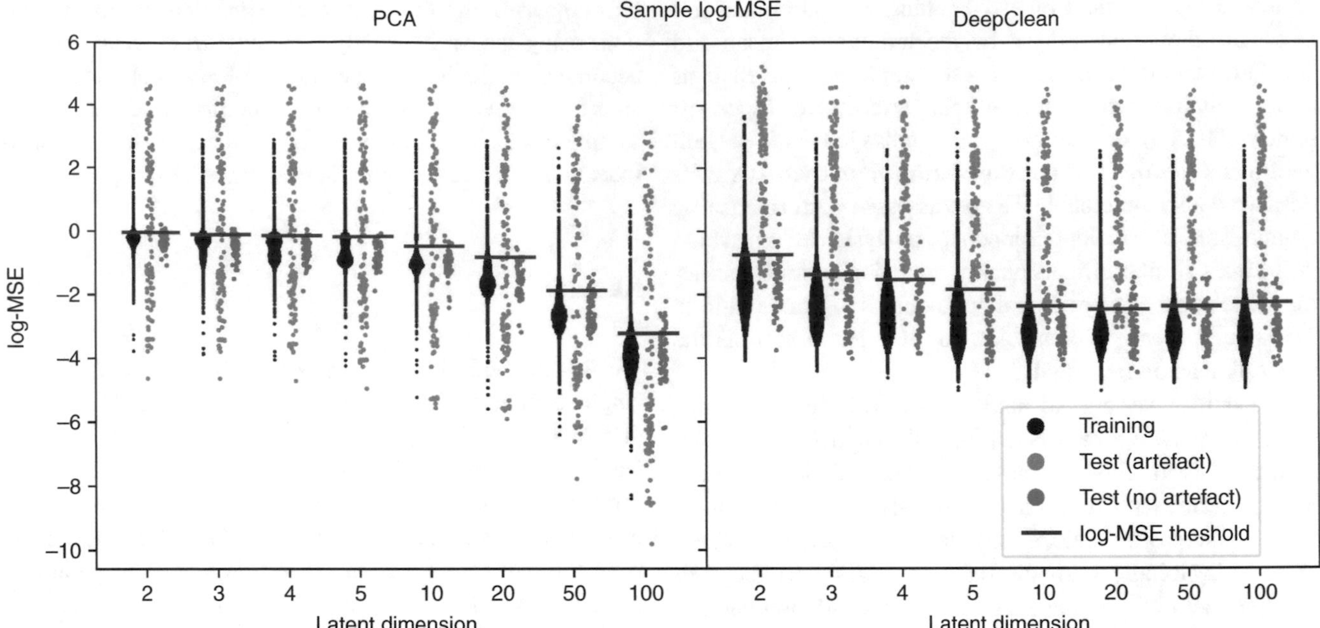

Fig. 2 Log-MSE values for both PCA and DeepClean, with increasing latent dimension. The distribution of training set log-MSE is shown with the training set 90th-percentile threshold. The test samples are split into two, shown separately: those annotated as containing an artefact and as not containing an artefact. The 'ground truth' artefacts that lie below the threshold and non-artefacts above the threshold were samples that were incorrectly identified and were false negatives and false positives respectively. Therefore, the proportion of test artefacts points above the threshold is the sensitivity and the proportion of test non-artefacts below the threshold is the specificity. Figure reproduced under creative commons licence from [18]

Table 1 Assessment of the classification of samples as containing an artefact or not, for both PCA and DeepClean (VAE). Both methods had comparable specificity, i.e. correctly identifying non-artefact data as such, with PCA performing slightly better. However, DeepClean alone can identify artefactual data as such, with high sensitivity

	Accuracy		Sensitivity		Specificity		ROC AUC	
Latent dim	PCA	VAE	PCA	VAE	PCA	VAE	PCA	VAE
2	0.61	0.88	0.454	0.854	0.9	0.929	0.471	0.967
3	0.615	0.925	0.462	0.977	0.9	0.886	0.478	0.984
4	0.62	0.945	0.462	0.977	0.914	0.886	0.482	0.987
5	0.62	0.945	0.462	0.992	0.914	0.857	0.487	0.994
10	0.62	0.86	0.470	0.869	0.9	0.843	0.496	0.953
20	0.63	0.855	0.470	0.877	0.929	0.814	0.528	0.96
50	0.605	0.905	0.454	0.931	0.886	0.857	0.474	0.976
100	0.58	0.895	0.446	0.908	0.828	0.871	0.478	0.969
Mean	0.613	0.901	0.460	0.919	0.896	0.868	0.487	0.973

Discussion

We have demonstrated the use of a VAE to clean ABP signals in a self-supervised manner, suggesting a clear potential role for deep generative learning in this clinical application. DeepClean requires only two basic steps alongside jointly training encoder and decoder neural networks: straightforward thresholding heuristics for preprocessing, which may even be omitted at the cost of a slightly weaker model, and a metric or decision rule for discriminating artefacts based on reconstruction error, which may include learning an acceptance threshold from the training data based on an approximate target false negative rate. Unlike a recent study [21], which employed a stacked convolutional autoencoder (SCAE) combined with a CNN, our approach does not require pulse pre-segmentation (which is in itself a difficult task requiring heuristics) or a supervised final classification network. Furthermore, since DeepClean functions in the time domain, it avoids the quadratic complexity of first mapping the pulse morphology to a two-dimensional space.

We decided to split the data into 10s samples for training and prediction, since such segments typically contain a small number of beats, and we do not expect physiology to vary significantly over this period from clinical experience. A sample of this length should include a sufficient number of beats that the model can learn so as to generalise the structure of the waveform and therefore distinguish artefacts that occur over similar or longer time scales. It is important that the model recognises clinical events as part of the same generative process and so does not classify these as artefacts. Failure to flag a clinical event that has been incorrectly identified as a signal artefact risks delayed intervention and treatment. Whilst such events are characterised by sudden changes across multiple frequency bands concurrently, the structure of the waveform during a clinical event is largely retained within a sample of this length, so it is a suitable choice.

Artefact detection is often only the first of two parts involved in handling invalid data because simply removing artefacts creates missing data that may also bias further analysis. One major advantage of a generative model is that it can be used to generate realistic, synthetic data by sampling directly from the latent distribution. An obvious solution, then, is to replace an artefact sample with its reconstruction, and further, we can also set missing data to a fixed non-viable value and similarly treat this as an artefact. This may only be suitable for a given sample if, for any artefacts within that sample, the reconstruction can approximate (with large enough reconstruction error such that it is classified as an artefact) the underlying waveform behaviour that would be expected in the absence of the artefact mechanism whilst simultaneously maintaining a small error for any non-artefact regions in the same sample (e.g. Fig. 3, left and third from top). For an artefact, the latent representation, described by the variational distribution $q_\phi(z|x)$, gives some hint as to when DeepClean is successful at this. In imposing the generative model on new data that does not come from the same process or mechanism as the training data, the probability that an artefactual sample will be generated by latent variables that are similar to those of valid data is very low, and as a result, the artefactual sample is forced to have a latent representation with vanishingly small probability mass in the average encoding distribution or the prior. Because the model has spent little or no time training this region of the latent space, the reconstruction is therefore very unlike that of any valid data, and we cannot impute using it. Density-based anomaly detection methods, which identify anomalies by the sparsity of the region of space in which they occupy, may be useful to recognise artefacts for which these imputations are not appropriate. An alternative is to track the trajectory of a patient in the latent space and sample at points close to this trajectory when an artefact has been identified, but further work is needed to understand the structure of the latent space. For example, β-VAEs [22, 23] can improve the ability of a network to disentangle meaningful features in the data via constrained optimisation.

We have considered expert manual mark-up for 'ground truth' artefact assignment. Some artefacts are clearly identifiable to clinicians because their signal profile is so extreme. For example, blood sampling or subsequent flushing of the arterial line may be highly variable in profile but will clearly contain signal excursions which are unphysiological. Other signals are not so clear-cut to categorically assign as artefact. Patient movement may introduce vibration, which in the extreme may render the signal unusable but in less severe cases often simply decreases the signal-to-noise ratio; whether such signals are identified as artefacts is to some extent arbitrary. Changes in the resonant properties of the ABP transduction system due to blood clots or bubbles represent another difficulty. This may occur as a result of 'over-damping' (mean pressure preserved) or attenuation [24] (mean pressure not preserved): in either case the pulse amplitude is reduced and high-frequency features are lost. Since the presence of high-frequency features varies with cardiac output, it is impossible to absolutely describe such regions as valid or otherwise. As a result of these considerations, a good gold standard is lacking and therefore imposes limitations on our ability to rigorously evaluate model performance.

We have focused little attention on optimising hyperparameter and architecture choices, using deep CNNs for both encoder and decoder that we have deliberately kept small relative to the deep generative learning literature. However, we expect the gains from increasing the network size or complexity, for example, to be marginal in this application domain. Indeed, increasing the learning capacity of the decoder may mean that the latent variables are ignored and do not encode information about the data. One hyperparameter we have investigated is the latent dimension. This is particularly interesting in view of unsupervised representation learning, provided we are able to learn disentangled interpretable features encoded in the latent space.

We chose the ABP signal as a test case for several reasons. Firstly, it is particularly artefact-prone due to the effects of movement and flushing on the fluid-filled catheter system typically employed. Secondly, ABP is of universal physiological importance, especially the extremes of ABP (hypo- and hypertension), which are particularly influenced by artefacts. Finally, ABP morphology tends to have good signal-to-noise properties. The performance of our model with other types of physiological signal is an area of future investigation and optimisation. We have trained and tested our system on available data from a patient in sinus rhythm, which is strongly periodic over the sample lengths considered. The performance of this framework on data from

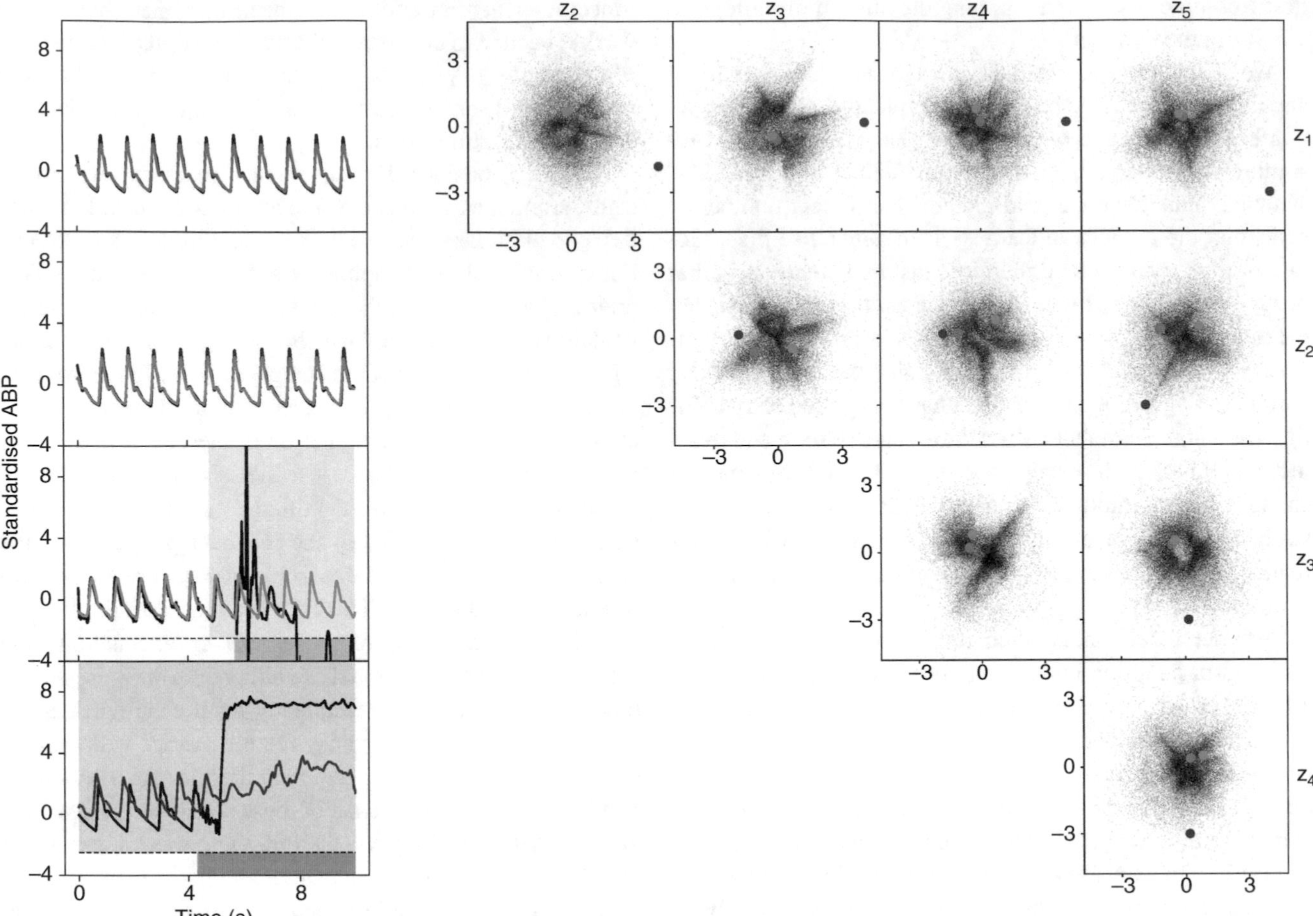

Fig. 3 Illustration of key principles involving the latent distribution, via examples. Each example test input is given in black (left) with the corresponding latent representation within the latent distribution (right) and reconstruction (left) in (matching) colour. The shaded region above the dotted line (left) shows where DeepClean identifies an artefact (within the artefactual sample, using a sliding 1-s window MSE calculation as in [18]), and the shaded region below the dotted line shows the artefactual region as defined by the manual annotation. The latent distribution is the average encoding distribution and is approximately equal to the distribution of the prior, a multivariate unit Gaussian [25]. It shows the latent representations of the training samples, where each subplot shows the marginal distribution of a pair of latent variables as a scatter plot, after marginalising over all other latent variables. First, almost identical inputs (the first two panels on the left, blue and orange) have almost identical latent representations (in fact, the blue marker corresponding to the first panel is barely visible because the orange marker has been overlaid on top) and, similarly, almost identical reconstructions. Second, inputs containing an artefact but with high probability mass in the latent distribution (third panel, green) have 'valid' reconstructions, synthetic waveforms that are of the underlying process described by the generative model, and we can therefore impute the section marked as artefact using this reconstruction. Conversely, an input with very low probability mass in the learnt latent distribution (fourth panel, red) does not have a valid reconstruction, and we must resort to using an alternative latent representation if we want to use the generative model for imputation in this case

patients with more irregular (e.g. patients with arrhythmias, such as atrial fibrillation or multiple ectopics) has not been determined and will be the subject of future work. It is important to establish whether a generative model trained on the waveforms from one patient is able to generalise to other patients and maintain similar performance. If retraining is required, it is possible to initialise from a previous model and so not necessary to train from scratch. Such transfer learning between patients requires either identical recording frequencies, which is common with standardised monitoring software, or an interpolation scheme such that the length of samples corresponding to a fixed time interval is constant.

This work offers a promising alternative to the identification of signal artefacts in physiological waveforms from intensive care multimodality monitoring. This study proposes DeepClean, a self-supervised deep generative learning approach to identify and reject these artefacts. This method demonstrated high sensitivity and specificity for the identification of samples containing an artefact from an ICU ABP waveform. High-frequency waveforms are central to clinical prognosis of patient state, and clinical parameters associated with outcome are derived from features of signals. Analysis that may inform care and treatment is susceptible to biases that arise from unidentified signal artefacts, and subsequent potential misdiagnosis of clinical events could result in aggressive yet unnecessary clinical intervention. Further, by removing artefacts within a signal, an improvement in the prognostic ability of a real clinical event will reduce the high false positive rate of alarms in ICU monitoring systems, improving the conditions in which clinical staff can provide the best possible care for patients. Real-time identification of artefacts and signal irregularities is absolutely critical, and DeepClean suggests that deep generative learning can play an important role in this task.

Data and Code Availability

The data used in this work were recorded as part of routine clinical care and not available for open access. However, the authors will consider requests for collaborative research projects. The code used in this study is available at https://github.com/tedinburgh/deepclean.

Acknowledgements We thank Jim Stone for helpful discussions. T.E. is funded by the Engineering and Physical Sciences Research Council (EPSRC) National Productivity Investment Fund (NPIF), reference 2089662, and Cantab Capital Institute for Mathematics of Information.

Author Contributions: T.E., S.E. and A.E. contributed to development of code and analysis. P.S., M.C. and M.C. contributed to the acquisition of data. T.E. prepared the manuscript, which was edited by S.E. and A.E. and approved by all authors. Correspondence requests should be made to T.E. and A.E.

Competing Interests **The authors declare no competing interests.**

References

1. Vincent J-L (2017) The coming era of precision medicine for intensive care. Crit Care 21(Suppl 3):314. https://doi.org/10.1186/s13054-017-1910-z
2. Aries MJH et al (2012) Continuous determination of optimal cerebral perfusion pressure in traumatic brain injury*. Crit Care Med 40(8):2456–2463. https://doi.org/10.1097/CCM.0b013e3182514eb6
3. Karmali SN, Sciusco A, May SM, Ackland GL (2017) Heart rate variability in critical care medicine: a systematic review. Intensive Care Med Exp 5(1):33. https://doi.org/10.1186/s40635-017-0146-1
4. Bishop SM, Yarham SI, Navapurkar VU, Menon DK, Ercole A (2012) Multifractal analysis of hemodynamic behavior: intraoperative instability and its pharmacological manipulation. Anesthesiology 117(4):810–821. https://doi.org/10.1097/ALN.0b013e31826a4aa2
5. Gao L, Smielewski P, Czosnyka M, Ercole A (2017) Early asymmetric cardio-cerebral causality and outcome after severe traumatic brain injury. J Neurotrauma 34(19):2743–2752. https://doi.org/10.1089/neu.2016.4787
6. Beqiri E et al (2019) Feasibility of individualised severe traumatic brain injury management using an automated assessment of optimal cerebral perfusion pressure: the COGiTATE phase II study protocol. BMJ Open 9(9):e030727. https://doi.org/10.1136/bmjopen-2019-030727
7. Sullivan AM, Xia H, Mc Bride JC, Zhao X (2010) Reconstruction of missing physiological signals using artificial neural networks. Comput Cardiol 37:317–320
8. Scalzo F, Hu X (2013) Semi-supervised detection of intracranial pressure alarms using waveform dynamics. Physiol Meas 34(4):465–478. https://doi.org/10.1088/0967-3334/34/4/465
9. Chambrin MC (2001) Alarms in the intensive care unit: how can the number of false alarms be reduced? Crit Care 5(4):184–188. https://doi.org/10.1186/cc1021
10. Sun JX, Reisner AT, Mark RG (2006) A signal abnormality index for arterial blood pressure waveforms. Comput Cardiol 33:13–16. https://doi.org/10.1097/CCM.0b013e3181930174
11. Megjhani M et al (2019) An active learning framework for enhancing identification of non-artifactual intracranial pressure waveforms. Physiol Meas 40(1):15002. https://doi.org/10.1088/1361-6579/aaf979)
12. Chandola V, Banerjee A, Kumar V (2009) Anomaly detection: a survey. ACM Comput Surv 41(3):15:1–15:58. https://doi.org/10.1145/1541880.1541882
13. Kingma DP, Welling M (2013) Auto-encoding variational Bayes. arXiv. https://arxiv.org/abs/1711.00464
14. An J, Cho S (2015) Variational autoencoder based anomaly detection using reconstruction probability. Spec Lect IE 2:1–18
15. Stone JV (2019) Artificial intelligence engines: a tutorial introduction to the mathematics of deep learning. Sebtel Press
16. Kingma DP, Welling M (2019) An introduction to variational autoencoders. arXiv. https://arxiv.org/abs/1906.02691
17. Doersch C (2016) Tutorial on variational autoencoders. arXiv. Preprint at https://arxiv.org/abs/1606.05908
18. Edinburgh T, Smielewski P, Czosnyka M, Eglen SJ, Ercole A (2019) DeepClean—self-supervised artefact rejection for intensive care waveform data using generative deep learning. arXiv. https://arxiv.org/abs/1908.03129
19. Chollet F et al (2015) Keras. https://keras.io
20. Abadi M et al (2016) TensorFlow: large-scale machine learning on heterogeneous distributed systems. arXiv. Preprint at https://arxiv.org/abs/1312.5663
21. Lee S-B et al (2019) Artifact removal from neurophysiological signals: impact on intracranial and arterial pressure monitoring in traumatic brain injury. J Neurosurg 132(6):1–9. https://doi.org/10.3171/2019.2.JNS182260
22. Higgins I et al (2017) Beta-VAE: learning basic visual concepts with a constrained variational framework. ICLR 2(5):6
23. Rezende DJ, Viola F (2018) Taming VAEs. arXiv. Preprint at https://arxiv.org/abs/1810.00597
24. Ercole A (2006) Attenuation in invasive blood pressure measurement systems. Br J Anaesth 96(5):560–562. https://doi.org/10.1093/bja/ael070
25. Hoffman MD, Johnson MJ (2016) ELBO surgery: yet another way to carve up the variational evidence lower bound. NIPS Workshop in Advances in Approximate Bayesian Inference

Comparison of Two Algorithms Analysing the Intracranial Pressure Curve in Terms of the Accuracy of Their Start-Point Detection and Resistance to Artefacts

Anna-Li Schönenberg-Tu, Benjamin Pätzold, Adam Lichota, Christa Raak, Ghaith Al Assali, Friedrich Edelhäuser, Dirk Cysarz, Martin Marsch, and Wolfram Scharbrodt

Abbreviations

ABP	Arterial blood pressure
BP	Blood pressure
CBF	Cerebral blood flow
CPP	Cerebral perfusion pressure
ECG	Electrocardiogram
GCS	Glasgow coma scale
GOS	Glasgow outcome scale
ICH	Intracranial haemorrhage
ICP	Intracranial pressure
ICU	Intensive care unit
MAP	Mean arterial blood pressure
PEEP	Positive end-expiratory pressure
SAH	Subarachnoid haemorrhage
TBI	Traumatic brain injury

The original version of this chapter has been revised. The correction to this chapter can be found at https://doi.org/10.1007/978-3-030-59436-7_71

A.-L. Schönenberg-Tu (✉) · B. Pätzold · A. Lichota · G. Al Assali
M. Marsch
Gemeinschaftskrankenhaus Herdecke (Community Hospital Herdecke), Herdecke, Germany
e-mail: a.tu@gemeinschaftskrankenhaus.de

C. Raak · D. Cysarz
Institute of Integrative Medicine, University of Witten, Herdecke, Germany

F. Edelhäuser
Gemeinschaftskrankenhaus Herdecke (Community Hospital Herdecke), Herdecke, Germany

Institute of Integrative Medicine, University of Witten, Herdecke, Germany

University of Witten, Herdecke, Germany

W. Scharbrodt
Gemeinschaftskrankenhaus Herdecke (Community Hospital Herdecke), Herdecke, Germany

University of Witten, Herdecke, Germany
e-mail: w.scharbrodt@gemeinschaftskrankenhaus.de

Introduction

Background

Intracranial pressure (ICP) monitoring-based care of both traumatic brain injury (TBI) and non-TBI has proven to produce favourable outcomes and is by now general practice [1] as elevated ICP serves as an independent predictor of outcome [2, 3], to the point that ICP monitoring is considered a useful technique even in less severe brain injury [4].

The effects of ICP-based care have been most extensively studied in TBI; however, there is ample evidence that increased ICP also adversely affects outcomes in, e.g., non-TBI such as in intracranial haemorrhage (CH), subarachnoid haemorrhage (SAH), ischemic stroke, and meningitis/encephalitis [5]. The influence of ICP monitoring-based care on clinical outcomes seems less robust here, but it remains useful in guiding therapeutic decisions.

Therapies to reduce ICP or prevent its further increase include hyperventilation, application of hyperosmolar and colloidal solutions as well as barbiturates, removal of focal mass lesions and (hemi) craniectomy [6].

All of these therapies can be classed as moderately to highly aggressive. Reduced cerebral perfusion pressure (CPP) and cerebral blood flow (CBF) themselves can lead to hypoperfusion, resulting in cerebral ischemia, and the procedures to reduce CPP and CBF are potentially dangerous to the rest of the organism because of their side effects. This means that an accurate estimation of ICP and its meaning for action is crucial.

So far ICP monitoring-based care is based on thresholds that have been defined as potentially damaging for the brain, at least in the long run, and are usually classed around 20–25 mmHg [7].

It can be assumed, though, not only that a peak of ICP over a certain threshold or an elevation of ICP over a certain duration of time might be damaging to the brain tissue but

B. Depreitere et al. (eds.), *Intracranial Pressure and Neuromonitoring XVII*, Acta Neurochirurgica Supplement 131,
https://doi.org/10.1007/978-3-030-59436-7_46,

also that the overall waveform and pressure elevation of the ICP curve might play an important role in guiding clinical decision-making. This has been partially investigated in the concepts of dose or burden of elevated ICP [8] and the correlation of elevated ICP with the Glasgow Outcome Scale (GOS) [9]. Both studies imply that not only the elevation of ICP over a certain threshold is relevant to the clinical outcome, but also the duration and frequency of the ICP increase.

Objective

New insights into the nature and especially the prognostic value of the ICP might be derived from the waveform itself. Studies suggest that not only a certain threshold of ICP, but also an increased amplitude of the ICP waveform [10] and a change in ICP curve morphology can serve as predictors of a general rise in ICP burden and, consequently, unfavourable outcomes. Such a morphologic change is the elevation of the second peak in the ICP curve, which can be detected by simple visual assessment, correlates with worsened outcome [11] and indicates compromised cerebrovascular pressure reactivity [12]. There is evidence to support the notion that complex pulse analysis combined with machine learning could help in forecasting elevated ICP and thus advance aggressive treatment of ICP in neurocritical care earlier [13].

For a profound analysis of the predictive qualities of the ICP waveform a recording of the ICP curve itself and a reliable identification of its components and characteristics is a prerequisite. If ICP waveform analysis is to be used on site to guide clinical decision-making, then the challenge is in recording and analysing the data with an acceptable runtime performance and in achieving an accurate and reliable detection of the peaks and troughs of the ICP curve.

The sheer amount of data involved requires an automated, computational analysis of ICP waveforms, which raises problems of accuracy, reliability and actually defining the ICP wave. This can be achieved by defining each individual ICP wave as one between the start point of the first wave and the start point of the second wave, and so on, so that the start point becomes the defining factor for the ICP wave and start-point identification accuracy the benchmark for computational analysis.

In physiological signals we are usually confronted with a lot of artefacts and having to cut through this noise, especially when dealing with inconsistent waveform morphology has been a rather common problem in waveform analysis [14]. In our data we tried to conquer these difficulties by linking the wave analysis of different vital parameters, specifically ICP and ECG, to each other.

Materials and Methods

Dataset

To establish an extensive dataset and allow for subsequent clinical substudies the monitoring data of all patients in our ICU that underwent ICP monitoring based care within a certain period of time were recorded on a Dell Workstation, Xeon W-2133, 32GB RAM external server.

The recording system registered not only the numerical values but also the respective waveforms of these biodata such as ICP and other vital parameters.

Patients included were those who had suffered brain injury severe enough that their further clinical management required ICP monitoring and justified invasive recording. ICP monitoring was done via invasive probe, often incorporated into a ventricular drainage catheter. The other vital parameters comprised electrocardiogram (ECG), pulsoxymetry, arterial blood pressure (ABP), mean arterial blood pressure (MAP), temperature and details of the ventilation parameters such as positive end-expiratory pressure (PEEP) and peak ventilating pressure. Furthermore, details of medication and applicational therapies were also recorded for future analysis.

The only other inclusion criteria besides brain injury severe enough to require ICP monitoring-based care according to the usual standards [5, 15] was age between 18 and 99 years. Exclusion criteria were accompanying intracranial infections during the monitoring period. Monitoring usually concluded only after either the patient could be referred to another department or died due to the severity of the illness. Informed consent was obtained from all patients included in the study either by themselves or by their legal representatives. After recording, the data were anonymised for further analysis. The study was approved by the ethical commission board of the University of Witten/Herdecke.

In the period from 27 January 2017 until 22 March 2019 we were able to obtain datasets from 55 patients via continuous monitoring over a period of at least 37 h up to 12 days. ECG was recorded at a frequency of 200 Hz, ICP and ABP at a frequency of 100 Hz.

Algorithm Design

To actually define and recognise the peaks and troughs in physiological signals such as the ICP wave, we resorted first to the modified Scholkmann algorithm (further referred to as AR[SA]), which detects peaks and troughs by scale analysis and which has been described by Bishop et al. [16]. However, we still faced the problem of having to deal with a high level of artefacts in our clinical biodata (see graph below).

To solve that problem, we developed a further modification of the modified Scholkmann algorithm, which analyses not only the ICP waveform itself but also the ICP waveform linked to the ECG. Henceforth this algorithm will be referred to as AR[ECG]. AR[ECG] applies feature extraction by multi-scale wavelet transform to the analysis of the ICP curve. Wavelet transform has already been applied successfully in the analysis of ECG waves [17] and has been shown to outperform other ECG analysing algorithms [18]. For AR[ECG] we specifically used the Daubechies wavelet filter [19]. It was designed based on the following strategy.

In a first step, it identified the R wave of the ECG, distinguishing it from movement artefacts by wavelet transform. In a second step, the modified Scholkmann algorithm AR[SA] was applied to the ICP curve to identify all of its peaks and mark specifically the first peak of the ICP wave after each R wave of the ECG. Thirdly, the peak of the R wave of the ECG and the peak of the ICP curve that directly follows that R wave were used to define the time interval in which the corresponding trough as the start point of each ICP wave could possibly be found. Lastly, the derivative of that interval of the ICP curve was used to calculate its peak values and consequently also the minimum of the ICP curve which represents the start point.

This start point could then be used to define the beginning and end of each ICP wave, so that the ICP curve could then be divided into its individual waves. The start point of the individual waves was then set to zero on the *y*-axis, and each ICP wave was depicted consecutively in a three-dimensional diagram, with the *z*-axis representing time (Fig. 1).

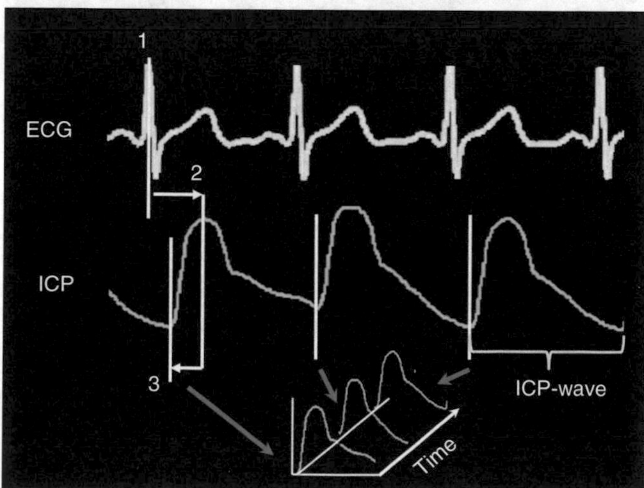

Fig. 1 By means of wavelet transform the algorithm AR[ECG] detects only those peaks of the ICP wave that directly follow the R wave of the ECG

Study Design

This new algorithm design now needed to be compared to the modified Scholkmann algorithm with regard to artefact resistance and proven, if possible, to at least not be significantly inferior. Since the single most distorting influence on an algorithm that is ECG based should be cardiac arrhythmia, we specifically wanted to analyse the performance of AR[ECG] in arrhythmic patients and sought a suitable subset in our patient cohort.

Because of the location of Herdecke Community Hospital, the main reason for referral to our ICU within the field of neurosurgery is non-TBI, especially due to ICH and SAH. In patients with SAH, cardiac arrhythmia is known to be rather common [20], so we decided to run our analysis first on patients who had suffered SAH.

In the analysis we compared start-point identification accuracy of the ECG-linked algorithm AR[ECG] to the modified Scholkmann algorithm AR[SA] in rhythmic patients first. Then we applied the same algorithms to the monitoring data of patients with cardiac arrhythmia. In both scenarios start-point identification accuracy was then compared to the manual start-point markings of a proficient physician as a point of reference.

Results

To estimate whether we could achieve any useful results with this strategy, we piloted the analysis of start-point identification accuracy on five rhythmic and four arrhythmic patients for 1 min. The results showed a sensitivity of 1.0 for both AR[SA] and AR[ECG] and a positive predictive value of 0.85 for AR[SA] and 0.99 for AR[ECG] in the five rhythmic patients. However, in the four patients with cardiac arrhythmia, sensitivity was 1.0 again for both AR[SA] and AR[ECG], but the positive predictive value was 0.9 for AR[SA] and 0.97 for AR[ECG].

These results supported the further analysis of our total cohort of patients who had suffered SAH. This subset consisted of 19 patients in total, 7 of which developed cardiac arrhythmia with an arrhythmic R wave, such as extra systoles or atrial fibrillation, within the first 48 h. Smaller changes in the ECG, such as lengthening of the QT time or amplitude changes of the Q wave that did not affect the R wave, were not taken into account to class a patient as arrhythmic. In each of these patients, we selected a representative period of 10 min on the second day of monitoring around 1:30 am middle european time (MET), when there was normally no manipulation by nurses or doctors on the patient, for the analysis.

In this second trial we again compared start-point identification accuracy in rhythmic patients first, which now showed a sensitivity of 95.14% for AR[SA] and 99.99% for AR[ECG], with a positive predictive value of 98.30% for AR[SA] and 99.76% for AR[ECG]. Overall error rates were 1.95 for AR[SA] and 0.49 for AR[ECG].

In patients with cardiac arrhythmia, sensitivity was 98.05% for AR[SA] and 99.73% for AR[ECG], with a positive predictive value of 100% for AR[SA] and 99.78% for AR[ECG].

Overall error rates were 7.03 for AR[SA] and 0.25 for AR[ECG] (Fig. 2).

Conclusion

Not only has AR[ECG] proven to be not inferior to AR[SA], but it has actually shown higher sensitivity, higher positive predictive value and lower overall error rates in rhythmic patients. In patients with cardiac arrhythmia, the positive predictive value of AR[ECG] was slightly lower than that of AR[SA], while the sensitivity of AR[ECG] was still higher than that of AR[SA], and the overall error rate of AR[ECG] was lower than that of AR[SA]. AR[ECG] is thus suitable for analysis in cases of more complex or irregular vital parameters. With these possibilities of accurate start-point detection

a

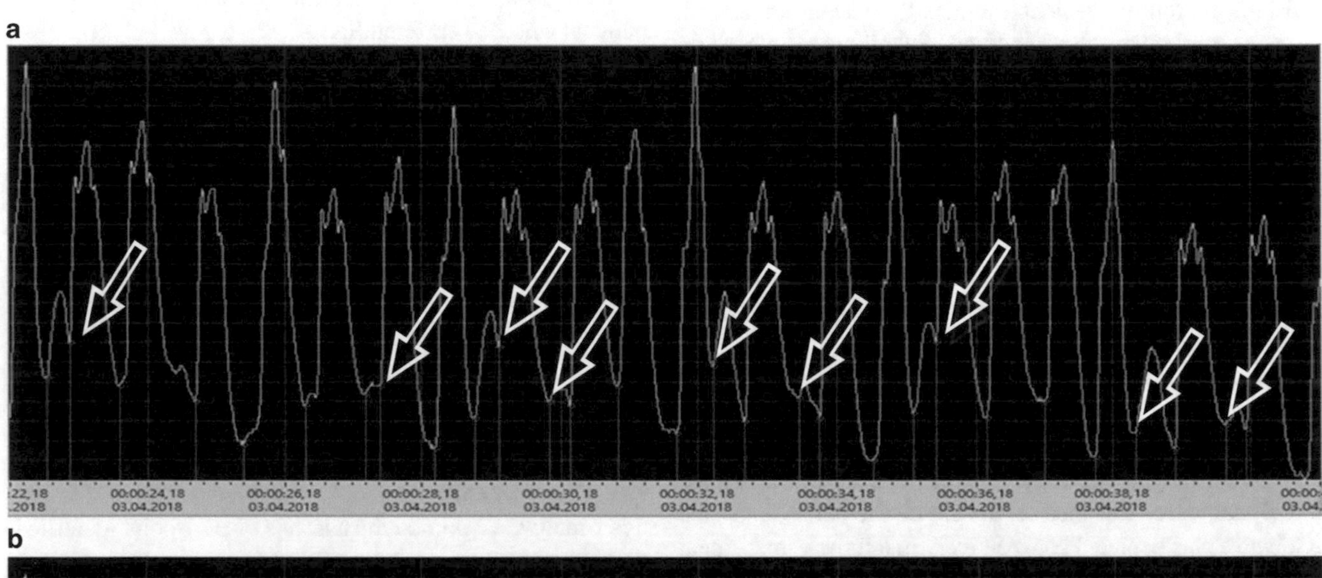

b

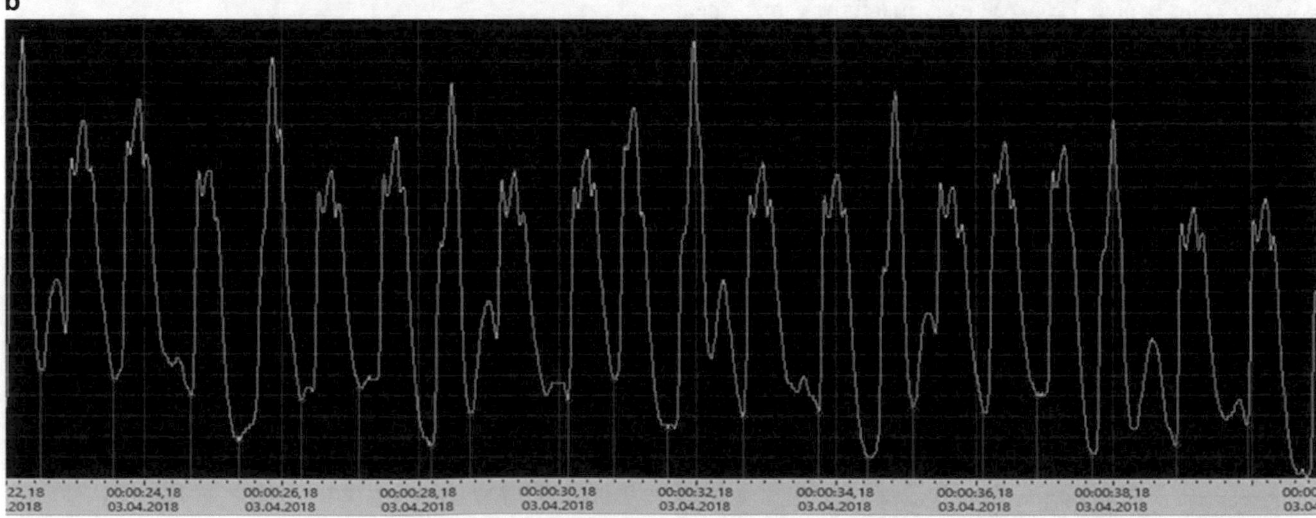

Fig. 2 Top graph shows AR[SA] (**a**), bottom graph shows AR[ECG] (**b**). The arrows mark those peaks of the ICP wave that are falsely identified as start points of an ICP wave by AR[SA]. The comparison illustrates how much more accurate AR[ECG] is for start-point detection and resistance to artefacts, even if vital parameters are irregular

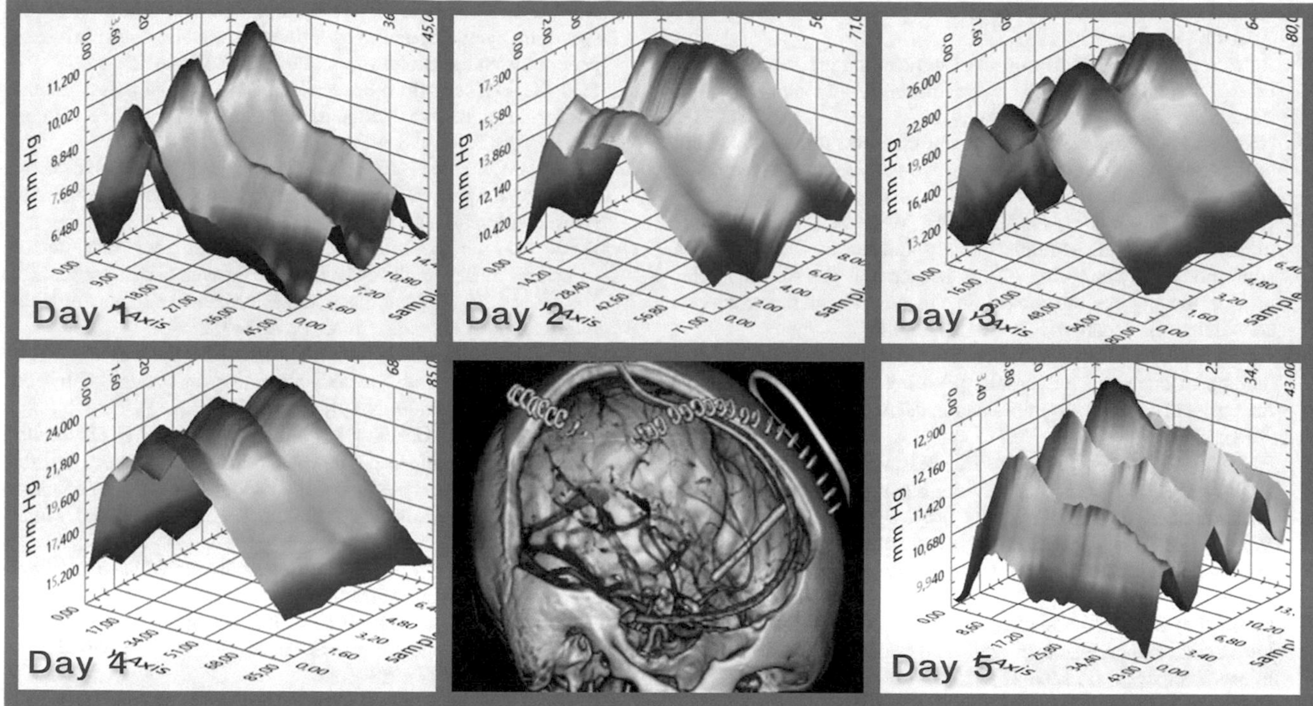

Fig. 3 Example of three-dimensional ICP diagram that visualizes time-dependent ICP-wave morphology. Each graph shows a representative period of approx. 10 s of ICP curve recording in a patient with SAH, WFNS IV over the course of several days. In the first row of graphs it can be noticed that on day 1 p1 is the highest peak within the single ICP waves, while on subsequent days p2 and p3 become higher than p1. In the second row of graphs the return of p1 as the highest peak after decompressive craniectomy becomes clearly visible

we can now receive reliable ICP diagrams with three-dimensional, time-dependent visualization of long-term changes in ICP-wave morphology (Fig. 3).

Discussion

Artefact resistance in signal processing is not a problem unique to physiological signals or ICP curves, which is why the previously discussed diverse strategies were created to counteract this problem [21]. Yet for waveform analysis of the ICP curve it represents a crucial issue since the ICP curve is often overlaid with a lot of noise due to its changing waveform morphology and its reactivity to other vital parameters.

This study reflects the performance of an ECG-dependent algorithm on actual biodata. Many of the algorithm designs that we found and considered to apply to our dataset had been developed on synthetized waveforms [16, 21]. When applied to our biodata, the algorithm AR[ECG], whose design is specifically intertwined with the ECG, proved to be significantly more resistant to artefacts than the algorithm AR[SA], even in cases when it could be most perturbed, such as with cardiac arrhythmia.

Cardiac arrhythmia, on the other hand, is a common and relevant problem in patients who have suffered SAH. In some studies, up to 90–100% of all patients with SAH developed some form of cardiac arrhythmia during the first 48 h [22, 23]. Cardiac arrhythmia is also a relevant issue in patients with other structural brain lesions [24], so an algorithm that can filter through the additional artefacts created by cardiac arrhythmia would be very useful in clinical application.

Altogether this study will allow for further in-depth investigation of the clinical implications and prognostic value of the ICP waveform in our dataset.

Acknowledgments We received research grants from Software AG Stiftung and would like to thank them for their generous funding of this work.

Conflict of Interest **The authors are employed by their institutions as stated above independently of this research. There are no conflicts of interest.**

References

1. Smith M (2008) Monitoring intracranial pressure in traumatic brain injury. Anesth Analg 106(1):240

2. Ross N, Eynon CA (2005) Intracranial pressure monitoring. Curr Anaesth Crit Care 16(4):255–261
3. Balestreri M et al (2006) Impact of intracranial pressure and cerebral perfusion pressure on severe disability and mortality after head injury. Neurocrit Care 4(1):8–13
4. Narayan RK et al (1982) Intracranial pressure: to monitor or not to monitor? A review of our experience with severe head injury. J Neurosurg 56(5):650–659
5. Helbok R, Olson DM, Le Roux PD, Vespa P, The Participants in the International Multidisciplinary Consensus Conference on Multimodality Monitoring (2014) Intracranial pressure and cerebral perfusion pressure monitoring in non-TBI patients: special considerations. Neurocrit Care 21(2):85–94
6. Grande P-O, Asgeirsson B, Nordstrom C-H (2002) Volume-targeted therapy of increased intracranial pressure: the Lund concept unifies surgical and non-surgical treatments. Acta Anaesthesiol Scand 46(8):929–941
7. Federico M, Matteo P, Matteo R, Alessia V, Giuseppe C (2015) High-resolution intracranial pressure burden and outcome in subarachnoid hemorrhage. Stroke 46(9):2464–2469
8. Vik A et al (2008) Relationship of 'dose' of intracranial hypertension to outcome in severe traumatic brain injury. J Neurosurg 109(4):678–684
9. Güiza F et al (2015) Visualizing the pressure and time burden of intracranial hypertension in adult and paediatric traumatic brain injury. Intensive Care Med 41(6):1067–1076
10. Czosnyka M et al (1996) Significance of intracranial pressure waveform analysis after head injury. Acta Neurochir 138(5):531–542
11. Kirkness CJ, Mitchell PH, Burr RL, March KS, Newell DW (2000) Intracranial pressure waveform analysis: clinical and research implications. J Neurosci Nurs 32(5):271–277
12. Balestreri M et al (2004) Intracranial hypertension: what additional information can be derived from ICP waveform after head injury? Acta Neurochir 146(2):131–141
13. Hu X, Xu P, Asgari S, Vespa P, Bergsneider M (2010) Forecasting ICP elevation based on prescient changes of intracranial pressure waveform morphology. IEEE Trans Biomed Eng 57(5):1070–1078
14. Du P, Kibbe WA, Lin SM (2006) Improved peak detection in mass spectrum by incorporating continuous wavelet transform-based pattern matching. Bioinformatics 22(17):2059–2065
15. Saul TG, Ducker TB (1982) Effect of intracranial pressure monitoring and aggressive treatment on mortality in severe head injury. J Neurosurg 56(4):498–503
16. Bishop SM, Ercole A (2018) Multi-scale peak and trough detection optimised for periodic and quasi-periodic neuroscience data. Acta Neurochir Suppl 126:189–195
17. Desai KD, Sankhe MS (2012) A real-time fetal ECG feature extraction using multiscale discrete wavelet transform. 2012 5th International Conference on BioMedical Engineering and Informatics, Chongqing, China, pp 407–412
18. Martinez JP, Almeida R, Olmos S, Rocha AP, Laguna P (2004) A wavelet-based ECG delineator: evaluation on standard databases. IEEE Trans Biomed Eng 51(4):570–581
19. Balachandran A, Ganesan M, Sumesh EP (2014) Daubechies algorithm for highly accurate ECG feature extraction, in 2014 International Conference on Green Computing Communication and Electrical Engineering (ICGCCEE), Coimbatore, India, pp 1–5
20. Chatterjee S (2011) ECG changes in subarachnoid haemorrhage: a synopsis. Neth Hear J 19(1):31–34
21. Scholkmann F, Boss J, Wolf M (2012) An efficient algorithm for automatic peak detection in noisy periodic and quasi-periodic signals. Algorithms 5(4):588–603
22. Andreoli A, di Pasquale G, Pinelli G, Grazi P, Tognetti F, Testa C (1987) Subarachnoid hemorrhage: frequency and severity of cardiac arrhythmias. A survey of 70 cases studied in the acute phase. Stroke 18(3):558–564
23. Vidal BE et al (1979) Cardiac arrhythmias associated with subarachnoid hemorrhageprospective study. Neurosurgery 5(6):675–680
24. Katsanos AH, Korantzopoulos P, Tsivgoulis G, Kyritsis AP, Kosmidou M, Giannopoulos S (2013) Electrocardiographic abnormalities and cardiac arrhythmias in structural brain lesions. Int J Cardiol 167(2):328–334

Plateau Waves of Intracranial Pressure: Methods for Automatic Detection and Prediction

Sofia Moreira, Maria Celeste Dias, and Miguel Velhote Correia

Introduction

As a closed box, the skull provides protection to the brain, the blood vessels and cerebrospinal fluid (CSF) against external damage, such as falls and accidents. According to the Monro-Kellie doctrine, these components occupy a constant volume, and any change in the volume of one of them will require changes in the other two. TBI, brain tumour, subarachnoid haemorrhage and space-occupying lesions [1–4] are acute brain lesions that can cause recurrent phenomena with increased intracranial pressure (ICP), designated as plateau waves. The ICP signal consists of the sum of the CSF pressure component with the vasogenic component related to the continuous fluctuations observed in cerebral blood volume (CBV) [5]. On the other hand, cerebral perfusion pressure (CPP) is the difference between the inflow and the outflow pressures that are represented by mean arterial blood pressure (ABP) and ICP, respectively (Eq. 1) [6]:

$$\text{CPP} = \text{ABP} - \text{ICP} \tag{1}$$

Abnormal tissue growth, difficulty in CSF absorption and the accumulation of liquid in the interstitial and intracellular spaces are some causes that may increase the volume inside the skull, a decrease in brain compliance and, therefore, an increase in ICP. Described for the first time in 1950 as 'sudden rises in ICP' by Lundberg, plateau waves, A waves or Lundberg A waves are typically characterised by an increase in ICP above 40 mmHg for a minimum period of 5 min [7].

S. Moreira (✉)
Faculty of Engineering, University of Porto, Porto, Portugal

M. C. Dias
Department of Intensive Care, Centro Hospitalar Universitário São João, Porto, Portugal

M. V. Correia
Faculty of Engineering, INESC-TEC and Department of Electrical and Computer Engineering, University of Porto, Porto, Portugal
e-mail: mcorreia@fe.up.pt

Plateau waves appear in patients with preserved autoregulation and a low cerebrospinal compensatory reserve. Such phenomena are triggered by a vasodilation cascade loop and can end naturally or in response to a treatment to activate the vasoconstriction mechanism, since it will decrease the amount of blood present in the brain. These events are characterised by a rise in ICP above 40 mmHg, for a minimal period of 5 min, along with a decrease in CPP, whereas the ABP signal remains almost constant during the occurrence.

In addition to the aforementioned signals, there is an important index of cerebrovascular pressure reactivity (PRx), calculated as the correlation coefficient between CPP and ICP, and the value provides information about the cerebrovascular reactivity status. In this regard, a value that is negative or below 0.2 indicates the presence of a normal cerebrovascular autoregulation (CAR), while a value that is positive and above 0.2 implies an impaired CAR [8].

In 2012, a study conducted by Oliveira et al. [9] showed that TBI incidence in the European Union was 235 in 100,000 individuals. Thus, the correct diagnosis and continuous multimodal monitoring can improve patients' health, since it may avoid the development of undesirable outcomes, namely secondary brain injuries, via the administration of the most adequate treatment to the patient. In this regard, the need arose for a tool that could detect automatically plateau waves to improve diagnosis. To address this need, the present study consists in the development of an algorithm to automatically detect plateau waves. As a first goal, it should be implemented on data already collected from patients.

This algorithm is more helpful if used with online data, as a software plugin used in neurocritical care units (NCCUs) for multimodal monitoring. With this, the data would be collected in real time and simultaneously provided to the algorithm to detect plateau waves, and that information could be used as a feedback for physicians. Thus, the purpose of this study consists in the creation of a tool that can facilitate the detection of plateau waves in order to allow a faster diagnosis by a physician about the state of the cerebral autoregulation mechanism of patients.

B. Depreitere et al. (eds.), *Intracranial Pressure and Neuromonitoring XVII*, Acta Neurochirurgica Supplement 131,
https://doi.org/10.1007/978-3-030-59436-7_47,

Materials and Methods

Available Data

The study was developed in partnership with the NCCU of Centro Hospitalar São João (CSHJ), which is responsible for providing anonymously the data that were used to create the algorithm. This NCCU uses ICM+ software to display all signals collected from patients in real time and simultaneously. It consists of software developed by the Clinical Neurosciences Department of the University of Cambridge [10]. ICM+ allows multimodal monitoring, which is important for monitoring patients, detecting physiological events and adjusting treatments.

Each ICM+ data file contains several signals, namely ICP, CPP, ABP, and some computed variables, such as PRx. In addition, there is a variable containing the date and time of the signal collection as the number of days combined with the number of seconds elapsed since 31 December 1899. In ICM+, each file was exported as a csv file, which was imported in MATLAB so that the data could be used to develop the algorithm. However, only the key variables for the mentioned goal were imported.

Plateau Wave Definition

Figure 1 shows the typical delineation of a plateau wave. In normal conditions, ICP values vary between 0 and 15 mmHg. Therefore, the mean of ICP in the 30 min before the occurrence of the wave is designated as the pre-wave baseline, defined by the 1–2 interval. However, the presence of a stimulus can change the stationarity of ICP, and the signal varies from 20 to 40 mmHg, which is represented by the 2–3 interval. ICP values above 40 mmHg define the plateau phase (3–4 interval). At the end, the signal reverts to the baseline values with oscillations between 40 and 20 mmHg, as shown in the 4–5 interval. Thus, the mean of ICP in the first 30 min after the episode correspond to the first post-wave baseline (5–6 interval), and along with the second 30 min it composes the 60-min post-wave baseline (5–7 interval).

Along with the rise in ICP, variations in other signals can be monitored to conclude the final diagnosis, namely the decrease observed in the CPP signal. This change occurs to compensate the oscillations in ICP, since the sum of these two latter signals equals the ABP value (Eq. 2). Thus, a plateau wave can be defined by an increase in ICP and ABP values which are nearly constant during the occurrence:

$$ABP = ICP + CPP \qquad (2)$$

Development of Algorithm for Plateau Wave Detection

The purpose of the development of the algorithm for plateau wave detection was focused on the creation of an extra and helpful tool to easily and automatically identify the presence of plateau waves in a patient file. Thus, this is a binary problem where the instances associated with the presence of waves were labelled 1 and the remaining instances 0.

To achieve the objective, the algorithm was designed based on the plateau wave definition given in the previous

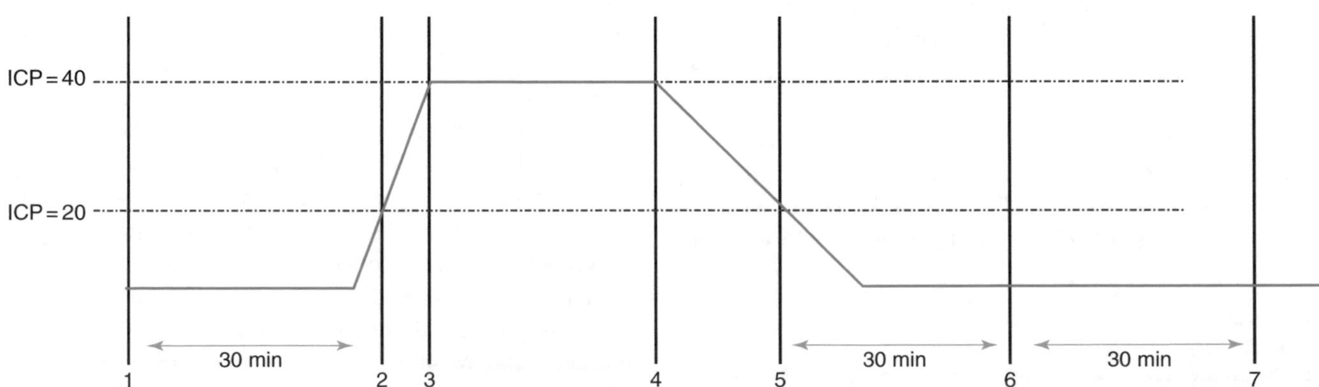

Fig. 1 Plateau wave delineation. ICP values below 20 mmHg before the occurrence of the wave define the baseline of the signal, as can be observed in 1–2, 5–6 and 6–7 intervals. The mean of ICP in the 30 min before the wave defines the pre-wave baseline (1–2 interval), whereas the first 30 min after the event composes the first post-wave baseline (5–6 interval), which combined with the second 30 min defines the 60 min post-wave baseline (5–7 interval). The changes in the stationarity of the ICP signal are characterised by oscillations in signal between 20 and 40 mmHg with an exponential behaviour in the 2–3 interval and a slower variation in the 4–5 interval. Finally, the plateau phase is defined by ICP values above 40 mmHg, as observed in the 3–4 interval

section. Therefore, all data instances were analysed and those with an ICP value above 40 mmHg were considered potential plateau waves. In addition, this variation must occur in at least two subsequent instances. The final classification as plateau wave was assigned if each set of instances considered a potential plateau wave had an ABP standard deviation lower than 10% of the mean of the total ABP signals, since, according to Eq. (2), the ABP should remained constant during the occurrence of the event.

Although the proposed algorithm could be an extra tool facilitating the identification of events by clinical staff, this algorithm would never invalidate the diagnosis made by physicians. Thus, the plateau waves identified should be used as guidance for the final diagnosis.

Results

For event detection, one patient data file was imported in MATLAB and the ICP and ABP signals were used to compute the final classification of all instances. The dashed lines in Fig. 2a correspond to a physician's classification, which was manually performed through the visualisation of ICP, ABP and PRx signals in ICM+. These lines determine the beginning of the many plateau waves present in this patient's data file. The white dashed lines correspond to all plateau waves correctly identified by the algorithm, whereas the pink dashed line shows the unique incorrectly classified plateau wave. The green dashed lines represent false plateau waves, i.e. instances that could be classified as plateau waves since they seem to meet both requirements, but the algorithm has not assigned a label of 1 to them (Fig. 2b), as expected. Thus, although those instances show an ICP value above 40 mmHg, the variation in the ABP signal is higher than 10% of the mean of all ABP signals.

Algorithm detection is shown in Fig. 2b (blue lines). Although the two panels are not completely aligned because of the scales used, a deeper analysis focused on comparing both sets of instances labelled 1, as shown in Table 1.

The data presented in Table 1 show that some episodes present a difference of seconds in the beginning of the detection, which is due to the data available to the algorithm. However, the similarity of time instances indicates that the algorithm may exhibit good performance for the proposed goal of the present study.

Discussion

Regarding Table 1, it is possible to assert that most of the plateau waves identified by the physician were also detected by the algorithm, although the timing does not match perfectly. Only one plateau wave was identified by the physician and the algorithm at the exact same time. The difference of seconds observed in the remaining episodes is due to the data export in ICM+, since only one instance per minute is

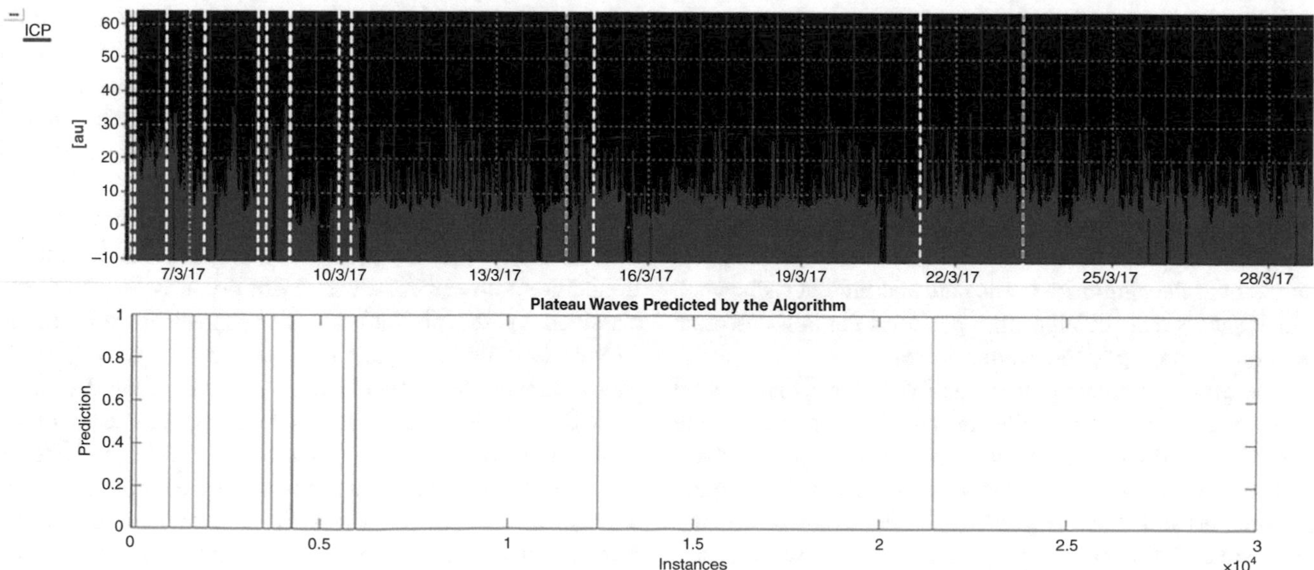

Fig. 2 (top) Event identification in ICM+ by a physician, with real plateau waves represented as white dashed lines. The pink dashed line corresponds to a plateau wave incorrectly detected by the algorithm, while the green dashed lines identify false plateau waves. (bottom) Representation of plateau waves identified by second version of the algorithm

Table 1 Comparison of date and time of each plateau wave identified by physician in ICM+ and algorithm

Number ofplateau wave	Physician identification	Algorithm detection
PW1	05/03/2017 23:05:51	05/03/2017 23:06:01
PW 2	06/03/2017 00:50:01	06/03/2017 00:51:01
PW 3	06/03/2017 15:41:01	06/03/2017 15:42:00
PW 4	07/03/2017 09:18:01	07/03/2017 09:19:00
		07/03/2017 09:27:01
		07/03/2017 09:29:01
PW 5	Not detected	08/03/2017 09:39:24
PW 6	08/03/2017 09:45:24	08/03/2017 09:46:24
PW 7	08/03/2017 13:35:24	08/03/2017 13:35:24
PW 8	09/03/2017 00:18:38	09/03/2017 00:19:38
PW 9	09/03/2017 00:53:05	09/03/2017 00:52:00
PW 10	09/03/2017 22:47:07	09/03/2017 22:44:00
PW 11	10/03/2017 04:18:33	10/03/2017 04:18:07
PW 12	14/03/2017 22:11:16	14/03/2017 22:10:38
PW 13	21/03/2017 06:54:18	21/03/2017 06:54:00

exported instead of each time instance. Therefore, the plateau wave detection performed by the algorithm begins at the first instance that meets both conditions defined, and it may result in a later detection than the actual occurrence estimated by the physician in ICM+. In this regard, it is important to note the similarity in the date and time of each event, which shows that the algorithm performs the best detection possible according to the available data.

The plateau wave identified as PW4 shows that several waves were identified while the physician detected only one. The reason associated with the identification of these multiple events relies on the fluctuations in ICP signal between 30 and 40 mmHg. Since the definition of the plateau wave in the algorithm requires an ICP value above 40 mmHg, any instance with a lower value results in a non-detection or interrupts the detection of the event, even if it happens between two instances with an ICP value higher than 40 mmHg. To overcome this problem, an additional step can be implemented in the code to ensure that these oscillations are classified as a unique episode instead of multiple waves.

The plateau wave denominated as PW5 consists of an event incorrectly classified as a plateau wave by the algorithm, because, clinically, it seems to be a unique episode of long duration. Thus, it is more correct to affirm that PW5 is associated with PW6, since it resulted from a one-off increase in ICP, and it can indicate that a plateau wave will happen soon, rather than the classification of an actual event. Along with ICP and ABP, the PRx coefficient can be added to improve the algorithm and to avoid the presence of misclassified instances as PW5, since PRx quantifies the cerebrovascular reactivity status to pressure.

The physician noticed two false plateau waves that were not classified by the algorithm. The set of instances contains an ICP value above 40 mmHg; however, the ABP variation is higher than 10% of the mean ABP, which underscores the good performance of the developed tool.

The results obtained showed that most of the events were detected correctly. The pink dashed line represents plateau waves incorrectly classified by the algorithm. Although those instances present ICP values above 40 mmHg, the physician considered that the variation observed in ABP during that potential plateau wave was higher than 10% of the mean of all ABP signals. Therefore, this misclassification could have resulted from the fact that the variation is compared against the mean value calculated for the entire signal, which can be biased by higher and lower ABP values. In this regard, a small window of ABP signal can be used to compare the variation during that period.

The false plateau waves (green dashed lines) consist of instances that seem to meet the conditions of the algorithm, namely those associated with ICP values. However, the variation in ABP is higher than the ABP variation observed during a plateau wave, and for that reason the algorithm did not detect them as plateau waves as well as the physician did.

To conclude, the results show that the proposed algorithm can be used as an extra, helpful tool to facilitate the detection of plateau waves since most events are correctly identified. In addition, false plateau waves are properly analysed and classified by the algorithm, which shows its robustness. Despite the misclassification of some instances as plateau waves, the algorithm would never invalidate the diagnosis made by a physician, and the misclassifications can be solved by the implementation of an additional step in the code. A deeper analysis of the results shows that the date and time of the beginning of plateau waves did not match in most of the events, which is due to the data extracted from ICM+ that contain minute-by-minute instances.

In this regard, as future work, the PRx coefficient can be implemented in the algorithm to avoid the detection of false plateau waves since PRx consists in the correlation between ICP and ABP and, thus, the effect that ABP variations have on ICP. Moreover, an additional step can also merge the multiple plateau waves as a unique event if they really reflect a single episode. This would increase the robustness of the algorithm, improving its performance and confidence in its use in a hospital environment, specifically in NCCUs.

Conclusion

The developed algorithm detects plateau waves automatically. Such events may result from a rise in ICP above 40 mmHg and a standard deviation of the ABP signal below 10% of the mean ABP signal. Because of the data structure available to the algorithm, although the time involved in physician and algorithm detection is not equal, the time of the first instance of each plateau wave classified by the algorithm can be considered correct. The algorithm can be used as an extra tool to facilitate and expedite the detection of plateau waves in offline patient data, without invalidating a physician's diagnosis. It can then be implemented subsequently as a software plugin to provide real-time feedback on the presence of these events in patients admitted to NCCUs.

References

1. Czosnyka M et al (1999) Hemodynamic characterization of intracranial pressure plateau waves in head-injured patients. J Neurosurg 91(1):11–19
2. Hayashi M et al (1991) Plateau-wave phenomenon (I) correlation between the appearance of plateau waves and CSF circulation in patients with intracranial hypertension. Brain 114(6):2681–2691
3. Luis A et al (2015) Heart rate variability during plateau waves of intracranial pressure: a pilot descriptive study. in Engineering in Medicine and Biology Society (EMBC), 2015 37th Annual International Conference of the IEEE. IEEE, New York
4. Varsos GV et al (2013) Critical closing pressure during intracranial pressure plateau waves. Neurocrit Care 18(3):341–348
5. Czosnyka M (2000) Association between arterial and intracranial pressures. Br J Neurosurg 14(2):127–128
6. Czosnyka M et al (2007) A synopsis of brain pressures: which? when? Are they all useful? Neurol Res 29(7):672–679
7. Dias C et al (2014) Pressures, flow, and brain oxygenation during plateau waves of intracranial pressure. Neurocrit Care 21(1):124–132
8. Donnelly J et al (2016) Regulation of the cerebral circulation: bedside assessment and clinical implications. Crit Care 20(1):129
9. Oliveira E et al (2012) Traumatismo crânio-encefálico: abordagem integrada. Acta Medica Port 25:3
10. Cambridge, U.O. About (2018) [cited 2018 December]. https://icmplus.neurosurg.cam.ac.uk/home/about/

Python-Embedded Plugin Implementation in ICM+: Novel Tools for Neuromonitoring Time Series Analysis with Examples Using CENTER-TBI Datasets

Michał M. Placek, Abdelhakim Khellaf, Benjamin L. Thiemann, Manuel Cabeleira, and Peter Smielewski

Introduction

Over the past 15 years, ICM+ [1–3] (https://icmplus.neurosurg.cam.ac.uk) has become a widely used tool for the collection, integration, and real-time processing of physiological data from patient bedside monitors. Multiple secondary metrics have been developed, e.g. cerebrovascular reactivity indices, relying on the inbuilt calculation engine from ICM+, which offers a range of general statistical and specialised functions to use in fully user-configurable analysis [2, 4–7]. However, there is growing interest in more advanced, custom calculations. This is driven to a large extent by the appearance of publicly available, high-resolution, physiological datasets, like Collaborative European NeuroTrauma Effectiveness Research in Traumatic Brain Injury (CENTER-TBI) [8] (https://www.center-tbi.eu), and by widespread understanding in the neurocritical care community of the need and importance for in-depth interrogation of information-rich clinical datasets. Furthermore, a new generation of clinical researchers is becoming much more familiar and comfortable with scripting languages and popular environments, e.g. Python, R, and MATLAB. In particular, Python is a simple-syntax, high-level interpreted programming language with numerous libraries available (https://www.python.org). For many years, there was a possibility of extending the ICM+ function list with custom functions, but that required writing and compiling low-level code into Microsoft Windows dynamic-link libraries (DLL), which is not trivial and necessitates a full programming environment, like Visual C++. The objective of this project was to develop a user-friendly interface in ICM+ that would provide a simple way of adding Python scripting functionality to the ICM+ calculation engine, thus exponentially expanding its capabilities for the clinical researcher.

M. M. Placek (✉)
Division of Neurosurgery, Department of Clinical Neurosciences, University of Cambridge, Cambridge, UK

Department of Biomedical Engineering, Faculty of Fundamental Problems of Technology, Wrocław University of Science and Technology, Wrocław, Poland
e-mail: mp963@cam.ac.uk

A. Khellaf
Division of Neurosurgery, Department of Clinical Neurosciences, University of Cambridge, Cambridge, UK

Faculty of Medicine, McGill University, Montreal, QC, Canada

B. L. Thiemann
Division of Neurosurgery, Department of Clinical Neurosciences, University of Cambridge, Cambridge, UK

Graduate Research Program, Mayo Clinic, Jacksonville, FL, USA

M. Cabeleira · P. Smielewski
Division of Neurosurgery, Department of Clinical Neurosciences, University of Cambridge, Cambridge, UK

Materials and Methods

Python Plugin for ICM+

The solution involves creating a plugin that works as a gateway (middleman) between ICM+ and Python scripts. Apart from this plugin, users willing to utilise Python functions in ICM+ will need to have the Python environment installed on their machine. Depending on whether custom Python functions which are to be used in ICM+ demand additional Python libraries, like *NumPy* (https://numpy.org) or *SciPy* (https://www.scipy.org) for scientific computing in Python, such libraries must also be included in the Python environment. Currently, only 32-bit release variants of Python are supported. This may change, however, once a 64-bit version of ICM+ is released.

Although the user may install a Python environment with all the necessary components independently, to ease the installation process, we provide a special installer which can be directly downloaded from the ICM+ website. The installer will first install the Python environment (version 3.x) with

B. Depreitere et al. (eds.), *Intracranial Pressure and Neuromonitoring XVII*, Acta Neurochirurgica Supplement 131,
https://doi.org/10.1007/978-3-030-59436-7_48,

the *Pip3* package manager. Next, up-to-date versions of *Numpy*, *SciPy*, and *StatTools* packages will be installed via *Pip3*. Since some commonly used statistical functions from *SciPy* require the Microsoft Visual C++ redistributable package (not to be confused with Microsoft Visual Studio integrated development environment), it will also be installed by the provided installer. Finally, this installer will need to place the Python plugin library file for ICM+ in the correct folder location, completing the environment required to use Python functions in ICM+.

The new ICM+ Python plugin scans the Python plugin folder and imports into ICM+ all the available Python scripts that have an associated eponymous configuration file in XML format. All the other files are ignored by the plugin; thus, they can be used to hold other functions imported and used internally inside the Python scripts. All Python functions successfully imported into ICM+ are available under their own names preceded by a '*Py*' prefix to differentiate them from the native functions. Apart from that, there is no difference in the use of those functions, native or Python-powered.

Facilitating Creation of Custom Python Functions for ICM+

To facilitate the creation of custom Python functions for ICM+, we provide within the new versions of ICM+ (8.6 and newer) a tool which generates a complete XML configuration file and a skeleton/template of a Python code file according to the user's specifications (Fig. 1). This tool allows users to provide a name and a description to their new function, which will appear in ICM+, and to specify on how many input variables the function operates (Fig. 1a). Users can also parametrise the function by an arbitrary number of options. There are four types of options: logical, categorical, integer, and numerical. (1) A logical option can only assume two values and is depicted in the user interface as a checkbox which can be ticked or unticked. (2) A categorical option can have one value from a custom set of labels. (3 and 4) Both integer and numerical options accept number values. An integer-type option is limited to integer values, whereas a numerical-type option can also assume decimal values. Users will have to specify available labels for categorical-type options (Fig. 1b) as well as minimal and maximal values for both integer- and numerical-type options. Note that it is possible to specify default values for all types of options.

All the information provided in the dialog window for defining the custom Python function will be exported to an XML configuration file which describes this function to ICM+ (Fig. 1c). Further, a skeleton of Python script will be created with dynamically generated comments advising about the number of input signals passed by ICM+ and the names of the available options (Fig. 1d). Users will need to include their own code inside the *calculate* method and import external modules, if required (Fig. 1e). The *set_parameter* function is part of the ICM+/Python interface; therefore, it should not be modified or deleted. It is responsible for initialising at the Python side options previously set by an end user in ICM+ and passing sampling frequency of input signals. If some custom code for initialisation and finalisation is needed, it can be added to the so-called constructor (*__init__*) and destructor (*__del__*), respectively. In the vast majority of cases, however, this will not be needed. The *calculate* method will be invoked by ICM+ repeatedly for each new data frame. Once initialised, the options remain set; however, each occurrence of the same Python function in the analysis calculation profile can have its own options selected independently.

Dealing with Missing Data

Generally, missing data points (NaN values) might be problematic. If an external function does not handle them properly, the result of calculations might be erroneous or, in extreme cases, the function could even result in the crash of the ICM+ calculation engine. To relieve the Python function developer from an obligation to deal with NaN values from the Python side, we offer a few streamlined ways to handle missing data from the ICM+ side.

A *Missing data treatment* option is included in all available Python functions. It tells ICM+ what should be done (if anything) with NaN values before passing a data frame to a given Python function. In the current version of the Python plugin, there are four possible actions: *ignore*, *replace by mean*, *delete*, and *return no value* (*NaN*) (Fig. 2). The *ignore* action means that data frames will not be checked for the presence of NaN values and will be passed unchanged to a Python function. In this scenario, it is expected that the Python function will not be affected by NaN values or that it will already have implemented some procedure for dealing with them. The *delete* action indicates that all NaN values in the data frame will be excluded. This will shorten the data frame and may introduce discontinuities. In the current version of the Python plugin, the *delete* action is the default one. The *replace by mean* action replaces all missing data points by a mean value obtained from remaining valid data points in the data frame. The *return no value* (*NaN*) action is the most restrictive. If it is selected, then NaN value will be returned immediately without passing any data to the Python function whenever the data frame contains at least one missing data point. It should be mentioned that in the case of functions operating on more than one input signal, the actions *replace by mean* and *delete* alter all inputs that are arguments of the current function call, when at least one input has missing data points.

a

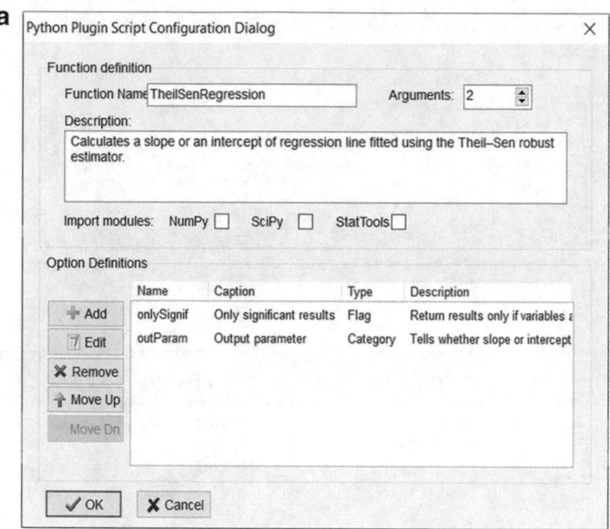

b

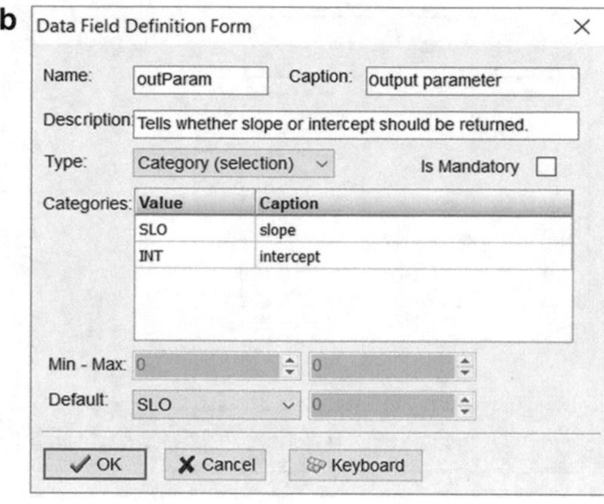

c

```
<?xml version = "1.0"?>

<PyToICMPlusConfig>
  <Function Name="TheilSenRegression" Type="Stats" SignalsCount="2">
    <GUID>{D4FE6333-0667-46D4-BA3A-607964BBF3BC}</GUID>
    <Description>
      Calculates a slope or an intercept of regression line fitted using the Theil-Sen robust estimator.
    </Description>
    <Parameter ShortName="onlySignif" IsMandatory="False">
      <Caption>Only significant results</Caption>
      <Description>Return results only if variables are significantly related.</Description>
      <Type Name="Bool" DefaultValue="False"/>
    </Parameter>
    <Parameter ShortName="outParam" IsMandatory="False">
      <Caption>Output parameter</Caption>
      <Description>Tells whether slope or intercept should be returned.</Description>
      <Type Name = "StringList">
        <Item Value="SLO" Caption="slope" IsDefault="True"/>
        <Item Value="INT" Caption="intercept"/>
      </Type>
    </Parameter>
  </Function>
</PyToICMPlusConfig>
```

d

```
#import ...

class TheilSenRegression:

    # DO NOT MODIFY THIS METHOD. It is a part of the ICM+--Python interface.
    def set_parameter(self, param_name, param_value):
        setattr(self, param_name, param_value)

    # You can append your own code to the constructor, if needed.
    # You should not set here values of parameters declared in your XML
    # configuration file because ICM+ will do it for you.
    # You will have to add your own code, only if you need to initialise some
    # extra data structures which were not declared in the XML config file.
    def __init__(self):
        self.sampling_freq = None

    # You can append your own code to the destructor but most likely
    # you will not need it.
    def __del__(self):
        pass

    # 'calculate' is the main work-horse function.
    # It is called with a data buffer (one or more) of size corresponding to the Calcu
    # It must return one floating-point number.
    # It take the following parameters:
    # sig1 - input variable/signal 1,
    # sig2 - input variable/signal 2,
    # ts_time - part of the data time stamp - number of milliseconds since midnight,
    # ts_date - Part of the data time stamp - One plus number of days since 1/1/0001.
    # It can also use the data sampling frequency:
    #     self.sampling_freq
    # and the following variables already set at the initialisation time (via function
    #     self.onlySignif - Return results only if variables are significantly related.
    #     self.outParam - Tells whether slope or intercept should be returned.
    def calculate(self, sig1,sig2, ts_time,ts_date):
        # my_own_code_here
        result = 0.0
        return result
```

e

```
from scipy.stats import theilslopes


def calculate(self, sig1,sig2, ts_time,ts_date):
    coeffs = theilslopes(sig1, sig2)
    slope = coeffs[0]
    intercept = coeffs[1]
    slope_lci = coeffs[2]
    slope_uci = coeffs[3]

    if self.onlySignif == True:
        if slope_lci * slope_uci <= 0:
            return float('nan')

    if self.outParam == 'SLO':
        return slope
    elif self.outParam == 'INT':
        return intercept
    else:
        return float('nan')
```

Fig. 1 Facilitating creation of custom Python functions for ICM+, illustrated by the example of Theil–Sen regression estimator. (**a**) ICM+ tool which allows users to characterise their new function. (**b**) Definition of a custom option associated with new function. (**c**) Generated XML configuration file. (**d**) Created skeleton of Python script with dynamically generated comments advising about number of input signals and names of available options. (**e**) Custom code which needs to be added manually

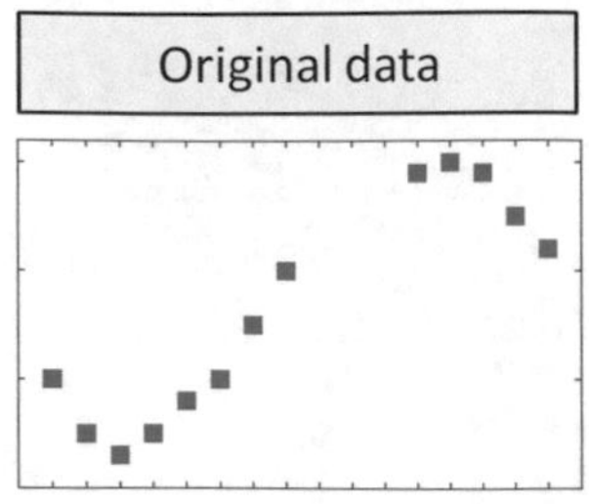

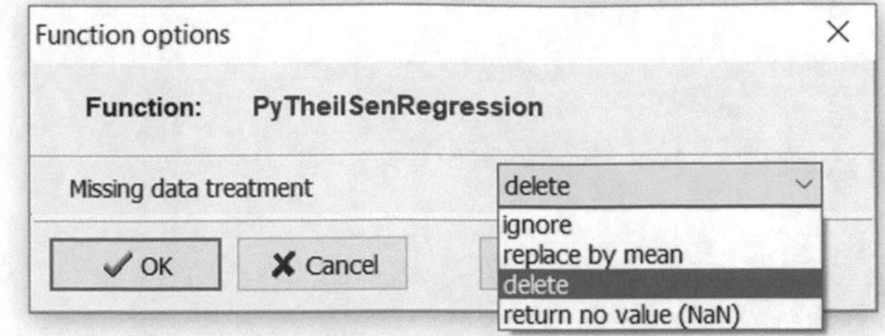

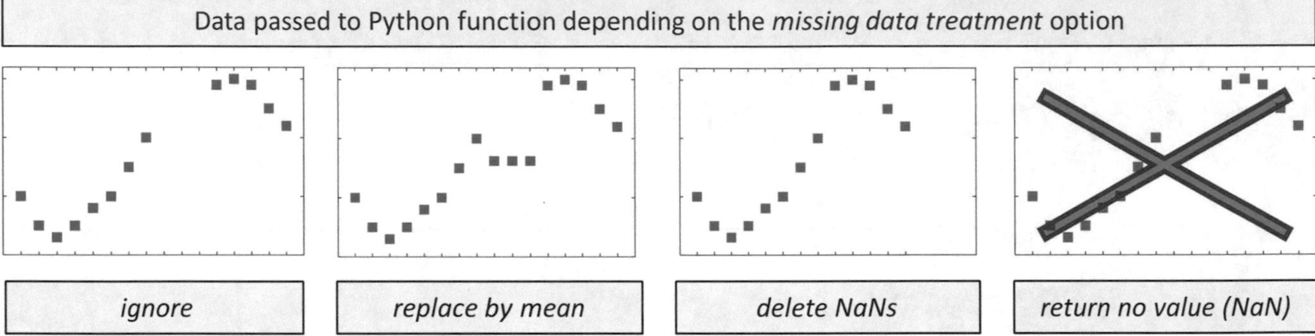

Fig. 2 Four simple strategies for handling missing data points (NaN values) on ICM+ side, before passing a data frame to a given Python function

Assessing Performance

To assess the performance of the Python extension, we first selected four native ICM+ basic functions (mean, median, standard deviation, and max) and implemented their Python counterparts returning the same output. Then, we compared the execution times of two batches of calculations—one with ICM+ functions only and one with Python functions only—performed on datasets from 20 patients, totalling 95 days of high-resolution data chosen randomly from the CENTER-TBI cohort. All the input data were resampled to 200 Hz (in the first calculation step, the Virtual Signals stage) and the calculation window was set to 60 s with no overlap.

Results

Example of a Python Function Extension for ICM+

Figure 1 refers to an example of a Python function that fits the regression line using the Theil–Sen estimator [9]. Unlike the common least-squares approach, the Theil–Sen regression estimator is a robust method against outliers. The presented ICM + -compatible implementation of the function is parametrised by two custom options: *onlySignif* (logical type) and *outParam* (categorical type). If the *onlySignif* option is ticked, it forces the function to return results only when the effect in the regression is significant. The *outParam* option allows selecting which regression line parameter should be returned: the slope or intercept.

Figure 3 shows how the implemented Python function can be used for calculations in ICM+. Each ICM+-compatible Python function can be configured in the same fashion as other ICM+ functions (Fig. 3a). The function options available in the user interface correspond to the function specification presented in Fig. 1. Additionally, there is also the *missing data treatment* option that instructs ICM+ how missing data should be dealt with. For the presented Theil–Sen linear regression example, the *delete* action is the most appropriate. Upon function configuration, the proper formula appears in the analysis configuration window (Fig. 3b). In this example, the function is used twice with two different values of the *outParam* option in order to return the slope and intercept of the regression line. Figure 3c shows an illustrative result of calculations defined in Fig. 3b using an example file from CENTER-TBI datasets. Time trends shown are fragmentary because the *onlySignif* option was ticked.

Performance

On average, Python functions were 15–60% slower than the inbuilt ICM+ functions. For the set of basic functions selected for this benchmark, the processing time of 24-h-long

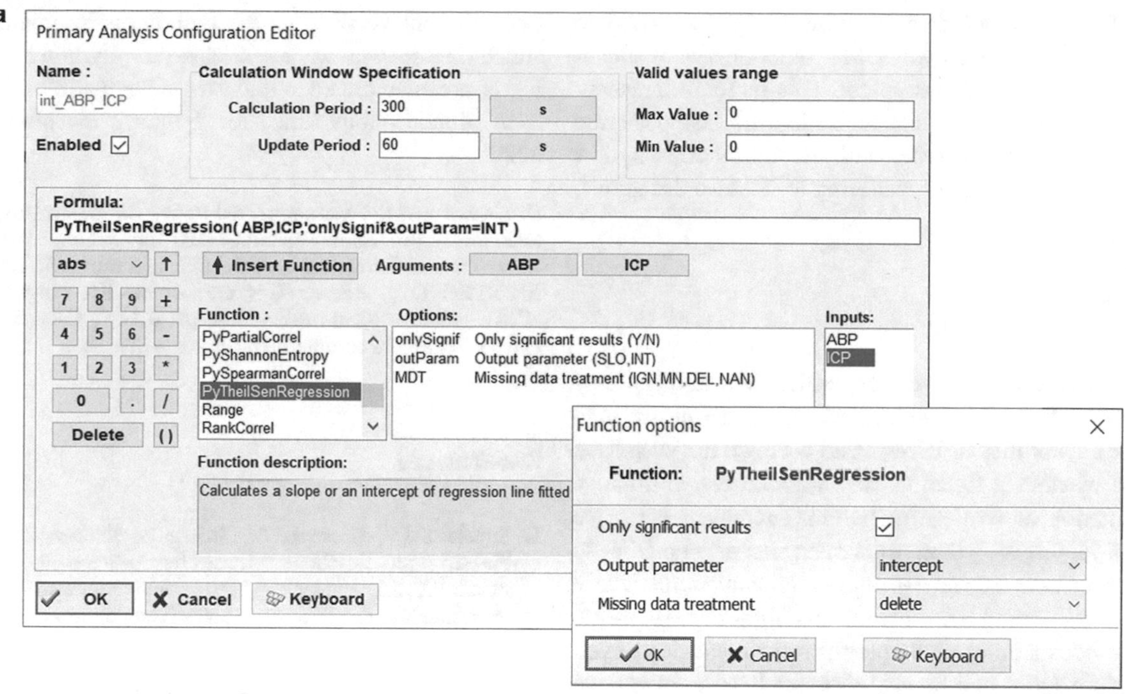

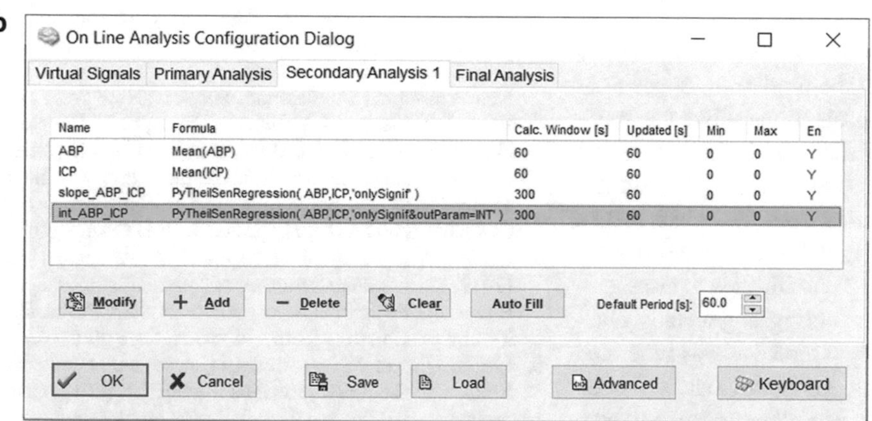

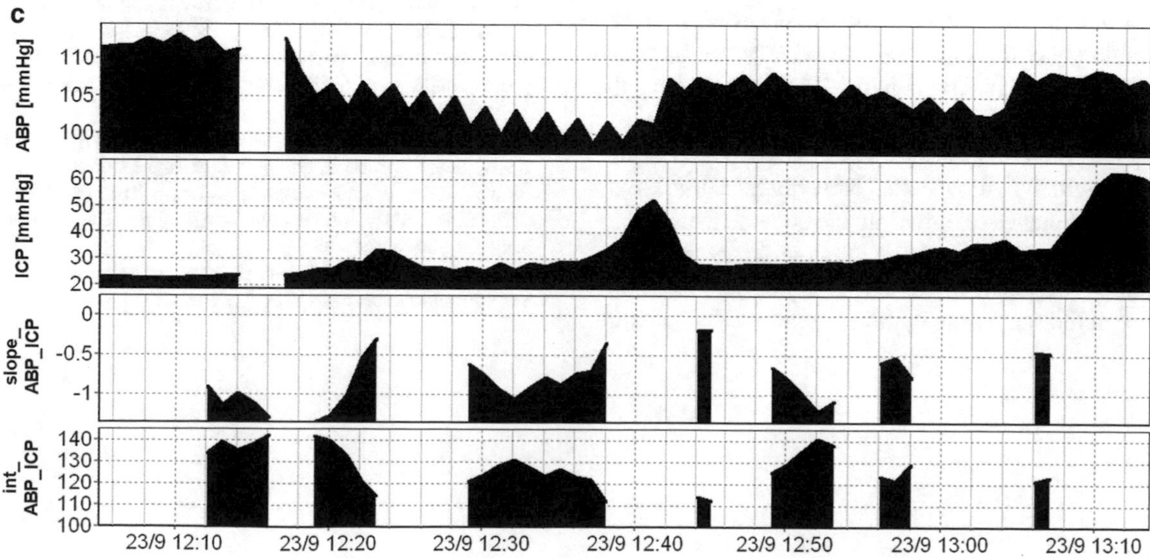

Fig. 3 Employing a custom Python function in ICM+. (**a**) Formula configuration with function options configuration window providing an interface to select and parametrise the function. (**b**) Analysis configuration dialog window showing two variables (*slope_ABP_ICP* and *int_ABP_ICP*) which are to be calculated via the Python function. (**c**) An illustrative result of calculations defined in (**b**)

blocks of single input data increased from 16.4–18.5 to 19.0–29.8 s, after the native ICM+ functions were substituted by their Python counterparts. This increase in execution time is a more-than-adequate trade-off for empowering the modern clinical researcher with the unlimited analytical freedom that Python scripts can bring to ICM+ calculations.

Discussion

The Python extension works very efficiently, and any user with some degree of experience in scripting can use it to enrich the capabilities of ICM+. End users do not even have to realise whether a function they want to use is a native ICM+ function or written in Python. Moreover, extensive libraries available to Python users open vast new horizons to ICM+ users. For those who work predominantly with Python and those who would like to learn this high-level language, ICM+ provides a tailor-made platform for managing physiological time series and for real-time application of custom Python scripts on data streamed from bedside patients' monitors.

So far, the new interface for importing Python functions into ICM+ has some limitations. The modern interface does not support intellectual property protection, unlike the previous plugin interface based on DLLs, which does so in two particular ways. First, within the previous plugin interface, the end user only requires a compiled DLL file, which is then imported by ICM+. Hence, the original source code does not have to be disseminated. There are possibilities to disassemble a DLL; however, reverse engineering is generally challenging in this context, particularly if the DLL was generated by C or C++ compilers, which generate machine code directly. Second, the previous interface allows custom licencing of third-party plugins. That is, the end user may be obliged to obtain an individual licence key to activate the plugin limitlessly or for a specified period. The new interface for importing Python functions into ICM+ does not have the aforementioned licensing support. Also, users who want to release their Python functions for ICM+ are expected to provide their original Python code. Nevertheless, users may apply some techniques to obfuscate the code on their own.

The Python plugin can work with an arbitrary version of the Python environment for ICM+. It is not possible, however, to use at the same time Python functions which require two different versions of the Python environment, e.g. 3.x and 2.7. Users who want to release their Python functions for ICM+ are encouraged to make them compatible with Python 3, as official maintenance for Python 2 is slated to end in 2020.

Disclosure **M.M.P. was supported by the European Union Seventh Framework Programme (grant 602150) for Collaborative European NeuroTrauma Effectiveness Research in Traumatic Brain Injury (CENTER-TBI). P.S. receives part of the licensing fees for the ICM+ software (Cambridge Enterprise Ltd., UK). A.K., B.L.T., and M.C. have no competing interests to disclose.**

References

1. Smielewski P, Czosnyka M, Steiner L, Belestri M, Piechnik S, Pickard J (2005) ICM+: software for on-line analysis of bedside monitoring data after severe head trauma. Intracranial pressure and brain monitoring XII. Springer, New York, pp 43–49
2. Smielewski P, Czosnyka Z, Kasprowicz M, Pickard JD, Czosnyka M (2012) ICM+: a versatile software for assessment of CSF dynamics. Intracranial Pressure and Brain Monitoring XIV. Springer, New York, pp 73–79
3. Smielewski P, Lavinio A, Timofeev I, Radolovich D, Perkes I, Pickard J, Czosnyka M (2008) ICM+, a flexible platform for investigations of cerebrospinal dynamics in clinical practice. Acta Neurochirurgica Supplements. Springer, New York, pp 145–151
4. Beqiri E, Smielewski P, Robba C, Czosnyka M, Cabeleira MT, Tas J, Donnelly J, Outtrim JG, Hutchinson P, Menon D (2019) Feasibility of individualised severe traumatic brain injury management using an automated assessment of optimal cerebral perfusion pressure: the COGiTATE phase II study protocol. BMJ Open 9:e030727
5. Kramer AH, Couillard PL, Zygun DA, Aries MJ, Gallagher CN (2019) Continuous assessment of "optimal" cerebral perfusion pressure in traumatic brain injury: a cohort study of feasibility, reliability, and relation to outcome. Neurocrit Care 30:51–61
6. Liu X, Donnelly J, Czosnyka M, Aries MJ, Brady K, Cardim D, Robba C, Cabeleira M, Kim D-J, Haubrich C (2017) Cerebrovascular pressure reactivity monitoring using wavelet analysis in traumatic brain injury patients: a retrospective study. PLoS Med 14:e1002348
7. Liu X, Maurits NM, Aries MJ, Czosnyka M, Ercole A, Donnelly J, Cardim D, Kim D-J, Dias C, Cabeleira M (2017) Monitoring of optimal cerebral perfusion pressure in traumatic brain injured patients using a multi-window weighting algorithm. J Neurotrauma 34:3081–3088
8. Maas AIR, Menon DK, Steyerberg EW, Citerio G, Lecky F, Manley GT, Hill S, Legrand V, Sorgner A (2014) Collaborative European NeuroTrauma Effectiveness Research in Traumatic Brain Injury (CENTER-TBI) a prospective longitudinal observational study. Neurosurgery 76:67–80
9. Ohlson JA, Kim S (2015) Linear valuation without OLS: the Theil-Sen estimation approach. Rev Acc Stud 20:395–435

Part VIII

Laboratory and Translational Research

Physical Model for Investigating Intracranial Pressure with Clinical Pressure Sensors and Diagnostic Ultrasound: Preliminary Results

Rikke von Barm, Isabel Martinez Tejada, Marianne Juhler, Morten Andresen, and Jens E. Wilhjelm

Introduction

Intracranial pressure (ICP) is a commonly monitored brain-specific parameter in neurocritical care. Despite its widespread use, aspects related to its genesis and factors contributing to the final waveform remain unsettled. Therefore, it is of interest to mimic clinical ICP signals in order to obtain an improved understanding of the ICP waveform and origin.

Several types of modelling can be used in an attempt to mimic clinical ICP; this study made use of a physical head model. The minimal level of complexity of the model needed to reach the final goal is unknown. For this reason, a simple physical head model was constructed as the first step towards mimicking clinical ICP, whose micro-patterns contain P1, P2, and P3 peaks.

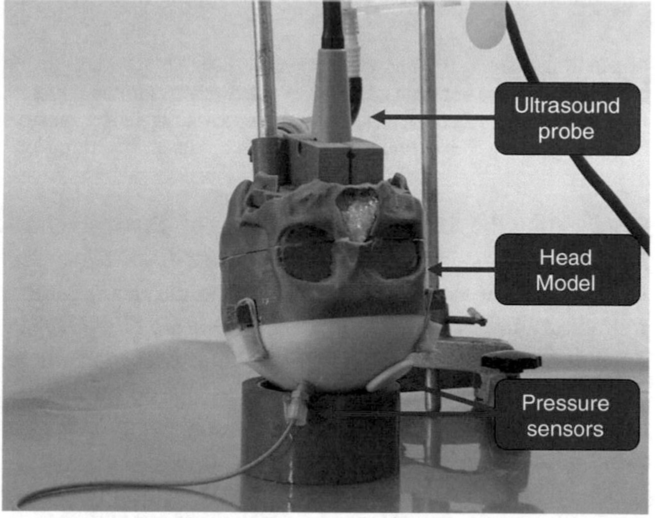

Fig. 1 Physical head phantom model, with ultrasound probe and pressure sensors

Materials and Methods

The simple physical head phantom (Fig. 1) consisted of a skull, a brain tissue substitute, and a pressure-generating balloon. The skull was segmented from a computed tomography (CT) scan of a human head that was remodelled into a three-dimensional (3D) structure. During the reconstruction, the spine, jaw, and non-homogeneous crooked underpart on the skull were removed. This model was modified to contain a holder for an ultrasound transducer and premade burr holes at Kocher's point bilaterally. Natural openings in the skull were closed and eyes were blinded such that structures supporting the eyes did not cover for the ultrasound visibility of the pressure sensors. Lastly, the skull was modelled as a tripartite construction and 3D-printed in either polylactic acid or acrylonitrile butadiene styrene with polycarbonate additives.

The cavity of the skull was filled with a brain tissue mimicking material and a balloon that served as a pressure-increasing device used to induce pressure in the enclosed skull by controlled volume changes. The brain tissue substitute consisted of 2% w/v agar, 1.2% w/v silica dioxide, 25% v/v evaporated milk, alcohol, and water [1–4]. Evaporated milk was full-cream milk (3.5% fat, 3.4% protein) condensed to 50% of its volume.

The volume of the balloon inside the brain tissue substitute was controlled by two different pressure generators,

R. von Barm (✉) · J. E. Wilhjelm
DTU Health Technology, Technical University of Denmark, Lyngby, Denmark

I. M. Tejada
DTU Health Technology, Technical University of Denmark, Lyngby, Denmark

CSF Study Group, Clinic of Neurosurgery, NK 2092, Copenhagen University Hospital, Copenhagen, Denmark

M. Juhler · M. Andresen
CSF Study Group, Clinic of Neurosurgery, NK 2092, Copenhagen University Hospital, Copenhagen, Denmark

B. Depreitere et al. (eds.), *Intracranial Pressure and Neuromonitoring XVII*, Acta Neurochirurgica Supplement 131,
https://doi.org/10.1007/978-3-030-59436-7_49,

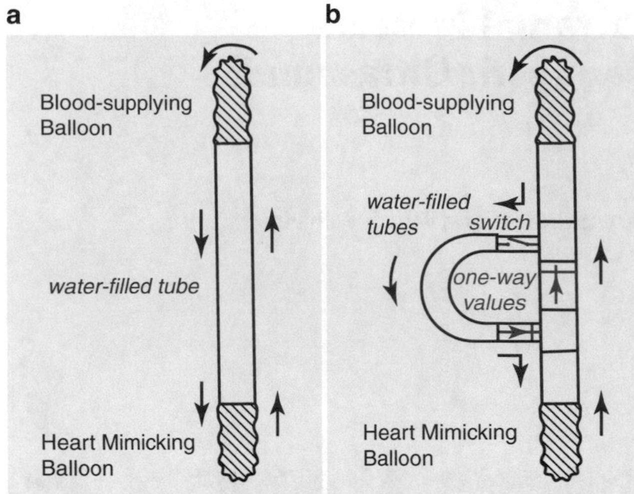

Fig. 2 Illustrations of (**a**) pressure generator 1 and (**b**) pressure generator 2, which were constructed of water-filled tubes and two balloons. Pressure generator 2 contains internal resistance introduced by a smaller tube and one-way valves and a switch. Arrows indicate flow direction

representing the first two generators of our physical model. Both generators were constructed of water-filled tubes with two balloons at each end: one mimicking the heart, another mimicking the blood supply within the brain (Fig. 2). The latter balloon was placed inside the brain tissue substitute, while the heart-mimicking balloon was placed outside the skull. A heart beat was imitated by quickly compressing the heart-mimicking balloon by hand.

Using the first pressure generator (Fig. 2a) the water moved towards the blood-supplying balloon and would instantaneously expand the balloon followed by a rapid volume reduction as the water would move back towards the heart-mimicking balloon again. A rapid sequential increase and decrease in intracranial pressure was expected. For improved imitation of clinical ICP, a second-generation pressure generator was developed. The second pressure generator incorporated internal resistance more closely related to human anatomy. The internal resistance imposed by water was forced through a smaller tube on its way back to the heart-mimicking balloon by use of one-way valves (Fig. 2b). In contrast to pressure generator 1, the heart-mimicking balloon was therefore slowly filled with water.

Multiple experiments were conducted to validate the usefulness of the physical head model and to obtain a better understanding of the generation of the ICP waveform, thereby reaching the goal of mimicking clinical ICP. The differences between the first and second pressure generator were investigated. The pressure was manually applied by single and continuous compressing of the heart-mimicking balloon. Single applied pressure refers to one isolated compression of the heart-mimicking balloon, whereas continuously applied pressure refers to repeated compressions of the heart-mimicking balloon within a small time window (several heart beats). The relationship between the measured pressure during pressure application and the associated tissue displacement around the pressure sensor was explored using diagnostic ultrasound.

Results

Analysis of the measured ICP demonstrated the usefulness of the constructed physical head model. The pressure waveform did not resemble the clinical ICP waveform; however, comparisons of the pressure waveform obtained with pressure generators 1 and 2 showed that the first produced a pressure with a rapid rise followed by small oscillations that debilitate around baseline (Fig. 3). The use of the second pressure generator with internal resistance showed the presence of two peaks.

The analysis of the speckle images measured with diagnostic ultrasound during pressure application enabled visualization of tissue displacement around the pressure sensor. A comparison with the measured ICP signals revealed that the tissue was displaced at the first peak, but smaller pressure patterns were not distinct in the ultrasound displacement images.

Discussion

Accurate modelling of ICP in a physical head model would allow for potentially interesting modifications to mimic different disease entities and function as an inspiration for subsequent clinical studies. Our results showed clear improvements due to progression from the first to the second pressure generator. The pressure generated with pressure generator 1 had one peak followed by rapid small oscillations that weakened around the baseline. Applying the second pressure generator, having incorporated internal resistance, improved our model as this generated two pressure peaks as part of the pressure waveform.

The experiment setup is still far from being comparable to a patient, for various reasons. For instance, the brain tissue substitute consists of a biodegradable substance (i.e. evaporated milk) whose physical properties change over time. Although kept under refrigeration to slow down material degradation, it must be taken into account that 75 days elapsed between the first and last experiment. The elasticity of both balloons and water-filled tubes used to build the pressure generators also changes over time. As a result, a larger

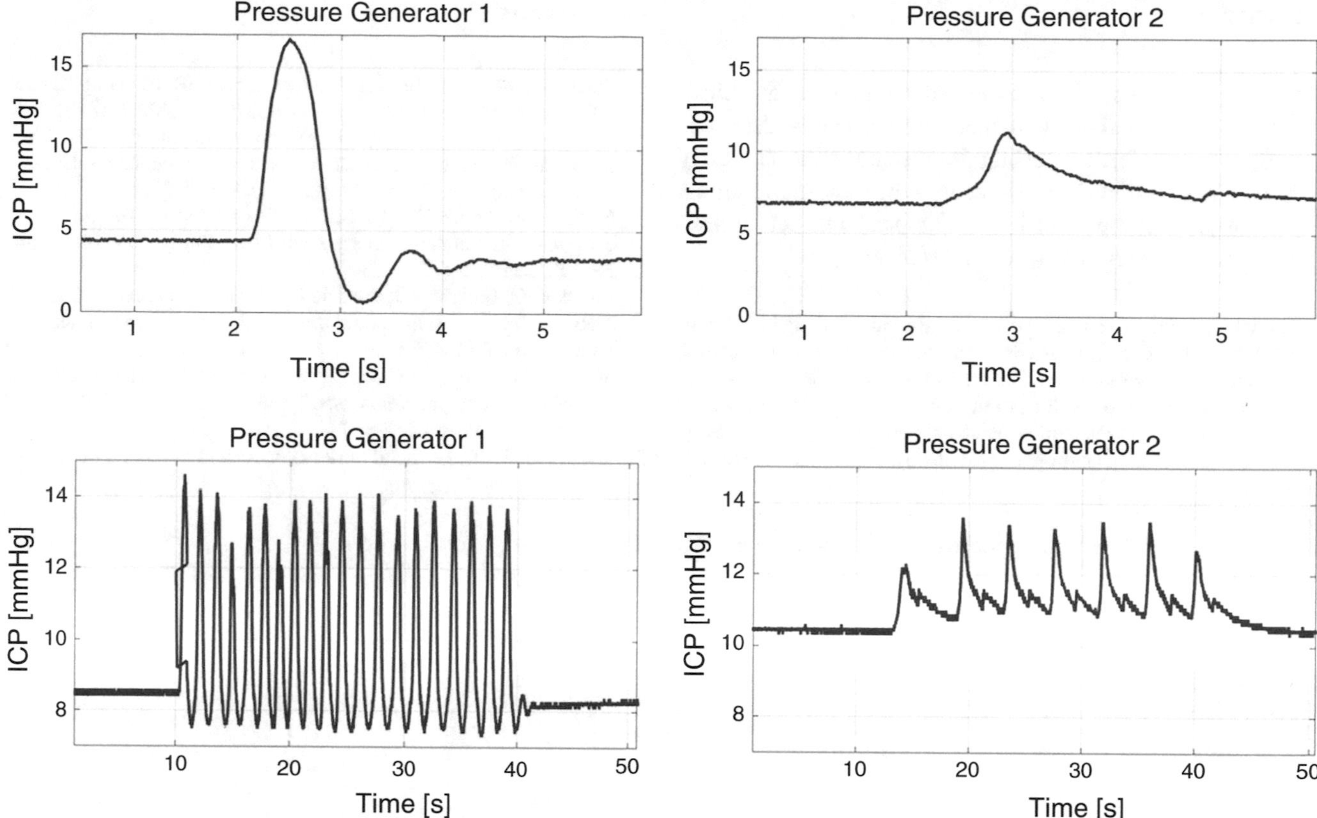

Fig. 3 Measured ICP during pressure application generated by pressure generator 1 (left column) or 2 (right column). Both single applied pressure (top) and continuously applied pressure (bottom) are shown. All pressure data were obtained within the same physical model in a 180° elevation from the supine position and measured at room temperature

expansion would influence the applied pressure by a rise in ICP. It must also be further noted that all experiments were carried out with the head in an upside-down position to ensure full contact between the tissue substitute and the pressure sensor, making it difficult to compare measured pressure values with those found in the literature. Thus, upright positioning of the physical head phantom together with further investigations in elasticity properties are to be considered.

In addition to the foregoing points, the complex brain consists of multiple anatomical compartments such as the spinal cord, ventricles, meninges, eyes, arterial tree, and so forth. The incorporation of these would help construct a more realistic head phantom. Spine phantoms could be 3D-printed using rubber-like material for the spinal cord, platinum-core silicone gel for the intervertebral disc, polymide for the intervertebral disc, and gelatin for the soft tissue [5]. The inclusion of the ventricles would make it possible to differentiate between ICP measurements at parenchymal and ventricular depths. The cerebrospinal fluid (CSF) within the ventricles could be mimicked using water. Pulsation in the meninges is also thought to influence ICP. Earlier researchers tried to mimic the dura mater using mixtures of silk cocoons [1], silicone, gelatine, collagen, and polymer sheets [5]. However, although the shape of the skull was thought at the beginning to be a potential factor influencing the resulting ICP, we believe that most influencing waveform factors giving rise to the three distinctive peaks have a vascular origin. Therefore, the next model will go one step backwards, using a box as a skull, and instead focus on the incorporation of the aforementioned anatomical compartments. This includes the addition of an arterial tree and a constant pressure generator. While a simple arterial tree could be constructed using various blood-supplying balloons, tubes, or similar expandable/compressible materials in various shapes and sizes, the pressure generator requires the same force to be applied at every mimicked heartbeat.

Regarding tissue displacement, it was possible to identify the high-pressure peaks, whereas minor peaks were not distinct. Increased ultrasound frame rate and improved spatial resolution might allow for this. Furthermore, it is likely that with higher-amplitude pressure peaks (closer to the clinical ICP) these smaller peaks might become visually distinct.

Conclusion

This study presented the first steps towards mimicking clinical ICP in a physical head phantom model. The model needs refinement and further testing to resemble the clinically obtained ICP. Future improvements will first and foremost focus on placing the skull in the clinically relevant upright positioning and includomg ventricles and a spine.

Acknowledgments The financial support for participating in this conference from the Otto Moensteds Foundation is greatly appreciated. Furthermore, a thanks go to BK Medical for the use of their transducer and transducer covers as well as to the Center for Fast Ultrasound for letting us use their ultrasound scanner bk5000 (BK Medical). Lastly, access to the software DataLogger provided by Raumedic Company is appreciated.

Conflict of Interest **The authors declare that they have no conflict of interest**.

References

1. Sang JH, Jinseu P, Dong HH, Seung SH, Hae LR, Haeyong K, Seok KW, Kwang LG, Youn CS, Hyoung JJ, Yong CJ, Soo CY, Dae KW, Won ES (2011) A transparent artificial dura mater made of silk fibroin as an inhibitor of inflammation in craniotomized rats: laboratory investigation. J Neurosurg 114(2):485–490
2. Madsen EL, Frank GR, Dong F (1998) Liquid or solid ultrasonically tissue-mimicking materials with very low scatter. Ultrasound Med Biol 24:535–542
3. Menikou G, Dadakova T, Pavline M, Bock M, Damianou C (2015) MRI compatible head phantoms used for ultrasound surgery. Ultrasonics 57:144–152
4. Menikou G, Damianou C (2017) Acoustic and thermal characterization of agar based phantoms used for evaluating focused ultrasound exposures. J Therap Ultras 5:14
5. Taira et al (1999) Artificial dura mater (Patent number 5,861,034)

Augmented Reality-Assisted Neurosurgical Drain Placement (ARANED): Technical Note

Frederick Van Gestel, Taylor Frantz, Mumtaz Hussain Soomro, Shirley A. Elprama, Cedric Vannerom, An Jacobs, Jef Vandemeulebroucke, Bart Jansen, Thierry Scheerlinck, and Johnny Duerinck

Introduction

Recent years have seen a boost in the development of innovative technologies, including virtual (VR) and *augmented reality* (AR). Once a vision of the future, these technologies are currently sufficiently advanced to be implemented in a variety of industries and disciplines, including medical practice and, more specifically, surgery. The main challenge in developing an AR solution for surgical use is to combine the required technical development in order to achieve maximal accuracy with attention to end-user requirements.

The *Surgical Augmented Reality Assistance (SARA)* project took shape through the interaction between a group of people with relevant expertise who are interested in the potential of this novel technology and clinicians (end users) expressing a clear clinical need. The project aims to investigate the feasibility of AR for preoperative planning, intraoperative visualisation and navigational support and assess its potential impact on surgical training. Clinical validation of technical solutions is a crucial step in assessing the real-world accuracy and usefulness of the AR holographic information provided to surgeons.

Other research groups have reported on small, single-surgeon trials in which the Microsoft HoloLens was used to plan or perform neurosurgical procedures [1, 2]. In these reports, generic open-source software for three-dimensional (3D) model creation and visualisation was used, which is typically not adapted for intuitive use by unfamiliar end users. Registration of the hologram to the patient was performed using manual positioning in 3D space and relying on the head-mounted display's (HMD) built-in simultaneous localisation and mapping (SLAM) algorithm for stability. Although it demonstrates the potential of AR for neurosurgical procedures, this approach provides insufficient accuracy. We previously reported on a proof of concept using red-green-blue (RGB) camera tracking instead of the built-in SLAM algorithm [3]. Although this method provided good navigational accuracy in our setup (1.41 ± 0.89 mm), use of the RGB camera in everyday surgical practice is hindered by several practical limitations, such as the narrow field of view, the necessity to create new operative hardware and a generally lower reliability when it comes to tracking instruments.

The aim of our project, targeted at Microsoft's HoloLens, is to address these shortcomings by developing a *customised software solution* for hologram creation, planning and visualisation that is continuous between the planning station and the AR device, as well as a proprietary application for inside-out infrared (IR) tracking and semi-automated hologram-to-patient registration, optimising both the accuracy and stability of the hologram relative to the physical world. Validation of the AR solution is provided through preclinical and *clinical testing*, focused on intracranial drain placement.

Intracranial drain placement is a frequent procedure that is used not only for patients with intracranial hypertension (ICH) but, more recently, also for intracranial haemorrhage (chronic subdural haematoma (CSDH) or intraparenchymal haemorrhage (IPH)) [4, 5]. The placement of an intracranial drain is most often performed freehand, following inspection and sometimes planning on computed tomography (CT) images of the patient. Additionally, literature-defined landmarks that are not patient-specific are used. Although it is an

F. Van Gestel (✉) · C. Vannerom · J. Duerinck
Department of Neurosurgery, UZ Brussel, Jette, Belgium
e-mail: frederick.vangestel@uzbrussel.be

T. Frantz · M. H. Soomro · J. Vandemeulebroucke · B. Jansen
Department of Electronics and Informatics (ETRO), Vrije Universiteit Brussel, Etterbeek, Belgium

Imec, Leuven, Belgium

S. A. Elprama · A. Jacobs
Imec, Leuven, Belgium

Department of Studies in Media, Innovation and Technology (SMIT), Vrije Universiteit Brussel, Etterbeek, Belgium

T. Scheerlinck
Department of Orthopedic Surgery, UZ Brussel, Jette, Belgium

B. Depreitere et al. (eds.), *Intracranial Pressure and Neuromonitoring XVII*, Acta Neurochirurgica Supplement 131,
https://doi.org/10.1007/978-3-030-59436-7_50,

oft-performed procedure, it has been demonstrated that optimal placement is only achieved in 60–80% of cases [5–7]. Having a 3D representation of relevant patient anatomy, along with planned trajectories or approaches, shown to the surgeon on top of the real-life patient, has the potential to vastly improve on these accuracy results.

Materials and Methods

Hardware and Software

The HoloLens, developed by Microsoft Corporation, was chosen as the development platform. It combines an unobstructed HMD with an integrated untethered computer and a multitude of sensors. Using accelerometers, gyroscopes and an inside-out tracking system, the real world around it can be registered and the position of the device itself, and thus of the wearer's head, can be tracked. Knowing the position and orientation of the user's head, it is possible to transform the displayed data into an appropriate position, rotation and scale which give the data an illusion of depth and pose. The HoloLens can interpret the real world around it and adjust its projected visuals accordingly, allowing for AR creation. The combination of the ability to triangulate positions in 3D space through tracking and an augmented display of visual information makes it suitable for the development of a surgical navigation platform.

Preclinical and Clinical Validation

Both phantom and patient trials for neurosurgical drain placement received ethical approval and are currently being performed at UZ Brussel. For the phantom trial a 3D-printed head and skullcap are created, along with agar-casted hemispheres and a silicone skin substitute. The phantom is scanned, after which a 3D model with eight virtual drain trajectories is created, which is displayed during the procedure. Drain placement is performed under IR tracking by surgeons of varying expertise levels, after which the performed placements are compared to the planned trajectories.

For the patient trial a clinical pilot study was initiated for patients requiring neurosurgical drain placement, comparing current practice to AR guidance. After a CT scan, a 3D model is created using the image processing pipeline. Minimal invasive drain placement in the cerebrospinal fluid (CSF) space (ventricle) or haematoma (for CSDH and IPH) is then performed in standard fashion, but with the aid of a 3D model of the patient and the specific compartment to be targeted displayed on top of the patient. To allow the surgeons to become accustomed to the HMD, the 3D model was displayed floating next to the patient in the first few cases to serve as a simple 3D visualisation.

Results

HoloLens Software Solution

Our consortium designed a HoloLens solution with proprietary hardware and software adaptations to optimise the HMD specifically for neurosurgical navigation. For this, a *comprehensive pipeline* was created allowing for the transformation of Digital Imaging and Communications in Medicine (DICOM) images into a 3D model containing multiple layers/objects, which can then be transferred to and displayed on the Microsoft HoloLens. Through sequential automated and semi-automated algorithms and additional software optimisation we are currently able to create valid 3D models of patients and display them on the HoloLens as anatomical overlays with several interaction functionalities in less than 30 min (Fig. 1). Because this sequence can be performed during the time of the CT scan, patient transfers and the operative installation and preparation, *little to no additional time is required* for the surgeon.

Remote Planning Station

The planning station has a *customised user interface* (UI), which takes the surgeon through the DICOM segmentation and 3D model creation in a stepwise manner. The UI is based on a sequence of semi-automated planning algorithms that run in the background, while maintaining a straightforward and organised foreground. The planning sequence guides the surgeon through the segmentation, layer by layer, after which the surgeon can verify and adjust even the slightest inaccuracy during every step of the process. The algorithms run in a *semi-automated* fashion, requiring a minimal amount of interactions for the creation of a valid 3D model, while simultaneously collecting several 3D landmark coordinates. In the second stage of the workflow, these landmarks will be used for the automation of both the procedure planning and patient registration. Following validation and confirmation of the entire 3D model by the surgeon, it is exported as a set of Wavefront OBJ files along with an Extensible Markup Language (XML) file that contains the essential patient data and the collected coordinates.

The complete planning and DICOM segmentation procedure took 5–10 min on average. The average duration per layer of interactions required from the surgeon is displayed

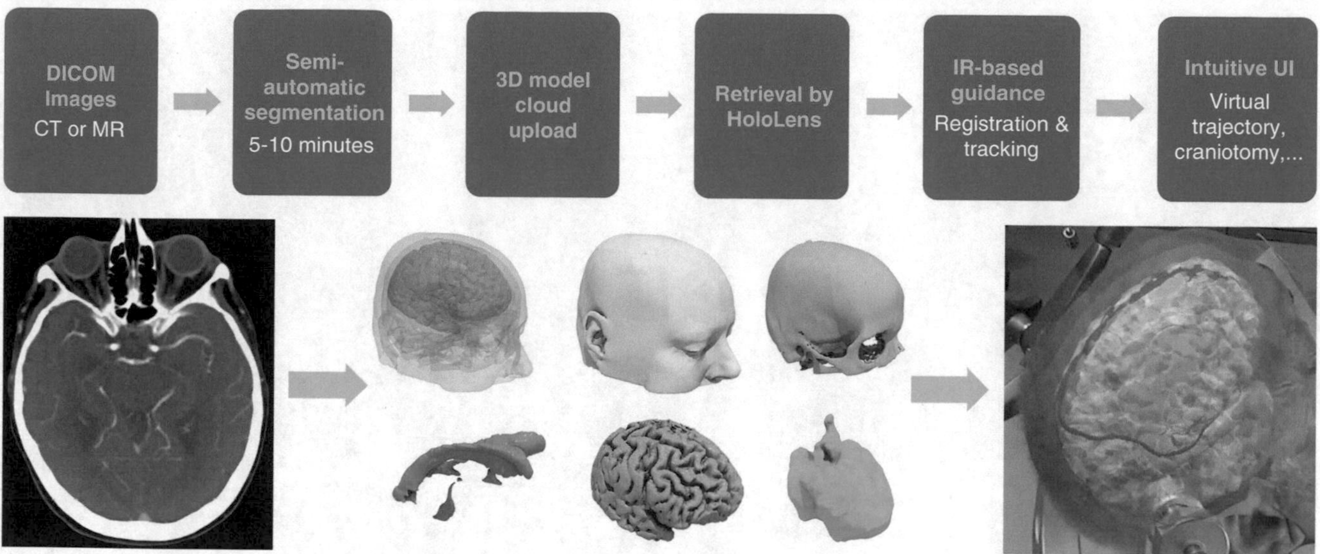

Fig. 1 Image processing pipeline: from left to right we laid out all key steps needed to go from a DICOM image to a 3D anatomical overlay as fast and efficiently as possible. Underneath an example of the resulting multi-layered hologram is shown before and after registration to the patient

Table 1 Average duration of interactions for planning and DICOM segmentation per layer

				Haemorrhage	
Layer	Skin (n = 20)	Skull (n = 20)	Ventricles (n = 20)	IPH (n = 10)	CSDH (n = 10)
Average duration (min)	0.00	0.00	1.18	2.80	8.00

in Table 1. For each of the three pathologies, skin, skull and ventricles were segmented, with an additional segmentation of the haemorrhage for the IPH and CSDH. This resulted in an average duration of 1.18 min for ICH, 3.98 min for IPH and 9.18 min for CSDH. The duration of the automated processes, such as the planning of trajectories which uses specific 3D coordinates collected during the segmentation phase, was not considered since their speed relied solely on the CPU capacities of the used planning station. In general, they never took longer than an additional minute.

Data Transfer to Device

The patient model, composed of multiple OBJ files and an XML file, is transferred to the HoloLens, which reads the OBJ files and reconstructs them as a single, multi-layered 3D model. This model is displayed for verification, along with the patient data retrieved from the XML file. The latter also contains several coordinates which are used for both the instant recreation of previously planned trajectories and the hologram-to-patient registration. After the surgeon confirms the correct identity of the patient, the software proceeds to tracking and registration.

HoloLens Functionalities and User Interface

Infrared Tracking

The initial RGB-tracked solution, created in our proof of concept [3], was replaced by an IR-based tracking system (Fig. 2a) to meet surgical requirements in terms of *accuracy, field of view* and *practical application* of the trackers without the need to create additional hardware. As such, a lightweight framework (adapted from [8, 9]) for the detection and tracking of surgical instruments (stylus and reference star) based on the integrated IR camera was developed (Fig. 2c). This was tested through post hoc analysis of three videos, recorded with the IR camera, simulating different movements and relative poses of the instruments (Fig. 2b). The instrument pose can be determined by iteratively solving the perspective-n-point problem between each instrument's model and the corresponding detections per frame [10]. Two methods of determining correspondence between the instruments' IR markers and the detections are used: if correspondence is unknown, an exhaustive search is performed to try and establish correspondence; however, if a recent correspondence is known, the current correspondence can be quickly re-established through a Hungarian algorithm method [11].

Run-time performance of the IR tracking algorithm was approximately 15 frames per second (FPS) on the HMD; however, since processing was offloaded from the main application thread, the application visuals could render at the recommended 60 FPS. During the post hoc video analysis, mean instrument detection latency over all video sequences using an exhaustive search was 122 ms, while the Hungarian-based method could be performed with a latency of 66 ms (Table 2). For the Hungarian-based method, tracking success for the world stable reference star was at 99.2% of all frames

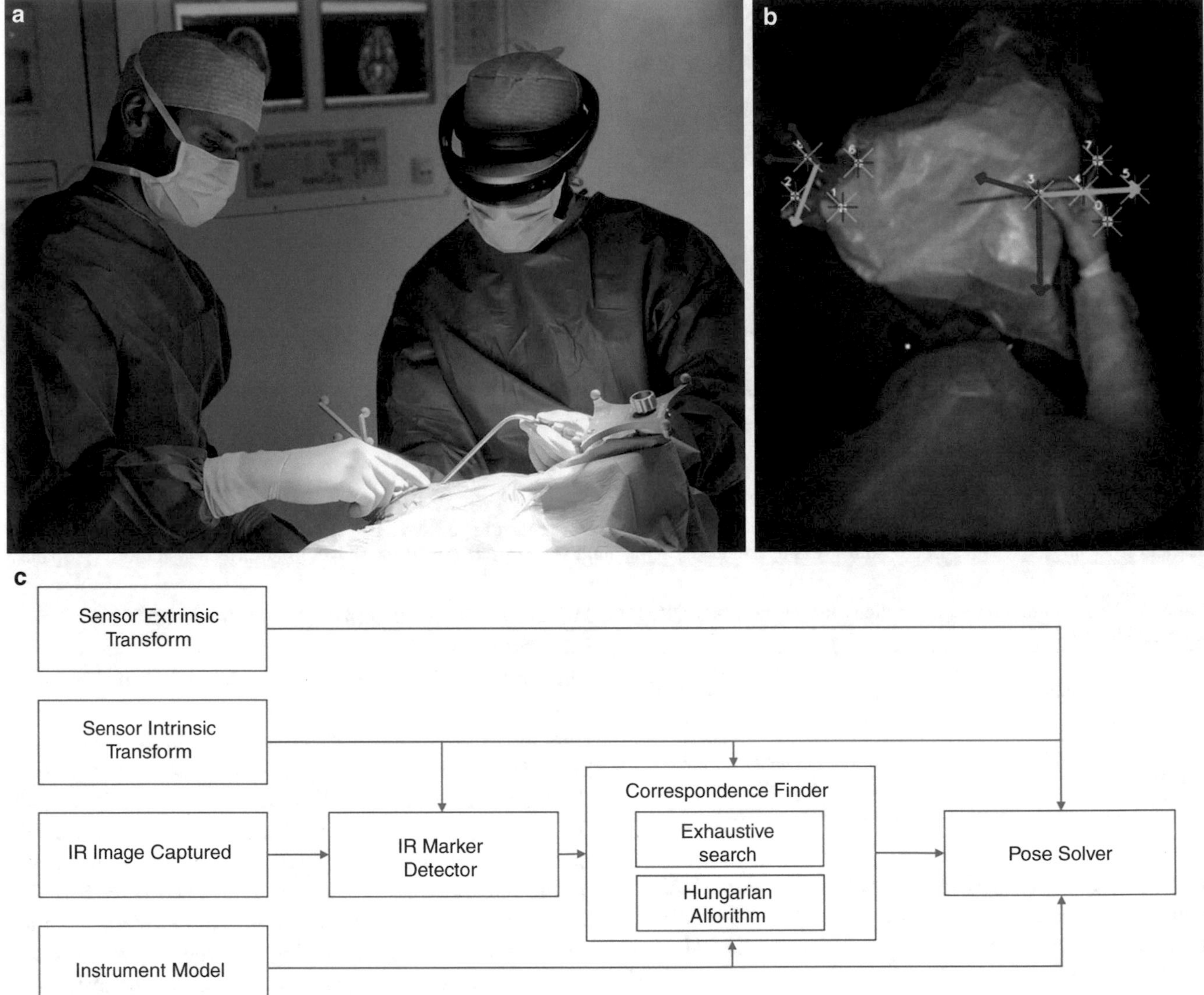

Fig. 2 Inside-out IR tracking on an AR-HMD: (**a**) surgeon wearing HoloLens using instruments that are tracked through reflective orbs; (**b**) tracked image from IR camera, on which pose and orientation of instruments (3D axes) are defined through recognition of reflective orbs (numbered crosshairs); (**c**) lightweight framework for real-time detection and tracking of instrumentation using integrated IR camera of HMD

Table 2 Per-frame run-time latency

Correspondence search method	Latency (ms)
Exhaustive search for both instruments	122.9
Hungarian search for both instruments	66.2

(Table 3). Similarly, the stylus, which was free to move in world space, could be tracked in 92.7% of frames without detection prediction, and 93.6% with. There existed a perceived shift between the tracked instrument and its augmented projection of approximately 1 cm. Since their correspondence relative to one another appeared correctly, this shift is assumed to result from the HMD's visualisation engine failing to account for the transform between the

Table 3 Overall binned instrument tracking results [# frames per tracking outcome]

Hungarian parameter	Last known location		Last known location and prediction	
	Stylus	Reference	Stylus	Reference
Successful exhaustive search	14	5	10	5
Successful Hungarian search	1155	1301	1168	1302
Recovered Hungarian search	4	2	7	2
Detection failed	81	5	70	4
Not enough points for detection	100	41	100	41

displays and the user's eyes. However, this could be accounted for through display-eye calibration [12].

Hologram-to-Patient Registration

The advanced registration feature uses the automated recognition of both the IR-tracked pointer and reference star. The software guides the user to indicate the previously defined landmarks with the pointer on the patient in order to match the virtual model with its corresponding anatomy. After verification of the accuracy, the reference star, connected to the patient's head in a fixed position, is used to establish a coordinate system as an anchor for accurate and stable hologram registration and visualisation (Fig. 1), even when the patient is covered with surgical drapes. Henceforth, the hologram's position is *continuously tracked and adjusted* to assure the multi-layered patient model remains in its true anatomical location.

User Interface

The proprietary HoloLens UI allows the user to intuitively interact with the virtual model using voice and gesture commands, as well as the IR-tracked tools. The surgeon can choose to display only certain structures, cycle through different anatomical layers, adjust predetermined trajectories and apply several advanced planning functions whenever necessary. An example of the latter is virtual craniotomy: using the tracked pointer, the surgeon can create a virtual opening in the skull around an indicated point through which (s)he can inspect the cortex and vasculature directly underneath. This allows the visualisation of the direct approach to any deep-seated structures or anomalies. By only displaying the AR view through the craniotomy window, the impression of an opening in the skull is created. Other surgical equipment, such as drills, can be tracked as well by mounting IR trackers directly on the instrument. The proportions of these instruments can be calibrated using the reference star. Through this type of instrument tracking, the system can not only estimate the surgical phase the surgeon is in, optimising its provided support, but it can also improve the accuracy and safety of the tracked instrument's use. When drilling a hole in the skull, for example, the optimal entry point and drilling angle, as well as the depth of the drill bit, can be indicated. This can *prevent unnecessary reiterations and damage* to the cortex directly underneath.

Preclinical and Clinical Validation

The first tests of AR-assisted intracranial drain placement on a phantom head using IR tracking (Fig. 3a, b) were performed and compared to their respective planned trajectories (Fig. 3c). The comparisons, however, showed mixed results due to line-of-sight issues with the tracked reference (Fig. 3d). This was recently improved by implementing a correction for possible occlusion during IR tracking. The accuracy of the results of newly performed phantom drain placements using IR tracking with occlusion correction will be reported on shortly.

In the patient trial, the first three intracranial drain placements with a simple 3D visualisation next to the patient were performed. The simple 3D visual aid, however, turned out to be distracting and overinformed the surgeon, causing mistakes in an otherwise easy procedure. All three procedures demonstrated misplaced drains, of which two were corrected per procedure and one required a second intervention. This conflict between customary guidelines and the 3D guidance did not appear in preliminary cases where the model was registered to the patient's anatomy (providing the surgeon with the impression of "see-through vision") (Fig. 1). We therefore committed to an exact anatomical overlay of the virtual 3D model with the real-life patient. Preliminary accuracy results of these drain placements will be reported on shortly.

Discussion

Rethinking the definition of surgical navigation using new technologies above all requires a uniform and straightforward UI that helps rather than challenges the surgeon throughout both planning and procedure. The customised, semi-automated planning station guides the user through the entire planning sequence in such a way that it can be performed *without expertise in image segmentation.* The step-by-step sequence supports verification and adjustments during every step of the process, providing the surgeon with an additional quality control of the entire model and preoperative planning. This procedure takes *less than 10 minutes* and is capable of accurately defining CSDHs with *minimal input* from the surgeon. Efficient, semi-automated segmentation of CSDHs is a unique feature that, to the best of our knowledge, has not been reported on previously.

Anticipating surgical implementation, the switch from RGB to IR tracking was essential. When solely focusing on its technical capabilities, the IR sensor already has three important advantages over the devices' colour sensor: first of all it allows robust identification of surgical instruments from the environment; second, its field of view of 120° is nearly three times that of the RGB sensor, considerably *improving overall tracking performance*; and third, its orientation is down-turned towards the wearer's hands, where one would expect an instrument to be held. What truly sets apart the IR from the RGB tracking, however, is the ability to *integrate and track existing surgical equipment*, supporting both preoperative and intraoperative tracking with high accuracy. We

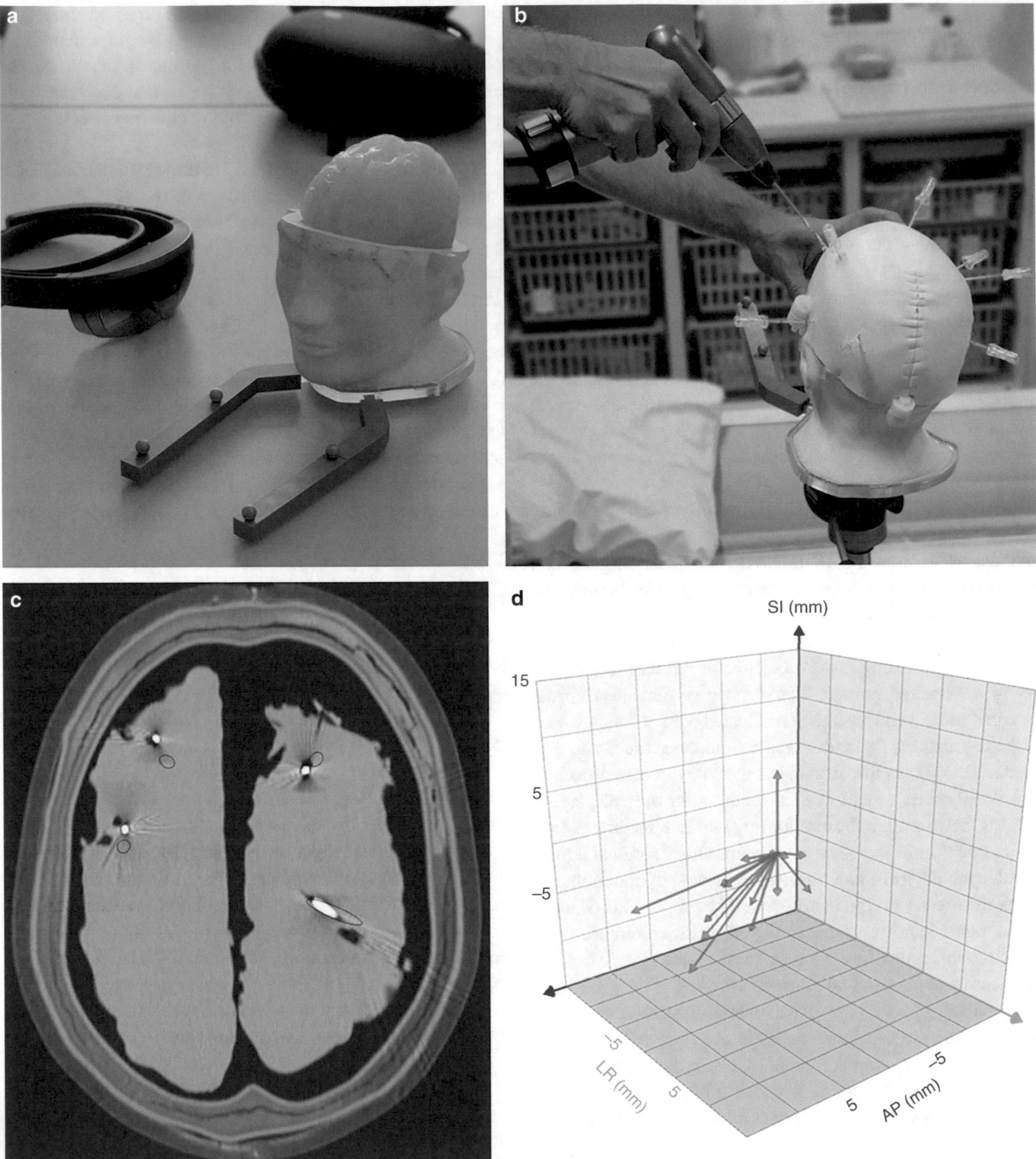

Fig. 3 Phantom trial setup: (**a**) 3D-printed phantom with agar-casted hemispheres on IR-tracked base; (**b**) AR-assisted drain placement; (**c**) comparison of performed placements (white) to planned trajectories (blue); (**d**) placed drain tip deviation plotted on 3D (*x*,*y*,*z*) graph (*SI* superior-inferior, *LR* left-right, *AP* anterior-posterior)

previously demonstrated in our proof of concept a navigational accuracy approaching that of current navigation systems [3]. With the newly developed solution, using continuous IR tracking, a *higher reliability* can be achieved. To the best of our knowledge, this is the first reported demonstration of a real-time, inside-out IR tracking workflow used on an AR-HMD for the establishment of a stable coordinate system and medical instrument tracking.

Preclinical and clinical trials are being performed at UZ Brussel. The first tests of both showed mixed results due to technical constraints, which have now been resolved. The results of newly performed drain placements, in both phantoms and patients, will be reported on shortly. The study by Li et al. [2], however, already demonstrated the potential of AR guidance for intracranial drain placement, despite the use of RGB tracking, improving their mean target deviation from 11.26 ± 4.83 mm in the control group to 4.34 ± 1.63 mm in the AR-guided group. So far, no publication has investigated the benefits of inside-out IR tracking on an AR-HMD as a navigation tool for intracranial drain placement.

Conclusion

The AR solution presented here provides a *fully integrated and completely mobile navigation setup*, allowing its use for everyday procedures that are frequently performed without imaging guidance but could still benefit from navigational support, such as intracranial drain placements. The solution offers a quick and intuitive image processing pipeline and requires little additional time and effort from the surgeons. The system's real-time, inside-out IR tracking supports mobility while maintaining accuracy. With a focus on both *optimal accuracy* and an *intuitive end-user experience* and simultaneous *clinical validation*, this AR solution has the potential to vastly improve the accuracy results of intracranial drain placement procedures.

Acknowledgements This project was funded by the Flemish government through the imec.icon research programme. The remote planning station and phantom head were created in conjunction with Materialise NV; the HoloLens UI was developed in conjunction with Roger Roll NV (part of the Cronos Group).

Conflict of Interest **The authors declare that they have no conflict of interest.**

References

1. Incekara F, Smits M, Dirven C, Vincent A (2018) Clinical feasibility of a wearable mixed-reality device in neurosurgery. World Neurosurg 118:e422–e427
2. Li Y, Chen X, Wang N et al (2018) A wearable mixed-reality holographic computer for guiding external ventricular drain insertion at the bedside. J Neurosurg 1:1–8
3. Frantz T, Jansen B, Duerinck J, Vandemeulebroucke J (2018) Augmenting Microsoft's HoloLens with Vuforia tracking for neuronavigation. Healthc Technol Lett 5(5):221–225
4. Sindou M, Ibrahim I, Maarrawi J (2010) Chronic sub-dural hematomas: twist drill craniostomy with a closed system of drainage, for 48 hours only, is a valuable surgical treatment. Acta Neurochir 152(3):545–546
5. Fam MD, Hanley D, Stadnik A et al (2017) Surgical performance in minimally invasive surgery plus recombinant tissue plasminogen activator for intracerebral hemorrhage evacuation phase III clinical trial. Neurosurgery 81(5):860–866
6. Kakarla UK, Kim LJ, Chang SW et al (2008) Safety and accuracy of bedside external ventricular drain placement. Neurosurgery 63(1 Suppl 1):ONS162-6; discussion ONS166-7
7. Patil V, Lacson R, Vosburgh KG et al (2013) Factors associated with external ventricular drain placement accuracy: data from an electronic health record repository. Acta Neurochir 155(9):1773–1779
8. Bilesan A, Owlia M, Behzadipour S et al (2018) Marker-based motion tracking using Microsoft Kinect. IFAC-PapersOnLine 51(22):399–404
9. Faessler M, Mueggler E, Schwabe K, Scaramuzza D (2014) A monocular pose estimation system based on infrared LEDs. IEEE Int Conf Robot Autom 2014:907–913
10. Bradski G (2000) The OpenCV Library. Dr Dobbs J 25:120–125
11. Kuhn HW (1955) The Hungarian Method for the assignment problem. Nav Res Logist 2:83–97
12. Azimi E, Qian L, Navab N, Kazanzides P. Alignment of the virtual scene to the tracking space of a mixed reality head-mounted display. IEEE. arXiv:1703.05834v4.

Lower Limit of Reactivity Assessed with PRx in an Experimental Setting

Erta Beqiri, Ken M. Brady, Jennifer K. Lee, Joseph Donnelly, Frederick A. Zeiler, Marek Czosnyka, and Peter Smielewski

Introduction

Individualising cerebral perfusion pressure (CPP) is a major issue after traumatic brain injury (TBI) patients. Monitoring cerebral autoregulation (CA) using the pressure reactivity index (PRx) has been suggested as a tool for identifying individual dynamic targets of CPP. This is because the PRx/CPP relationship over time describes a U-shaped curve, with its nadir identifying a CPP value at which CA is best preserved (CPPopt). Moreover, values of CPP corresponding to a certain threshold of PRx above which CA is impaired identify the lower (LLR) and upper limit of reactivity. Large retrospective studies [1, 2] have shown that patients managed with CPP close to CPPopt had better outcomes, suggesting CPPopt as a suitable individualised CPP target. The first prospective randomised controlled trial assessing the feasibility and safety of managing patients according to CPPopt is currently ongoing (COGiTATE) [3]. However, CPPopt describes the centre of the CA range and does not provide information about the behaviour of the whole range of autoregulation in terms of width and stability. The range might be very narrow, making CPPopt a desired target, or very large, in which case keeping CPP above LLR could possibly be sufficient, without needing to push for a high CPP to reach CPPopt and making it possible to concentrate on other clinical issues of the patient. The range might vary in the same patient according to the progression of the disease. In fact, a strong correlation with mortality was shown when CPP was below LLR derived with PRx [4]. This confirms that PRx statistically agrees with autoregulation, suggesting once more its added value in TBI patients' management. However, the reliability of the method when applied to individual cases deserves to be studied in greater details, before making it possible to use it as a tool at the bedside prospectively.

The objective of this project was to establish on an individual basis how curve fit–derived LLR (dynamic autoregulation) compares with the experimentally determined real lower limit of autoregulation (LLA-static autoregulation).

Methods

We present a retrospective analysis of intracranial pressure (ICP), arterial blood pressure (ABP) and laser Doppler flow (LDF) signals recorded in nine piglets (at 200 Hz) undergoing controlled, terminal hypotension (Fig. 1). Details about the experimental setting are described in a previously published manuscript by Brady et al. [5] and here are briefly

E. Beqiri (✉)
Brain Physics Laboratory, Division of Neurosurgery, Department of Clinical Neurosciences, University of Cambridge, Cambridge, UK

Department of Physiology and Transplantation, Milan University, Milan, Italy

K. M. Brady
Pediatric Cardiology, Texas Children's Hospital, Baylor College of Medicine, Houston, TX, USA

J. K. Lee
Department of Anesthesiology and Critical Care Medicine, Johns Hopkins, Baltimore, MD, USA

J. Donnelly · M. Czosnyka · P. Smielewski
Brain Physics Laboratory, Division of Neurosurgery, Department of Clinical Neurosciences, University of Cambridge, Cambridge, UK

F. A. Zeiler
Department of Surgery, Rady Faculty of Health Sciences, University of Manitoba, Winnipeg, MB, Canada

Department of Human Anatomy and Cell Science, Rady Faculty of Health Sciences, University of Manitoba, Winnipeg, MB, Canada

Biomedical Engineering, Faculty of Engineering, University of Manitoba, Winnipeg, MB, Canada

Division of Anaesthesia, Department of Medicine, University of Cambridge, Cambridge, UK

B. Depreitere et al. (eds.), *Intracranial Pressure and Neuromonitoring XVII*, Acta Neurochirurgica Supplement 131,
https://doi.org/10.1007/978-3-030-59436-7_51,

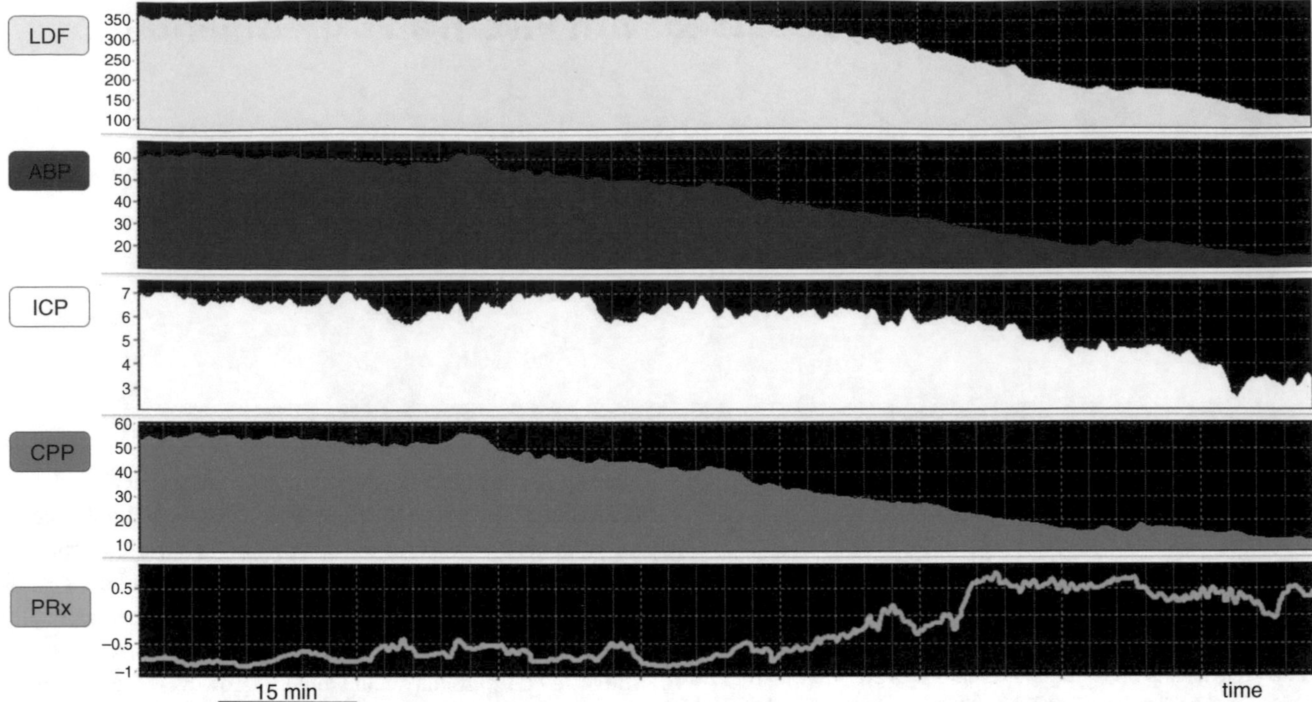

Fig. 1 Example of section with monotonous decrease in CPP. LDF, ABP and ICP were monitored at 200 Hz. The data were cleaned and down-sampled at 0.1 Hz (as presented in the picture). CPP was calculated as ABP-ICP. PRx was calculated as moving coefficient correlation between slow changes in ABP and in ICP. After hypotension is induced, LDF is constant until CPP crosses LLA. When CPP decreases below LLA, LDF decreases and PRx increases. *LDF* laser Doppler flow, *ABP* arterial blood pressure, *ICP* intracranial pressure, *CPP* cerebral perfusion pressure, *PRx* pressure reactivity index

mentioned. The data were collected and analysed with ICM+ software (https://icmplus.neurosurg.cam.ac.uk/). Ventilator-imposed positive end-expiratory pressure (PEEP) waves (5–10 cm H_2O, sine-wave pattern, period 60 s) increased the variability in ABP, facilitating the brain vascular reactivity monitoring [5]. Only sections of the recordings with stable experimental conditions where a clear breakpoint of LDF/CPP characteristic (LLA) could be identified, using piecewise linear regression, were studied (Fig. 2). The behaviour of PRx in the PRx/CPP plots (LLR defined by breakpoint) and in the PRx/CPP error bar chart (LLR defined as CPP at PRx 0.3) was examined (Fig. 2).

Results

Over the nine experiments, one was excluded because of the bad quality of the signals in the period with a monotonous decrease of CPP. In the remaining eight experiments, the following pattern was observed (Fig. 2): when CPP had a monotonous decrease, the relationship PRx/CPP showed two breakpoints (LLR_1 > LLR_2); LLA was between them; LLR (CPP at PRx 0.3 in the error bar chart) was close to LLR_2. In Table 1 the values of LLA, LLR, LLR_1 and LLR_2 are shown for each experiment.

Discussion

When CPP has a monotonous decrease, the pressure reactivity starts worsening (PRx starts to increase) before CPP crosses the LLA, a point marked LLR_1 in Fig. 2. A further decrease in CPP below the LLA would cause a decrease in CBF, even if the pressure reactivity is not completely lost, which happens at point LLR_2 in Fig. 2. This pattern suggests two important features that should be taken into account and investigated when PRx is used to detect LLA continuously and when fixed thresholds for PRx are used for this purpose.

First of all, our results highlight the difference between dynamic and static autoregulation. Static autoregulation is the mechanism that describes the regulation of cerebral blood flow, which cannot be kept constant below LLA, and is explored with a continuous monotonous decrease in CPP. Such a decrease in CPP cannot be used in TBI patients, given their fragility. Therefore, dynamic autoregulation is used instead. Oscillations in the diameter of the vessels, which happen continuously in the range of the slow waves (0.005–0.05 Hz), are considered the autoregulatory response to changes in CPP. The oscillations are transmitted to the ICP. These slow wave variations are assessed by PRx to probe the mechanism of dynamic autoregulation, which is

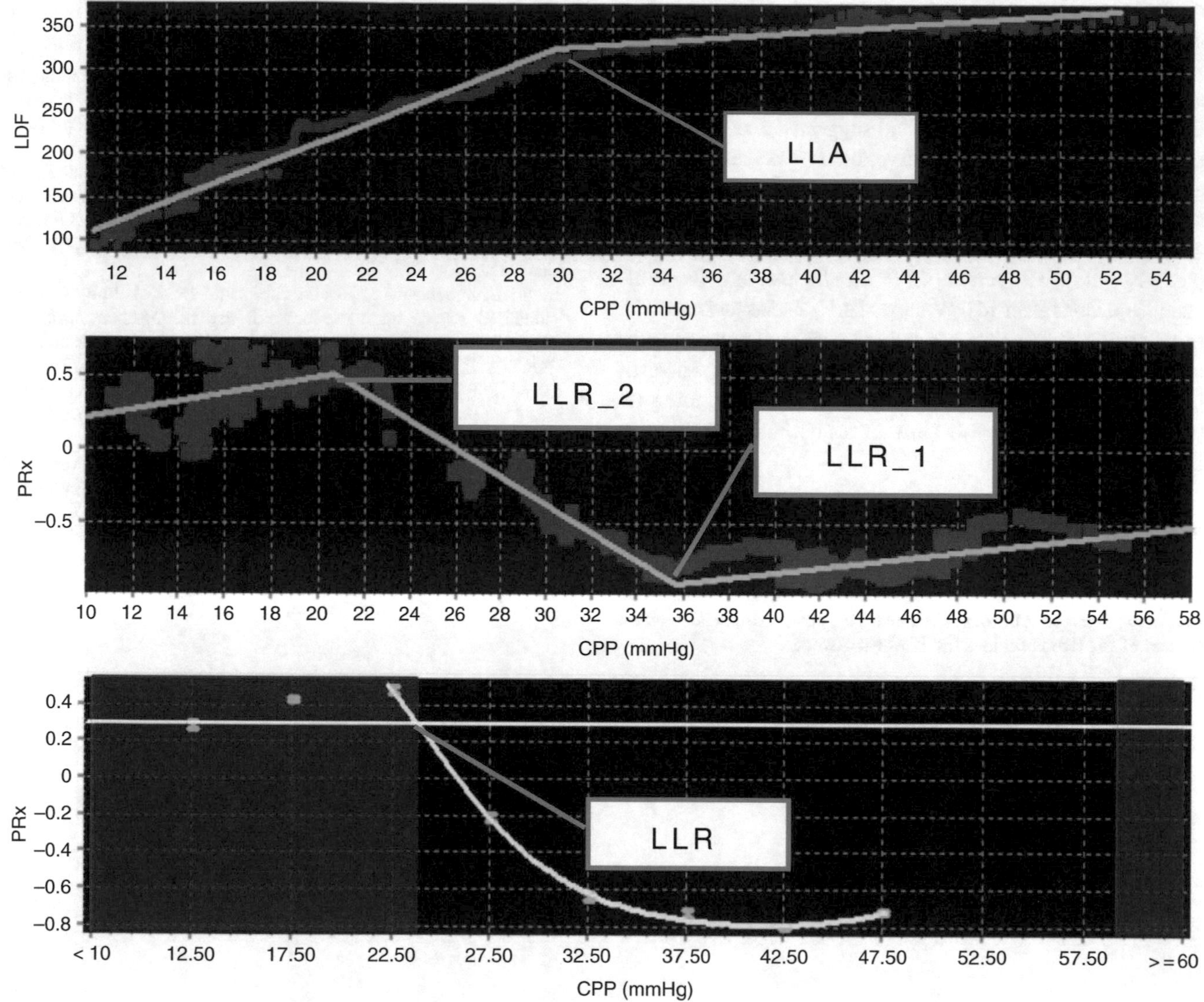

Fig. 2 Difference between static (flow) and dynamic (pressure and volume) assessment of lower limit of autoregulation. The relationships between flow and CPP (top chart) and between PRx and CPP (middle chart) are shown and compared to the error bar chart PRx/CPP. *LDF* laser Doppler flow, *PRx* pressure reactivity index, *CPP* cerebral perfusion pressure. Note that because of the CPP binning process in the error bar chart and its U-shaped curve fit, the exact location of LLR_1 and LLR_2 are impossible to ascertain from this presentation

Table 1 Values of studied variables are reported

N	LLA (mmHg)	LLR (mmHg)	LLR_1 (mmHg)	LLR_2 (mmHg)
1	38	29	40	28
2	35	34	42	28
3	20	19	36	16
4	29	20	34	10
5	30	22	35	20
6	26	28	35	22
7	38	25	49	30
8	32	21	35	20
9	NA	NA	NA	NA

LLA LDF-based lower limit of autoregulation, *LLR* CPP at PRx = 0.3 in error bar plot PRx/CPP, *LLR_1* CPP at first breakpoint in PRx/CPP scatterplot, at which PRx starts worsening, *LLR-2* CPP at second breakpoint in PRx/CPP scatterplot, at which PRx reaches worse status

pressure related, as opposed to static autoregulation, which is flow related. A preserved pressure reactivity is related to a preserved flow regulation, but it is not the same.

Second, the PRx/CPP plot shows an interesting behaviour compared to the LDF/CPP plot in our study. In fact, while the LDF/CPP relationship shows only one clear breakpoint, identifying LLA, the PRx/CPP plot shows two breakpoints. When the relationship between PRx and CPP is explored in a boxplot, the LLR is defined by a threshold. None of these values corresponds to LLA (Fig. 2), but they could possibly describe different features of the same phenomenon. The first breakpoint in the PRx/CPP plot (LLR_1) identifies the CPP at which the pressure reactivity switches from a good autoregulation to a status of lost autoregulation. At this point, though, flow regulation is still maintained, showing that other mechanisms are working. The second PRx/CPP breakpoint is at a lower CPP when compared to LLA. This suggests that for a certain range of CPP (between LLA and LLR_2), vessel reactivity is still partially conserved but not sufficient to ensure flow regulation. Using transcranial Doppler (TCD), Varsos et al. had suggested a second breakpoint of the autoregulatory curve, below the classical LLA, as a point when diastolic ABP reaches the critical closing pressure (CrCP). At this point the diastolic closing margin (diastolic ABP—CrCP) equals 0, and below it, the pressure passivity of CBF versus CPP accelerates and ischemic changes occur faster [6]. Whether LLR_2 is associated with the diastolic closing margin being equal to 0 remains to be demonstrated. These features also need to be further investigated for assessing PRx reliability (and the correct interpretation) in identifying the LLA in a continuous fashion in individual patients.

Acknowledgments M.C. is supported by NIHR Cambridge Biomedical Research Centre.

Conflict of Interest **Authors M.C. and P.S. have a financial interest in part of the licensing fees for ICM+ software.**

References

1. Aries MJH, Czosnyka M, Budohoski KP et al (2012) Continuous determination of optimal cerebral perfusion pressure in traumatic brain injury. Crit Care Med 40(8):2456–2463. https://doi.org/10.1097/CCM.0b013e3182514eb6
2. Steiner LA, Czosnyka M, Piechnik SK, Smielewski P, Chatfield D, Menon DK, Pickard JD (2002) Continuous monitoring of cerebrovascular pressure reactivity allows determination of optimal cerebral perfusion pressure in patients with traumatic brain injury. Crit Care Med 30(4):733–738
3. Beqiri E, Smielewski P, Robba C et al (2019) Feasibility of individualised severe traumatic brain injury management using an automated assessment of optimal cerebral perfusion pressure: the COGiTATE phase II study protocol. BMJ Open 9(9):e030727
4. Donnelly J, Czosnyka M, Adams H et al (2018) Pressure reactivity-based optimal cerebral perfusion pressure in a traumatic brain injury cohort. Acta Neurochir Suppl 126:209–212
5. Brady KM, Easley RB, Kibler K et al (2012) Positive end-expiratory pressure oscillation facilitates brain vascular reactivity monitoring. J Appl Physiol 113(9):1362–1368
6. Varsos GV, Richards HK, Kasprowicz M, Reinhard M, Smielewski P, Brady KM, Pickard JD, Czosnyka M (2014) Cessation of diastolic cerebral blood flow velocity: the role of critical closing pressure. Neurocrit Care 20(1):40–48

Analysis of Intracranial Pressure Pulse–Pressure Relationship: Experimental Validation

Katarzyna Kaczmarska, Piotr Śmielewski, Magdalena Kasprowicz, Agnieszka Kazimierska, Antoni Grzanka, Zofia H. Czosnyka, and Marek Czosnyka

Introduction

The increase in intracranial pressure (ICP) amplitude along with increases in mean ICP is a well-known feature of ICP physiology and has been explained by increased pulse wave transmission due to an increase in intracranial rigidity [1]. A pulse wave is the most characteristic repetitive component of the ICP signal. There is strong interest in the evaluation of the pulse amplitude (AMP) of ICP as well as the slope of the AMP-ICP curve to explain the dynamic aspects of normal pressure hydrocephalus (NPH).

In simplification, the amplitude of ICP can be considered a result of the difference between arterial inflow and venous outflow phase-shifted in time. It was thought that determining the pulse-pressure relationship (PPR) and the shape of pressure volume curve would allow for continuous monitoring of intracranial elasticity and that it may reflect the status of ICP better than the mean value of ICP [2]. However, changes in the PPR slope were observed to occur rapidly from 1 h to another without any appreciable change in the patient's condition [2].

Materials and Methods

Animals and Experimental Paradigms

The experiments were conducted in accordance with the rules provided by the UK Animals Scientific Procedures Act, under a UK Home Office licence and with permission from the Institutional Animal Care and Use Committee at Cambridge University.

We retrospectively analysed the experimental material collected under a wide range of conditions affecting cerebrovascular tone and ICP. Data from 29 anaesthetised New Zealand white rabbits (weighing from 2.7 to 3.7 kg) were collected, including recordings of arterial blood pressure (ABP), ICP, and basilar artery cerebral blood flow velocity (CBFV). All details about the animal preparation and experimental protocols have been described elsewhere [3, 4]. CBFV was monitored by an 8-MHz Doppler ultrasound probe (PcDop 842, SciMed, Bristol, UK) positioned over the basilar artery. A catheter placed in the femoral artery was used for ABP recording (GaelTec, Dunvegan, UK) and for regular sample collection for blood gas analysis.

K. Kaczmarska (✉)
Department of Neurosurgery, Mossakowski Medical Research Centre Polish Academy of Sciences, Warsaw, Poland

Faculty of Electronics and Information Technology, Institute of Electronic Systems, Warsaw University of Technology, Warsaw, Poland
e-mail: kkaczmarska@imdik.pan.pl

P. Śmielewski · Z. H. Czosnyka
Division of Neurosurgery, Department of Clinical Neurosciences, University of Cambridge, Cambridge, UK

M. Kasprowicz · A. Kazimierska
Faculty of Fundamental Problems of Technology, Department of Biomedical Engineering, Wroclaw University of Science and Technology, Wroclaw, Poland

A. Grzanka
Faculty of Health Sciences, Medical University of Warsaw, Warsaw, Poland

M. Czosnyka
Faculty of Electronics and Information Technology, Institute of Electronic Systems, Warsaw University of Technology, Warsaw, Poland

Division of Neurosurgery, Department of Clinical Neurosciences, University of Cambridge, Cambridge, UK

B. Depreitere et al. (eds.), *Intracranial Pressure and Neuromonitoring XVII*, Acta Neurochirurgica Supplement 131,
https://doi.org/10.1007/978-3-030-59436-7_52,

In all rabbits, under various conditions of ABP and arterial carbon dioxide tension ($PaCO_2$), ICP was increased by infusion of Hartmann's solution into the lumbar subarachnoid space with an infusion rate from 0.1 to 0.2 mL/min ($n = 43$).

Arterial hypotension ($n = 19$) was induced by intravenous administration of the short-termautonomic ganglia blocker trimetaphan (0.5 mg/kg).

Changes in $PaCO_2$ ($n = 17$) were achieved by decreasing or increasing the respiratory tidal volume to obtain hypocapnia or hypercapnia, respectively.

We investigated whether the slope of the AMP–ICP line depended on $PaCO_2$ and ABP changes.

Data Acquisition and Analysis

The signals were analysed using ICM+ software (Cambridge Enterprise, Cambridge, UK, http://www.neurosurg.cam.ac.uk/icmplus/).

Raw signals were digitised using a 12-bit analogue–digital converter (DT 2814, Data Translation, Marlboro, MA) and sampled at a frequency of 50 Hz. Fundamental amplitudes of CBFV and ABP pulse waveforms were calculated using spectral analysis (the discrete Fourier transforms performed for 20-s-long data segments). The heart rate was calculated by finding a frequency of the spectral peak associated with the first harmonic of ABP. Mean values of ABP, ICP, CBFV and CPP were calculated in ICM+ by averaging values in a moving 10-s time window.

Pulse amplitude was expressed as a fundamental harmonic of ICP pulse waveform using spectral analysis within the range of the rabbit's heart rate 150–400 bpm. The AMP-ICP line was determined using linear regression. The points above the lower breakpoint of AMP-ICP were taken into account, where the AMP starts to rise with increasing ICP (Fig. 1).

Statistical Analysis

Statistica data analysis software (StatSoft, Inc., Tulsa, OK, USA) was used to perform the statistical analysis. To determine whether the data were normally distributed, the Shapiro–Wilk test was used. The hypothesis of normality was rejected for most of the analysed parameters, so the non-parametric Wilcoxon signed-rank test was used to examine the significance of a difference in analysed variables between baseline and plateau phases of the infusion test. Spearman correlation was used to determine the relationship between the slope of the AMP-ICP and arterial wall tension (WT). The significance level of all tests was set at 0.05

Results

The physiological variables in a total group of animals at three different levels of $PaCO_2$ and two levels of ICP are presented in Table 1 and at two different levels of ABP and ICP in Table 2.

We found a linear correlation between AMP and ICP with positive slope having a mean value of 0.043 with a standard deviation of 0.022. Regression of slope against mean ABP shows negative dependence with a correlation coefficient equal to $R = -0.35$, $p = 0.02$ (Fig. 2a). In contrast, the rela-

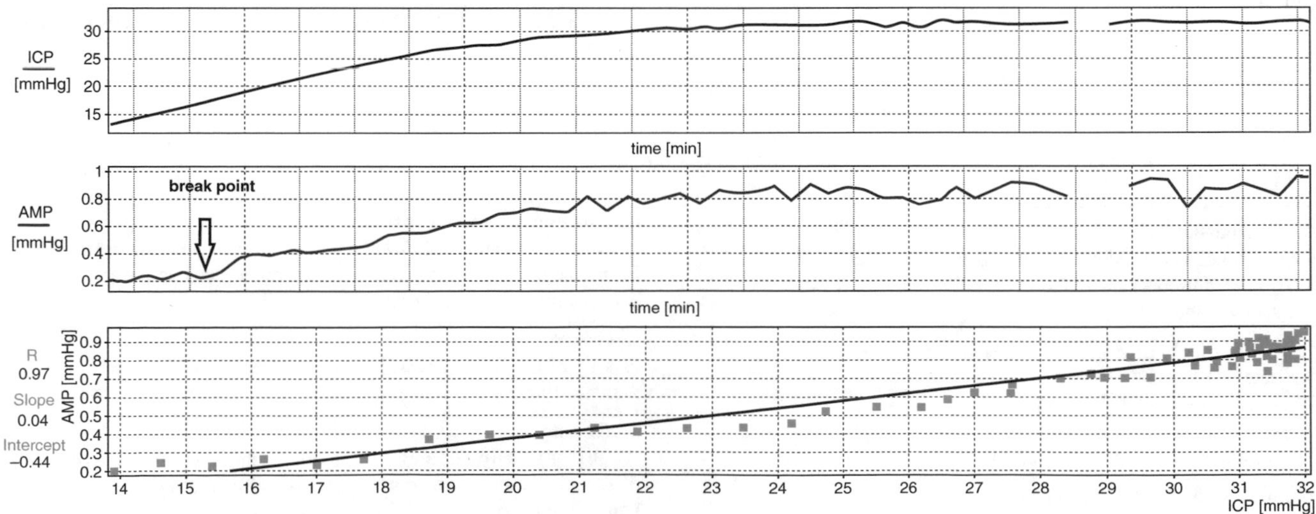

Fig. 1 Example of ICP signal (top) with evaluated amplitude (middle) and their relationship to linear fitting (bottom; AMP is plotted along *y*-axis and ICP along the *x*-axis) during infusion test

Table 1 Median values (25th–75th percentiles) of measured variables at baseline and during plateau phase of ICP elevation for three different levels of $PaCO_2$: hypo-, normo- and hypercapnia

$PaCO_2$	Hypocapnia 25.50 mmHg (23.00–28.00 mmHg)			Normocapnia 35.00 mmHg (34.00–36.00 mmHg)			Hypercapnia 45.45 mmHg (41.00–48.00 mmHg)		
ICP	Baseline	Plateau	*p*-Value	Baseline	Plateau	*p*-Value	Baseline	Plateau	*p*-Value
CBFV (cm/s)	17.12 (10.93–22.26)	11.59 (10.57–17.77)	0.004	18.76 (13.57–22.10)	13.49 (11.40–16.76)	<0.001	23.50 (15.84–27.00)	20.79 (16.23–25.76)	0.285
ABP (mmHg)	81.73 (75.47–95.27)	84.21 (69.74–92.07)	0.657	96.27 (81.50–103.10)	91.46 (80.71–104.90)	0.136	103.80 (102.20–107.10)	103.70 (100.80–107.10)	0.508
ICP (mmHg)	6.96 (5.58–11.65)	29.16 (17.09–36.40)	0.003	7.28 (5.06–11.40)	30.46 (26.39–35.81)	<0.001	11.47 (8.75–14.66)	34.44 (27.11–45.10)	0.005
CPP (mmHg)	75.42 (67.09–86.36)	51.97 (48.92–65.18)	0.003	86.27 (72.23–99.54)	62.47 (49.04–69.12)	<0.001	92.55 (89.59–102.10)	69.23 (60.09–74.84)	0.005

Table 2 Median values (25th–75th percentile) of measured variables at baseline and during plateau phase of ICP elevation for two different levels of ABP: normal pressure and arterial hypotension

ABP	Normal pressure 97.01 mmHg (81.50–105.00)			Arterial hypotension 46.84 mmHg (44.81–55.24)		
ICP	Baseline	Plateau	*p*-Value	Baseline	Plateau	*p*-Value
CBFV (cm/s)	19.21 (13.97–25.77)	14.31 (11.46–21.64)	<0.001	10.46 (9.58–11.33)	10.70 (8.74–12.73)	0.594
ABP (mmHg)	97.01 (81.50–105.00)	97.14 (82.51–107.10)	0.304	46.84 (44.81–55.24)	65.44 (58.79–68.65)	0.007
ICP (mmHg)	6.88 (4.38–11.40)	30.31 (26.39–35.81)	<0.001	9.79 (9.46–11.11)	24.79 (20.95–26.65)	0.007
CPP (mmHg)	87.20 (72.23–99.54)	63.68 (51.11–71.84)	<0.001	36.60 (34.21–42.39)	37.42 (35.48–44.50)	0.594

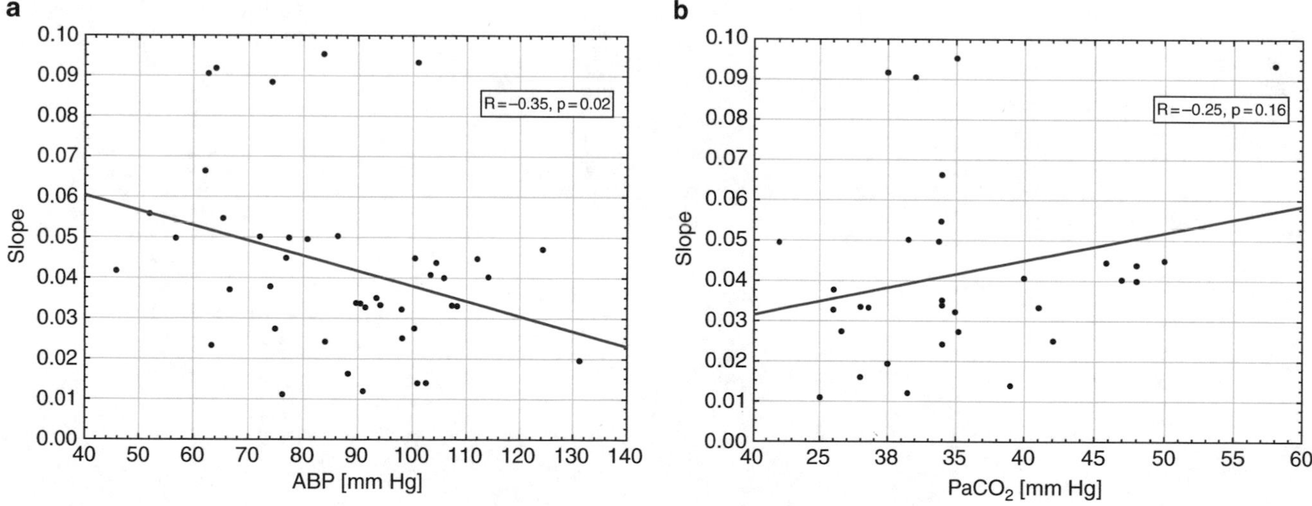

Fig. 2 Scatterplots showing relationships between slope of AMP-ICP line and (**a**) ABP and (**b**) arterial carbon dioxide tension ($PaCO_2$). Data combined from all manoeuvres

tionship between slope and $PaCO_2$ was positive, although it did not reach statistical significance ($R = 0.25$, $p = 0.16$) (Fig. 2b). The slope of the AMP-ICP line was not correlated with the arterial WT calculated during the infusion test ($p > 0.1$).

Discussion

Theoretically, the slope of the amplitude-pressure line is dependent on the product of cerebrospinal elasticity and cerebral fraction of arterial blood stroke volume. While elasticity is a craniospinal parameter, and arterial blood stroke volume is a cerebral haemodynamic parameter. Changes in cerebral haemodynamic conditions are stronger and faster than changes in elasticity. Therefore, a clear relationship between MAP and the slope and a less strong one between slope and $PaCO_2$ were recorded. The slope of the AMP-ICP line is dependent on vascular parameters and should be interpreted with caution as a parameter guiding decision on shunting in patients suffering from NPH.

During intracranial hypertension induced by the infusion of extra fluid volume into the lumbar cerebrospinal space, ABP does not change, while the CBFV decreases significantly ($p < 0.05$). This is due to failing autoregulation and decreases in CPP during infusion.

Acknowledgments *Disclosure:* Authors M.C. and P.S. have a financial interest in part of the licensing fees for ICM+ software.

Funding: **This work was supported by the National Science Centre (Poland) under Grant UMO-2016/23/N/ST7/01364. M.C. is supported by NIHR, Biomedical Research Centre, Cambridge, UK.**

References

1. Hoffmann O, Zierski JT (1982) Analysis of the ICP pulse-pressure relationship as a function of arterial blood pressure. Clinical validation of a mathematical model. Acta Neurochir 66(1–2):1–21
2. Szewczykowski J, Sliwka S, Kunicki A et al (1977) A fast method of estimating the elastance of intracranial system. J Neurosurg 47:19–26
3. Czosnyka M, Piechnik S, Richards HK et al (1997) Contribution of mathematical modelling to the interpretation of bedside tests of cerebrovascular autoregulation. J Neurol Neurosurg Psychiatry 63(6):721–731
4. Czosnyka M, Richards HK, Czosnyka Z et al (1999) Vascular components of cerebrospinal fluid compensation. J Neurosurg 90(4):752–759

Cerebrovascular Impedance During Hemodynamic Change in Rabbits: A Pilot Study

Agnieszka Kazimierska, Magdalena Kasprowicz, Michał M. Placek, and Marek Czosnyka

Introduction

Cerebrovascular impedance describes the relationship between pulsatile arterial blood pressure (ABP) and pulsatile cerebral blood flow (CBF), i.e., the input and response of the cerebral vascular bed [1]. As a complex function of frequency, it is defined by modulus and phase shift, which represent respectively the amplitude ratio and phase difference between components of pressure and flow signals of corresponding frequency [2]. An impedance model of cerebral vascular bed that recognizes the frequency dependence of its parameters has been successfully used in studies on pulsatility index [3, 4] and critical closing pressure [5, 6]; however, while the link between vascular properties and impedance has been widely explored for most major vascular beds, relatively little is known about cerebrovascular impedance patterns [7, 8].

Traditionally, cerebrovascular impedance estimates are derived from Fourier spectra of CBF velocity (CBFV) and ABP [8], and the analysis is limited to steady-state conditions, fulfilling the signal stationarity requirements of Fourier transform. In this study, we propose an approach to calculate cerebrovascular impedance using heartbeat-to-heartbeat analysis and time-frequency methods, which allowed for the assessment of cerebrovascular impedance during controlled changes in ABP and intracranial pressure (ICP) in rabbits.

A. Kazimierska (✉) · M. Kasprowicz
Department of Biomedical Engineering,
Faculty of Fundamental Problems of Technology, Wroclaw University of Science and Technology, Wroclaw, Poland
e-mail: agnieszka.kazimierska@pwr.edu.pl

M. M. Placek
Department of Biomedical Engineering,
Faculty of Fundamental Problems of Technology, Wroclaw University of Science and Technology, Wroclaw, Poland

Brain Physics Laboratory, Division of Neurosurgery,
Department of Clinical Neurosciences,
University of Cambridge, Cambridge, UK

M. Czosnyka
Brain Physics Laboratory, Division of Neurosurgery,
Department of Clinical Neurosciences,
University of Cambridge, Cambridge, UK

Institute of Electronic Systems, Faculty of Electronics and Information Technology, Warsaw University of Technology, Warsaw, Poland

Materials and Methods

Material and Data Acquisition

A retrospective analysis of experiments conducted in New Zealand white rabbits between 1993 and 1997 was performed. The experiments were carried out in accordance with the standards established by the United Kingdom Animals (Scientific Procedures) Act of 1986. The experimental protocol is described in detail in [1, 9].

In short, the animals were anesthetized and supported in a sphinx position. The full group of 20 rabbits was divided into three subgroups, with each of the subgroups undergoing a different procedure: (a) in 8 rabbits a step decrease in ABP was induced by administration of trimetaphan, (b) in 5 rabbits a transient increase in ABP was induced by administration of dopamine, and (c) in 7 rabbits ICP was raised using constant-rate infusion (0.2 mL/min) of normal saline into the lumbar cerebrospinal fluid space.

ABP was recorded in the femoral artery with a direct pressure monitor inserted via a polyethylene cannula. CBFV was recorded in the basilar artery with an 8-MHz transcranial Doppler ultrasound probe positioned over a posterior frontal burr hole. In selected rabbits, ICP was recorded with a subarachnoid microsensor introduced through a second burr hole. The signals were collected using customized software at a sampling frequency ranging from 50 to 100 Hz.

B. Depreitere et al. (eds.), *Intracranial Pressure and Neuromonitoring XVII*, Acta Neurochirurgica Supplement 131,
https://doi.org/10.1007/978-3-030-59436-7_53,

Data Analysis

All analyses were performed using programs custom-written in MATLAB® (MathWorks®, Natick, MA, USA). Prior to analysis, all signals recorded at sampling frequencies under 100 Hz were upsampled to 100 Hz to ensure uniform sampling frequency across the whole data set. Phase-shift analysis was performed on signals bandpass filtered with cutoff frequencies of 1 and 20 Hz.

Selection of analysis period. First, signals were divided into individual heartbeats based on local minima of the CBFV signal. Duration of the analysis period extracted from each recording was expressed in heartbeats to account for variations in heart rate between the animals and during measurements. Due to the contrasting patterns of hemodynamic changes, different analysis periods were selected in each group: (a) for rabbits with arterial hypotension, 800 heartbeats before and 800 heartbeats after trimetaphan injection; (b) for rabbits with arterial hypertension, 100 heartbeats before and 1500 heartbeats after dopamine injection; and (c) for rabbits with intracranial hypertension, 200 heartbeats before and 2000 heartbeats after infusion onset. The time points corresponding to the administration of drugs or infusion onset were annotated manually. Extracted parts of the recording were subsequently used to obtain estimates of cerebrovascular impedance.

Modulus of cerebrovascular impedance. The modulus of cerebrovascular impedance ($|Z|$) describes the ratio of amplitudes of corresponding frequency components of ABP and CBFV [10]. At heart rate frequency, the modulus of cerebrovascular impedance (denoted $|Z(f_{HR})|$) is calculated as

$$\left|Z\left(f_{\text{HR}}\right)\right| = \frac{\text{AMP}_{\text{ABP}}}{\text{AMP}_{\text{CBFV}}} \tag{1}$$

where AMP_{ABP} and AMP_{CBFV} are the amplitudes of the fundamental harmonics of ABP and CBFV, respectively. In this work, to reduce the effect of changes in heart rate, amplitude estimates were calculated on a heartbeat-to-heartbeat basis as the difference between the systolic and the diastolic value of each signal.

Phase shift of cerebrovascular impedance. The phase shift of cerebrovascular impedance (PS) describes the time delay between corresponding frequency components of ABP and CBFV [2]. To follow PS in both time (i.e., during hemodynamic changes) and frequency (i.e., taking into account the changes in heart rate occurring during the experiment), a method of nonstationary signal processing called the joint time and frequency (TF) approach was used. In the TF approach, signals are represented on the two-dimensional time-frequency plane, which makes it possible to track their time-variant spectral content [11]. Here, the Zhao-Atlas-Marks (ZAM) distribution [12] was chosen to obtain estimates of TF phase shift (TFPS) between ABP and CBFV. This distribution is characterized by relatively high suppression of so-called interference cross-terms and limited trade-off between time and frequency resolution. The framework is described in detail in our previous work on the subject of cerebral autoregulation [13].

TFPS in the ZAM-distribution-based approach is calculated as [14]

$$\text{TFPS}(t,f) = \arg\left[S_{\text{ZAM},xy}(t,f)\right] \tag{2}$$

where $S_{\text{ZAM},xy}(t, f)$ is the cross spectrum of signals x and y (here: ABP and CBFV). The cross spectrum (and, similarly, auto spectra of signals x and y, denoted by $S_{\text{ZAM},xx}(t, f)$ and $S_{\text{ZAM},yy}(t, f)$, respectively) is in turn described by the equation [15]

$$S_{\text{ZAM},xy}(t,f) = \int_{-\infty}^{\infty} h(\tau) e^{-j2\pi f\tau} \left[\int_{t-|\tau|/2}^{t+|\tau|/2} g(u-t)\, x\left(u+\frac{\tau}{2}\right) y^*\left(u-\frac{\tau}{2}\right) du\right] d\tau \tag{3}$$

In the preceding equation, g and h are window functions responsible for smoothing the representation in time and frequency domain.

Here the TFPS representation obtained from Eq. (2) was further processed using a two-step masking procedure to extract areas that are both related to heart rate frequency and characterized by significant coupling between ABP and CBFV. To estimate the extent of coupling between the signals in the TF domain, magnitude-squared TF coherence (TFCoh) was used. TFCoh is described as [16]

$$\text{TFCoh}(t,f) = \frac{\left|S^{(c)}_{\text{ZAM},xy}(t,f)\right|^2}{S^{(c)}_{\text{ZAM},xx}(t,f) \cdot S^{(c)}_{\text{ZAM},yy}(t,f)} \tag{4}$$

where the superscript (c) indicates smoothing of the cross and auto spectra required to ensure that TFCoh is bounded to the range <0,1>. Only the (t, f) points of the TFPS representation where the corresponding TFCoh values exceeded the threshold value of 0.9 were included in further analysis [13]. Then a binary mask based on the fundamental frequency of ABP (i.e., the heart rate frequency) was applied to the coherence-filtered TFPS. A 3-decibel mask was obtained using the procedure proposed in [16] by first finding the maximum value in the TF representation of ABP around the heart rate frequency at each time instant and then locating the frequencies at which the value in the representation drops by 3 dB on either side of the maximum. Final time courses of PS at heart rate frequency ($\text{PS}(f_{HR})$) were derived by averaging TFPS values along the frequency axis within the combined coherence- and ABP-based mask at each time instant. Time in seconds was then converted to dimensionless time expressed in heartbeats. Illustrative TF representations used to obtain $\text{PS}(f_{HR})$ are presented in Fig. 1.

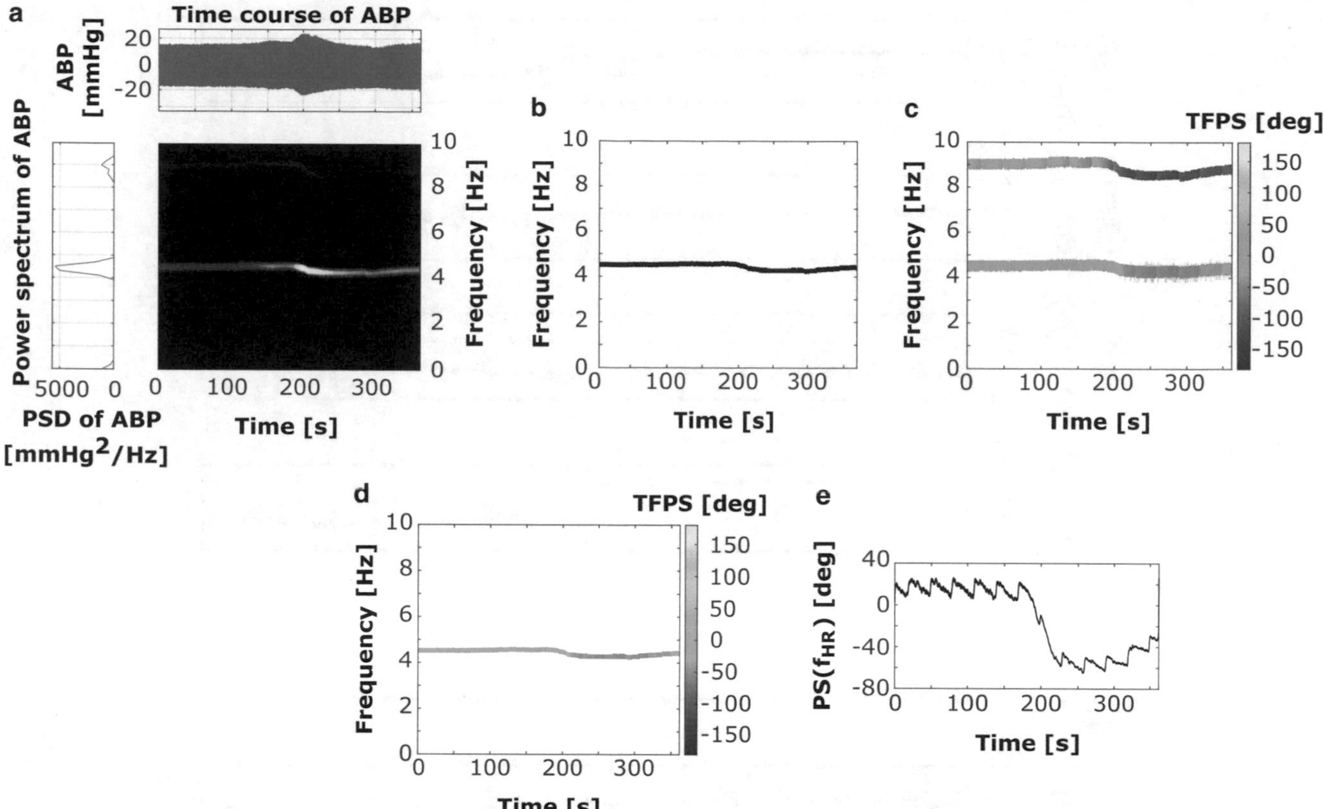

Fig. 1 Illustrative time-frequency representations used to obtain time course of phase shift of cerebrovascular impedance at heart rate frequency (PS(f_{HR})). (**a**) Bandpass-filtered time course (upper plot), power spectrum (left plot), and time-frequency auto spectrum (center graph) of arterial blood pressure (ABP). Note the fundamental harmonic of ABP around 4.5 Hz. (**b**) Binary mask based on the fundamental harmonic of ABP. Black areas indicate parts of the representation included in subsequent analyses. (**c**) Coherence-masked time-frequency phase shift (TFPS) between ABP and cerebral blood flow velocity (CBFV). White areas indicate parts of the representation where coherence between ABP and CBFV is lower than 0.9, which are excluded from subsequent analyses. (**d**) Coherence- and ABP-masked TFPS between ABP and CBFV obtained by overlaying mask presented in (**b**) on representation presented in (**c**). (**e**) Time course of PS(f_{HR}) values obtained from representation presented in (**d**)

Time courses of cerebrovascular impedance estimates. The time courses of $|Z(f_{HR})|$ and PS(f_{HR}) were compared with the time courses of mean ABP, ICP, and cerebral perfusion pressure (CPP; where available, estimated as CPP = ABP − ICP) calculated by averaging the signals over the period of one heartbeat. Illustrative time courses for one rabbit are presented in Fig. 2.

Results

Figure 3 shows the group-averaged time courses of impedance estimates and available parameters (ICP—and, consequently, CPP—was not recorded in the arterial hypertension group).

Following the injection of trimetaphan, mean ABP and mean CBFV both decreased (from the first 200 heartbeats to the last 200 heartbeats: ABP, decrease to 53% [52–57%] of baseline value; CBFV, decrease to 78% [52–96%]; values are presented as median [first-third quartile]). Similarly, CPP fell (to 45% [43–47%]) as mean ICP increased slightly (to 108% [93–172%]). $|Z(f_{HR})|$ decreased to 60% [45–74%] while PS(f_{HR}) changed from 25° [14°–66°] to −26° [−54° to 23°].

Conversely, following administration of dopamine, mean ABP increased (from the first 100 heartbeats to 100 heartbeats around the maximum of group-averaged mean ABP: an increase to 208% [119–214%]), as did mean CBFV (an increase to 117% [104–138%]). $|Z(f_{HR})|$ rose to 141% [123–168%] and PS(f_{HR}) changed from −34° [−50° to -27°] to −27° [−39° to −20°].

Saline infusion resulted in a mean ICP increase to 330% [315–370%] (from the first 200 heartbeats to the last 200 heartbeats), a mean CBFV decrease to 86% [80–98%], and a CPP decrease to 70% [67–82%]. No significant change was observed in either mean ABP or PS(f_{HR}), but $|Z(f_{HR})|$ dropped on average to 76% [69–109%].

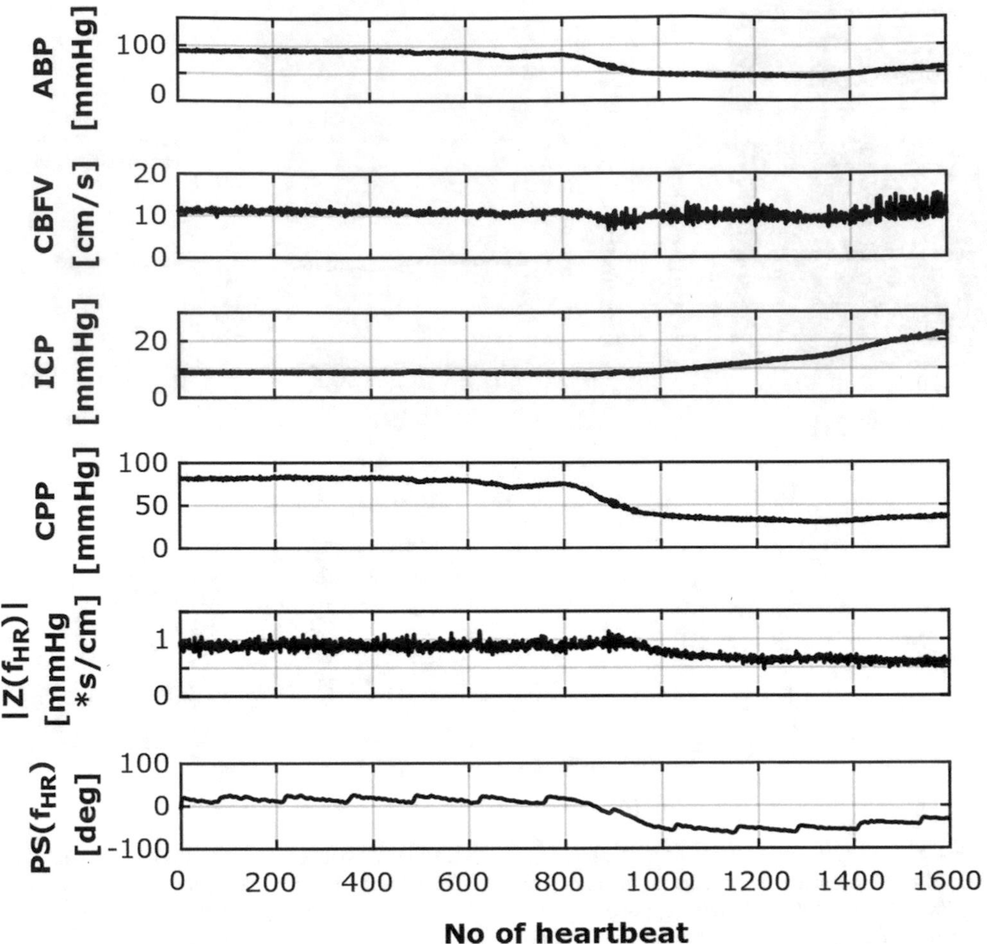

Fig. 2 Illustrative time courses for one rabbit from arterial hypotension group. Top to bottom: mean arterial blood pressure (ABP), mean cerebral blood flow velocity (CBFV), mean intracranial pressure (ICP), cerebral perfusion pressure (CPP), modulus of cerebrovascular impedance at heart rate frequency ($|Z(f_{HR})|$), and phase shift of cerebrovascular impedance at heart rate frequency ($PS(f_{HR})$)

Discussion

Frequency-dependent parameters describing cerebral hemodynamics are traditionally estimated using Fourier analysis [8]. However, the applicability of classical Fourier transform is restricted to steady-state conditions where the signals can be assumed to be stationary, significantly limiting the range of experiments where this approach is valid. On the other hand, the nonstationarity of biomedical signals, including those related to the cardiovascular system, has been widely recognized in recent years, leading to a rise in prominence of more advanced signal processing tools such as time-frequency methods [17]. The approach presented in this study was chosen specifically to offer the possibility of monitoring changes in cerebrovascular impedance estimates in time. In particular, the method of extracting heart-rate-related components of phase shift between ABP and CBFV, which takes into account the degree of coupling between them, uniquely supports tracking related changes despite the time-varying spectral content of the signals. Potential insights into phenomena governing cerebral hemodynamics offered by impedance analysis have been suggested by a number of studies that emphasized the importance of including frequency-dependent properties when interpreting indices describing the state of cerebral circulation in various conditions [3, 4, 8, 18]. In an attempt to extend cerebrovascular impedance analysis to transient hemodynamic changes, we have demonstrated that the proposed procedure allows for the assessment of modulus and phase shift of cerebrovascular impedance during controlled changes in systemic ABP and ICP.

Our results show that both $|Z(f_{HR})|$ and $PS(f_{HR})$ change during alterations in systemic ABP and follow the direction of changes in CPP, with increases observed in the hypertension and decreases in the hypotension group, while only $|Z(f_{HR})|$ is affected by changes in ICP. Interestingly, alterations in $PS(f_{HR})$ appear to depend not only on the magnitude but also the direction of change in ABP and its initial level, since we observed that baseline values of $PS(f_{HR})$ differ

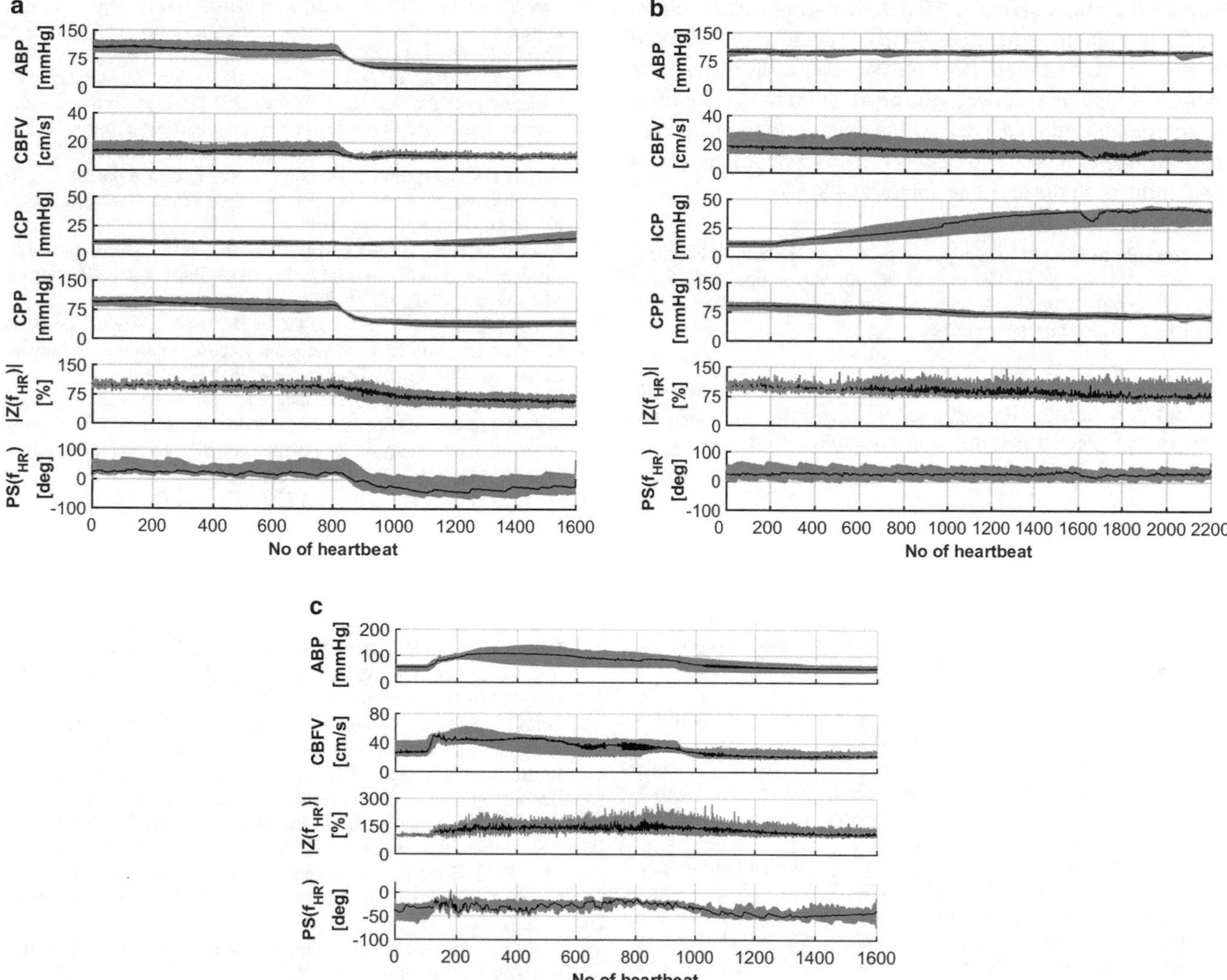

Fig. 3 Group-averaged time courses from (**a**) arterial hypotension, (**b**) intracranial hypertension, and (**c**) arterial hypertension group. Top to bottom: mean arterial blood pressure (ABP), mean cerebral blood flow velocity (CBFV), mean intracranial pressure (ICP; not included in part (**c**)), cerebral perfusion pressure (CPP; not included in part (**c**)), modulus of cerebrovascular impedance at heart rate frequency ($|Z(f_{HR})|$), and phase shift of cerebrovascular impedance at heart rate frequency ($PS(f_{HR})$). $|Z(f_{HR})|$ is presented as a percentage of baseline value. Black lines: median, gray area: interquartile range

between groups. The latter can be, at least in part, explained by the fact that the mean absolute ABP at baseline in the hypertension group (Fig. 3) corresponds to end rather than baseline level in the hypotension group. However, a comparable level of mean ABP reached after dopamine injection still did not produce positive $PS(f_{HR})$, which could be expected by comparison with the hypotension group. So far, phase relationships between ABP and CBFV have primarily been used to assess the state of cerebral autoregulation based on low-frequency components (i.e., below respiration frequency) [19], and little attention has been given to phase shift between signals related to cerebral pulsations in general. One previous study investigated the phase shift between the fundamental harmonics of CBFV and ICP during infusion tests and its relationship with diminished compensatory reserve at higher ICP levels [20]. This study, on the other hand, suggests an influence of the level of CPP on the characteristics of the cerebrovascular bed regarded as a system transferring pressure pulsations to pulsatile flow.

Limitations. In this study, transcranial Doppler measurements of CBFV in the basilar artery were used as estimates of pulsatile CBF, and ABP recordings in the femoral artery were used as substitutes for arterial pressure at brain level. It should be noted that CBFV is not a direct equivalent of the CBF waveform due to its dependence on the diameter of insonated vessels and the properties of the vascular bed, and femoral ABP is only an approximation of input cerebral pressure waveform (although it has been shown that in humans the use of systemic ABP in modeling studies allows for fairly reliable estimation of CBF waveforms when used to replace cerebral pressure [21]). Moreover, the differences in pulse transit time between the heart and femoral and basilar arteries in individual recordings were not compensated, and the physical distance between measurement sites may have influenced the absolute values of PS(f_{HR}).

Acknowledgments M.C. is supported by NIHR Biomedical Research Centre, Cambridge, UK. The authors acknowledge support from the Polish National Agency for Academic Exchange under the International Academic Partnerships programme.

Conflicts of Interest **M.C. has a financial interest in the licensing fees of ICM+ software (https://icmplus.neurosurg.cam.ac.uk). The other authors declare that they have no conflict of interest.**

References

1. Czosnyka M, Richards H, Pickard JD, Harris N, Iyer V (1994) Frequency-dependent properties of cerebral blood transport—an experimental study in anaesthetized rabbits. Ultrasound Med Biol 20:391–399
2. O'Rourke MF (1982) Vascular impedance in studies of arterial and cardiac function. Physiol Rev 62:570–623
3. de Riva N, Budohoski KP, Smielewski P, Kasprowicz M, Zweifel C, Steiner LA, Reinhard M, Fabregas N, Pickard JD, Czosnyka M (2012) Transcranial Doppler pulsatility index: what it is and what it isn't. Neurocrit Care 17:58–66
4. Michel E, Zernikow B (1998) Gosling's Doppler pulsatility index revisited. Ultrasound Med Biol 24:597–599
5. Varsos GV, de Riva N, Smielewski P, Pickard JD, Brady KM, Reinhard M, Avolio A, Czosnyka M (2013) Critical closing pressure during intracranial pressure plateau waves. Neurocrit Care 18:341–348
6. Varsos GV, Richards HK, Kasprowicz M, Reinhard M, Smielewski P, Brady KM, Pickard JD, Czosnyka M (2014) Cessation of diastolic cerebral blood flow velocity: the role of critical closing pressure. Neurocrit Care 20:40–48
7. Tzeng YC, Chan GS (2011) Unraveling the human cerebral circulation: insights from cerebral blood pressure and flow recordings. J Appl Physiol (1985) 111:349–350
8. Zhu YS, Tseng BY, Shibata S, Levine BD, Zhang R (2011) Increases in cerebrovascular impedance in older adults. J Appl Physiol (1985) 111:376–381
9. Czosnyka M, Richards HK, Reinhard M, Steiner LA, Budohoski K, Smielewski P, Pickard JD, Kasprowicz M (2012) Cerebrovascular time constant: dependence on cerebral perfusion pressure and end-tidal carbon dioxide concentration. Neurol Res 34:17–24
10. Varsos GV, Kasprowicz M, Smielewski P, Czosnyka M (2014) Model-based indices describing cerebrovascular dynamics. Neurocrit Care 20:142–157
11. Wacker M, Witte H (2013) Time-frequency techniques in biomedical signal analysis. A tutorial review of similarities and differences. Methods Inf Med 52:279–296
12. Zhao Y, Atlas LE, Marks RJ (1990) The use of cone-shaped kernels for generalized time-frequency representations of nonstationary signals. IEEE Trans Acoust 38:1084–1091
13. Placek MM, Wachel P, Iskander DR, Smielewski P, Uryga A, Mielczarek A, Szczepanski TA, Kasprowicz M (2017) Applying time-frequency analysis to assess cerebral autoregulation during hypercapnia. PLoS One 12:e0181851
14. Orini M, Laguna P, Mainardi LT, Bailon R (2012) Assessment of the dynamic interactions between heart rate and arterial pressure by the cross time-frequency analysis. Physiol Meas 33: 315–331
15. Auger F, Flandrin P, Goncalves P, Lemoine O (1996) Time-frequency toolbox. http://tftb.nongnu.org/ Accessed 9 Nov 2020
16. Muma M, Iskander DR, Collins MJ (2010) The role of cardiopulmonary signals in the dynamics of the eye's wavefront aberrations. IEEE Trans Biomed Eng 57:373–383
17. Orini M, Laguna P, Mainardi LT, Bailon R (2017) Time-frequency analysis of cardiovascular signals and their dynamic interactions. In: Barbieri R, Scilingo EP, Valenza G (eds) Complexity and non-linearity in cardiovascular signals. Springer, Cham, pp 257–287
18. Varsos GV, Richards H, Kasprowicz M, Budohoski KP, Brady KM, Reinhard M, Avolio A, Smielewski P, Pickard JD, Czosnyka M (2013) Critical closing pressure determined with a model of cerebrovascular impedance. J Cereb Blood Flow Metab 33:235–243
19. Diehl RR (2002) Cerebral autoregulation studies in clinical practice. Eur J Ultrasound 16:31–36
20. Kim DJ, Czosnyka M, Kim H, Baledent O, Smielewski P, Garnett MR, Czosnyka Z (2015) Phase-shift between arterial flow and ICP pulse during infusion test. Acta Neurochir 157: 633–638
21. Zamir M, Moir ME, Klassen SA, Balestrini CS, Shoemaker JK (2018) Cerebrovascular compliance within the rigid confines of the skull. Front Physiol 9:940

Improved Cerebral Perfusion Pressure and Microcirculation by Drag Reducing Polymer-Enforced Resuscitation Fluid After Traumatic Brain Injury and Hemorrhagic Shock

Denis E. Bragin, Olga A. Bragina, Alex Trofimov, Lucy Berliba, Marina V. Kameneva, and Edwin M. Nemoto

Introduction

A serious complication of traumatic brain injury (TBI) in polytrauma is arterial hypotension due to hemorrhagic shock (HS) that impairs cerebral autoregulation and reduces cerebral perfusion pressure (CPP) and cerebral blood flow (CBF), increasing hypoxia and doubling mortality [1–3]. The duration of hypotension is inversely associated with outcome in TBI patients [4]. TBI + HS occurs more frequently on the battlefield because of extremity or penetrating injuries from shrapnel and has taken on even greater importance owing to the increased incidence of improvised explosive devices [5]. Current treatments for HS are based on volume expansion with resuscitation fluids (RFs) with the goal of rapidly restoring blood pressure and, potentially, CPP, followed by transfusion of donor blood at the hospital. In the case of TBI, this approach is controversial because it does not adequately alleviate impaired cerebral microcirculation and is thus not neuroprotective. Moreover, *crystalloids*, standard civilian RFs, rapidly move into the extravascular compartment, requiring large infused volumes that could exacerbate pulmonary and brain edema and lead to increased bleeding, dilution coagulopathy, and increased mortality [6]. *Colloid solutions*, such as hydroxyethyl starch, are preferred for resuscitation in *combat casualty* settings due to lower volume and weight. However, the use of colloids is controversial due to increased rates of coagulopathies, kidney failure, and mortality [7]. Thus, novel types of RF and approaches are needed. One of the new possible approaches we propose is an addition of drag-reducing polymers (DRPs) to the RF. DRPs are linear, blood-soluble, nontoxic macromolecules that in nanomolar concentrations substantially improve the rheological properties of blood flow. In our previous studies in a rat TBI model, we showed that nanomolar concentrations of DRP significantly enhanced microvascular perfusion and tissue oxygenation in pericontusional areas and protected neurons [8]. It has also been demonstrated that DRP additives to RF (DRP-RF) reduced the required fluid amount and improved hemodynamics, blood chemistry, and survival in various animal models of HS [9]. We hypothesized that a small amount of DRP, added to isotonic Hetastarch (HES 6%; 0.9% NaCl), would improve cerebral microcirculation and oxygen supply but not induce ICP increase. The HES was chosen as a first-choice non-blood-derived RF for TBI + HS in combat casualty settings [10].

D. E. Bragin (✉)
Lovelace Biomedical Research Institute, Albuquerque, NM, USA

Department of Neurosurgery, University of New Mexico School of Medicine, Albuquerque, NM, USA
e-mail: dbragin@lrri.org

O. A. Bragina · L. Berliba · E. M. Nemoto
Lovelace Biomedical Research Institute, Albuquerque, NM, USA

A. Trofimov
Department of Neurosurgery, Privolzhsky Research Medical University, Nizhniy Novgorod, Russia

M. V. Kameneva
McGowan Institute for Regenerative Medicine, University of Pittsburgh, Pittsburgh, PA, USA

Methods

All procedures were performed as previously described in earlier studies [6]. Protocol 200640 was approved by the Institutional Animal Care and Use Committee of the University of New Mexico, and the studies were conducted according to the NIH Guide for the Care and Use of Laboratory Animals.

Overall Study Design

TBI was induced after baseline physiological recording and followed by a 1-h *hemorrhagic phase*, where blood was slowly

B. Depreitere et al. (eds.), *Intracranial Pressure and Neuromonitoring XVII*, Acta Neurochirurgica Supplement 131,
https://doi.org/10.1007/978-3-030-59436-7_54,

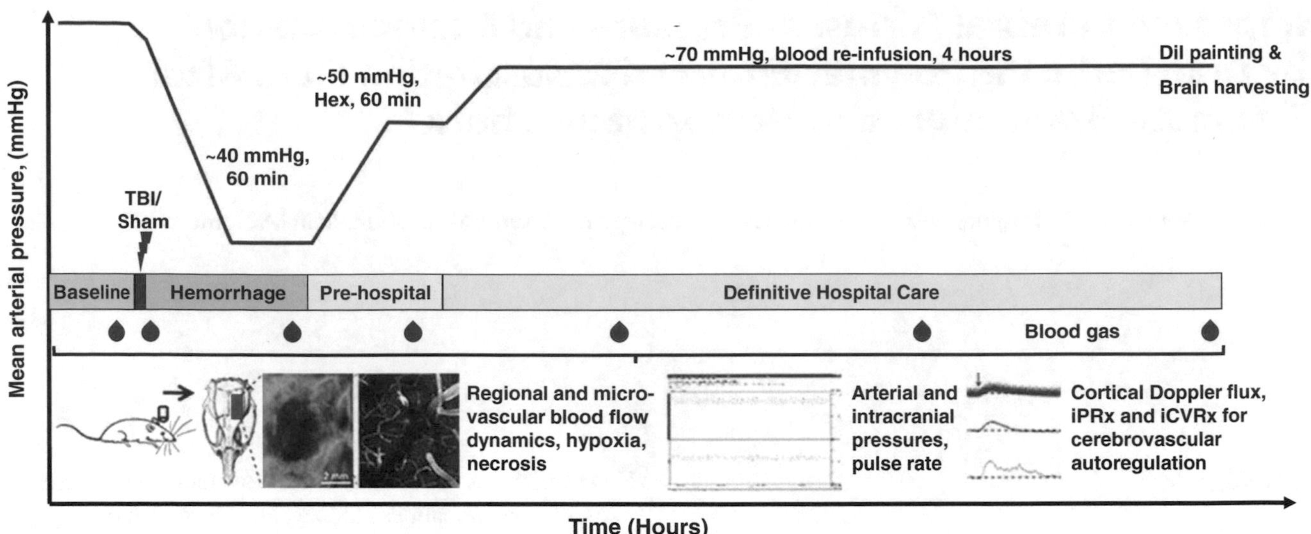

Fig. 1 Experimental design

withdrawn through the femoral vein to decrease mean arterial pressure (MAP) to 40 mmHg. In the subsequent 1-h *prehospital care phase*, isotonic RFs (HES 6%; 0.9% NaCl) or (HES-DRP) were gradually infused intravenously to increase MAP to ~55 mmHg and CBF (Doppler flux) to ~65% of baseline. In the subsequent 3-h *definitive hospital care phase*, shed blood was reinfused to a MAP of 70 mmHg and CBF of ~75% of baseline (Fig. 1). Arterial and intracranial pressures were continuously monitored using the Biopac system (Goleta, CA). In vivo two-photon laser scanning microscopy (2PLSM) over the pericontusional area of the parietal cortex of the rat brain was performed during the whole study. Monitored variables included cerebral microvascular blood flow velocity, number of perfused capillaries, tissue oxygen supply (Nicotinamide adenine dinucleotide (NADH) autofluorescence) and neuronal necrosis (intravenous propidium iodide). The laser Doppler flux (LDF) was measured via a lateral temporal window using a 0.9-mm-diameter probe (DRT4, Moor Inst., Axminster, UK) in the same region of the brain studied by 2PLSM. Brain and rectal temperatures were monitored and maintained at 38 ± 0.5 °C. Arterial blood samples for gases, electrolytes, hematocrit, base excess, and pH, as well as kidney function (creatinine), were measured hourly (epoc Blood Analysis System, Alere Inc., Waltham, MA, USA). At the end of the experiments, animals were subjected to perfusion with vessel painting.

Surgical Preparation

Acclimatized male Sprague-Dawley rats (250–300 g) were ventilated on isoflurane (2%), nitrous oxide (69%), and oxygen (29%) anesthesia. Femoral venous and arterial catheters (PE 50) were inserted for fluid and drug administration, controlled hemorrhage, arterial pressure monitoring, and blood sampling, respectively. A catheter (PE 50) inserted into the cisterna magna through the atlanto-occipital membrane was used to monitor intracranial pressure (ICP). For TBI and imaging, a craniotomy (5 mm) over the left parietal cortex was filled with agarose in saline (2%) and sealed by a glass cover. The fluid percussion TBI was induced by a pulse from the pneumatic impactor connected to the brain through a transducer filled with artificial cerebrospinal fluid (1.5 atm, 50 ms). For HS, blood was slowly withdrawn through the femoral vein.

DRP Preparation

Polyethylene oxide (PEO) (MW ~4000 kDa) was dissolved in saline to 0.1% (1000 ppm), dialyzed against saline using a 50-kD cutoff membrane, diluted in saline to 50 ppm, slow rocked for ~2 h, and then sterilized using a 0.22-μm filter [6]. HES-DRP was prepared before infusion by adding DRP to the Hetastarch to reach the final DRP concentration of 0.0005% (5 ppm).

Two-Photon Laser Scanning Microscopy

Fluorescent serum (intravenous fluorescein isothiocyanate (FITS) dextran, 150 kDa in physiological saline, 5% wt/vol) was visualized using an Olympus BX 51WI upright microscope and water-immersion LUMPlan FL/IR 20×/0.50 W objective. Excitation was provided by a Prairie View Ultima multiphoton microscopy laser scan unit powered by a Millennia Prime 10 W diode laser source pumping a Tsunami Ti:Sapphire laser (Spectra-Physics, Mountain View, CA, USA) tuned to 750-nm center wavelength. Bandpass-filtered epifluorescence (510–530 nm for FITS, 445–475 nm for NADH, and 565–600 for Ethidium bromide (ET)) was collected by photomultiplier tubes of the Prairie View Ultima system. Images (512 × 512 pixels, 0.15 μm/pixel on the x- and y-axes) or line scans were acquired using Prairie View software. Red blood cell flow velocity was measured in microvessels ranging from 3 to 50 μm in diameter up to 500 μm below the surface of the parietal cortex, as described previously [5]. Tissue hypoxia was assessed by NADH autofluorescence measurement. In an offline analysis, using NIH ImageJ software, a three-dimensional anatomy of the vasculature in areas of interest were reconstructed from two-dimensional (planar) scans of the fluorescence intensity obtained at successive focal depths in the cortex (XYZ stack).

Animal Perfusion and Vessel Painting

At the end of the study, cerebral vessels were painted by cardiac perfusion with 1,1′-dioctadecyl-3,3,3′,3′-tetramethylindocarbocyanine perchlorate (DiI, Invitrogen, USA), which binds preferentially to endothelial cells. The sequential order for infusion of solutions was as follows: (a) Phosphate-buffered saline (PBS) (150 mL), (b) 50 mL DiI (13 μg/mL), and (c) paraformaldehyde (4%, 200 mL). Then the brain was extracted from the skull and all meninges removed. Imaging was done by 2PLSM in a custom-made fixed tissue imaging chamber.

Statistical analysis was done with GraphPad Prism software 6.0 (La Jolla, CA, USA) by Kolmogorov-Smirnov test or Student's t-test where suitable. Intergroup differences were evaluated using a two-way analysis of variance (ANOVA) for multiple comparisons and post hoc testing with the Mann-Whitney U-test. Data are presented as mean ± standard error, statistical significance was preset to $p < 0.05$.

Results

Moderate TBI did not induce significant changes in MAP, ICP, and CPP, while cortical flux, measured by surface laser Doppler probe in the pericontusional area, fell to 86.9 ± 5.1 a.u. from the baseline ($p < 0.05$). In the pericontusional area after TBI, microvascular CBF, measured by in vivo 2PLSM, showed a reduction in capillary flow velocity to 0.62 ± 0.04 mm/s from 0.87 ± 0.06 mm/s and approximately 18% reduction in the number of functioning capillaries due to microthrombosis, leading to tissue hypoxia, reflected by an approximately 23% increase in NADH autofluorescence ($p < 0.05$ from baseline) (Fig. 2), which agrees with our previous observations [6].

Subsequent hemorrhagic shock reduced MAP to 42.5 ± 7 mmHg and ICP to 5.4 ± 5 mmHg and calculated CPP to 37.5 ± 5 mmHg (Fig. 2). This caused further cortical LDF reduction to 46 ± 6 a.u. from baseline (Fig. 2d), a, additional twofold reduction in capillary flow velocity, microthrombosis, and tissue oxygenation, leading to neuronal necrosis.

In the prehospital phase, HES, slowly infused in the amount of 4.5 ± 1.8 mL, restored MAP to 59.4 ± 6 mmHg and cortical LDF to 58.9 ± 6.8 a.u. (Fig. 2a, d). However, ICP increased to 32.6 ± 8 mmHg and further decreased CPP to 26.8 ± 4.5 mmHg (Fig. 2b, c), while capillary perfusion and tissue oxygen supply remained the same.

HES-DRP, infused during the prehospital phase in the smaller amount of 1.9 ± 0.8 mL, increased MAP to 60.3 ± 6 mmHg, while cortical LDF increased to 67.3 ± 6.1% (Fig. 2a, d). The infusion of HES-DRP did not induce such an increase in ICP (15.4 ± 7.9 mmHg) or a decrease in CPP (44.9 ± 4.6 mmHg) as in the HES group ($p < 0.05$ from HES) (Fig. 2b, c). As a result, capillary perfusion and tissue oxygen supply substantially increased.

During the hospital phase in the HES group, the reinfusion of blood increased MAP to 71.4 ± 7 mmHg and cortical LDF to 72.8 ± 8.4 a.u. (Fig. 2a, d). However, ICP remained high (34.8 ± 6.1 mmHg), while CPP increased insignificantly to 36.6 ± 4.5 mmHg because the MAP rise remained low (Fig. 2b, c). As in the prehospital phase, microcirculation and tissue oxygenation in the pericontusional regions did not change significantly; however, there was a trend toward improvement. The number of dead neurons by the end of the hospital phase was 185.5 ± 10.3 per 0.075 mm^3 of tissue, while the microvascular density was 3.2 ± 0.3% vessel/total area×100 (Fig. 3). The contusion volume reached 42 mm^3 (Fig. 3).

In the HES-DRP group, the reinfusion of blood *during the hospital phase* increased MAP to 73.2 ± 6.7 mmHg and cortical LDF to 81.8 ± 6.8 a.u. (Fig. 2a, d). The ICP level unchanged, while CPP increased to 56.4 mmHg because of the MAP increase ($p < 0.05$ from the HES) (Fig. 2b, c). Perfusion in capillaries and tissue oxygenation further improved, which protected neurons from necrosis, as the number of dead neurons was significantly less than in the HES group: 67.1 ± 8.8 per 0.075 mm^3 ($p < 0.01$ from the HES group) (Fig. 3). DiI vessel painting showed less reduction in microvascular density compared to the HES group as percentage of vessel/total area×100 was 5.1 ± 0.4 ($p < 0.05$)

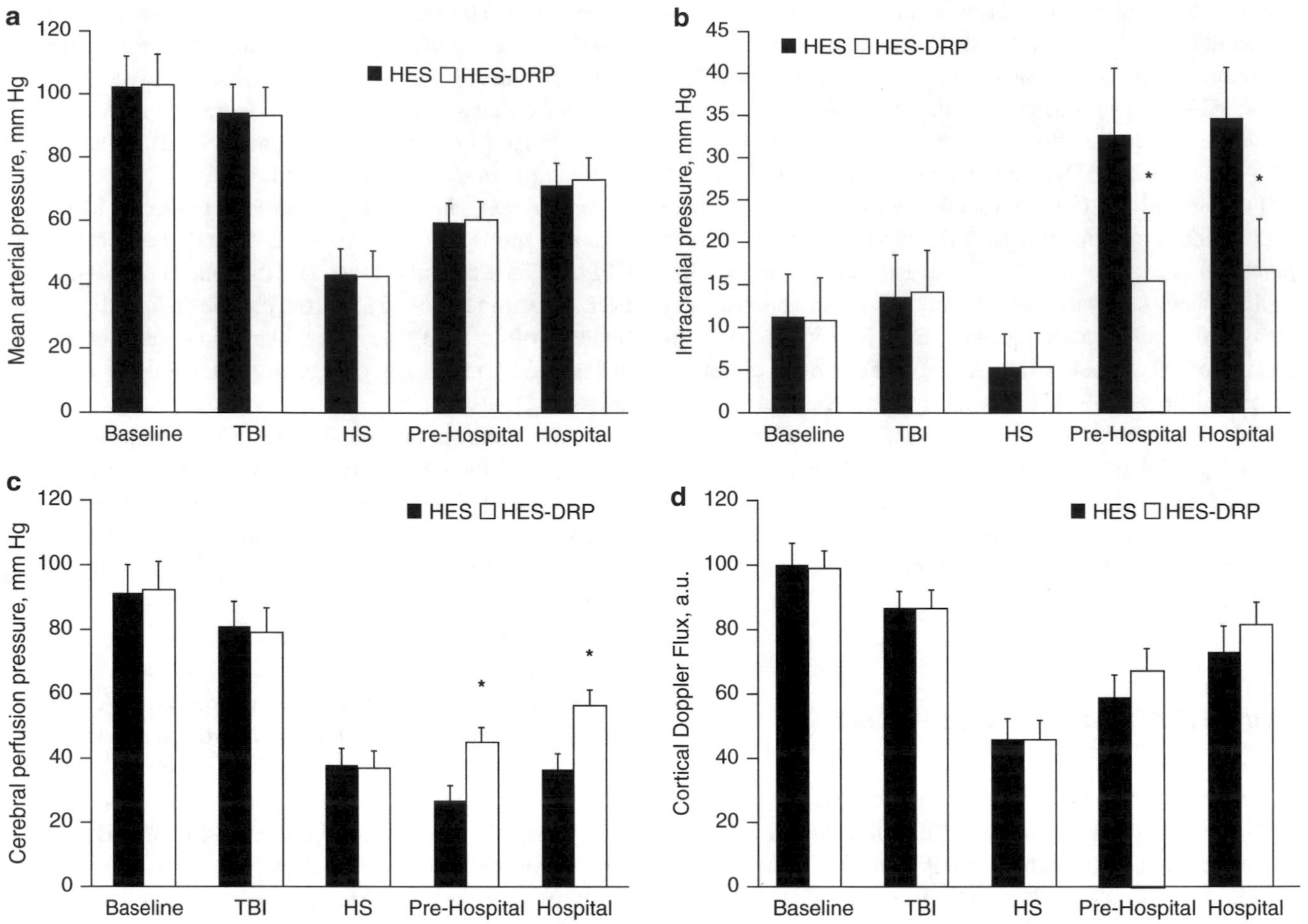

Fig. 2 Changes in arterial pressure, intracranial pressure, cerebral perfusion pressure, and cortical Doppler flux at resuscitation with Hetastarch (HES) and with drag-reducing polymer addition (HES-DRP) after TBI with hemorrhagic shock. (**a**) Arterial pressure; (**b**) intracranial pressure; (**c**) cerebral perfusion pressure; and (**d**) cortical Doppler flux. $n = 10$, $^*p < 0.05$ between HES and HES-DRP

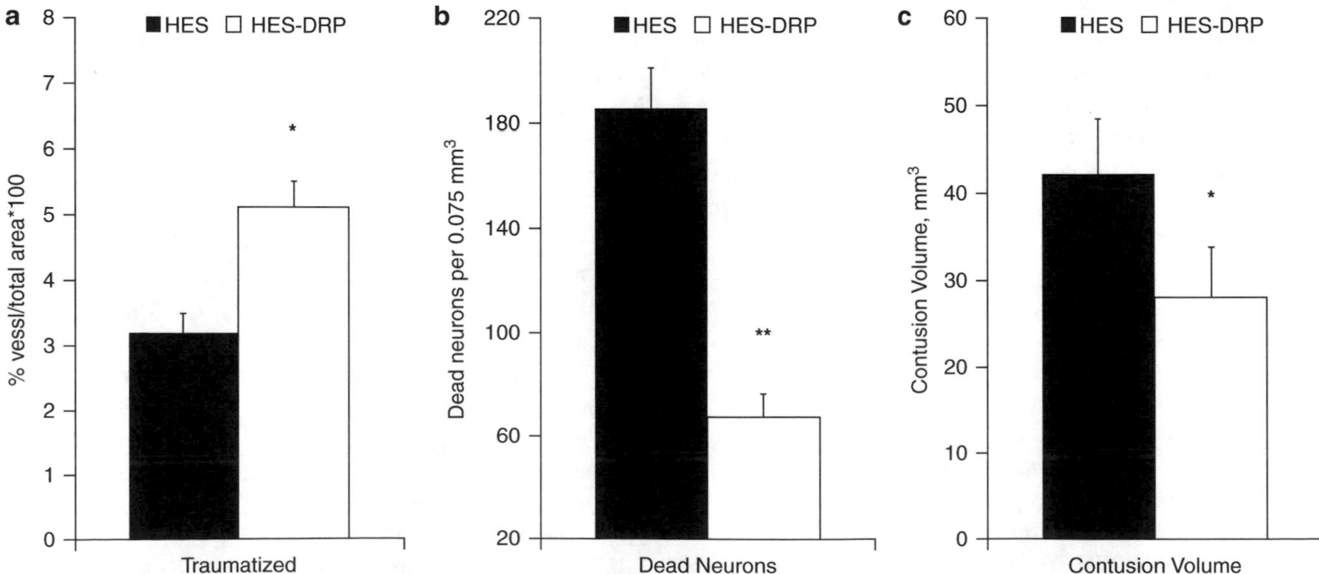

Fig. 3 HES-DRP better than HES (**a**) Prevents microthrombosis; (**b**) protects neurons; and (**c**) reduces contusion volume. $n = 10$, $^*p < 0.05$, $^{**}p < 0.05$ between HES and HES-DRP

(Fig. 3). The contusion volume was also less than in the HES group: 28 ± 5.7 mm^3 ($p < 0.05$) (Fig. 3).

Discussion

In this and previous studies [8, 9] we have shown that DRP addition to RF improves cerebral microcirculation by increasing the blood flow rate in arterioles by the flow velocity increase due to reduction of flow vortices and separations at vessel bifurcations, leading to pressure loss decrease across the arterial tree. All of these mechanisms lead to an increase in the precapillary pressure, enhancing capillary flow, reducing capillary thrombosis, increasing the number of functioning capillaries and the number of red blood cells flowing through, which improves tissue oxygenation. Thus, DRP addition transforms ordinary RF to a neuroprotective fluid through the decrease in cerebral ischemia. In addition, HES-DRP requires a lower volume to be infused, which is especially important to avoid edema expansion in a traumatized brain. This is of particular importance as large volumes of infused current RFs move into the extravascular space, aggravating brain edema [11], intracranial hypertension, and reduction in CPP, thereby decreasing the oxygen-carrying capacity of blood, which exacerbates tissue hypoxia in the injured brain [12]. Restored by HES-DRP, capillary perfusion is crucial to sustain homeostasis, remove metabolites that may exert toxic effects, and improve oxygen supply.

The limitation of the study is the lack of a specific evaluation of HES and HES-DRP effects on kidney function and the coagulation system. However, we were able to estimate kidney function by creatinine level in arterial blood samples. Creatinine is a breakdown product of creatine phosphate from muscle and protein metabolism that filters continuously through healthy kidneys and is excreted in urine. Creatinine level in the blood is a useful marker of kidney function, with a critical level of >4–5 mg/dL. In the HES-DRP group, arterial blood creatinine was significantly lower than in the HES group (1.37 ± 0.29 vs. 2.41 ± 0.34 mg/dL, respectively, $p < 0.05$), compared to the baseline of 0.67 ± 0.24 mg/dL, which reflects better-preserved kidney function. Future research will seek to determine whether this effect is due to a possible nephroprotective effect of DRP additive or reduced infused volume, as well as an impact on the coagulation system. Nevertheless, even in the HES group, arterial blood creatinine levels did not reach the critical level.

Conclusions

Resuscitation after TBI/HS using HES-DRP restores CBF and reduces tissue hypoxia and neuronal necrosis compared to HES. HES-DRP requires an infusion of smaller volume, resulting in lower ICP and brain edema but higher CPP compared to HES.

Acknowledgments This work was supported by the US Department of Defense Grant DOD CDMRP DM160142-W81XWH-17-2-0053.

References

1. Manley G, Knudson MM, Morabito D et al (2001) Hypotension, hypoxia, and head injury: frequency, duration, and consequences. Arch Surg 136(10):1118–1123
2. Navarro JC, Pillai S, Cherian L et al (2012) Histopathological and behavioral effects of immediate and delayed hemorrhagic shock after mild traumatic brain injury in rats. J Neurotrauma 29(2):322–334
3. Chesnut RM, Marshall SB, Piek J et al (1993) Early and late systemic hypotension as a frequent and fundamental source of cerebral ischemia following severe brain injury in the Traumatic Coma Data Bank. Acta Neurochir Suppl 59:121–154
4. Pietropaoli JA, Rogers FB, Shackford SR et al (1992) The deleterious effects of intraoperative hypotension on outcome in patients with severe head injuries. J Trauma 33(3):403–407
5. Fabrizio KS, Keltner NL (2010) Traumatic brain injury in operation enduring freedom/operation Iraqi freedom: a primer. Nurs Clin North Am 45(4):569–580
6. Ramming S, Shackford SR, Zhuang J et al (1994) The relationship of fluid balance and sodium administration to cerebral edema formation and intracranial pressure in a porcine model of brain injury. J Trauma 37(5):705–713
7. Adamik KN, Yozova ID (2019) Starch wars-new episodes of the saga. changes in regulations on hydroxyethyl starch in the european union. Front Vet Sci 18(5):336
8. Bragin DE, Kameneva MV, Bragina OA et al (2017) Rheological effects of drag-reducing polymers improve cerebral blood flow and oxygenation after traumatic brain injury in rats. J Cereb Blood Flow Metab 37(3):762–775
9. Kameneva MV, Wu ZJ, Uraysh A et al (2004) Blood soluble drag-reducing polymers prevent lethality from hemorrhagic shock in acute animal experiments. Biorheology 41(1):53–61
10. US Department of Defense Center of Excellence for Trauma. Joint Trauma System Tactical Combat Casualty Care Guidelines (2019). https://www.deployedmedicine.com/market/11/content/40
11. Falk JL (1995) Fluid resuscitation in brain-injured patients. Crit Care Med 23(1):4–6
12. Lee EJ, Hung YC, Lee MY (1999) Anemic hypoxia in moderate intracerebral hemorrhage: the alterations of cerebral hemodynamics and brain metabolism. J Neurol Sci 164(2):117–123

Critical Closing Pressure by Diffuse Correlation Spectroscopy in a Neonatal Piglet Model

Leah I. Elizondo, Eric L. Vu, Kathleen K. Kibler, Danielle R. Rios, R. Blaine Easley, Dean Andropoulos, Sebastian Acosta, Craig Rusin, Kenneth Brady, and Christopher J. Rhee

Background

Premature infants have an overall increased risk of mortality and neurodevelopmental deficits compared to infants born at term or near term. Acquired brain injury, especially in extremely low birth weight (ELBW) infants, is highest during the first week of life and includes hypoxic-ischemic injury, periventricular leukomalacia (PVL), and intraventricular hemorrhage (IVH) [1, 2]. These various insults can result from alterations in cerebral blood flow (CBF) and arterial blood pressure (ABP). Ischemia can result when the blood flow falls below the level necessary to support normal function. Alternatively, IVH may occur when blood flow exceeds the capacity of the blood vessels in the brain, typically within the germinal matrix. CBF is, in part, influenced by ABP; however, an optimal ABP required to maintain adequate brain perfusion is currently unknown despite the continued use of ABP as the proxy for CBF in the neonatal intensive care unit (NICU).

In adults and healthy infants, cerebral perfusion pressure (CPP) is maintained by cerebrovascular pressure autoregulation. When CPP falls below the lower limit of autoregulation, CBF becomes pressure passive where decreases in ABP result in decreases in CBF and place the brain at risk for injury. Cerebral pressure passivity has been seen in the first week of life and in sick preterm infants and is associated with IVH [3]. The reduction of CPP even further leads to a cessation of CBF. The ABP at which CBF ceases is the critical closing pressure (CrCP).

Using transcranial Doppler (TCD) ultrasonography, Rhee et al. utilized a novel brain-specific perfusion parameter, the diastolic closing margin (DCM), which is the difference between diastolic ABP and CrCP [4]. This parameter normalizes ABP to the CrCP, thereby rendering an effective CPP. In this study, a high DCM was strongly associated with severe IVH when ABP alone was not predictive of neurological injury. The ability to prevent acquired brain injury in ELBW infants is hindered by the lack of complete understanding of the pathophysiology of disease combined with a lack of reliable bedside monitoring approaches available for recognizing hemodynamic risk factors.

TCD ultrasound and near-infrared spectroscopy (NIRS) are the currently available modalities available at the bedside for estimating CBF in preterm infants. TCD ultrasound measures macrovascular blood flow velocity, usually in the cerebral arteries [5]. It has been used to measure CBF velocity by measuring the frequency shift of scattering of moving red blood cells in response to acoustic waves. TCD ultrasound has been used to study CBF, CrCP, and DCM in animal models and humans [6, 7]. It is often difficult, however, to maintain continuous measurements using TCD ultrasonography due to the heat generated by the ultrasound probe. NIRS is also noninvasive and utilizes nonionizing near-infrared light to measure tissue oxy- and deoxyhemoglobin concentrations [8]. It calculates CBF indirectly based on Fick's principle and also reports regional oxygen saturation for the interrogated organ. Hence, NIRS is limited by the assumption that CBF, cerebral blood volume, and cerebral oxygen extraction remain constant, which is not always the case in clinical scenarios.

Diffuse correlation spectroscopy (DCS) is a promising optical modality that uses near-infrared light to noninvasively quantify CBF by measuring the microvascular flow of deep tissue [3, 9]. The study of the microvascular component of cerebrovasculature is promising because

L. I. Elizondo · K. K. Kibler · R. B. Easley · D. Andropoulos
S. Acosta · C. Rusin · C. J. Rhee (✉)
Baylor College of Medicine, Texas Children's Hospital, Houston, TX, USA
e-mail: cjrhee@texaschildrens.org

E. L. Vu · K. Brady
Northwestern University, Lurie Children's Hospital, Chicago, IL, USA

D. R. Rios
University of Iowa, Stead Family Children's Hospital, Iowa City, IA, USA

B. Depreitere et al. (eds.), *Intracranial Pressure and Neuromonitoring XVII*, Acta Neurochirurgica Supplement 131,
https://doi.org/10.1007/978-3-030-59436-7_55,

the microvasculature controls oxygen and nutrient delivery to tissues. The advantages of DCS are that it is portable and continuous and can be used at any location of the patient's head without exposing the patient to ionizing radiation. Additionally, it can measure cerebral oxygenation, CBF, and oxygen metabolism similarly to combining NIRS and TCD into one instrument [9]. Multiple validation studies in animal models have shown that absolute and relative changes in CBF as measured by DCS correlate with multiple studied modalities, including NIRS, spin-labeled magnetic resonance imaging, and invasive laser Doppler flowmetry [9]. At present, there are limited studies comparing measures of CBF by DCS to TCD ultrasonography.

DCS may be an ideal tool to ultimately monitor cerebral hemodynamics in premature infants at the bedside and has favorable characteristics for continuous monitoring in this population. The objective of this study was to compare and validate the CrCP calculated using DCS measurements versus TCD ultrasound in a neonatal piglet model of hemorrhagic shock.

Materials and Methods

Approval was obtained by the Animal Care and Use Committee at Baylor College of Medicine. All procedures conformed to the standards of animal experimentation of the National Institutes of Health.

Anesthesia

Thirteen neonatal piglets arrived within 1 week of life and were housed in the animal facility for at least 24 h prior to the studies to allow for acclimation to their new environment. The piglets were anesthetized with inhaled 5% isoflurane and 50% oxygen via facemask for induction. Tracheostomy was performed and mechanical ventilation was initiated using a cuffed endotracheal tube. Ventilation was adjusted to maintain arterial pH between 7.35 and 7.45. Maintenance anesthesia consisted of 0.8% isoflurane, 50% nitrous oxide, 50% oxygen, fentanyl (25-μg bolus followed by 25-μg/h infusion), and vecuronium (5-mg bolus followed by 2-mg/h infusion) to maintain a heart rate less than 160 bpm and to maintain a normal blood pressure during baseline recordings. This anesthetic technique ensured the animals' comfort while minimizing the cerebrovascular response to volatile anesthetic.

Surgery and Physiologic Data Processing

The femoral veins were cannulated bilaterally for placement of central venous lines for drug infusion and central venous pressure (CVP) monitoring. The femoral arteries were cannulated bilaterally for placement of an arterial line for arterial blood pressure and blood gas monitoring and for active removal of blood. Middle cerebral artery CBF velocity was recorded by TCD ultrasound (Nicolet Vascular/Natus Medical Incorporated, San Carlos, CA) using a 2-MHz probe. Microvascular blood flow of the cerebral cortex was measured with DCS (MetaOx/ISS Inc., Champaign, IL). Measurements of TCD and DCS were made concurrently and continuously throughout the experiment.

Signal Sampling

Arterial and CVPs, as well as laser-Doppler signals and DCS signals, were sampled at 200 Hz using an analog-to-digital converter (Data Translation, Marlboro, MA, USA) and ICM+ software (Cambridge University, Cambridge, UK). CrCP was determined using an impedance-based model [7]. Data were analyzed using MATLAB (Mathworks Inc., Natick, MA).

Statistical Analyses

Lower limit of autoregulation was determined by piecewise regression analysis. Comparisons of CrCP measured by DCS and TCD ultrasound were made using linear regression and Bland-Altman analysis.

Results

Neonatal piglets had an average weight, age, and starting hemoglobin of 2.8 kg (±0.5), 12 days (±3), and 8.2 g/dL (±0.8), respectively. The complete baseline piglet characteristics can be seen in Table 1. There were no significant differences in the baseline characteristics of the piglets.

ABP was slowly lowered via continuous hemorrhage. Lower limit of autoregulation was determined for each piglet using piecewise regression analysis, and then behavior was observed both above and below the lower limit of autoregulation. For each piglet a linear regression and Bland-Altman

Table 1 Baseline piglet characteristics

Pig#	Weight (kg)	Age (days)	pH	pCO_2	pO_2	Hct	Hb	HCO_3-	Base excess
1	2.7	10	7.413	44.4	261.9	25.0	8.4	28.6	4.2
2	2.7	13	7.339	47.7	307.7	22.0	7.5	25.9	0.7
3	2.6	14	7.379	52.6	260.1	21.0	7.2	31.3	6.2
4	3.58	14	7.367	45.8	256.6	26.0	8.6	26.6	1.6
5	3.52	15	7.420	38.3	356.8	25.0	8.5	25.1	1.3
6	3.25	16	7.450	37.4	243.9	19.0	6.4	26.4	2.9
7	2.0	14	7.468	36.0	371.1	25.0	8.4	26.3	2.3
8	3.4	16	7.359	49.3	340.8	24.0	8.1	28.1	2.4
9	2.2	07	7.364	35.7	278.3	28.0	9.3	20.6	−5.1
10	2.5	08	7.342	49.5	293.9	24.0	8.2	27.1	1.1
11	2.7	09	7.360	39.9	340.8	25.0	8.4	22.8	−3.0
12	2.2	10	7.394	37.6	330.9	25.0	8.3	23.2	−2.0
13	2.8	11	7.380	39.6	286.3	28.0	9.4	23.6	−1.7
Avg	**2.8**	**12**	**7.390**	**42.6**	**302.0**	**24.4**	**8.2**	**25.8**	**0.83**
SD	**± 0.52**	**± 3**	**± 0.04**	**± 5.8**	**± 42**	**± 2.5**	**± 0.8**	**± 2.8**	**± 3.10**

Table 2 Comparison of critical closing pressure between transcranial Doppler and diffuse correlation spectroscopy by linear regression and Bland-Altman analysis

	Linear regression	Bland-Altman analysis
Piglet #	r^2	Bias ±1.96 SD
1	0.72	−6.4 ± 3.2
2	0.95	−4.2 ± 2.5
3	0.97	−3.2 ± 5.1
4	0.87	11.0 ± 20.0
5	0.80	4.3 ± 10.7
6	0.64	−3.6 ± 6.4
7	0.48	−1.5 ± 13.5
8	0.87	−3.5 ± 6.0
9	0.88	−0.28 ± 8.5
10	0.71	−5.6 ± 6.4
11	0.71	0.95 ± 6.5
12	0.16	−13.0 ± 8.0
13	0.86	−4.6 ± 8.4
Average all	0.74	−2.3 ± 8.1

analysis was performed to determine the agreement of CrCP measured by both DCS and TCD ultrasound.

Across all piglets, CrCP determined by the two modalities showed good correlation by linear regression, median $r^2 = 0.8$ (interquartile range (IQR) 0.71–0.87), and Bland-Altman analysis showed a median bias of −3.5 (IQR −4.6 to −0.28). Results are shown in Table 2.

Discussion

The results of the experiments presented here have two implications. First, DCS and TCD ultrasonography can be used concurrently to measure the CrCP to better understand cerebral hemodynamics in a piglet model of hemorrhagic shock. The two signals were continuous, and signal acquisition was not hindered by using both concurrently. Second, we found strong agreement in CrCP measured between DCS and TCD ultrasound; however, their values were not identical across the experiments. These differences between measured CrCP may be a result of the different behavior of the cerebral vasculature measured by the two modalities. Thus, because DCS measures CBF in the microvasculature of the cerebral cortex compared to the TCD ultrasound measurements of the macrovasculature of the cerebral arteries, we believe the measurements reported here demonstrate the similar but contrasting physiology of those vascular beds.

ELBW infants remain at risk for brain injury in the early postnatal period [10, 11]. ABP may not be a good surrogate for CBF in this population despite its use in guiding hemodynamic measurement in this at-risk population. However, the tools available to monitor CBF at the bedside in preterm infants remain limited. TCD ultrasound and NIRS are the most commonly used modalities at the bedside in the NICU to assess cerebral perfusion and oxygenation. DCS provides an alternative to TCD ultrasound and NIRS.

DCS is a continuous, noninvasive optical technique that utilizes light intensity fluctuations to measure microvascular blood flow in the cerebral cortex [11]. DCS may be a more useful alternative to TCD ultrasound and NIRS because it provides more comprehensive cerebral hemodynamic data as it monitors tissue oxygenation, CBF, and oxygen metabolism concurrently. DCS measures CBF using a blood flow index (BFI), in units of square centimeters per second (cm^2/s), that relies on an effective Brownian diffusion coefficient of red blood cells and is proportional to tissue microvascular blood flow [12]. In contrast, TCD ultrasound measures blood flow velocity in large vessels (in mL/100 g/min). Thus, comparison of the two measurements is difficult and not straightforward.

A recent study by Giovannella et al. in neonatal piglets validated the DCS measurements against positron emission tomography ^{15}O-labeled water, a more accurate and accepted measurement of regional CBF [13]. The authors reported excellent correlation between BFI measured by DCS and regional CBF measured by positron emission tomography ($R = 0.94$, $p < 0.0001$) and derived a calibration formula to convert the BFI measurement into flow units. This important animal work similar to the findings in this study can therefore be used to further inform studies in human infants.

At this time, there are a limited number of studies using DCS in human preterm and term infants. A study by Buckley et al. showed that DCS correlated well with TCD ultrasound [14]. In this feasibility study, DCS and TCD ultrasound were performed in four very low birth weight preterm infants during a 12° positional change and showed that this minor postural change did not significantly affect CBF. However, these positional changes were not expected to result in changes in CBF. In another study by Busch et al., DCS was used to continuously monitor CBF during deep hypothermic circulatory arrest during cardiac surgery in a term infant [15]. They demonstrated that DCS was capable of measuring changes in CBF from a normal, physiological range of blood flow to near zero blood flow. This work highlighted the feasibility of continuous, real-time optical measurement of CBF. Further, a more recent study by Baker et al. compared CrCP calculations by the Windkessel model using DCS versus TCD ultrasound in healthy adults and found good agreement [16]. They also measured cerebrovascular arteriole compliance, which supported the idea that the DCS measures microvasculature vs. the macrovasculature. Finally, Andresen et al. used DCS in normal term infants at rest to demonstrate that DCS measurements were comparable to other expected values for the estimation of CBF [17].

In our study, CrCP measured by DCS and TCD ultrasound had good correlation but were not identical in value. As previously indicated, this difference may simply be due to the type of vascular bed that was being monitored because the behavior of the microvasculature compared to the macrovasculature is different. The hemodynamics of a premature infant is changing constantly, and being able to monitor the CrCP continuously and easily at the bedside may have great advantages to the neonatologist in using brain-specific metrics to define the goals of care.

In conclusion, this is the first comparison of CrCP determined by DCS compared to TCD ultrasound in a neonatal piglet model of hemorrhagic shock. We found strong agreement between DCS and TCD ultrasound in their ability to estimate CrCP; however, their values were not identical across the experiment. The difference between the two modalities may be due to the differences in vasomotor tone within the microvasculature of the cerebral arterioles as measured by DCS compared to the microvasculature of a major cerebral artery by TCD ultrasound. The results from this study will provide pilot data to serve as a basis for the application of DCS to human infants.

Acknowledgments C.J.R. is supported by the National Institutes of Health (1K23NS091382). D.R.R. is supported by the National Institutes of Health (1K23HLI130522). The technical assistance of Leticia McGuffey was greatly appreciated.

Conflict of Interest **Dr. Rusin has an significant financial interest in Medical Informatics Corp. MIC has no financial interests in this work.**

References

1. du Plessis A, Volpe JJ (2002) Perinatal brain injury in the preterm and term newborn. Curr Opin Neurol 15(2):151–157
2. Perlman J (1998) White matter injury in the preterm infant: an important determination of abnormal neurodevelopment outcome. Early Hum Dev 53(2):99–120
3. O'Leary H, Gregas MC, Limperopoulos C et al (2009) Elevated cerebral pressure passivity is associated with prematurity-related intracranial hemorrhage. Pediatrics 124:302–309
4. Rhee CJ, Kaiser JR, Rios DR et al (2016) Elevated diastolic closing margin is associated with intraventricular hemorrhage in premature infants. J Pediatr 174:52–56
5. Romagnoli C, Giannantonio C, De Carolis MP, Gallini F, Zecca E, Papacci P (2006) Neonatal color Doppler US study: normal values of cerebral blood flow velocities in preterm infants in the first month of life. Ultrasound Med Biol 32:321–331
6. Rhee CJ, Fraser CD, Kibler K et al (2015) The ontogeny of cerebrovascular critical closing pressure. Pediatr Res 78(1):71–75
7. Varsos GV, Kolias AG, Smielewski P et al (2015) A noninvasive estimation of cerebral perfusion pressure using critical closing pressure. J Neurosurg 123:638–648
8. Wolfberg AJ, du Plessis AJ (2006) Near-infrared spectroscopy in the fetus and neonate. Clin Perinatol 33:707–728. viii
9. Buckley EM, Parthasarathy AB, Grant PE, Yodh AG, Franceschini MA (2014) Diffuse correlation spectroscopy for measurement of cerebral blood flow: future prospects. Neurophotonics 1(1):011009
10. Perlman J, Volpe JJ (1986) Intraventricular hemorrhage in extremely small premature infants. Am J Dis Child 140(11):1122–1124

11. Volpe JJ (1997) Brain injury in the premature infant. Neuropathology, clinical aspects, pathogenesis, and prevention. Clin Perinatol 24(3):567–587
12. Diop M, Verdecchia K, Lee T-Y et al (2012) Calibration of diffuse correlation spectroscopy with a time-resolved near-infrared technique to yield absolute cerebral blood flow measurements. Biomed Opt Express 3:1476
13. Giovannella M, Adnresen B, Andersen JB et al (2019) Validation of diffuse correlation spectroscopy against 15O-water PET for regional cerebral blood flow measurement in neonatal piglets. JCBFM 2019:271678X19883751. https://doi.org/10.1177/0271678X19883751
14. Buckley EM, Cook NM, Durduran T et al (2009) Cerebral hemodynamics in preterm infants during positional intervention measured with diffuse correlation spectroscopy and transcranial Doppler ultrasound. Opt Express 17:12571–12581
15. Busch DR, Rusin CG, Miller-Hance W et al (2016) Continuous cerebral hemodynamic measurement during deep hypothermic circulatory arrest. Biomed Opt Express 7:3461–3470
16. Baker WB, Parthasarathy AB, Gannon KP et al (2017) Noninvasive optical monitoring of critical closing pressure and arteriole compliance in human subjects. J Cereb Blood Flow Metab 37:2691–2705
17. Andresen B, De Carli A, Fumagalli M et al (2019) Cerebral oxygenation and blood flow in normal term infants at rest measured by a hybrid near-infrared device (BabyLux). Pediatr Res 86(4):515–521. https://doi.org/10.1038/s41390-019-0474-9

Part IX

Hydrocephalus and Cerebrospinal Fluid Biophysics

Diffusion and Flow MR Imaging to Investigate Hydrocephalus Patients Before and After Endoscopic Third Ventriculostomy

Olivier Balédent, Cyrille Capel, Serge Metanbou, and Roger Bouzerar

Introduction

Infusion test procedures have shown that increased pulsatile intracranial pressure (ICP) and impaired intracranial compliance characterize patients with noncommunicating hydrocephalus who respond clinically to cerebrospinal fluid (CSF) diversion surgery even though static ICP was not increased [1, 2]. In such patients, fluid-structure interactions lead to ventricular dilation that stresses the white matter fibers and alters the cerebral blood flow and CSF dynamics [3].

Magnetic Resonance Imaging (MRI) appears to be an excellent non-invasive technique to monitor these disorders. To detect and quantify white matter (WM) alterations, diffusion tensor imaging (DTI) is widely employed [4–6], while phase contrast MRI (PCMRI) is a reference for CSF and blood flow measurements [7–9].

The purpose of this work was to noninvasively investigate how endoscopic third ventriculostomy (ETV) could impact white matter bundles, CSF oscillations, and cerebral blood flow.

Materials and Methods

Eleven patients presenting with chronic headaches and noncommunicating hydrocephalus due to aqueductal stenosis, who were successfully treated by ETV, were included in the study (mean ± SD age, 63 ± 10 years [48–78]). The subjects underwent the same MR exam before and after surgery.

Magnetic Resonance Imaging was performed on a 3 T Signa HDx MR scanner (GE Healthcare, Milwaukee, WI, USA). In addition to the classical morphological MRI sequences, PCMRI and DTI sequences were added to the standard radiological protocol (Fig. 1).

DTI data were acquired along 12 directions using a 128 × 128 matrix and a b-value of 1000 s/mm^2. Regions of interest (ROI) were manually delineated in the corona radiata (CR) and the genu of the corpus callosum (CC). DTI parameters were then processed using Functool Software (GE healthcare) on a dedicated vendor console. Three eigenvalues (L1, L2, L3), obtained after diagonalization of the diffusion tensor, permitted calculation of the apparent diffusion coefficient (ADC) and the fractional anisotropy (FA) coefficients, defined as follows:

- $ADC = (L1 + L2 + L3)/3$
- $FA = \{(3/2)[(L1\text{-}ADC)^2 + (L2\text{-}ADC)^2 + (L3\text{-}ADC)^2]/(L1^2 + L2^2 + L3^2)\}^{1/2}$

PCMRI measurements were performed using a fast 2D cine PC sequence with retrospective peripheral gating. Thirty-two velocity images covering one cardiac cycle (CC) were obtained.

O. Balédent (✉)
Department of Medical Image Processing, Amiens University Hospital, Amiens, France

Chimère Research Team EA7516, Amiens Jules Verne University, Amiens, France
e-mail: olivier.baledent@chu-amiens.fr

C. Capel
Chimère Research Team EA7516, Amiens Jules Verne University, Amiens, France

Department of Neurosurgery, Amiens University Hospital, Amiens, France

S. Metanbou
Department of Radiology, Amiens University Hospital, Amiens, France

R. Bouzerar
Department of Medical Image Processing, Amiens University Hospital, Amiens, France

B. Depreitere et al. (eds.), *Intracranial Pressure and Neuromonitoring XVII*, Acta Neurochirurgica Supplement 131,
https://doi.org/10.1007/978-3-030-59436-7_56,

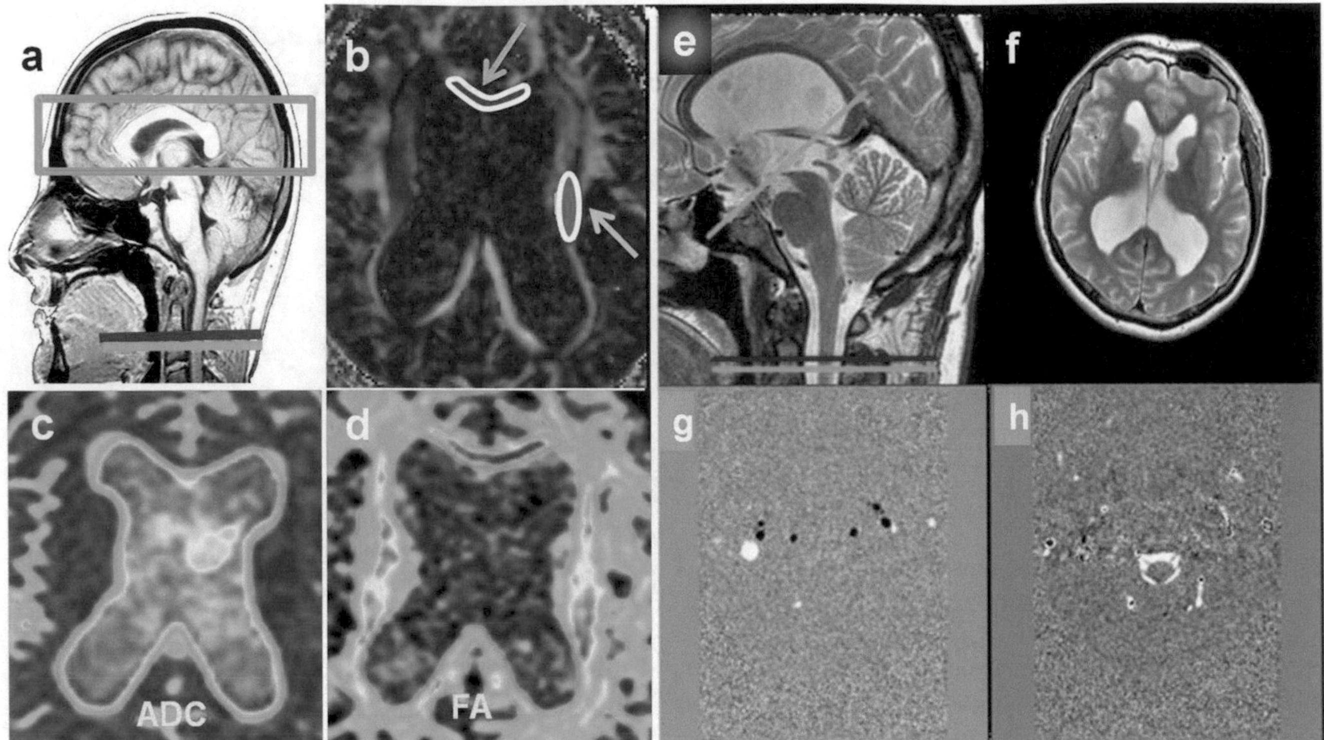

Fig. 1 Diffusion tensor imaging (DTI) and phase-contrast imaging (PCMRI). (**a**) Sagittal view showing the rectangular slab used for DTI acquisition. (**b**) RGB Cartography of fibers orientations. Regions of interest are delineated in the Corona Radiata and the Corpus Callosum (arrows). (**c**, **d**) Cartography of apparent diffusion coefficient (ADC) and fractional anisotropy (FA). Phase contrast MRI (PC-MRI) can measure CSF and blood flow in the cranio-spinal system during a cardiac cycle. (**e**, **f**) Classical morphological images. Green lines and red line show the levels of PC-MRI acquisitions. One of the planes passes through the flow void resulting from the aperture in the third ventricle. (**g**) Grayscale intensities in the arterial and venous vessels crossing the slice (red line) at the cervical level. Pixel intensities represent blood velocities. (**h**) Hyper-intensities at the image center represent CSF flow velocities in the subarachnoid spaces around the spine

Measurement planes were placed on sagittal views perpendicularly to the presumed direction of fluid flow. For CSF, planes were selected at the aqueduct level, C2–C3 spinal level, and at the roof of the third ventricle. For arterial blood flow (carotid + vertebral arteries) assessment, the plane was set at the C2–C3 level. Post-processing of the velocity images was performed using a homemade software [10]. ETV success was confirmed after quantification of the CSF oscillations through the aperture of the third ventricle roof. The same PCMRI measurements were also performed in 12 healthy volunteers.

Statistics

Data were expressed as mean ± SD. Comparison between values of DTI or flow parameters before and after ETV were performed using Wilcoxon's test for paired samples. Statistical significance was reached for p values inferior to 0.05.

Results

All patients improved after surgery.

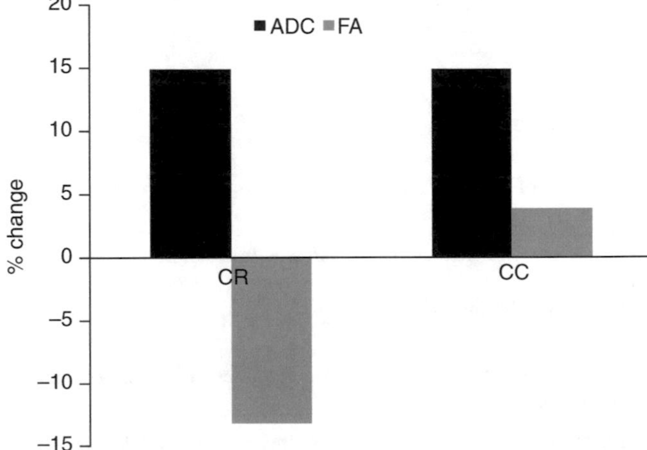

Fig. 2 Percentage change of ADC and FA parameters before and after ETV

DTI Analysis

For the WM CR fibers, we observed a significant increase in ADC ($+15 \pm 9\%$, $p < 0.001$), while FA significantly decreased ($-13 \pm 8\%$, $p < 0.001$) after ETV (Fig. 2).

Table 1 CSF and blood flow measurements

Population	CBF (mL/min)	Cervical CSF (μL/CC)	Ventricular CSF (μL/CC)
Healthy ($n = 12$)	700 ± 135	430 ± 190	40 ± 20
Before ETV ($n = 11$)	555 ± 123	594 ± 250	0
After ETV ($n = 11$)	670 ± 105	496 ± 147	210 ± 100

Note: *CC* cardiac cycle

For the CC fibers, a significant increase in ADC was also observed (+15 ± 15%, $p < 0.01$), while FA did not change (+4 ± 13%, $p = 0.37$) after ETV (Fig. 2).

Flow Analysis

In one patient, a CSF flow considered as normal was observed in the aqueduct of Sylvius after ETV. Mean values of CSF and blood flow, before and after surgery, are synthesized in Table 1. The mean CSF stroke volume through the third ventricle aperture was five times larger than the average normal aqueductal stroke volume. A decrease in cervical CSF oscillations was observed: 594 and 496 μL per cardiac cycle before and after ETV, respectively. Concomitantly, a significant 15% increase ($p < 0.05$) in mean cerebral blood flow before and after ETV was highlighted (555 and 670 mL/min, respectively).

Discussion

In this study, we explored the impact of endoscopic third ventriculostomy on white matter structures, blood flow, and CSF oscillations. We observed that MRI can be a useful noninvasive tool that allowed us to easily study flow of cerebral fluids and mechanical stresses of the brain in hydrocephalus. Image acquisition can be performed in a limited time, e.g., only 10 min for the whole sequence.

After ETV, the CSF flow observed through the third ventricle aperture was larger than a standard aqueductal flow. This seems obviously related to the drastically lower resistance to flow offered by this orifice, which therefore generates a reorganization of the circulation of cranio-spinal fluids in the different compartments. As a result, spinal CSF flow decreased, while CBF concomitantly increased after ETV. These results could be explained either by an increase in the global intracranial compliance or by an ICP decrease, which are, in any case, intimately related parameters; indeed, by definition, the compliance represents the change in volume per unit change in pressure. This compliance gives the intracranial compartment the ability to accommodate to an increase in volume without a large increase in intracranial pressure. The subsequent CSF recirculation changes also lead to a reorganization of the white matter fiber bundles, which is supported by the variations of the DTI parameters. The increase in ADC for both CC and CR can be interpreted as a structural decompression since the water molecules are more freely diffusible. This is clearly confirmed by the decrease in anisotropy at the CR level, but it remains less obvious at the CC level: this could be mainly be explained by the location of the fiber structures that may reside near regions with various ventricle curvature. Indeed, several authors showed that a gradient of compression is observed in HCA subjects and conclude that the mechanical stresses depended on the location of the anatomical structure [11, 12].

All the structural changes observed after surgery also impact the arterial cerebral inflow, which increases significantly. This change may contribute to global enhancement of the cerebral perfusion, which corroborates patient improvement after surgery.

In conclusion, PCMRI and DTI can provide useful noninvasive information to evaluate brain biomechanics and help neurosurgeons select patients with a good chance to improve after ETV and shunt.

Conflict of Interest **The authors declare that they have no conflict of interest.**

References

1. Eide PK, Sorteberg W (2010) Diagnostic intracranial pressure monitoring and surgical management in idiopathic normal pressure hydrocephalus: a 6-year review of 214 patients. Neurosurgery 66(1):80–91
2. Smielewski P, Czosnyka M, Steiner L, Belestri M, Piechnik S, Pickard JD (2005) ICM+: Software for on-line analysis of bedside monitoring data after severe head trauma. Acta Neurochir Suppl 95:43–49
3. Balédent O, Gondry-Jouet C, Meyer ME, De Marco G, Le Gars D, Henry-Feugeas MC, Idy-Peretti I (2004) Relationship between cerebrospinal fluid and blood dynamics in healthy volunteers and patients with communicating hydrocephalus. Investig Radiol 39(1):45–55
4. Daouk J, Chaarani B, Zmudka J, Capel C, Fichten A, Bouzerar R, Gondry-Jouet C, Jouanny P, Balédent O (2014) Relationship between cerebrospinal fluid flow, ventricles morphology, and DTI properties in internal capsules: differences between Alzheimer's disease and normal-pressure hydrocephalus. Acta Radiol 55(8):992–999
5. Keong NC, Pena A, Price SJ, Czosnyka M, Czosnyka Z, DeVito EE, Housden CR, Sahakian BJ, Pickard JD (2017) Diffusion tensor imaging profiles reveal specific neural tract distortion in normal pressure hydrocephalus. PLoS One 12(8):e0181624
6. Le Bihan D, Breton E, Lallemand D, Grenier P, Cabanis E, Laval-Jeantet M (1986) MR imaging of intravoxel incoherent motions:

application to diffusion and perfusion in neurologic disorders. Radiology 161(2):401–407
7. Bhadelia RA, Bogdan AR, Kaplan RF, Wolpert SM (1997) Cerebrospinal fluid pulsation amplitude and its quantitative relationship to cerebral blood flow pulsations: a phase-contrast MR flow imaging study. Neuroradiology 39(4):258–264
8. Enzmann DR, Pelc NJ (1991) Normal flow patterns of intracranial and spinal cerebrospinal fluid defined with phase-contrast cine MR imaging. Radiology 178(2):467–474
9. Feinberg DA, Mark AS (1987) Human brain motion and cerebrospinal fluid circulation demonstrated with MR velocity imaging. Radiology 163(3):793–799
10. Balédent O, Henry-Feugeas MC, Idy-Peretti I (2001) Cerebrospinal fluid dynamics and relation with blood flow: a magnetic resonance study with semiautomated cerebrospinal fluid segmentation. Investig Radiol 36:368–377
11. Dutta-Roy T, Wittek A, Miller K (2008) Biomechanical modelling of normal pressure hydrocephalus. J Biomech 41:2263–2271
12. Taylor Z, Miller K (2004) Reassessment of brain elasticity for analysis of biomechanisms of hydrocephalus. J Biomech 37:1263–1269

Lower Breakpoint of Intracranial Amplitude-Pressure Relationship in Normal Pressure Hydrocephalus

Zofia H. Czosnyka, Afroditi D. Lalou, Eva Nabbanja, Matthew Garnett, Nicole C. Keong, Eric A. Schmidt, D. J. Kim, and Marek Czosnyka

Introduction

The relationship between intracranial pulse amplitude (AMP) and mean intracranial pressure (ICP) has been previously described [1–3]. In general, AMP increases proportionally to rises in ICP. Such an increase in AMP can be observed particularly often (but not exclusively) if the rise in ICP is provoked by controlled cerebrospinal fluid (CSF) volume increase during the infusion test.

In patients suffering from normal pressure hydrocephalus (NPH), we studied the lower breakpoint (LB) of the amplitude-pressure relationship below which the pulse amplitude stays constant when ICP varies (Fig. 1). Theoretically, below this breakpoint, the pressure-volume relationship is linear (good compensatory reserve), and above the breakpoint it is exponential (brain compliance decreasing with rising ICP) (Fig. 2).

As a matter of interest, the amplitude–pressure relationship has two breakpoints. In head-injured patients, when the rise in ICP can be much higher than during an infusion test (we usually limit a pressure rise to 40 mmHg; after this level infusion is terminated), an upper breakpoint can be also seen [4]. Above this point, AMP starts to decrease, with mean ICP rising further.

Z. H. Czosnyka · A. D. Lalou · E. Nabbanja · M. Garnett
M. Czosnyka (✉)
Academic Neurosurgery, Cambridge University Hospital, Cambridge, UK
e-mail: Mc141@medschl.cam.ac.uk

N. C. Keong
Department of Neurosurgery, National Neuroscience Institute and Duke-NUS Medical School, Singapore, Singapore

E. A. Schmidt
Neurosurgery, Purpan Hospital, Toulouse, France

D. J. Kim
Department of Brain and Cognitive Engineering, Korea University, Seoul, South Korea

Materials and Methods

Infusion tests performed in 169 patients diagnosed for idiopathic NPH (2004–2013) were available for analysis. Inclusion: patients had a lumbar infusion test performed before surgery, the raw data of ICP were digitally recorded (ICM+ software, Cambridge Enterprise Ltd., UK) and available for post-hoc processing, and the response to shunting was assessed in the follow-up clinic.

The lumbar infusion test requires a patient to lie in bed on his or her side. The skin should be adequately cleaned. A single-wide (gauge 19) lumbar puncture needle is inserted in the lumbar CSF space. The pressure transducer and a syringe infusion pump are connected through a three-way tap. After monitoring baseline pressure for 10 min, the infusion, with a constant rate (typically 1.5 mL/min), begins. Pulse amplitude of ICP (AMP) and mean ICP are calculated by computer software and updated with 10 s period. After the test, all compensatory parameters (resistance to CSF outflow, elasticity, CSF production rate, reference pressure, and sagittal sinus pressure) are calculated. AMP is plotted against mean ICP values (as in Fig. 1) and examined (bi-linear regression between AMP and ICP) for detection of a LB.

Results

A lower breakpoint was observed in 62 patients diagnosed for NPH. In the majority of cases, therefore, LB cannot be seen. It may be interpreted that in those cases the baseline ICP was higher than the pressure of the lower breakpoint (Plb).

Post-shunting improvement (either permanent or temporary) in patients in whom a lower breakpooint was recorded was 77% versus 90% in patients where LB was not recorded ($p < 0.02$) (Fig. 3).

B. Depreitere et al. (eds.), *Intracranial Pressure and Neuromonitoring XVII*, Acta Neurochirurgica Supplement 131,
https://doi.org/10.1007/978-3-030-59436-7_57,

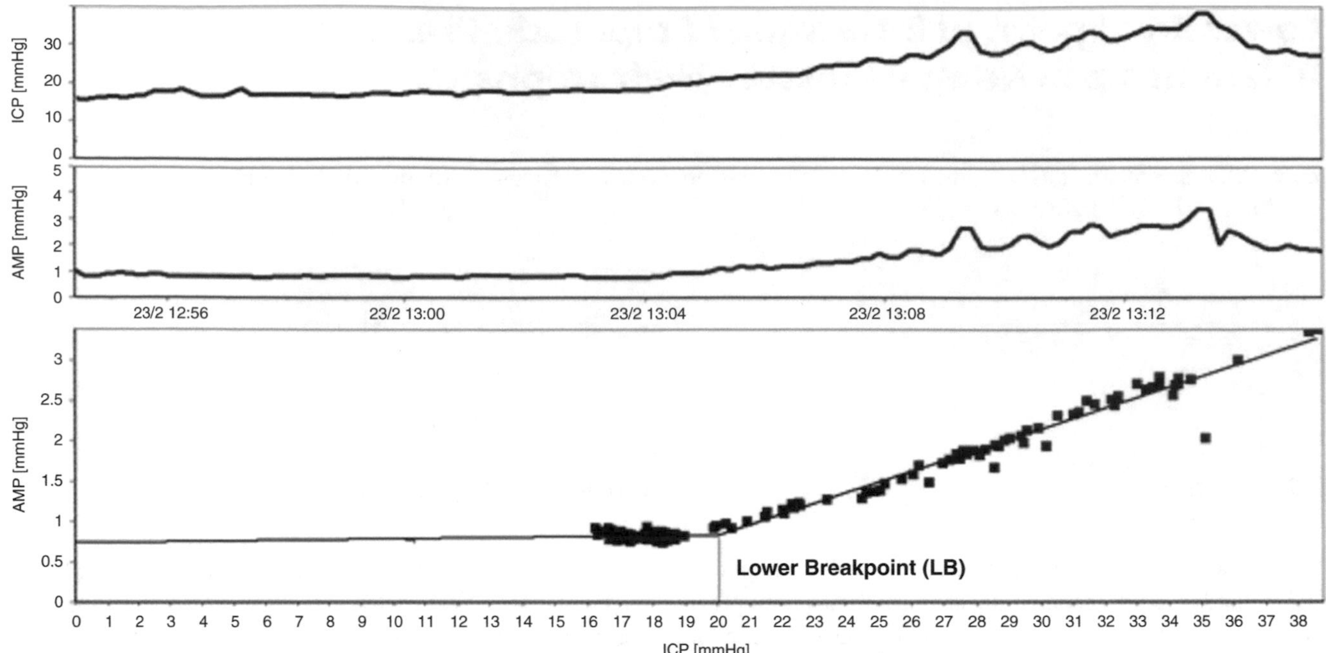

Fig. 1 Bi-linear shape of the relationship between pulse amplitude of ICP (AMP) and mean intracranial pressure (ICP) recorded during an infusion test. LB is its lower breakpoint. Below this point the curve is horizontal; above it shows a positive gradient

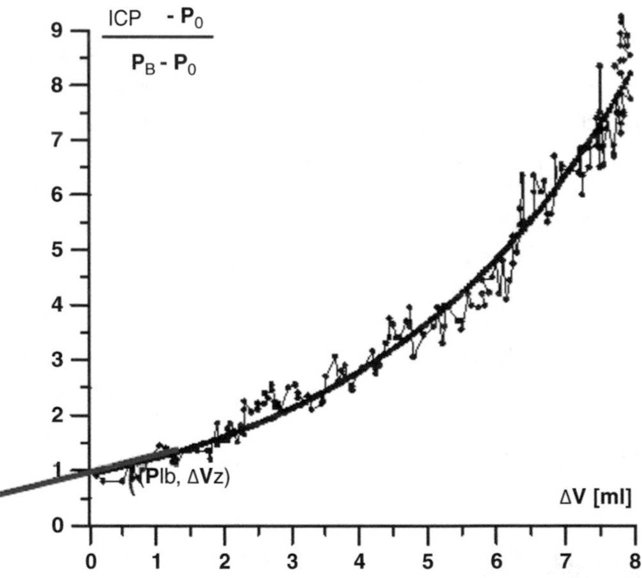

Fig. 2 The same breakpoint can be seen on the Pressure-Volume curve. Below the pressure of the lower breakpoint (Plb), the curve is linear. Above it is exponential

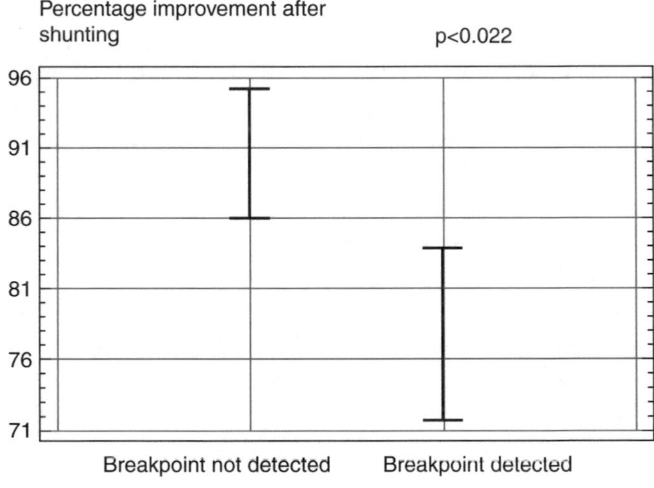

Fig. 3 The improvement rate in patients in whom LB was recorded was 77%. In patients where LB was not recorded, the improvement rate was 90% ($p < 0.02$)

In patients with a detected LB, the distance between Plb and baseline ICP was lower in patients who improved (no improvement: 4.1 ± 2.1 mmHg versus improved: 1.2 ± 2.7 mmHg; $p < 0.02$).

Despite a previous report [5], there was no correlation between the rate of improvement and the slope of the amplitude-pressure characteristic above the LB.

Discussion

The presence of a lower breakpoing is associated with less frequent improvement after shunting in NPH.

It may be interpreted that CSF pressure-volume compensatory reserve of patients working on the flat (linear) part of the pressure-volume curve is more generous and frequently associated with brain atrophy. Atrophy per se is less remediable with shunting.

The intracranial pressure-volume curve is a mathematical model, which is, relatively speaking, seldom identified in clinical practice. Fundamental experimental work of Zwetnow and Lofgren [6] and of Shapiro and Marmarou [7] laid foundations for the current understanding of CSF dynamics. Infusion tests give a unique opportunity to follow its shape. The amplitude-pressure relationship (or 'pulsatility curve' [2]) is a technique complementary to the pressure-volume curve plotting and can be identified in many clinical conditions. It is not limited to hydrocephalus.

References

1. Marmarou A, Shulman K, Rosende RM (1978) A nonlinear analysis of the cerebrospinal fluid system and intracranial pressure dynamics. J Neurosurg 48(3):332–344
2. Qvarlander S, Lundkvist B, Koskinen LO, Malm J, Eklund A (2013) Pulsatility in CSF dynamics: pathophysiology of idiopathic normal pressure hydrocephalus. J Neurol Neurosurg Psychiatry 84(7):735–741
3. Szewczykowski J, Sliwka S, Kunicki A, Dytko P, Korsak-Sliwka J (1977) A fast method of estimating the elastance of the intracranial system. J Neurosurg 47(1):19–26
4. Czosnyka M, Price DJ, Williamson M (1994) Monitoring of cerebrospinal dynamics using continuous analysis of intracranial pressure and cerebral perfusion pressure in head injury. Acta Neurochir 126(2–4):113–119
5. Anile C, De Bonis P, Albanese A, Di Chirico A, Mangiola A, Petrella G, Santini P (2010) Selection of patients with idiopathic normal-pressure hydrocephalus for shunt placement: a single-institution experience. J Neurosurg 113(1):64–73
6. Löfgren J, von Essen C, Zwetnow NN (1973) The pressure-volume curve of the cerebrospinal fluid space in dogs. Acta Neurol Scand 49(5):557–574
7. Shapiro K, Fried A, Marmarou A (1985) Biomechanical and hydrodynamic characterization of the hydrocephalic infant. J Neurosurg 63(1):69–75

Single Center Experience in Cerebrospinal Fluid Dynamics Testing

Zofia H. Czosnyka, Marek Czosnyka, Piotr Smielewski, Afroditi D. Lalou, Eva Nabbanja, Matthew Garnett, Slawomir Barszcz, Eric A. Schmidt, Shahan Momjian, Magda Kasprowicz, Gianpaolo Petrella, Brian Owler, Nicole C. Keong, Peter J. Hutchinson, and John D. Pickard

Introduction

Although normal pressure hydrocephalus (NPH) is more complex than simple failure of the cerebrospinal fluid (CSF) circulation, disturbed CSF dynamics are an important component of the disease. The original Katzman-Hussey [1] lumbar infusion test was based on Davson's steady-state model of CSF absorption. Marmarou [2] added a dynamic component, a computerized model of which was designed at the Warsaw University of Technology and used in the Child's Health Centre in Warsaw, Poland in 1985 [3]. Since then the procedure has gained in popularity in some centers, but not in all. The reason for this is multifactorial: It is considered an invasive procedure, it requires specialized hardware and software, and the results may be ambiguous, particularly if they are compared with clinical improvement after shunting. Finally, shunt technology, which remains based on pressure-passive drainage, may be not be sufficient to correct complex CSF circulatory failure in all cases.

Materials and Methods

Since 1992, 4473 infusion studies have been performed in both shunted and non-shunted patients at Cambridge University Hospital NHS Foundation Trust, UK.

All shunt-naïve patients had a working diagnosis of primary or secondary NPH, with documented ventriculomegaly, baseline intracranial pressure (ICP) below 18 mmHg, and at least two of the three cardinal symptoms of NPH, including gait disturbance. They attended the CSF Clinic, and an infusion test was indicated as part of their workup according to hospital protocols and in line with the National Institute of Clinical Excellence guidelines. All patients were provided with appropriate information and signed individual consent forms. In shunt-naïve patients, access was gained either via lumbar puncture (LP) or via a previously placed Ommaya reservoir (this is a reservoir placed under the scalp alone, with no associated shunt). Connection of a fluid-filled pressure transducer (Edwards LifesciencesTM) and pressure amplifier (Spiegelberg or Philips) to the LP needle facilitated pressure recording at a frequency of 30–100 Hz, with subsequent processing by software called ICM+ (University of Cambridge Enterprise Ltd). Once adequate CSF pressure with a detectable pulse waveform was recorded, baseline

Z. H. Czosnyka · M. Czosnyka (✉) · P. Smielewski · A. D. Lalou
E. Nabbanja · M. Garnett · P. J. Hutchinson · J. D. Pickard
Division of Neurosurgery, University of Cambridge, Addenbrooke's Hospital, Cambridge, UK
e-mail: Mc141@medschl.cam.ac.uk

S. Barszcz
Neurosurgery, Medical Academy Pediatric Hospital, ul Zwirki I Wigury, Warsaw, Poland

E. A. Schmidt
Neurosurgery, Pourpan Hospital, University of Toulouse, Toulouse, France

S. Momjian
Department of Neurosurgery, Geneva University Hospital, Geneva, Switzerland

M. Kasprowicz
Department of Biomedical Engineering, Wroclaw University of Science and Technology, Wroclaw, Poland

G. Petrella
Department of Neurosurgery, Hospital Santa Maria Goretti, Latina, Italy

B. Owler
Paediatrics and Child Health, The Children's Hospital at Westmead Clinical School, Sydney, NSW, Australia

N. C. Keong
National Neuroscience Institute, Duke-NUS Medical School, Singapore, Singapore

B. Depreitere et al. (eds.), *Intracranial Pressure and Neuromonitoring XVII*, Acta Neurochirurgica Supplement 131, https://doi.org/10.1007/978-3-030-59436-7_58, © Springer Nature Switzerland AG 2021

measurements were taken for 10 min, followed by infusion of Hartmann's solution at 1.5 mL/min until the pressure had plateaued for 5–10 min or had increased to 40 mmHg, at which point the infusion was stopped as a safety measure. The total duration of the infusion test was approximately 30–45 min.

Shunt-infusion studies were performed with two needles inserted into a pre-chamber for CSF pressure recording and CSF infusion. After baseline pressure recording, constant rate infusion was started until a new plateau was reached. ICM+ software contains the shunt's resistance characteristics. It compares them to the measured baseline CSF pressure and its amplitude, outflow resistance, and critical shunt pressure.

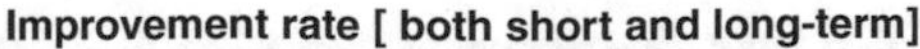

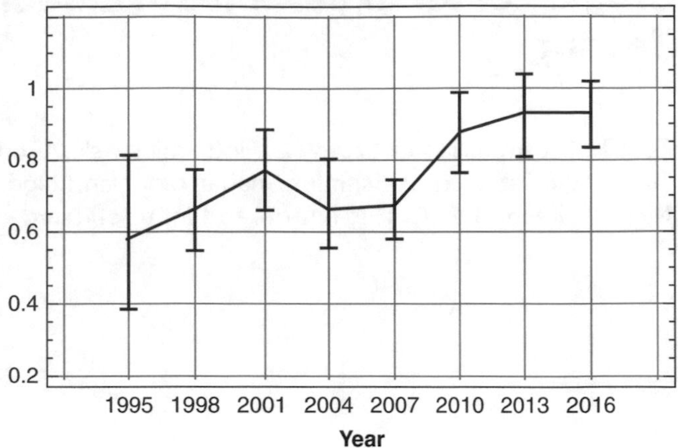

Fig. 1 Good outcome after shunting patients with confirmed normal-pressure hydrocephalus (rate of, along *y* axis) increased from year 1995 until 2015 ($p < 0.013$; ANOVA)

Results

Our Cambridge single center experience may be summarized as follows:

- The CSF infusion test is safe. There were no serious complications over 25 years. The infection rate was less than 1% in the years 1999–2015, and according to a very recent internal audit (2016–2018), there were no infections associated with a test at all.
- Knowledge of compensatory parameters helps in making decisions about the patient's management. Increased resistance to CSF outflow (Rout) is positively correlated with better outcome following shunting ($p < 0.014$; based on a study done in a sample of 310 patients with NPH and known follow up of shunt improvement: 79% improved, 21% did not improve [4]). The optimal threshold for increased Rout, which maximizes the improvement rate after shunting, is 13 mmHg/(mL/min) [4]. The inclusion of a correction for age (elderly patients should have a greater threshold), and for autoregulatory capacity, increases the sensitivity and specificity of outcome prediction (according to recent studies presented during the ICP 2019 symposium).
- In adults, Rout increases with age, while the estimated CSF production rate decreases ($p < 0.0001$). Elasticity of the CSF space also increases with age. The full set of data is available in Czosnyka et al. [5].
- The response to shunting in our center has improved over the past 25 years ($R = 0.205$; $p < 0.0003$) from 62% to nearly 90% at present (Fig. 1).
- In shunted patients, a reservoir infusion study helps to assess shunt function objectively and therefore avoids unnecessary revisions [6]. Yearly savings are estimated to amount to £one million, according to a paper accepted by Acta Neurochirurgica (2020).
- Defective CSF dynamics may coexist with cerebrovascular disease. In such cases both may contribute to a poor clinical status [7]. It has been shown that in patients with normal CSF circulation (Rout<10 mmHg/(mL/min)), global autoregulation of CBF, as estimated with transcranial Doppler, was worse ($p < 0.02$) than in patients with increased Rout (>13 mmHg/(mL/min)).
- In adults with idiopathic NPH, white matter cerebral blood flow (CBF) as estimated with PET imaging decreases toward the surface of the lateral ventricles. Autoregulation of CBF is also worse in this region (Fig. 2). This may reflect a reversal of the transependymal CSF flow (increased mean diffusivity) and its interference with periventricular CBF [8, 9].
- During increase and subsequent decrease of CSF pressure using a constant rate of infusion, the cerebrospinal pressure-volume curve shows hysteresis (Fig. 3) [10]. The width of the hysteresis positively correlates with cerebrospinal elasticity ($p < 0.0032$).
- Even a low elevation of CSF pressure (up to 20 mmHg) during the infusion study tends to increase arterial blood pressure and heart rate variability ($p < 0.05$) [11]. This is probably related to a central neuronal baro-sensitivity, suggesting the presence of an intracranial baroreflex [12]. The possible interplay between hypothalamus, basal ganglia, and NPH needs further study.

Discussion

Normal-pressure hydrocephalus is one of the very few reversible causes of dementia. Studies of CSF dynamics continue to advance our management of patients and the understanding of their pathophysiology. The definition of what

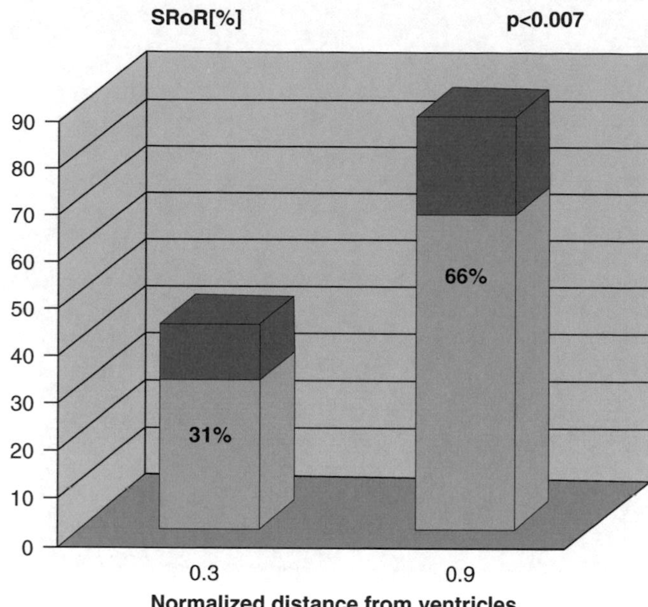

Fig. 2 Static rate of autoregulation (mean—light bar and 95% CI—dark bar) studied across white matter. SRoR at maximal distance from ventricles is significantly better than the SRoR close to surface of ventricles

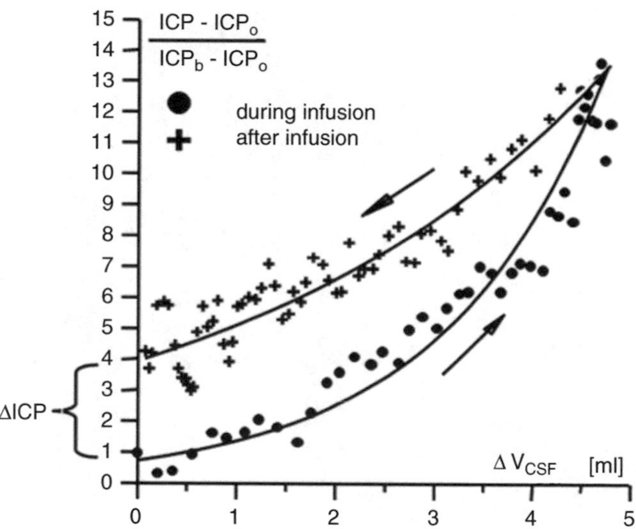

Fig. 3 The pressure-volume curve, detected from the ascending and descending phase of an infusion study, shows in most cases a hysteresis

constitutes a normal CSF circulation [13] is evolving. Phase-contrast MRI, when combined with pressure and flow dynamics [14], promises to produce a more precise delineation of normal and abnormal CSF compensation and circulation. Importantly, noninvasive methods such as MRI [8] will permit long-term serial studies to identify how NPH develops and how effective pressure-passive shunts are at correcting CSF dynamics in relation to cognition and gait.

A comprehensive interdisciplinary approach is required.

Acknowledgments P.J.H. is supported by the NIHR: Research Professorship, Biomedical Research Centre and Global Health Research Group on Neurotrauma and the Royal College of Surgeons of England. J.D.P. supported by the MRC (Programme Grants) and the NIHR (Senior Investigator 2009–2014; Brain Injury Medtech cooperative 2013–2022). E.A.S. is supported by the Clinical Research Hospital Program from the French Ministry of Health (PHRC 2011-A01091-40) and by the Occitania Region research funding (RPBIO 2015 n°14054344). ZC, MC, PS are supported by EC INterreg program (REVERT).

References

1. Katzman R, Hussey F (1970) A simple constant-infusion manometric test for measurement of CSF absorption. I. Rationale and method. Neurology 20(6):534–544
2. Marmarou A, Shulman K, LaMorgese J (1975) Compartmental analysis of compliance and outflow resistance of the cerebrospinal fluid system. J Neurosurg 43(5):523–534
3. Czosnyka M, Czosnyka ZH, Whitfield PC, Donovan T, Pickard JD (2001) Age dependence of cerebrospinal pressure-volume compensation in patients with hydrocephalus. J Neurosurg 94(3):482–486
4. Nabbanja E, Czosnyka M, Keong NC, Garnett M, Pickard JD, Lalou DA, Czosnyka Z (2018) Is there a link between ICP-derived infusion test parameters and outcome after shunting in normal pressure hydrocephalus? Acta Neurochir Suppl 126:229–232
5. Czosnyka M, Wollk-Laniewski P, Batorski L, Zaworski W (1988) Analysis of intracranial pressure waveform during infusion test. Acta Neurochir 93(3–4):140–145
6. Petrella G, Czosnyka M, Smielewski P, Allin D, Guazzo EP, Pickard JD, Czosnyka ZH (2009) In vivo assessment of hydrocephalus shunt. Acta Neurol Scand 120(5):317–323
7. Czosnyka ZH, Czosnyka M, Whitfield PC, Donovan T, Pickard JD (2002) Cerebral autoregulation among patients with symptoms of hydrocephalus. Neurosurgery 50(3):526–532
8. Keong NC, Pena A, Price SJ, Czosnyka M, Czosnyka Z, DeVito EE, Housden CR, Sahakian BJ, Pickard JD (2017) Diffusion tensor imaging profiles reveal specific neural tract distortion in normal pressure hydrocephalus. PLoS One 12(8):e0181624. https://doi.org/10.1371/journal.pone.0181624. eCollection 2017. PMID:28817574
9. Momjian S, Owler BK, Czosnyka Z, Czosnyka M, Pena A, Pickard JD (2004) Pattern of white matter regional cerebral blood flow and autoregulation in normal pressure hydrocephalus. Brain 127(Pt 5):965–972
10. Kasprowicz M, Czosnyka Z, Czosnyka M, Momjian S, Juniewicz H, Pickard JD (2004) Slight elevation of baseline intracranial pressure after fluid infusion into CSF space in patients with hydrocephalus. Neurol Res 26(6):628–631
11. Schmidt EA, Czosnyka Z, Momjian S, Czosnyka M, Bech RA, Pickard JD (2005) Intracranial baroreflex yielding an early cushing response in human. Acta Neurochir Suppl 95:253–256
12. Schmidt EA, Despas F, Pavy-Le Traon A, Czosnyka Z, Pickard JD, Rahmouni K, Pathak A, Senard JM (2018) Intracranial pressure is a determinant of sympathetic activity. Front Physiol 9:11. https://doi.org/10.3389/fphys.2018.00011. eCollection 2018
13. Ekstedt J (1978) CSF hydrodynamic studies in man: 2. Normal hydrodynamic variables related to CSF pressure and flow. J Neurol Neurosurg Psychiatry 41:345–353
14. Unnerbäck M, Ottesen JT, Reinstrup P (2018) ICP curve morphology and intracranial flow-volume changes: a simultaneous ICP and cine phase contrast MRI study in humans. Acta Neurochir 160(2):219–224

Why Hydrocephalus Patients Suffer When the Weather Changes: A New Hypothesis

Andreas Spiegelberg, Lennart Stieglitz, and Vartan Kurtcuoglu

Introduction

Hydrocephalus patients complain about symptoms related to weather changes, especially changes in atmospheric pressure (p_{at}). The symptoms described when the pressure decreases are comparable to those caused by intracranial hypotension. Weather changes associated with rising atmospheric pressure also cause complaints from these patients. The aims of this study were to identify physical, physiological, and pathophysiological effects that explain the described symptoms.

To this end, we established the following hypothesis: Arterial CO_2 partial pressure ($paCO_2$) is influenced by p_{at}, causing autoregulatory changes in the diameters of cerebral arteries. Changes in cerebral arterial diameter affect the intracranial blood volume and, consequently, ICP is altered. In hydrocephalus patients with reduced craniospinal compliance, the described dependence is amplified.

The typical difference in p_{at} between a high-pressure weather system and a low-pressure system is in the range of 50 hPa, as can be seen in any weather chart. To result in noticeable effects as described by patients, a change in p_{at} of 50 hPa should result in a change in ICP of >1 mmHg.

The original version of this chapter has been revised. The correction to this chapter can be found at https://doi.org/10.1007/978-3-030-59436-7_72

A. Spiegelberg (✉)
The Interface Group, Institute of Physiology, University of Zurich, Zurich, Switzerland
e-mail: andreas.spiegelberg@uzh.ch

L. Stieglitz
Department of Neurosurgery, University Hospital Zurich, Zurich, Switzerland

V. Kurtcuoglu
The Interface Group, Institute of Physiology, University of Zurich, Zurich, Switzerland

Zurich Center for Integrative Human Physiology and Neuroscience Center, University of Zurich, Zurich, Switzerland

Methods

We consulted the literature for data on the dependence of $paCO_2$ on p_{at}, and found data in Furian et al., Fan et al. and Crapo et al. [1–3]. For data points for which the atmospheric pressures were not provided, we calculated them from the elevations using the barometric formula [4].

We measured $paCO_2$ capnometrically on six healthy volunteers under varying p_{at}. Variation in p_{at} of approximately 50 hPas was achieved by change in elevation on a route from Zurich (elevation 490 m) to Einsiedeln (elevation 933 m). Written informed consent was obtained from the volunteers before participation in the study. We measured atmospheric pressure with a barometer (Manufacturer: Eurochron, Germany, REF: IB9015). Then we measured end-tidal CO_2 ($etCO_2$) as a surrogate for $paCO_2$ for 10 min at a sample rate of 1/s. For each volunteer we compared $etCO_2$ before and after each change in p_{at}. To assess whether the resulting change in $etCO_2$ was significant, we performed a Mann-Whitney U test. We then determined the slope of the $etCO_2$ vs. p_{at} relationship for each observed change in p_{at} and the resulting change in $etCO_2$.

Finally, we estimated the effect of the change in p_{at} on intracranial pressure (ICP). From the published data and our measurements, we quantified the relationship of ICP vs. p_{at} to assess whether symptoms reported by hydrocephalus patients during weather changes could be caused by changes in ICP as a result of changes in p_{at} of approximately 50 hPa.

Results

Published values for $paCO_2$ at different elevations are given in Table 1, along with measured or calculated atmospheric pressures. The data are further illustrated in Fig. 1.

Our own measurements yielded twelve pairs of data points on the change of $etCO_2$ with change of p_{at} by approximately 50 hPa. In eleven of these pairs, there was a significant differ-

https://doi.org/10.1007/978-3-030-59436-7_59,

Table 1 $paCO_2$ at different elevations

Elevation	p_{at}	$paCO_2$	Elevation	p_{at}	$paCO_2$	$\Delta paCO_2/\Delta\ p_{at}$	Source
(m)	(hPa)	(hPa)	(m)	(hPa)	(hPa)		
0	1013.3*	56.0	5050	536.6*	38.7	0.036	[2]
760	925.23*	52.0	3100	692.3*	46.0	0.026	[1]
0	1005.25	49.8	1400	859.9	44.5	0.037	[3]
						0.033	Mean

Data from [1–3]. Each row corresponds to one experimental condition where measurements were first made at a low elevation (first column) and then at a high elevation (fourth column). p_{at} values calculated using the barometric formula are marked by *

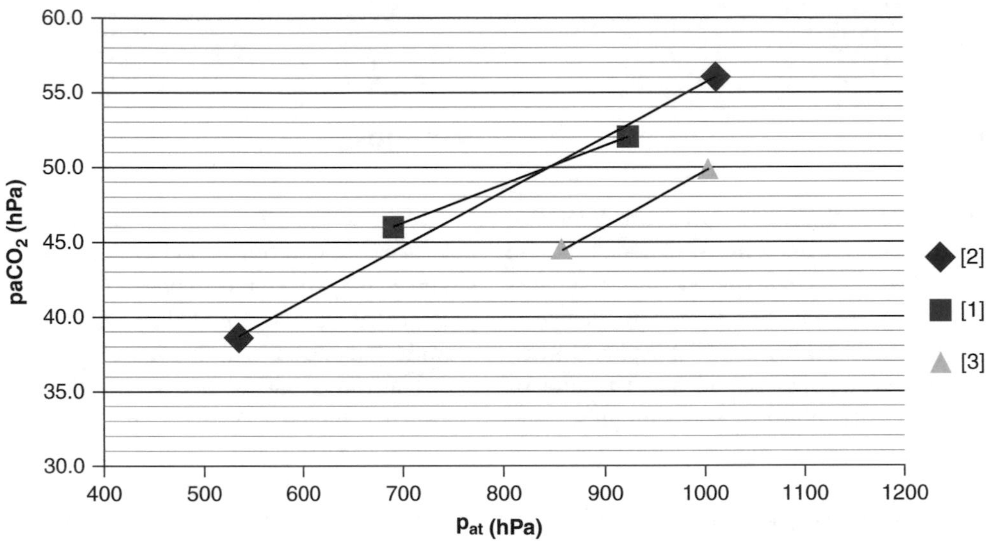

Fig. 1 Arterial partial pressure ($paCO_2$) vs. atmospheric pressure (p_{at}). Literature data [1–3]

ence between the $etCO_2$ values at either elevation ($p < 0.05$) with a positive ratio $etCO_2/p_{at}$. Table 2 shows the results. The mean ratio $etCO_2/p_{at}$ was 0.089, which is higher than the ratio described in Furian et al., Fan et al. and Crapo et al. [1–3], but still in the same order of magnitude.

Relying on the published data summarized in Fig. 1 and Table 1, we obtain

$$\Delta paCO_2 = 0.033 \bullet \Delta p_{at}. \quad (1)$$

With $\Delta p_{at} = 50$ hPa substituted into Eq. (1) we determine

$$\Delta paCO_2 = 1.65\,hPa. \quad (2)$$

While it is well known that ICP depends on $paCO_2$, there is no direct quantitative relationship given in the literature. However, for CO_2 breathing tests, the resulting change of $paCO_2$ vs. the volume-percentage of CO_2 (%CO_2) in the breathing gas is indicated in Diehl et al. [5] to be

$$\Delta paCO_2 = 2.3\,kPa / \%CO_2. \quad (3)$$

Furthermore, in Puppo et al. [6], the resulting ΔICP vs. the volume-percentage of CO_2 in the breathing gas is indicated to be

$$\Delta ICP = 0.43\,mmHg / \%CO_2 \text{ in patients with normal compliance} \quad (4)$$

and

$$\Delta ICP = 2.29\,mmHg / \%CO_2 \text{ in patients with reduced compliance.} \quad (5)$$

Substituting the value for $\Delta paCO_2$ from Eq. (2) into Eqs. (3) and (4) results in

$$\Delta ICP = 0.3\,mmHg \left(\text{with normal compliance}\right).$$

Substituting the value for $\Delta paCO_2$ from Eq. (2) into Eqs. (3) and (5) results

$$\Delta ICP = 1.65\,mmHg \left(\text{with reduced compliance}\right).$$

Performing the same calculations but using as input our own experimental data summarized in Table 2, we obtain changes in ICP that are approximately three times as large.

Table 2 Capnometrically measured end-tidal CO_2 ($etCO_2$) and atmospheric pressure (p_{at}) at different elevations on six healthy volunteers

Observation no.	Pers. no.	Elevation	p_{at}	$etCO_2$	Elevation	p_{at}	$etCO_2$	$etCO_2/p_{at}$
		(m)	hPa	hPa	(m)	hPa	hPa	
1	1	490	947.7	61.62	933	904.0	53.10	0.195
2	1	933	904.0	53.10	490	947.4	59.21	0.141
3	7	490	947.7	44.57	933	904.0	43.98	0.014
4	7	933	904.0	43.98	490	947.4	51.91	0.183
5	8	490	947.7	49.85	933	904.0	48.53	0.03
6	8	933	904.0	48.53	490	947.4	50.08	0.036
7	9	490	947.7	45.88	933	904.0	46.63	−0.017
8	9	933	904.0	46.64	490	947.4	50.19	0.082
9	10	490	947.7	49.45	933	904.0	42.21	0.166
10	10	933	904.0	42.21	490	947.4	46.45	0.098
11	4	490	930.3	55.03	933	880.3	51.16	0.077
12	1	933	889.5	54.62	490	942.2	58.02	0.064
							Mean	0.089

Person number (Pers. no.) is the identifier of the respective volunteer from a pool of volunteers. Each row corresponds to one experimental condition where measurements were first made at one elevation (second column) and then at another elevation (fifth column). For all but observation no. 7, the Mann-Whitney test resulted in $p < 0.05$ when applied to the respective change in $etCO_2$

Discussion

Our calculations, based on both published and our own data, support the hypothesis that ICP is influenced by changes of intracranial blood volume caused by autoregulatory changes in arterial diameter as a reaction to changing levels of $paCO_2$ due to changes in p_{at}. A decrease of atmospheric pressure would result in a decrease of intracranial pressure, possibly explaining the overdrainage-like symptoms described by patients. An increase of atmospheric pressure would result in an increase of intracranial pressure, possibly explaining overpressure symptoms.

Very limited data could be found in the literature on the association between p_{at} and $paCO_2$ (six data points). Likewise, the quantification of the well-known dependence of ICP on $paCO_2$ is only sparsely described in the literature (one publication, 13 patients).

We assumed linear relationships for our approximate calculations. Our own experiments resulted in only 12 observations of $etCO_2$ vs. p_{at} and they cannot be considered exhaustive. More experiments and possible determination of other factors that might have an influence on $paCO_2$ could shed further light on the interrelation between ICP and p_{at}.

Conclusion

Variations of p_{at} of 50 hPa typically observed during weather changes may result in a change of ICP of >1.65 mmHg in patients with impaired compliance. This might explain weather-related symptoms reported by hydrocephalus patients.

Conflict of Interest **The authors declare that they have no conflict of interest.**

References

1. Furian M, Lichtblau M, Aeschbacher SS et al (2018) Efficacy of dexamethasone in preventing acute mountain sickness in COPD patients. Chest 154:788–797
2. Fan JL, Burgess KR, Basnyat R, Thomas KN et al (2010) Influence of high altitude on cerebrovascular and ventilatory responsiveness to CO2. J Physiol 588:539–549
3. Crapo RO, Jensen RL, Hegewald M, Tashkin DP (1999) Arterial blood gas reference values for sea level and an altitude of 1,400 meters. Am J Respir Crit Care Med 160:1525–1531
4. Berberan-Santos MN, Bodunov EN, Pogliani L (1997) On the barometric formula. Am J Phys 65:404–412
5. Diehl RR, Berlit P, Aaslid R (2013) Funktionelle Dopplersonographie in der Neurologie. Springer-Verlag, Berlin
6. Puppo C, Fariña G, Franco LL, Caragna E, Biestro A (2008) Cerebral CO_2 reactivity in severe head injury. A transcranial Doppler study. Acta Neurochir Suppl 102:171–175

Transcranial Doppler Plateau Wave in a Patient with Pseudo-Chiari Malformation

Leandro Moraes, Mayda Noble, Bernardo Yelicich, Federico Salle, Karina DiCienzo, Alberto Biestro, and Corina Puppo

Introduction

Pseudotumor cerebri (PTC) is a syndrome caused by an increase in intracranial pressure (ICP) with normal cerebrospinal fluid (CSF) morphologic and cytochemical characteristics, without evidence of parenchymal injury in imagenologic studies.

The incidence of this medical condition is relatively frequent. In the general population it is around 0.9 per 100,000 persons. It is more frequent in women (approximately 8:1) at fertility ages, who present with obesity or weight increase during the last year, and who exhibit smoking and polycystic ovary syndrome. When obesity was considered, this increased to 13–15/100,000 for women 20–44 years of age who were 10% or more over ideal weight [1]. Furthermore, the incidence became 19.3/100,000 for women in the same age range when they were 20% or more over ideal weight. No single theory has been able to provide a comprehensive answer, and there is no consensus about the exact cause of PTC. Most of the evidence suggests increased resistance to CSF outflow as being pivotal to the syndrome [2–4].

PTC can be primary or secondary. In the first case, there is not an established pathophysiologic mechanism. In the second case, the pathophysiology is known. It can be secondary to drugs, venous sinus thrombosis, or other medical conditions.

Diagnosis is based on modified Dandy's criteria [5]:

1. Intracranial hypertension (ICH) symptoms such as headaches, nausea, vomiting, visual deficit, papilledema.
2. Absence of neurological focal signs.
3. Increased CSF pressure with normal cytochemical characteristics.
4. Normal or diminished size of cerebral ventricles.

Magnetic resonance imaging (MRI) helps to confirm or discard (extensive intracranial processes and ventricular disturbances leading to hydrocephalus) ICH causes. It also shows suggestive imaging characteristics [6, 7].

Chiari malformation is an anomaly characterized by the ectopia of tonsils, which are descended below the Foramen Magnum. This medical condition can be subdivided in primary or secondary cases. The former is congenital, and it has different genetic alterations based on embryonic development. Secondary conditions are due to cranioencephalic disproportion, chronic infratentorial space volume decrease, or cerebrospinal fluid leak leading to spinal liquor hypotension [8].

Case Report

A 26-year-old obese female patient was diagnosed with a superior sagittal and transverse sinus thrombosis with venous infarction in February 2012. No particular thrombophilic disorder was found responsible. In the next 6 months anticoagulation with warfarin was indicated but no improvement occurred. She developed progressive visual acuity impairment with peripheral campimetry deficit and fundoscopy papilledema. Lumbar puncture confirmed CSF hypertension (38 cm H_2O) compatible with ICH, and the patient was diagnosed with a secondary PTC syndrome. Cerebral digital subtraction angiography showed incom-

L. Moraes (✉) · M. Noble · B. Yelicich · K. DiCienzo
A. Biestro · C. Puppo
Intensive Care Unit, Clinicas Hospital School of Medicine, University of the Republic, Montevideo, Uruguay

F. Salle
Intensive Care Unit, Clinicas Hospital School of Medicine, University of the Republic, Montevideo, Uruguay

Neurosurgery Department, Institute of Neurology, Clinicas Hospital, School of Medicine, University of the Republic, Montevideo, Uruguay

B. Depreitere et al. (eds.), *Intracranial Pressure and Neuromonitoring XVII*, Acta Neurochirurgica Supplement 131,
https://doi.org/10.1007/978-3-030-59436-7_60,

plete sinus recanalization despite anticoagulant treatment. A lumbo-peritoneal shunt (LPS) was inserted. In 2013 symptoms recurred and a pseudo-Chiari malformation was diagnosed with MRI, showing 17 mm tonsillar descent. Intracranial hypotension as a complication of LPS was suspected. The LPS was removed and the cerebellar tonsils partially ascended, from 17 to 11 mm. After a short period of time without symptoms, she started to suffer from headaches and dizziness. A 30-min transcranial Doppler (TCD) monitoring session, including changing the height of the head of the bed, was performed in June 2018. TCD monitoring was started with the patient in a horizontal position and with the head of the bed elevated 45°. When the head of bed was lowered to 0°, dizziness and tinnitus appeared at the same time as a decrease in Cerebral Blood Flow Velocity (FV) and an increase in pulsatility index (PI) with the ultrasonographic characteristics of a plateau wave of ICH, lasting for 6 min.

A ventriculo-peritoneal shunt (VPS) was inserted, after which the patient began to improve clinically. Studies also showed signs of resolution. Specifically, the right visual field made a significant recovery (Figs. 1, 2, and 3).

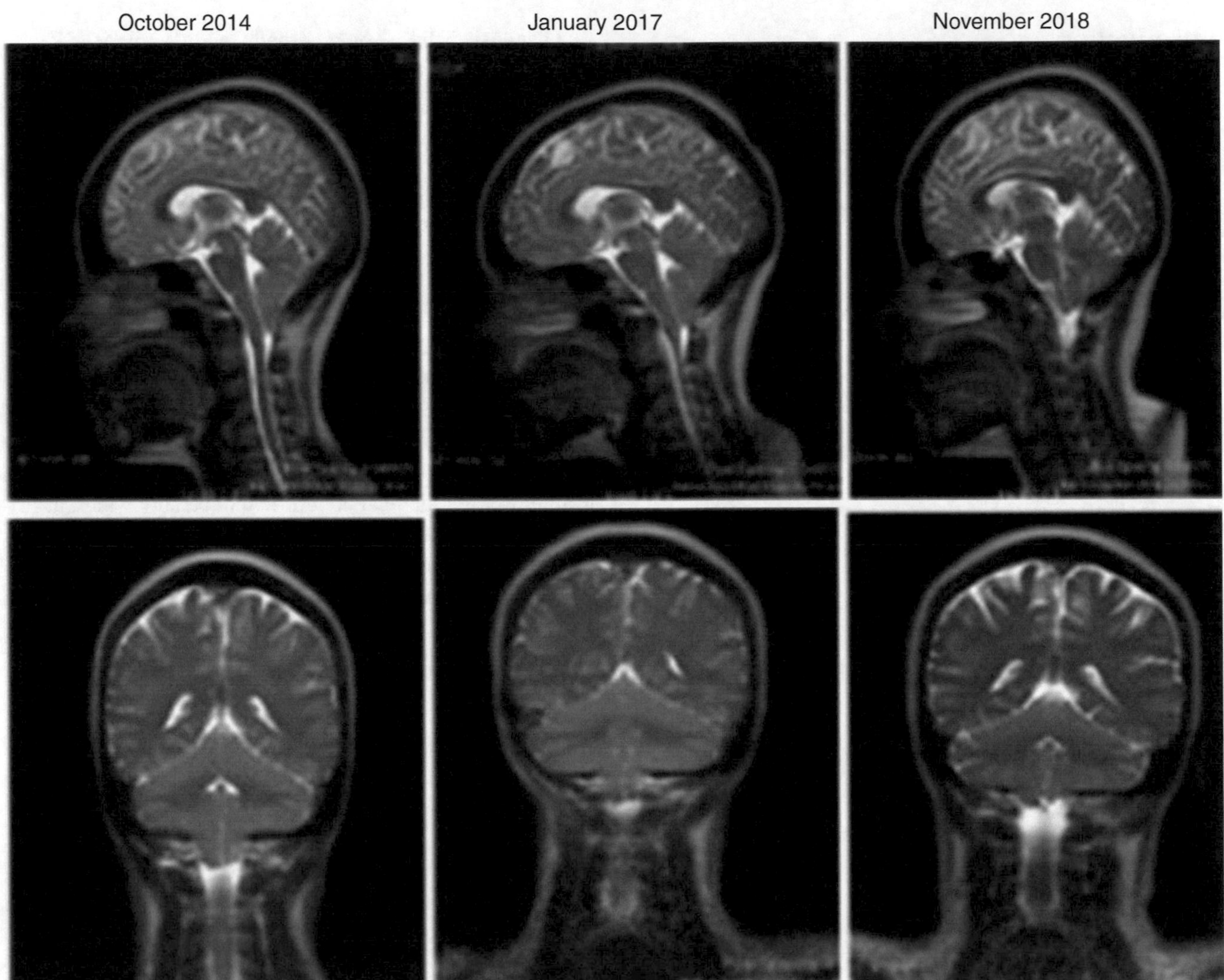

Fig. 1 Brain Magnetic Resonance Images in October 2014, January 2017 and November 2018

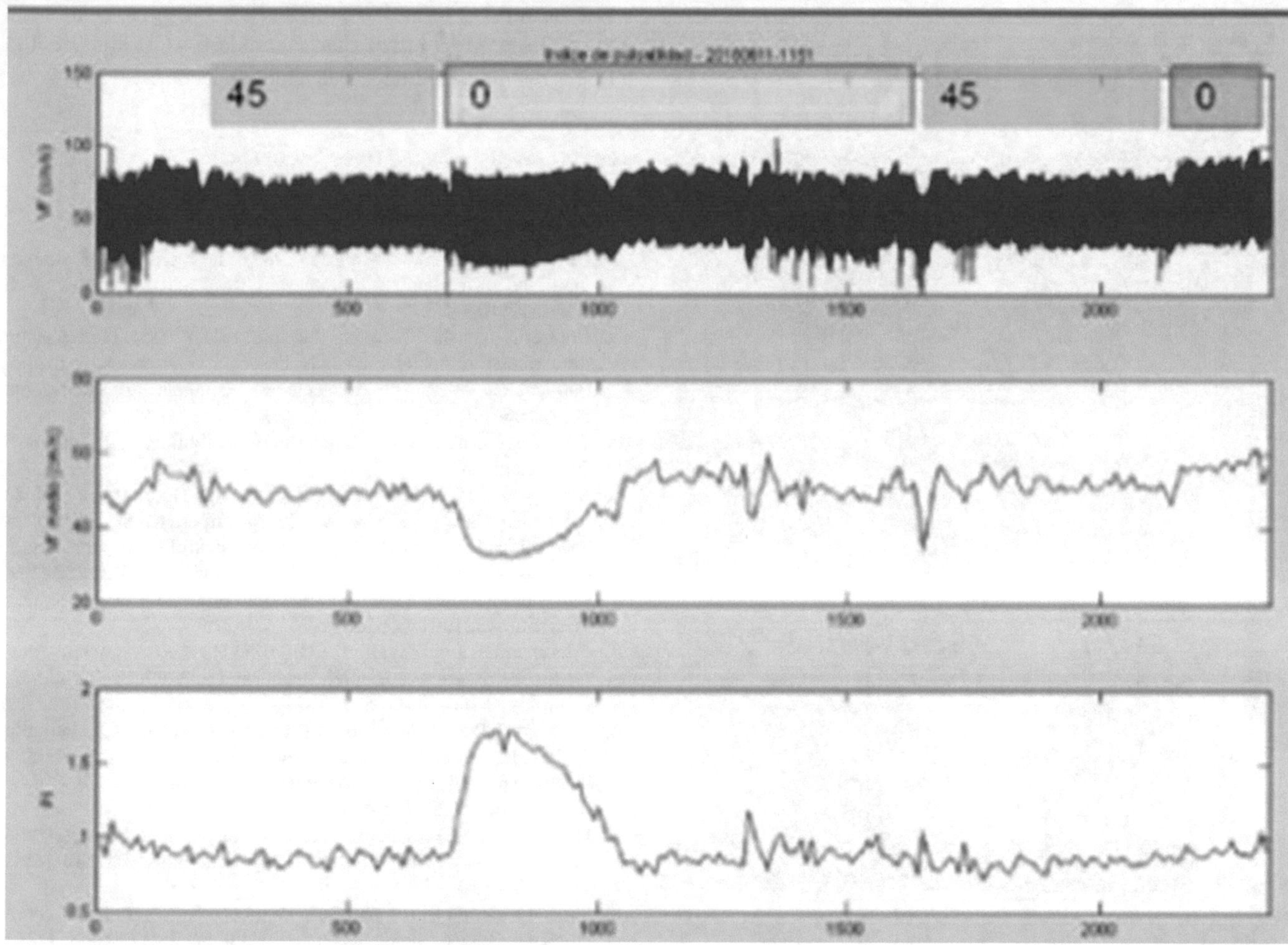

Fig. 2 Time sequence plot of cerebral blood flow velocity (FV) and pulsatility index (PI) evolution during changes in head of bed position (in green and orange bars). Upper line: FV raw signals; middle panel: FV mean; Bottom panel: PI

Discussion

Cerebral venous thrombosis is a well-known cause of Secondary PTC Syndrome [9]. Usually, anticoagulation facilitates thrombus resolution and venous circulation normalizes. Although a strict nutrition plan with weight reduction and targeted INR (2–3) were achieved, our patient did not respond to these measures and developed ICH. Typically, bilateral visual field compromise appeared, leading the neurosurgery team to indicate an LPS. Intracranial hypotension developed as an LPS complication, with a 17-mm transforaminal downward cerebellar (tonsillar) herniation (Pseudo-Chiari Malformation); therefore, LPS was removed. Symptomatology reappeared after removing the LPS, leading to high risk of bilateral visual field compromise and blindness. A noninvasive TCD continuous neuromonitoring was performed. Interestingly, the trigger maneuver (lowering the head of the bed) was critical to reach the final diagnosis. We hypothesize that when the position of the head of the bed was changed to zero, the descended cerebellar tonsils, already obstructing CSF flow at the cranio-cervical junction, would change their position, increasing the obstruction to CSF passage and thus generating ICH.

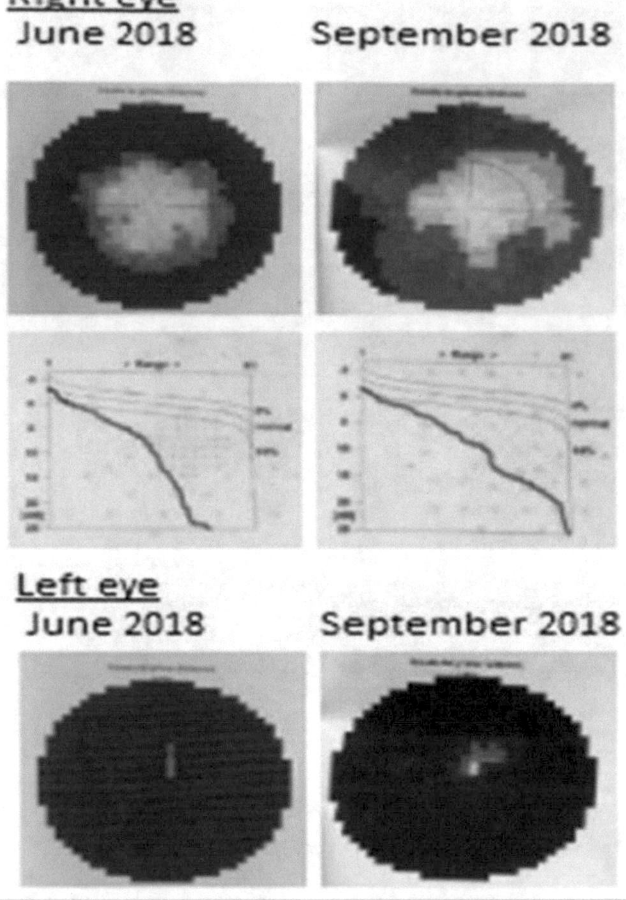

Fig. 3 Digital campimetry before and after ventriculo-peritoneal shunt

This 30-min totally noninvasive monitoring session highly suggested ICH during changes of head of bed height (trigger maneuver) and helped the neurosurgeon to decide on surgery. Considering the short time period required for TCD neuromonitoring (30–60 min including a trigger maneuver), use of this process rather than a standard TCD study could add interesting data in difficult clinical scenarios [10].

References

1. Durcan FJ, Corbett JJ, Wall M (1988) The incidence of pseudotumor cerebri: population studies in Iowa and Louisiana. Arch Neurol 45:875–877
2. Contreras Martin Y, Bueno Perdomo JH (2015) Hipertensión intracraneal idiopática: análisis descriptivo en nuestro medio. Publicación oficial de la sociedad Española de Neurología 30(2):106–110
3. Gaye Saavedra A (2016) Pseudotumor cerebral. Revista uruguaya de medicina interna 3:52–61
4. Rodriguez Pupo JM, Diaz Rojas YV, Rojas Rodriguez Y, Nuñez Arias E, Garcia Gomez A (2015) Hipertension intracraneana idiopática: principales aspectos neurofisiológicos, diagnosticos y terapéuticos. Articulos de revisión 19(2):282–299. Disponible en http://scielo.sld.cu/scielo.php?script=sci_arttext&pid=S1560-43812015000200010
5. Friedman DI, Liu GT, Digre KB (2013) Revised diagnostic criteria for the pseudotumor cerebri syndrome in adults and children. Neurology 81:1159–1165
6. Moncho D, Poca MA, Minoves T, Ferré A, Rahnama K, Sahuquillo J (2013) Potenciales evocados auditivos del tronco cerebral y somatosensoriales en los pacientes con malformación de Chiari. Rev Neurol 56(12):623–634
7. Panerai R (1998) Assessment of cerebral pressure autoregulation in humans—a review of measurement methods. Physiol Meas 19(3):305–338
8. Sanchez-Zuñiga M d J (2007) Tratamiento de hypertension endocraneana. Revista Mexicana de anestesiología 20(1):346–351
9. Bjornson A, Tapply I, Nabbanja E, Lalou AD, Czosnyka M, Czosnyka Z, Muthusamy B, Garnett M (2019) Ventriculoperitoneal shunting is a safe and effective treatment for idiopathic intracranial hypertension. Br J Neurosurg 33:62–70
10. Czosnyka M, Smielewski P, Piechnik S, Schmidt EA, Ai-Rawi PG, Kirkpatrick PJ, Pickard JD (1999) Hemodynamic characterization of intracranial pressure plateau waves in head-injury patients. J Neurosurg 91(1):11–19

Telemetric Intracranial Pressure: A Snapshot Does not Give the Full Story

Maya Kommer, Richard G. Boulton, Lynette Loi, Sophie Robinson, Christopher Hawthorne, Martin Shaw, Ian Piper, Laura Moss, Anthony Amato-Watkins, Emer Campbell, Meharpal Sangra, and Roddy O'Kane

Introduction

Complex hydrocephalus remains one of the major challenges of neurosurgical practice. Patients with this condition often have multiple admissions and procedures to assess and optimize shunt function. Historically these patients had multiple shunt revisions and valve adjustments with a high associated risk of morbidity due to infection, malposition, and blockage. The assessment of shunt function on purely clinical and radiological grounds is notoriously unreliable in this group of patients. Ventricular caliber may not always increase when there is shunt dysfunction and many of these patients also have a chronic headache disorder unrelated to their hydrocephalus. Intracranial pressure (ICP) monitoring can be used to assess shunt function and aid in the process of determining optimal valve settings. Traditional cabled monitors require a new surgical procedure with its risk of intraparenchymal hemorrhage and infection. In addition, the period of monitoring is limited and requires connection to a recording device. Telemetric ICP monitors have been developed to overcome some of these challenges. The device can remain in situ for several months and this can allow for multiple periods of shunt assessment and adjustment. Some neurosurgeons would use a one-off reading to exclude shunt dysfunction in situations where there is uncertainty about the clinical presentation. We sought to determine whether short recordings were reflective of longer periods of monitoring and thereby assess the safety of one-off measurements.

M. Kommer (✉) · R. G. Boulton · L. Loi · S. Robinson
C. Hawthorne · M. Shaw · I. Piper · L. Moss · A. Amato-Watkins
E. Campbell · M. Sangra · R. O'Kane
Institute of Neurological Sciences, Royal Hospital for Children, Glasgow, UK
e-mail: maya.kommer@ggc.scot.nhs.uk

Materials and Methods

We identified patients who had telemetric ICP monitors inserted between 2016 and 2019 at a single institution. Under a general anesthetic we made a frontal incision, performed a craniostomy, punctured the dura, and inserted an intraparenchymal Raumedic® telemetric ICP probe. The wound was closed, and the device was read to ensure it was functioning correctly. Data was downloaded from the device using Raumedic® datalog software, and this was subsequently processed using a custom python script. The data sampling frequency was one point per second. The first 60 s of continuous recording were compared to the overall trace for mean, median, maximum, and minimum values using the Wilcoxon signed rank test. The data was analyzed using R.

Results

Eleven patients were identified who underwent thirty periods of ICP recording. Seven were female and four were male. The median age at time of recording was 14.2 (range 2.4 years to 46.2 years). The underlying etiology of the CSF disturbance was idiopathic intracranial hypertension (IIH) in four, arachnoid cyst in two, spina bifida in two, one patient had a craniopharyngioma, one had Pfeiffer's syndrome, and one had aqueduct stenosis. The clinical indication for monitoring was for shunt assessment in 17 (57.7%), post new telemetric monitor insertion in six (16.7%), four post removal of shunt to assess shunt independence (13.3%), and three for investigation of IIH (10%). There were no complications of telemetric device insertion. The median length of the overall recording was 17.3 h (range 139.4 min to 41.4 h). The median value and interquartile ranges for the series of median ICP, mean ICP, maximum ICP, and minimum ICP for the full study and the first 60 s of continuous recording are shown in Table 1. The median ICP for the full recordings was

B. Depreitere et al. (eds.), *Intracranial Pressure and Neuromonitoring XVII*, Acta Neurochirurgica Supplement 131,
https://doi.org/10.1007/978-3-030-59436-7_61, © Springer Nature Switzerland AG 2021

Table 1 ICP values comparing the full study with the first 60 s of continuous recording

	Full study (n =30) IQR median (low, high)	60 s (n = 30) IQR median (low, high)	Z-score (p value)
ICP Median (mmHg)	2.33 (−5.19, 8.04)	−2.42 (−8.51, 4.16)	2.91 (0.0018)
ICP Mean (mmHg)	2.80 (−5.28, 8.29)	−2.42 (−8.51, 4.16)	2.94 (0.0016)
ICP Max (mmHg)	15.20 (9.08, 23.03)	−0.45 (−7.53, 10.15)	4.39 (<0.001)
ICP Min (mmHg)	−8.80 (−16.88, −4.20)	−1.25 (−7.65, 8.58)	−4.62 (<0.001)

The Z-score and p value were determined using the Wilcoxon signed rank test

2.33 mmHg compared with −2.42 mmHg for the first 60 s of recording ($p = 0.0018$). The mean ICP for the full recordings was 2.8 mmHg compared with −2.42 mmHg for the first 60 s of recording ($p = 0.0016$). The median of the maximum values of ICP for the full recordings was 15.2 mmHg compared with −0.45 mmHg for the first 60 s of recording ($p = <0.001$). The median of the minimum values of ICP for the full recordings was −8.8 mmHg compared with −1.25 for the first 60 s of recording ($p = <0.001$). Following the period of ICP monitoring the trace was felt to be reassuring in 24 instances of recording, and six patients had their programmable shunt valve setting changed. The telemetric ICP recording caused no suspicion of shunt dysfunction in any of the patients.

Discussion

ICP monitoring remains an essential assessment tool for any neurosurgical service; it has a wide range of indications, including the management of severe head injuries, as well as in the diagnosis and management of more chronic neurosurgical conditions. Despite their usefulness in clinical assessment, traditional cabled intracranial pressure monitors have significant limitations. They do not allow for extended periods of monitoring because there would be significant concerns about introducing infection. Each admission for assessment would require a new general anesthetic and new insertion of a probe with its associated risk of infection and intraparenchymal hemorrhage. The first preliminary design report of a telemetric ICP monitor came in 1977 [1], but it is only over the past decade that the neurosurgical community has embraced the use of these devices. More recent reports in the literature suggest that these devices are being used mainly in the management of complex hydrocephalus. Although all our patients were inpatients for their ICP monitoring, there are also reports in the literature of the device being used in the patients' home or school [2, 3]. This allows the assessment of these complex patients in their usual environment and may reduce the amount of time spent in hospital. This is of great benefit because many of these patients miss much time in school or at work. Many of the reports of the use of telemetric devices seem to support the one-off measurement of ICP when guiding shunt valve adjustment or even as a way to avoid hospital admission where there is diagnostic uncertainty [3, 4]. In our study we found that even a measurement lasting 60 s was not reflective of the overall trace, and as such we feel it would be unsuitable for clinical decision-making. This was statistically significant for median, mean, maximum, and minimum values. Although most of our patients were discharged, 20% had valve adjustments made based on their overall recording.

The limitation of this work is the small number of patients and the fact that none of our patients went on to require shunt revision based on their telemetric recording. In the setting of a completely blocked shunt the ICP reading should be high; even as a one-off recording. Overall, we feel that telemetric devices are extremely useful in the management of complex hydrocephalus and IIH, but the readings should be continuous to achieve the most accurate picture of the underlying pathophysiology.

Conflict of Interest **The authors declare no conflict of interest.**

References

1. Zervas NT, Cosman ER, Cosman BJ (1977) A pressure-balanced radio-telemetry system for the measurement of intracranial pressure. J Neurosurg 46(6):899–911
2. Tschan CA, Velazquez Sanchez VF, Heckelmann M, Antes S (2019) Home telemonitoring of intracranial pressure. Acta Neurochir 161(8):1605–1617
3. Barber J, Pringle CJ, Raffalli-Ebezant H, Pathmanaban O, Ramirez R, Kamaly-Asl ID (2016) Telemetric intra-cranial pressure monitoring: clinical and financial considerations. Br J Neurosurg 31(3):300–306
4. Freimann FB, Schulz M, Haberl H, Thomale UW (2013) Feasibility of telemetric ICP-guided valve adjustments for complex shunt therapy. Childs Nerv Syst 30(4):689–697

Noninvasive Intracranial Pressure Assessment in Patients with Suspected Idiopathic Intracranial Hypertension

Bernhard Schmidt, Marek Czosnyka, Danilo Cardim, and Bernhard Rosengarten

Introduction

Idiopathic intracranial hypertension (IIH), also called pseudotumour cerebri [1], usually occurs in obese women of childbearing age. The typical symptoms are headache, sight disorders, and vertigo. Besides ophthalmoscopy and MRI, lumbar puncture is a common procedure in IIH. It is used for both diagnosis, by assessing the lumbar pressure (LP) through height of column of cerebrospinal fluid (CSF), and for therapy, by draining some volume of CSF. Due to its invasive and painful nature, lumbar puncture is not always tolerated by patients. In this study, noninvasively assessed intracranial pressure (nICP) (Fig. 1) was used as a surrogate metric for LP. Comparison to LP should clarify the suitability of nICP assessment for diagnosis of IIH. nICP was calculated using continuous measures of noninvasive arterial blood pressure and flow velocity of middle cerebral artery (CBFV), a method previously introduced [2] and validated by the authors [3–6] in patients with traumatic brain injuries.

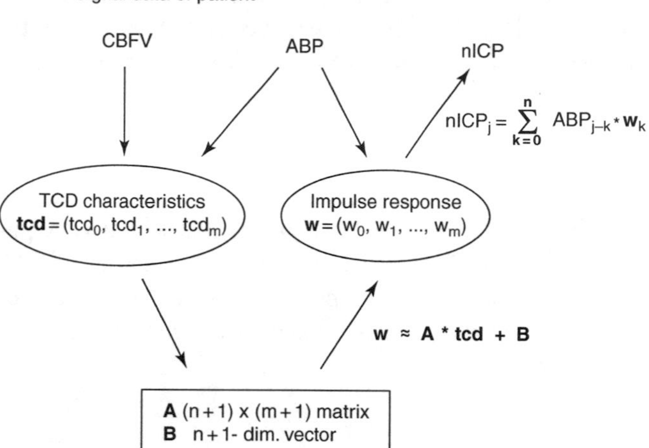

Fig. 1 Calculation of nICP. From measured CBFV and ABP the TCD characteristics are derived and multiplied with a matrix **A**. After adding vector **B** this results in the ABP → ICP impulse response, a function which transforms the ABP signal into the nICP signal. The TCD characteristics essentially consist of ABP → CBFV impulse response together with additional ICP related parameters. Matrix **A** and vector **B** have been formerly calculated using a signal database of approximately 200 reference patients (traumatic brain injuries: ~75%, stroke and other non-traumatic brain diseases: ~25%). The stored signals consisted of CBFV, ABP, and ICP (invasively assessed by intraparenchymal or intraventricular pressure probes). Multiple regressions were used to express the relationship between TCD characteristic and ABP → ICP impulse response in terms of **A** and **B**

Materials and Methods

Patients

In this prospective, ongoing study, thirteen patients with suspected IIH (f = 11, m = 2; age = 36 ± 10 years) treated between 2017 and 2019 in Chemnitz Medical Centre have been included so far. nICP was assessed 1 h prior to lumbar

B. Schmidt (✉) · B. Rosengarten
Department of Neurology, Chemnitz Medical Centre, Chemnitz, Germany
e-mail: b.schmidt@skc.de

M. Czosnyka
Brain Physics Laboratory, Division of Neurosurgery, Department of Clinical Neurosciences, University of Cambridge, Cambridge, UK

D. Cardim
Department of Neurology and Neurotherapeutics, University of Texas Southwestern Medical Center, Dallas, TX, USA

B. Depreitere et al. (eds.), *Intracranial Pressure and Neuromonitoring XVII*, Acta Neurochirurgica Supplement 131, https://doi.org/10.1007/978-3-030-59436-7_62, © Springer Nature Switzerland AG 2021 puncture. If LP was above 20 cmH_2O (~15 mmHg) a lumbar drainage of 10–30 ml of CSF was performed. LP was then measured again, immediately after drainage, and nICP was reassessed 2 h later.

The study was approved by the Local Ethics Committee. All patients agreed to participation to the study by informed consent. Lumbar puncture was part of the clinical routine in cases of suspected IIH.

Monitoring

CBFV was assessed by transcranial Doppler (TCD) ultrasound technique. A two-MHz pulsed Doppler device (Multidop-P, DWL, Sipplingen, Germany) was used for bilateral assessment of TCD signal. ABP was continuously measured, noninvasively, with a tonometric sensor device placed on radial artery (Colin CBM 7000, ScanMed Medical Instruments, Moreton-in-Marsh, UK), which regularly calibrates by a standard arm cuff using oscillometric techniques [7]. A personal computer fitted with data acquisition systems (Daq 112B, Iotech, Inc., Cleveland, OH, USA) and software developed in-house [2] was used for recording and analyzing TCD and ABP signals and for calculation of nICP.

Results

Due to measured high LP (above 20 cmH_2O), immediate lumbar drainage was performed in eight patients. In six of these patients LP was measured again directly after the drainage and compared to nICP, which was reassessed 2 h later. In three patients, one additional assessment of nICP versus LP was performed during control visits with time lags of 3 weeks, 3 months, and 9 months between initial and control assessments. In total, 22 data pairs of LP and nICP were compared. They correlated with $R = 0.82$ ($p < 0.001$; $N = 22$). Bivariate normal distribution was tested by Mudholkar test ($p = 0.08$; $N = 22$). Mean difference of ICP-nICP was 0.8 ± 3.7 mmHg, mean absolute difference was 3.0 mmHg. Presuming 15 mmHg as critical threshold for a need of lumbar drainage, the clinical implications would have been the same in both methods in 20 of 22 cases (Fig. 2).

Discussion

The nICP showed a good agreement with LP pressure readings in terms of absolute pressure values. Moreover, both methods largely coincide if used as a diagnostic tool for indication of CSF drainage. In view of its suitability to indicate

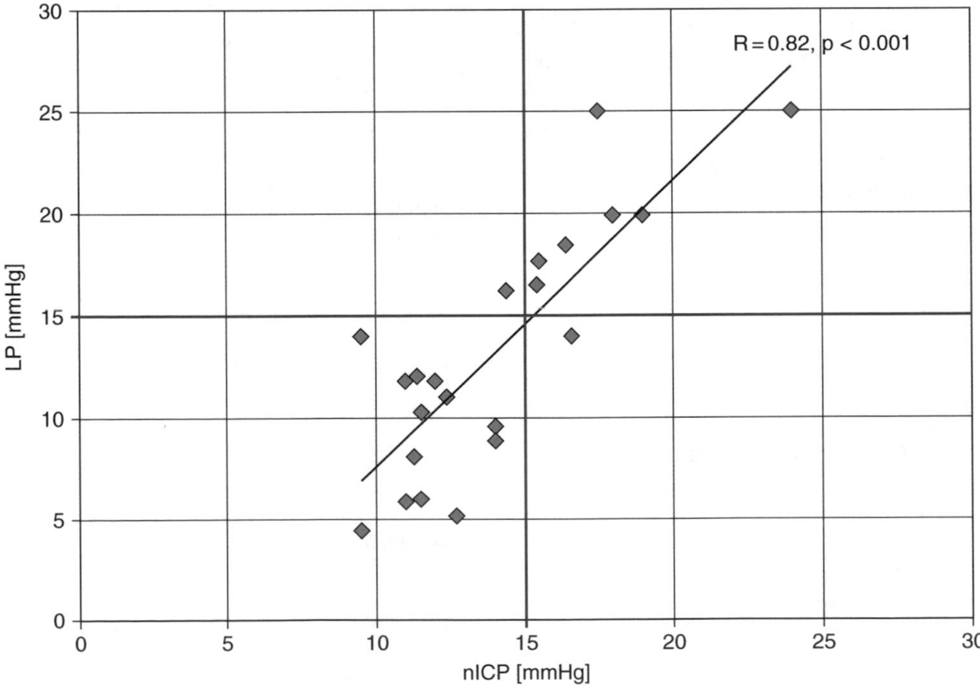

Fig. 2 LP versus nICP in 22 cases of 13 patients. LP significantly correlates with nICP with $R = 0.82$ ($p < 0.001$). The red lines highlight the critical threshold of 15 mmHg for clinical indication of lumbar drainage. The dots which are either in area upper right or lower left represent cases with concordant clinical implications in both methods. In only two cases the results were contradictive

both increased as well as normal ICP, it was important to compare nICP to LP before and, if applicable, after lumbar drainage, when ICP had decreased to normal values. Decrease of ICP causes a change of status in the investigated system; therefore, both observations could be assumed to be independent.

Limitations

The number of patients included in the study is small. More patients need to be included to enable more solid conclusions.

In some patients we also insonated the optic nerve sheath and estimated its diameter (ONSD) as a well-known ICP-sensitive parameter [8]. Up to this point, however, this has not been done systematically, so we did not mention any results here. Further exploration of this issue will be subject to the ongoing study. In three patients, LP and nICP assessment was repeated after readmission. Due to large time lags between their visits, the cases were treated as independent cases in our evaluation.

Conclusion

TCD-based assessment of ICP seems to be a promising method for a pre-diagnosis of increased LP, which might prevent the need for an invasive lumbar puncture in cases of low nICP. Moreover, the method might allow patient-friendly long-term monitoring. Further study is necessary to increase the number of included patients.

Conflict of Interest **B.S. and M.C. have financial interest in a part of licensing fee for noninvasive ICP plugin of ICM+ software.**

References

1. Wakerley BR, Tan MH, Ting EY (2015) Idiopathic intracranial hypertension. Cephalalgia 35(3):248–261. https://doi.org/10.1177/0333102414534329
2. Schmidt B, Klingelhöfer J, Schwarze JJ, Sander D, Wittich I (1997) Noninvasive prediction of intracranial pressure curves using transcranial Doppler ultrasonography and blood pressure curves. Stroke 28:2465–2472
3. Schmidt B, Czosnyka M, Klingelhöfer J (2002) Clinical applications of a non-invasive ICP monitoring method. Eur J Ultrasound 16(1–2):37–45
4. Schmidt B, Czosnyka M, Smielewski P, Plontke R, Schwarze JJ, Klingelhöfer J, Pickard JD (2016) Noninvasive assessment of ICP: evaluation of new TBI data. In: Ang BT (ed) Intracranial pressure and brain monitoring XV, Acta Neurochir Suppl, vol 122. Springer, Cham, pp 69–73. https://doi.org/10.1007/978-3-319-22533-3_14
5. Cardim D, Robba C, Donnelly J, Bohdanowicz M, Schmidt B, Damian M, Varsos GV, Liu X, Cabeleira M, Frigieri G, Cabella B, Smielewski P, Mascarenhas S, Czosnyka M (2016) Prospective study on noninvasive assessment of intracranial pressure in traumatic brain-injured patients: comparison of four methods. J Neurotrauma 33:792–802. https://doi.org/10.1089/neu.2015.4134
6. Cardim D, Robba C, Schmidt E, Schmidt B, Donnelly J, Klinck J, Czosnyka M (2019) Transcranial Doppler non-invasive assessment of intracranial pressure, autoregulation of cerebral blood flow and critical closing pressure during orthotopic liver transplant. Ultrasound Med Biol 45(6):1435–1445. https://doi.org/10.1016/j.ultrasmedbio.2019.02.003
7. Zorn EA, Wilson BM, Angel JJ, Zanella J, Alport BS (1997) Validation of an automated arterial tonomtry monitor using Association for the Advancement of Medical Instrumentation standards. Blood Press Monit 2:185–188
8. Koziarz A, Sne N, Kegel F, Alhazzani W, Nath S, Badhiwala JH, Rice T, Engels P, Samir F, Healey A, Kahnamoui K, Banfield L, Sharma S, Reddy K, Hawryluk GWJ, Kirkpatrick AW, Almenawer SA (2017) Optic nerve sheath diameter sonography for the diagnosis of increased intracranial pressure: a systematic review and meta-analysis protocol. BMJ Open 7(8):e016194. https://doi.org/10.1136/bmjopen-2017-016194

Should the Impact of Postural Change of Intracranial Pressure After Surgical Repair of Skull Base Cerebrospinal Fluid Leaks Be Considered? A Preliminary Survey

Valentin Favier, Louis Crampette, Laurent Gergelé, Generoso De Cristofaro, Emmanuel Jouanneau, and Romain Manet

Introduction

Skull base cerebrospinal fluid (CSF) leaks can result from cranio-facial trauma or from skull base surgery. Endoscopic endonasal skull base surgery (ESBS) for minimally invasive resection of skull base tumours, using the nasal fossae pathway, often requires a concomitant meningeal resection (when the tumour has an intracranial extension or adherence the dura). In such cases, cerebrospinal fluid (CSF) leaks may occur and must be closed at the same time. ESBS is also used to manage spontaneous or traumatic CSF leaks.

Surgical options to repair skull base osteomeningeal defects are numerous and have been widely described, including local pedicled flaps [1], free flaps [2], and autologous [3] or synthetic [4] grafts. The major principle is to achieve a watertight closure that can also support the brain (and avoid brain sagging) in the case of extensive skull base defects. Many clinical factors may influence the success rate of the reconstruction. Surprisingly, the influence of postural adaptation of intracranial pressure (ICP) [5, 6] has been rarely discussed in this context.

V. Favier · L. Crampette
Department of ENT—Head and Neck Surgery, Gui de Chauliac Hospital, University Hospital of Montpellier, Montpellier, France

L. Gergelé
Intensive Care, Ramsay Générale de Santé, Hôpital Privé de la Loire, Saint Etienne, France

G. De Cristofaro
Department of Mental and Physical Health and Preventive Medicine, ENT Unit of University of Campania "Luigi Vanvitelli"—University Hospital "Luigi Vanvitelli", Naples, Italy

E. Jouanneau · R. Manet (✉)
Skull Base Unit, Department of Neurosurgery B, Neurological Hospital Pierre Wertheimer, University Hospital of Lyon, Lyon, France
e-mail: romain.manet@neurochirurgie.fr

In this study we aimed to gather the opinion of skull base surgeons on postoperative posture restrictions of patients treated for skull base CSF leaks, and to evaluate their relevance from a physiological point of view.

Materials and Methods

An anonymous opinion survey on postoperative management of patients managed with ESBS was created in December 2018, then reviewed and accepted by the board of the French Association of Rhinology (AFR). An electronic questionnaire (Google Form, Google, Mountain View, California, U.S.A.) was submitted by e-mail to AFR members and to French College of Neurosurgery members in January 2019 and March 2019, respectively. This consisted of a single mail-out with no reminders sent subsequently. Responses from January 2019 through April 2019 were aggregated using Excel 2010 software (Microsoft Corp., Redmond, Washington, U.S.A.).

Statistical analysis was performed to determine if significant differences existed between the proportions or means of response data. A free website (https://biostatgv.sentiweb.fr/) was used for all data analysis. Descriptive statistics were used to analyse demographic data of respondents, case numbers, and proportions of various practice patterns. Continuous variables were described using means while categorical variables were presented as frequencies/percentages. Univariate analyses were conducted using two-tailed independent sample t-tests or Fisher's exact tests, as applicable. For all tests, P values <0.05 were considered as statistically significant.

This study was approved by the institutional review board of the Montpellier University Hospital (2019_IRM-MTP_10-12) and was registered on clinicaltrials.gov (RECHMPL19_0468).

B. Depreitere et al. (eds.), *Intracranial Pressure and Neuromonitoring XVII*, Acta Neurochirurgica Supplement 131,
https://doi.org/10.1007/978-3-030-59436-7_63,

Results

Thirty-nine surgeons completed the electronic survey in its entirety: 28 rhinologists and 11 neurosurgeons. The response rate was 28.2% of the AFR members; it was not possible to estimate the response rate among the French neurosurgical community (survey submitted through the domain @neurochirurgie.fr that accounts for approximately 600 addresses, with no possibility of knowing how many of these are routinely used). The demographic data for respondents are presented in Table 1. Postoperative CSF leak management was formally protocoled in 25.7% (written protocol, $n = 10$), protocoled but non-written in 35.9% ($n = 14$), and non-protocoled in 38.4% ($n = 15$). Only 7.7% ($n = 3$) of respondents never recommended a resting position regardless of the size or site of the leak. 46.15% ($n = 18$) systematically recommended a resting position following an ESBS CSF leak closure and 46.15% ($n = 18$) recommended a resting position according to the size or site of the leak.

Table 1 Demographic data of respondents

	Rhinologists *n* (%)	Neurosurgeons *n* (%)	Total *n* (%)
N	28 (100%)	11 (100%)	39 (100%)
Country			
France	25 (**89.3%**)	11 (100%)	36 (**92.3%**)
Switzerland	1 (**3.6%**)	0 (0%)	1 (**2.6%**)
Belgium	1 (**3.6%**)	0 (0%)	1 (**2.6%**)
Marocco	1 (**3.6%**)	0 (0%)	1 (**2/6%**)
Practice			
University Hospital	24 (**85.7%**)	11 (100%)	35 (**89.7%**)
Public Non-Academic Hospital	2 (**7.1%**)	0 (0%)	2 (**5.13%**)
Private practice	1 (**3.6%**)	0 (0%)	1 (**2.6%**)
Private/public practice	1 (**3.6%**)	0 (0%)	1 (**2.6%**)
Otorhinolaryngology and Neurosurgery Units			
Yes—same building	11 (**39.3%**)	8 (**72.7%**)	19 (**48.7%**)
Yes—other building	11 (**39.3%**)	3 (**27.3%**)	14 (**35.9%**)
No	6 (**21.4%**)	0 (**0%**)	6 (**15.4%**)
Experience in endoscopic skull base surgery			
<5 years	5 (**17.9%**)	3 (**27.3%**)	8 (**20.5%**)
5–9 years	6 (**21.4%**)	3 (**27.3%**)	9 (**23.1%**)
10–14 years	4 (**14.3%**)	2 (**18.2%**)	6 (**15.4%**)
15–19 years	2 (**7.1%**)	2 (**18.2%**)	4 (**10.3%**)
20 years or more	11 (**39.3%**)	1 (**9.1%**)	12 (**30.8%**)

Resting Position

The resting positions that were recommended, according to the location and size of the leak, are summarized in Table 2. Most of the respondents recommended a half-sitting position (Fowler's position) for all categories of CSF leak: 16/39 for

Table 2 Duration and type of resting position according to the site and size of the leak

	No*N* (%)	Supine *N* (%)	Fowler's position*N* (%)	Sitting *N* (%)	Total of respondents
Small CSF leaks of the ASB	16 (41%)	6 (15.4%)	16 (41.0%)	1 (2.6%)	39
24 h	NA	0	5	1 (2.6%)	6 (15.4%)
48 h	NA	5 (12.8%)	9 (23.1%)	0	14 (35.9%)
72 h	NA	1 (2.6%)	2 (5.1%)	0	3 (7.7%)
96 h	NA	0	0	0	0
120 h	NA	0	0	0	0
Large CSF leaks of the ASB	6 (15.8%)	10 (26.3%)	21 (55.3%)	1 (2.6%)	38
24 h	NA	0	2 (5.3%)	0	2 (5.3%)
48 h	NA	4 (10.5%)	8 (21.1%)	1 (2.6%)	13 (34.2%)
72 h	NA	2 (5.3%)	7 (18.4%)	0	9 (23.7%)
96 h	NA	2 (5.3%)	1 (2.6%)	0	3 (7.9%)
120 h	NA	1 (2.6%)	2 (5.3%)	0	3 (7.9%)
Variable	NA	1 (2.6%)	1 (2.6%)	0	0
Small CSF leaks of the sphenoid	19	5 (13.2%)	13 (34.2%)	1 (2.6%)	38
24 h	NA	0	3 (7.9%)	1 (2.6%)	4 (10.5%)
48 h	NA	4 (10.5%)	7 (18.4%)	0	11 (29%)
72 h	NA	1 (2.6%)	3 (7.9%)	0	4 (10.5%)

Table 2 (continued)

	No*N* (%)	Supine *N* (%)	Fowler's position*N* (%)	Sitting *N* (%)	Total of respondents
96 h	NA	0	0	0	0
120 h	NA	0	0	0	0
Large CSF leaks of the sphenoid	6 (16.2% [4.3–28.1])	10 (27%)	21 (56.8%)	0	37
24 h	NA	0	0	0	0
48 h	NA	4 (10.8%)	10 (27%)	0	14 (37.8%)
72 h	NA	3 (8.1%)	10 (27%)	0	13 (35.1%)
96 h	NA	1 (2.7%)	0	0	1 (2.7%)
120 h	NA	1 (2.7%)	1 (2.7%)	0	2 (5.4%)
Variable	NA	1 (2.7%)	0	0	1 (2.7%)
CSF leaks of the clivus	7 (20.6% [7–34.2])	7 (20.6%)	20 (58.8%)	0	34
24 h	NA	0	2 (5.9%)	0	2 (5.9%)
48 h	NA	4 (11.8%)	10 (29.4%)	0	14 (41.2%)
72 h	NA	0	7 (20.6%)	0	7 (20.6%)
96 h	NA	2 (5.9%)	0	0	2 (5.9%)
120 h	NA	1 (2.9%)	1 (2.9%)	0	2 (5.9%)

CSF Cerebrospinal fluid, *ASB* anterior skull base

small CSF leaks of the anterior skull base, 21/38 for large CSF leaks of the anterior skull base, 13/38 for small CSF leaks of the sphenoid, 21/37 for large CSF leaks of the sphenoid and 20/34 for CSF leaks of the clivus. The sitting position was recommended by only 1 respondent in the case of CSF leaks of the anterior skull base and small CSF leaks of the sphenoid. Other respondents recommended the supine position.

For small CSF leaks of the sphenoid or the anterior skull base, 41% of the respondents did not recommend any resting position (n = 16/39) versus 10% for large CSF leaks (n = 4/39) (p = 0.0103). For CSF leaks of the clivus, 20.6% of the respondents did not recommend any resting position (n = 7/34). Finally, 3 respondents (7.7%) never recommended a postoperative resting position, regardless of the location or size of the defect, while 18 respondents (46.2%) systematically recommended a resting position.

Exceptions to Resting Position

When a resting position was prescribed, in the case of small CSF leaks of the anterior skull base, 65% (15/23) of respondents allowed at least one exception among activities such as going to the toilet, taking a shower, or sitting up for meals; 56% (18/32) of respondents in the case of large CSF leaks of the anterior skull base; 63% (12/19) in the case of small CSF leaks of the sphenoid; 55% (17/31) in the case of large CSF leaks of the sphenoid; and 59% (16/27) in the case of CSF leaks of the clivus. Results are summarized in Table 3. Respondents allowed patients all of the exceptions mentioned during the rest period in 26% (6/23) of the small CSF leaks of the anterior skull base, 13% (5/32) of the large CSF leaks of the anterior skull base, 21% (4/19) of the small CSF leaks of the sphenoid, 16% (5/31) of the large CSF leaks of the sphenoid, and 19% (5/27) of the CSF leaks of the clivus.

There was no significant difference observed in postoperative practices between rhinologists and neurosurgeons.

Discussion

The postoperative management of CSF leaks remains controversial. Only weak evidence on this topic is available and most of the literature is based on case series or expert opinions. A recent large review of the literature [7] on endoscopic skull base surgery has been published by an international consensus of experts. Unfortunately, the role of postoperative resting position was not explored in this review. Two American-based opinion studies on ESBS practices were also recently published [8, 9], but these did not focus specifically on CSF leaks. The response rate was also low, being 3.2% of members of the American Rhinologic Society in Wannemuhler's study [9]. In the present study, the response rate was 28.2% of members of the AFR, but was difficult to estimate in the case of neurosurgeons, as the French College of Neurosurgeons mailing list includes both trainees and expert surgeons, as well as all subspecialties of neurosurgery. It is likely that ESBS surgeons are a minority among them. To the best of our knowledge, this study is the first to gather the opinions of skull base surgeons concerning the postoperative resting position after ESBS closure of CSF leaks.

In an American survey conducted among skull base surgeons [8], 19% recommended bedrest after all ESBS procedures without a CSF leak. In the case of "low-flow" leaks, 59% recommended bedrest, increasing to more than 78% in the case of "high-flow" leaks (including clival leaks). In our study, more than 92% of surgeons recommended a resting

Table 3 Exceptions allowed from the resting position, according to the site and size of the leak

	No exception *N* (%)	Exception: toilet *N* (%)	Exception: shower *N* (%)	Exception: meals *N* (%)	Prescription of resting position: total
Small CSF leaks of the ASB	8 (30.8%)	14 (53.9%)	6 (23.1%)	10 (38.5%)	26
Large CSF leaks of the ASB	14 (43.8%)	14 (43.8%)	5 (15.6%)	11 (34.4%)	32
Small CSF leaks of the sphenoid	7 (36.8%)	10 (52.6%)	4 (21.1%)	7 (36.8%)	19
Large CSF leaks of the sphenoid	14 (45.2%)	14 (45.2%)	5 (16.1%)	11 (35.5%)	31
CSF leaks of the clivus	11 (40.7%)	13 (48.2%)	5 (18.5%)	10 (37%)	27

CSF cerebrospinal fluid, *ASB* anterior skull base

position after closure of CSF leaks according to their size and location. Large defects were statistically associated with a greater percentage of recommendation for postoperative resting position (90%) compared to small defects (59%). CSF leaks of the clivus, regardless of size, were associated with a greater percentage of resting position recommendation (79%).

Postural changes, from supine to sitting or upright positions, results in a biphasic decrease of ICP: specifically a proportional decrease during phase 1 (0 to 30°–45° tilt); and stabilization during phase 2 (above 30°–45° tilt). This postural regulation of ICP remains controversial. We have summarized current knowledge regarding this topic in another contribution to this supplement (Gergelé L, Manet R. Postural regulation of intracranial pressure: a critical review of the literature). In brief, two major factors have been proposed to explain this decrease: I) Phase 1 corresponds to CSF transfer from the non-distensible cranial compartment to the distensible spinal compartment, where maximal expansion corresponds to the second phase of the decrease in ICP; II) the gravitational effect within the venous system is transferred to the CSF system according to Davson's equation, modulated by jugular collapse that would be responsible for the second phase of ICP decrease. The main clinical application of these observations has led to the recommendation of a semi-sitting position in head injury patients to lower ICP and improve cerebral perfusion pressure (CPP) [5]. Magnaes defined a so-called "hydrostatic indifference point," corresponding to a point located in the upper thoracic region (with interindividual differences) in which CSF pressure remains equal regardless of body position [10]. Above this point, CSF pressure will be lower in the sitting/upright position than in the supine position. Until recently, negative ICP values were interpreted as artefactual. Recent studies, however, have confirmed that head elevation can physiologically lower ICP to negative values [11–14].

Surprisingly, these observations of postural changes of ICP have never been integrated into discussions about the postoperative management of patients operated for a CSF leak with ESBS focused on avoiding leak recurrence. This risk is clearly increased if the ICP is raised [15]. Thus, patients must avoid Valsalva-type straining, especially when going to the toilet [16]. Laxative therapy or stool softeners should be used to decrease the strain and potential increase in ICP associated with bowel movements [17]. In this context, the sitting/upright position is preferable to also lower ICP. On the other hand, a decrease in ICP can result in negative pressure (pressure inferior to atmospheric pressure), that can induce a "ball-valve mechanism" resulting in the development of pneumocephalus [18]. It has been shown that head elevation could lead to negative pressure only at greater than 30° of tilt [19]. Moreover, rapid changes of position (e.g., quickly sitting up or lying down) could induce an instantaneous change of ICP range. Nevertheless, a slow change to vertical position for 15 min would not generate major changes in ICP [10].

Overall, bedrest restrictions are paradoxically recommended to avoid recurrence of CSF leaks, whereas the sitting/upright position actually lowers this risk. In fact, bedrest restrictions should be evaluated according to the risk of pneumocephalus, which is increased in the upright position and is probably more prevalent in the case of large skull-base defects. Considering the different aspects of the problem, Fowler's position (20°–30° sitting) seems to be a good compromise in this context. This position lowers ICP and thus limits the risk of recurrence of a CSF leak, but maintains a positive ICP, which lower the risk of pneumocephalus.

Conclusion

This study is the first to collect opinions from members of French skull base surgical societies on the postoperative management of patients treated for CSF leaks using ESBS. It emphasizes the role of postoperative bedrest that is commonly recommended but has not been studied extensively in the literature and whose role thus remains equivocal. Fowler's position may represent a good compromise by lowering ICP, and thus limiting the risk of recurrence of CSF leaks, while also limiting the risk of pneumocephalus. Future clinical protocols to study the efficacy and safety of this practice are required.

Conflict of Interest **All authors declare that no conflict of interest exists for this publication.**

References

1. Hadad G, Bassagasteguy L, Carrau RL, Mataza JC, Kassam A, Snyderman CH, Mintz A (2006) A novel reconstructive technique after endoscopic expanded endonasal approaches: vascular pedicle nasoseptal flap. Laryngoscope 116(10):1882–1886
2. Wang W, Vincent A, Sokoya M, Kohlert S, Kadakia S, Ducic Y (2019) Free-flap reconstruction of skull base and orbital defects. Semin Plast Surg 33(01):072–077
3. Gjuric M, Goede U, Keimer H, Wigand ME (1996) Endonasal endoscopic closure of cerebrospinal fluid fistulas at the anterior cranial base. Ann Otol Rhinol Laryngol 105(8):620–623
4. Kaptain GJ, Vincent DA, Laws ER Jr (2001) Cranial base reconstruction after transsphenoidal surgery with bioabsorbable implants: technical note. Neurosurgery 48(1):232–234
5. Kenning JA, Toutant SM, Saunders RL (1981) Upright patient positioning in the management of intracranial hypertension. Surg Neurol 15(2):148–152
6. Magnaes B (1976) Body position and cerebrospinal fluid pressure. Part 1: clinical studies on the effect of rapid postural changes. J Neurosurg 44(6):687–697
7. Wang EW, Zanation AM, Gardner PA et al (2019) ICAR: endoscopic skull-base surgery. Int Forum Allerg Rhinol 9(S3):S145–S365
8. Roxbury CR, Lobo BC, Kshettry VR, D'Anza B, Woodard TD, Recinos PF, Snyderman CH, Sindwani R (2018) Perioperative management in endoscopic endonasal skull-base surgery: a survey of the North American Skull Base Society. Int Forum Allerg Rhinol 8(5):631–640
9. Wannemuehler TJ, Rabbani CC, Burgeson JE, Illing EA, Walgama ES, Wu AW, Ting JY (2018) Survey of endoscopic skull base surgery practice patterns among otolaryngologists. Laryngosc Investig Otolaryngol 3(3):143–155
10. Magnaes B (1976) Body position and cerebrospinal fluid pressure. Part 2: clinical studies on orthostatic pressure and the hydrostatic indifferent point. J Neurosurg 44(6):698–705
11. Antes S, Tschan CA, Heckelmann M, Breuskin D, Oertel J (2016) Telemetric intracranial pressure monitoring with the raumedic neurovent P-tel. World Neurosurg 91:133–148
12. Holmlund P, Eklund A, Koskinen L-OD, Johansson E, Sundström N, Malm J, Qvarlander S (2018) Venous collapse regulates intracranial pressure in upright body positions. Am J Phys Regul Integr Comp Phys 314(3):R377–R385
13. Petersen LG, Petersen JCG, Andresen M, Secher NH, Juhler M (2016) Postural influence on intracranial and cerebral perfusion pressure in ambulatory neurosurgical patients. Am J Phys Regul Integr Comp Phys 310(1):R100–R104
14. Qvarlander S, Sundström N, Malm J, Eklund A (2013) Postural effects on intracranial pressure: modeling and clinical evaluation. J Appl Physiol Bethesda Md 115(10):1474–1480
15. Teachey W, Grayson J, Cho D-Y, Riley KO, Woodworth BA (2017) Intervention for elevated intracranial pressure improves success rate after repair of spontaneous cerebrospinal fluid leaks. Laryngoscope 127(9):2011–2016
16. Haykowsky MJ, Eves ND, R Warburton DE, Findlay MJ (2003) Resistance exercise, the Valsalva maneuver, and cerebrovascular transmural pressure. Med Sci Sports Exerc 35(1):65–68
17. Yadav YR, Parihar V, Janakiram N, Pande S, Bajaj J, Namdev H (2016) Endoscopic management of cerebrospinal fluid rhinorrhea. Asian J Neurosurg 11(3):183–193
18. Goldmann RW (1986) Pneumocephalus as a consequence of barotrauma. JAMA 255(22):3154–3156
19. Chapman PH, Cosman ER, Arnold MA (1990) The relationship between ventricular fluid pressure and body position in normal subjects and subjects with shunts: a telemetric study. Neurosurgery 26(2):181–189

Assessment of Pressure-Volume Index During Lumbar Infusion Study: What Is the Optimal Method?

Alexandra Vallet, Laurent Gergelé, Emmanuel Jouanneau, Eric A. Schmidt, and Romain Manet

Introduction

Assessment of cerebrospinal fluid (CSF) dynamics, by measuring intracranial pressure (ICP) variations during lumbar infusion study (LIS), can give precious information in patients suspected of CSF disorders, particularly cases of chronic hydrocephalus. Resistance to CSF outflow (Rout), has been the most studied hydrodynamic parameter. A high Rout (cutoff generally accepted >12 mmHg/mL/min) is considered as a good marker of hydrocephalus [1]. However, Rout assessment cannot detect impairment of cerebral compliance, which is also considered as an important marker of hydrocephalus [2, 3]. Unlike compliance ($C = dV/dP$) or its inverse, elastance ($E = dP/dV$), which both evaluate the cranio-spinal characteristics at a particular state of the system, the pressure-volume index (PVI), is deemed to characterize the craniospinal volume–pressure relationship over the whole physiological range of ICP. Marmarou et al. [4] showed that the craniospinal volume–pressure relationship can be considered as mono-exponential (Fig. 1a). For a given volume change ΔV, the resulting pressure change ΔP is linearly related to the pressure Pb before bolus injection (Fig. 1b). A constant term P_0 has been introduced in order to mathematically explain the shift along the abscissa axis of the curve ΔP versus Pb [5, 6]. PVI is calculated as

$$\mathrm{PVI} = \frac{\Delta V}{\log_{10}\left(\dfrac{\mathrm{Pp}-\mathrm{Pb}}{\mathrm{Pb}-P_0}+1\right)},$$

where ΔV corresponds to the bolus volume, Pb to the basal pressure before the bolus, Pp to the maximal ICP following the bolus, and P_0 is the intersect with the abscissa axis of the linear fit of ΔP versus P_0. Thus, the evaluation of P_0 necessitates several measures of ΔP with different values of the basal pressure Pb in order to fit a regression line. However, the physiological meaning of P_0 is still the subject of debate, even if it is thought to be strongly influenced by venous pressure [7].

In routine clinical practice, P_0 is often considered negligible and PVI is calculated according to the simplified formula:

$$\mathrm{PVI} = \frac{\Delta V}{\log_{10}\left(\dfrac{\mathrm{Pp}}{\mathrm{Pb}}\right)}.$$

In this case, the PVI can be assessed from only one bolus injection. A more robust evaluation can be obtained by averaging PVI evaluations from repeated bolus injections.

In this study, we have evaluated P_0 and compared the two methods for PVI assessment, in adult patients suspected of normal pressure hydrocephalus.

Material and Methods

In our department we retrospectively analyzed results of LIS performed in adult patients suspected of normal pressure hydrocephalus (Neurosurgery B, neurological hospital Pierre Wertheimer, Lyon university hospital, France). LIS are performed under strict aseptic conditions, within the operating theatre, in a lateral recumbent position, and under local

A. Vallet
Institute of Fluid Mechanics CNRS UMR 5502 & INSERM ToNIC, Toulouse, France

L. Gergelé
Department of Intensive Care, Ramsay Générale de Santé, Hôpital Privé de la Loire, Saint Etienne, France

E. Jouanneau · R. Manet (✉)
Department of Neurosurgery B, Neurological Hospital Pierre Wertheimer, University Hospital, Lyon, France
e-mail: romain.manet@neurochirurgie.fr

E. A. Schmidt
Institute of Fluid Mechanics CNRS UMR 5502 & INSERM ToNIC, Toulouse, France

Department of Neurosurgery, Purpan University Hospital, Toulouse, France

B. Depreitere et al. (eds.), *Intracranial Pressure and Neuromonitoring XVII*, Acta Neurochirurgica Supplement 131,
https://doi.org/10.1007/978-3-030-59436-7_64, © Springer Nature Switzerland AG 2021

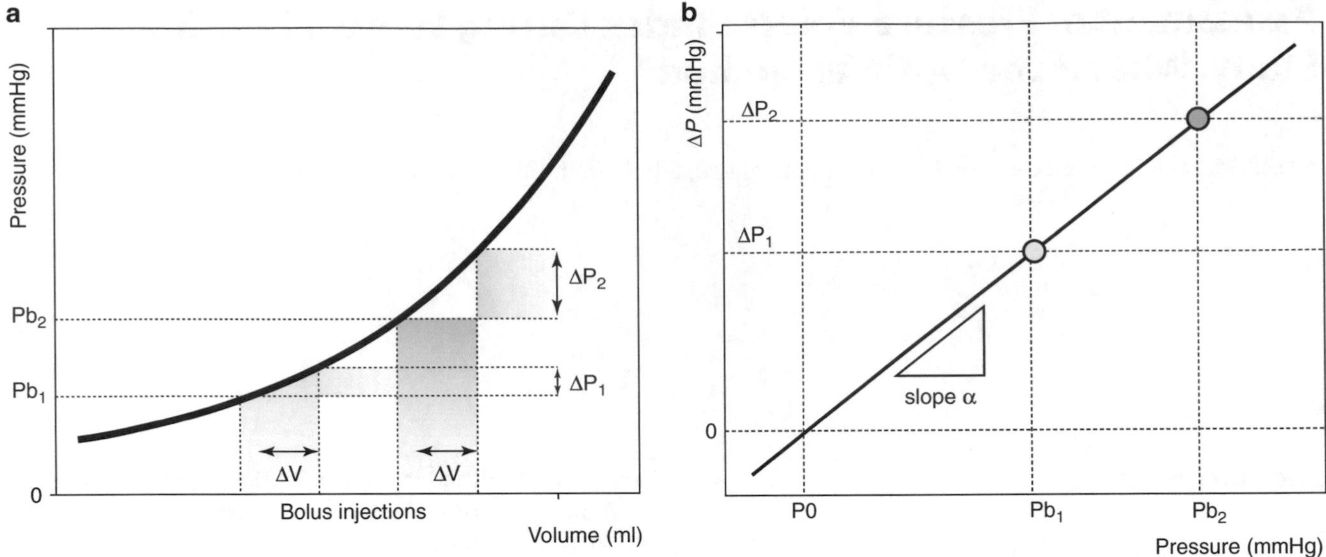

Fig. 1 Illustration of the Pressure-Volume exponential relationship (**a**) and the corresponding ΔP—pressure linear relationship for a constant bolus injection ΔV. The reference pressure P_0 and slope α are indicated on the plot (**b**)

anesthesia. The pressure transducer, the head of the patient, and the lumbar needle are placed at the same reference level. Thus, lumbar CSF pressure can be considered similar to ICP [8]. Both ICP recording and mock CSF (0.9% saline) infusion are performed through a single needle (20 GA—correction of related pressure artefacts are made during data processing). LIS includes a sequence dedicated to the assessment of PVI, consisting of a series of three fast bolus (1 mL/s) injections of 3 mL of saline at different levels of CSF pressure. ICP data are sampled at 100 Hz using a multimodal vital sign Philips IntelliVue MP70 (Koninklijke Philips N.V., Amsterdam, Netherlands) and recorded using an in-house software.

For this study, data were processed using Python computing language (Python Software Foundation, Beaverton, USA) and the scikit-learn library [9]. For each patient, a linear regression was performed to assess the slope (α) and the abscissa axis intersect (P_0), from the ΔP versus Pb data (Fig. 1b). The PVI evaluated using the $\text{PVI}_{\text{slope}}$ method was then calculated using the formula PVI = $\Delta V/\log_{10}(\alpha + 1)$. For each PVI evaluation, a coefficient of determination (r^2) was calculated to evaluate the "accuracy" of the result. Regressions with $r^2 < 0.7$ were considered as unreliable. We then evaluated the PVI using the classical method in routine use, PVI_{mean}, where the mean value of PVI is calculated using independent PVI evaluations from each bolus injection, with the simplified formula $\text{PVI} = \dfrac{\Delta V}{\log_{10}\left(\dfrac{\text{Pp}}{\text{Pb}}\right)}$ (assuming $P_0 = 0$).

In statistical analysis, the normality of distributions was tested with the omnibus test of normality. The correlation between the results from the two methods was assessed by Pearson analysis. A graphical comparison was performed by plotting the difference scores against the mean of the two PVI evaluations for each patient. Following the Bland-Altaman methodology [10], we added to the plot: the mean difference between the methods, i.e., the evaluation of the bias, and the 95% limit thresholds (1.96 times the standard deviation).

Results

PVI was assessed using both methods $\text{PVI}_{\text{slope}}$ and PVI_{mean} in the 18 consecutive LIS. The $\text{PVI}_{\text{slope}}$ evaluations were found to be reliable ($r^2 > 0.7$) in 82% of cases. Over the corresponding sample of 14 patients, both $\text{PVI}_{\text{slope}}$ and PVI_{mean} results showed a normal distribution with mean values 14.31 ± 6.51 mL and 18.25 ± 7.23 mL, respectively. The correlation between the results from the two methods (Fig. 2a) was small, with a correlation coefficient r = 0.52 and a p-value $p = 0.05$ (see Fig. 2a). We found that 95% of the difference scores between $\text{PVI}_{\text{slope}}$ and PVI_{mean} fall between the range −16.64 and 8.77 mL, with a mean value of −3.93 mL, which is elevated compared to the mean PVI values (Fig. 2b). The basal ICP before bolus injections had a normal distribution with a mean value of 6.50 ± 2.31 mmHg. The P_0 values evaluated had a normal distribution with a mean value of 2.12 ± 3.42 mmHg.

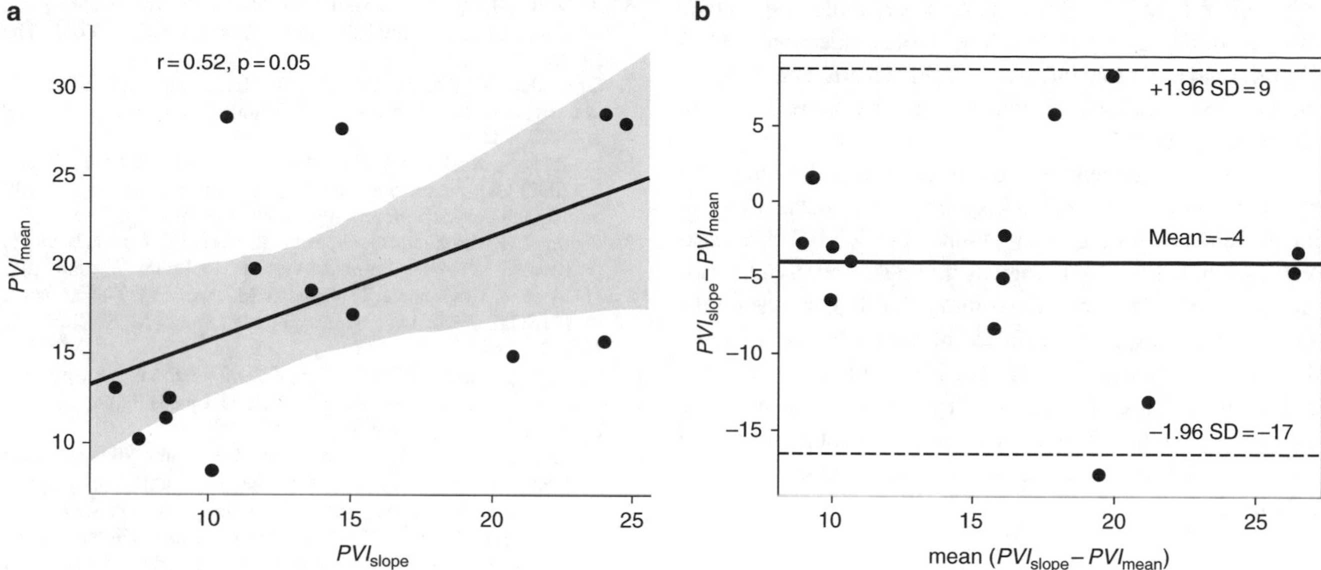

Fig. 2 (a) Correlation and (b) Bland Altman plot comparing PVI_{slope} and PVI_{mean} methods

Discussion

With the exception of Rout, which has been well documented and proposed in clinical guidelines as a good marker of hydrocephalus [1, 11], CSF hydrodynamics and brain biomechanics remain poorly investigated. Parameters related to "brain compliance," in particular to the PVI, were described many decades ago in only a few publications [4, 12, 13]. "Brain compliance" describes how the contents of the craniospinal space (central nervous system, CSF, and vasculature) can adapt to a change of volume. However, its exact significance remains uncertain. It probably reflects a mixture of different compartments (CSF, neural tissue, cerebral and spinal vasculature) with specific biomechanical properties, which have rarely been modelled and remain poorly characterized.

In clinical practice, reduced PVI has been reported to be associated with higher ICP values, ICP instability, and worse outcome in head-injured patients [14], and has also been described as a good marker of hydrocephalus [2, 3]. PVI is improved by head elevation, concomitantly with a decrease in ICP [15].

The optimal methods for calculation of PVI remain equivocal. Our methodology, using a series of fast bolus injections during LIS, is directly derived from Marmarou's work [4]. Assessment of PVI with LIS in communicating hydrocephalus provides similar results as intraventricular infusion studies [16]. In routine practice, P_0 (for which the clinical significance remains dubious/hazardous) is commonly considered negligible. Raabe et al. [15] found no difference in PVI calculations, with or without P_0 correction, using the method of Avezaat et al. [5], in patients examined in the recumbent position. The authors, however, recommend this correction if patients are examined in different body positions. However, P_0 has been reported in other publications to influence PVI assessment [16, 17]. In fact, the P_0 correction is needed to accurately assess PVI from data of one bolus injection, but its value is not used with the PVI_{slope} method. The generally accepted PVI cutoff is <25 mL when assessed with bolus injections (such as in this study) [18]. However, our results suggest that the interpretation of PVI must also consider the methodology used to process the data. The PVI_{slope} method provides results, independent of P_0. In our study, the PVI_{mean} method (assuming $P_0 = 0$) generally led to higher values than the PVI_{slope} method (on average, 3.93 mL higher). This difference could jeopardize the interpretation, especially in the case of moderately impaired compliance, close to cutoff values (e.g., PVI = 27 mL evaluated with the PVI_{mean} method, interpreted as "normal compliance" could actually correspond to PVI = 23 mL with the PVI_{slope} method, reflecting "impaired compliance"); the higher the P_0, the greater the difference between the two methods. Swallow et al. showed that the parameters for CSF dynamics assessed from infusion studies should be presented as ranges in which the actual patient values lie rather than fixed values (e.g., the estimated 95% confidence interval for Rout was ±3 mmHg/mL/min) [19]. This consideration is also adapted to PVI assessment, and confidence interval should always be provided in addition to the actual result value.

It should also be noted that PVI assessment can also be carried out during a constant slow infusion test (generally performed at the rate of 1–2 mL/min) with a lower cutoff (13 mL) [18]. However, this method for assessment of PVI seems less accurate than the bolus method because the determination of P_0 is more difficult and less reliable [16]. In fact, this important gap between the "bolus injection" cutoff (25 mL) and the "slow infusion" cutoff (13 mL) suggests that the two examinations do not explore the same aspect of "brain compliance."

Overall, assessment of "brain compliance" using PVI should always be interpreted keeping in mind the assessment method and integrating other parameters of CSF dynamics as well as clinical and radiological findings. The clinical reliability of PVI assessment, assuming $P_0 = 0$, depends on the value of P_0. Thus, *caution should* be used when *interpreting* these *results*, especially when the PVI value is close to the pathological cutoff. Further studies are needed to improve the calculation of PVI, to define a pathological range of PVI and to better understand the fundamental meaning of "brain compliance."

Conflict of Interest **The authors state that no conflict of interest exists regarding this study.**

References

1. Marmarou A, Bergsneider M, Klinge P, Relkin N, Black PM (2005) The value of supplemental prognostic tests for the preoperative assessment of idiopathic normal-pressure hydrocephalus. Neurosurgery 57(3 Suppl):S17–S28; discussion ii–v
2. Czosnyka M, Whitehouse H, Smielewski P, Simac S, Pickard JD (1996) Testing of cerebrospinal compensatory reserve in shunted and non-shunted patients: a guide to interpretation based on an observational study. J Neurol Neurosurg Psychiatry 60(5):549–558
3. Marmarou A, Foda MA, Bandoh K, Yoshihara M, Yamamoto T, Tsuji O, Zasler N, Ward JD, Young HF (1996) Posttraumatic ventriculomegaly: hydrocephalus or atrophy? A new approach for diagnosis using CSF dynamics. J Neurosurg 85(6):1026–1035
4. Marmarou A, Shulman K, LaMorgese J (1975) Compartmental analysis of compliance and outflow resistance of the cerebrospinal fluid system. J Neurosurg 43(5):523–534
5. Avezaat CJJ, van Eijndhoven JHM, de Jong DA, Moolenaar WCJ (1976) A new method of monitoring intracranial volume/pressure relationship. In: Beks JWF et al (eds) Intracranial pressure III. Springer, Berlin, Heidelberg, New York, pp 308–313
6. Avezaat CJJ, van-Eijndhoven JH (1984) Cerebrospinaluid pulse pressure and craniospinal dynamics. A Jongbloed en Zoon, The Hague
7. Czosnyka M, Pickard JD (2004) Monitoring and interpretation of intracranial pressure. J Neurol Neurosurg Psychiatry 75(6):813–821
8. Lenfeldt N, Koskinen L-OD, Bergenheim AT, Malm J, Eklund A (2007) CSF pressure assessed by lumbar puncture agrees with intracranial pressure. Neurology 68(2):155–158
9. Pedregosa F, Varoquaux G, Gramfort A, Michel V, Thirion B, Grisel O, Blondel M, Prettenhofer P, Weiss R, Dubourg V, Vanderplas J, Passos A, Cournapeau D, Brucher M, Perrot M, Duchesnay É (2011) Scikit-learn: machine learning in python. J Mach Learn Res 12:2825–2830
10. Bland JM, Altman DG (1986) Statistical methods for assessing agreement between two methods of clinical measurement. Lancet Lond Engl 1(8476):307–310
11. Halperin JJ, Kurlan R, Schwalb JM, Cusimano MD, Gronseth G, Gloss D (2015) Practice guideline: idiopathic normal pressure hydrocephalus: response to shunting and predictors of response: report of the Guideline Development, Dissemination, and Implementation Subcommittee of the American Academy of Neurology. Neurology 85(23):2063–2071
12. Shapiro K, Marmarou A (1982) Clinical applications of the pressure-volume index in treatment of pediatric head injuries. J Neurosurg 56(6):819–825
13. Sullivan HG, Miller JD, Becker DP, Flora RE, Allen GA (1977) The physiological basis of intracranial pressure change with progressive epidural brain compression. An experimental evaluation in cats. J Neurosurg 47(4):532–550
14. Maset AL, Marmarou A, Ward JD, Choi S, Lutz HA, Brooks D, Moulton RJ, DeSalles A, Muizelaar JP, Turner H (1987) Pressure-volume index in head injury. J Neurosurg 67(6):832–840
15. Raabe A, Czosnyka M, Piper I, Seifert V (1999) Monitoring of intracranial compliance: correction for a change in body position. Acta Neurochir 141(1):31–36; discussion 35–36
16. Tans JT, Poortvliet DC (1985) CSF outflow resistance and pressure-volume index determined by steady-state and bolus infusions. Clin Neurol Neurosurg 87(3):159–165
17. Tans JT, Poortvliet DC (1989) Relationship between compliance and resistance to outflow of CSF in adult hydrocephalus. J Neurosurg 71(1):59–62
18. Gergelé L, Baledent O, Manet R, Lalou A, Barszcz S, Kasprowicz M, Smielewsk P, Pickard JD, Czosnyka M (2019) Dynamics of cerebrospinal fluid: from theoretical models to clinical applications. In: Miller K (ed) Biomechanics of the brain. Biological and Medical Physics, Biomedical Engineering. Springer, Cham
19. Swallow DMA, Fellner N, Varsos GV, Czosnyka M, Smielewski P, Pickard JD, Czosnyka Z (2014) Repeatability of cerebrospinal fluid constant rate infusion study. Acta Neurol Scand 130(2):131–138

Postural Regulation of Intracranial Pressure: A Critical Review of the Literature

Laurent Gergelé and Romain Manet

Introduction

Intracranial pressure (ICP) plays a crucial role in the regulation of brain physiology. Since the first recordings 70 years ago [1, 2], ICP has been extensively explored. However, most of the data have been reported from patients investigated in the supine position, giving values of 5–15 mmHg, considered as the normal range in adults. The influence of body position on ICP has also been well-documented for many years: for example, head elevation results in lowering of ICP [3, 4] and raising cerebral compliance [5]. The main clinical application of these observations has been to recommend the semi-sitting position in head injury patients, to thus lower ICP and improve cerebral perfusion pressure [6]. Until recently, negative ICP values were interpreted as artefactual. Recent studies, however, have confirmed that ICP decreases with head elevation and can physiologically become negative in the upright position [7–10].

Postural regulation of ICP is incompletely understood. In this study, we aim to summarize current knowledge regarding the physiological mechanisms and interactions underlying postural regulation of ICP.

Method

A literature search was performed using the Medline database, from 1900 to 2019, using combinations of the following key words: "Intracranial pressure," "Posture," "Jugular vein," "Collapse," "Regulation," and "Physiology." In addition, a search by hand was undertaken of the references from retrieved articles for possible related studies.

The titles and abstracts of all papers were screened by both coauthors of the study. All studies selected by one of the two observers were double-checked by the other observer. Our study included only original articles published in English, describing physiological and pathophysiological data concerning postural regulation of ICP.

A total of 48 articles were completely reviewed; 40 were referenced in this work.

Results

ICP Behaviour During Postural Changes

ICP reflects a mixture of different compartments—cerebrospinal fluid (CSF), neural tissue, cerebral and spinal vasculature—with specific biomechanical properties, which have still been modelled to only a small degree and remain poorly understood. The pulsatility of ICP is mainly influenced by heart rate (first harmonic), but also by respiratory cycle (second harmonic), and by vasogenic phenomena (third harmonic) [11].

ICP is also influenced by posture. A postural transition from the supine to upright position results in a biphasic decrease in ICP [4, 12, 13] (Fig. 1b): a rapid decrease proportional to tilt (phase 1: low tilt angle, between 0° and 30°–45°), followed by a stabilization (phase 2: high tilt, above 30°–45°).

The Spinal Buffer

The cranial cavity is non-distensible and the Monro-Kelly doctrine states that the intracranial volume thus remains constant:

L. Gergelé
Department of Intensive Care, Ramsay Générale de Santé, Hôpital Privé de la Loire, Saint Etienne, France

R. Manet (✉)
Department of Neurosurgery B, Neurological Hospital Pierre Wertheimer, University Hospital of Lyon, Lyon, France
e-mail: romain.manet@neurochirurgie.fr

B. Depreitere et al. (eds.), *Intracranial Pressure and Neuromonitoring XVII*, Acta Neurochirurgica Supplement 131,
https://doi.org/10.1007/978-3-030-59436-7_65, © Springer Nature Switzerland AG 2021

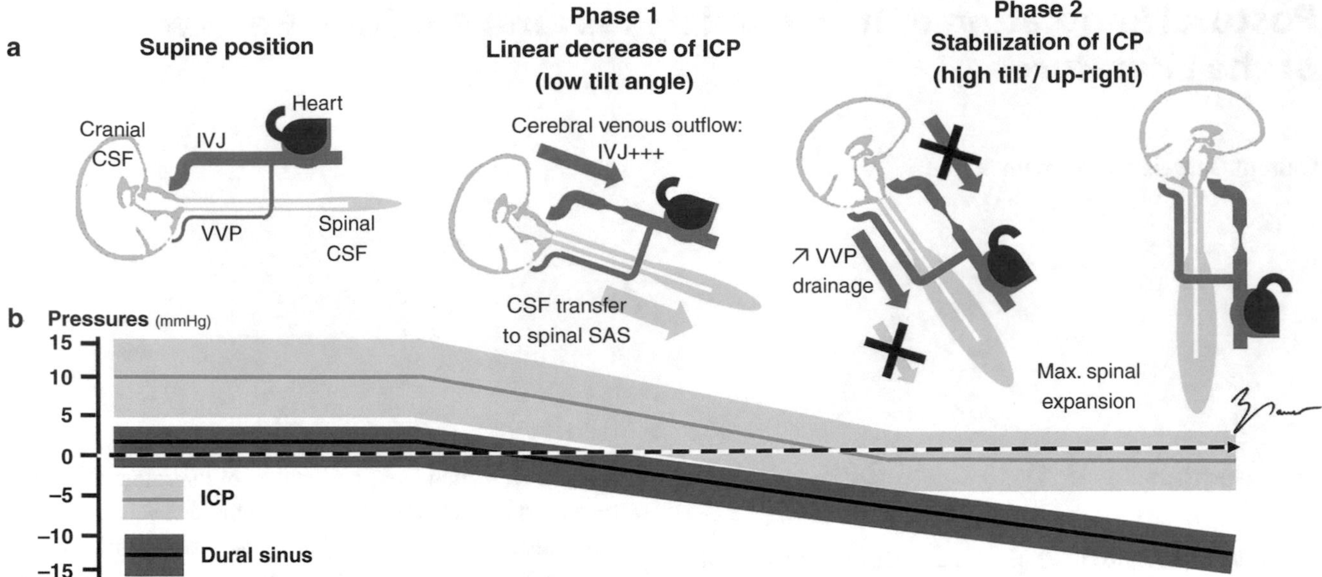

Fig. 1 Schematic representation of postural regulation of ICP. (**a**) Schematic representation of CSF compartments and cerebral venous outflow pathways, according to postural changes. *IVJ* internal jugular veins, *SAS* subarachnoid space, *VVP* vertebral venous plexus. (**b**) Schematic representation of ICP and venous pressure within intracranial dural sinus

$$V_{\text{brain}} + V_{\text{CSF}} + V_{\text{blood}} = \text{Constant}.$$

However, this compartment is connected to the spinal compartment, in which the Monro-Kelly doctrine cannot be applied. This latter compartment would contain about 50 mL of CSF in the supine position, with important inter-individual variability, which would be inversely correlated to body mass index (BMI) [14]. Contrary to the cranial dura, which is closely adherent to the cranial bone, the spinal dura is only partially attached to the spinal canal. Due to its elastic and collagenous structures, the spinal dura can be distended, especially in perpendicular directions [15]. The surrounding epidural space is composed of fat tissue and a venous plexus. Epidural venous blood volume is influenced by downstream venous pressures, themselves particularly influenced by thoracic and intra-abdominal pressure (IAP) [16]. IAP has been measured to be higher in the semi-sitting position than in the supine position, in both children [17] and adults [18]. Spinal compartment capacity is also influenced by modulation of the spinal canal volume in relation to vertebral flexion/extension: that is, the volume is increased in flexion and decreased in extension [19, 20]. These properties result in an important capacity for modulation of the spinal CSF volume (up to 40%) [14, 21].

By allowing fast withdrawal of CSF from the cranial compartment to spinal compartment [4, 22], the spinal buffer can explain the initial rapid postural decrease in ICP (phase 1). When the expansion of spinal dura reaches its maximal capacity, the spinal compliance decreases [13, 23–25], slowing the postural ICP decrease (phase 2) (Fig. 1a). Overall, the spinal compartment would provide up to 35% of the total CSF compliance in the supine position and 10% in upright posture [22].

The spinal buffer is also very important during acute brain insult, compensating for 30–80% of cranial pressure increase [26, 27].

Jugular Collapse

The close relationship between CSF pressure and venous pressure was outlined almost 100 years ago [28], and has been described by Davson et al. using the following equation [29]:

$$\text{ICP} = \text{Rout} \cdot Q_{\text{CSF}} + \text{SSP}$$

where Rout corresponds to resistance to CSF outflow, QCSF to CSF resorption and SSP to sagittal sinus venous pressure. In healthy humans lying in a supine position, the internal jugular veins (IJVs) support the major cerebral venous outflow. However, in the sitting/upright position, their position above the level of the heart induces progressive collapse in IJV, increasing their resistance and decreasing blood flow [10, 30, 31]. This phenomenon has been proposed as a factor in decoupling hydrostatic pressures of the intracranial venous compartment from the rest of the venous system [10], with a possible anti-siphoning effect in the erect position [32]. According to this theory, these gravitational effects within the venous system would be transferred to the CSF system

[8, 10, 22]. Thus phase 1 (low tilt angle) would correspond to free return of cerebral venous blood, and phase 2 (higher tilt angle) corresponds to a regulation of cerebral venous blood pressure by jugular collapse occurring grossly above an angle of 30°.

Discussion

The published literature provides extensive support to the role of the spinal buffer in postural regulation of ICP. Spinal compliance, which has been assessed by MRI studies [33], probably depends on multiple factors, including (1) height, which influences pressure gradients; (2) weight and BMI, which influence the IAP (and thus spinal venous flows); and (3) tissues properties, in particular their elasticity, which may be altered in some tissue pathologies (e.g., patients with Ehler-Danlos disease can suffer from orthostatic intracranial hypotension). When the compliance capacity is exceeded, CSF flow transfer decreases and ICP stabilizes (during the second phase). In a model of CSF spaces composed of a non-distensible compartment (mimicking the cranial cavity), and a distensible compartment (mimicking the spinal cavity), decoupled from any venous system, CSF pressure in the cranial compartment and in the spinal compartment were similarly affected by postural changes as CSF pressures measured in the ventricle and spinal SAS of animals submitted to similar postural changes [34]. In a large prospective cohort of 376 patients explored for various CSF disorders, Poca et al. showed that ICP, maximum ICP gradients, and mean ICP gradients, in supine vs. sitting position, were significantly greater in patients with free CSF flow through the craniospinal junction ($n = 299$) than in those with Chiari malformation ($n = 77$) [35]. Interestingly, the authors did not find a significant difference regarding ICP gradients in patients with communicating hydrocephalus, suggesting that the greater part of the postural change in ICP is due to CSF transfers between the cranial and spinal compartments.

Models that support the major contribution of IJV collapse to predict the postural change of ICP are quite sophisticated, but largely underestimate the role of alternative venous pathways [8, 10, 22, 36]. Indeed, IJVs provide the main pathway for venous return in the supine position. However, in erect posture, the role of alternative pathways for cerebral blood outflow have been described in early publications, in particular the role of the vertebral venous plexus (VVP) [37]. In addition to these anatomical observations, it has been shown that the reduction of venous blood flow within the IJVs were exactly counterbalanced by an increased blood flow within VVP [24, 38, 39] (Fig. 1a).

Moreover, according to Pascal's law, as the IJVs do not completely collapse and VVP take over, blood pressure within the venous compartment, and particularly in the SSP, is not impacted by jugular collapse. Blood pressure within the intracranial venous sinuses has been measured in humans and shown to decrease proportionally with head tilt without any stabilization above 30°, reaching values around −15 mmHg at 90° (Fig. 1b) [40].

Finally, Davson's equation supports slow CSF transfers from the subarachnoid spaces to the venous system (a few mL/min) and thus does not explain fast postural modulation of ICP (a few seconds): e.g., ICP = 10 mmHg, SSP = −5 mmHg, Rout = 5 mmHg/mL/min, CSF resorption rate = (ICP − SSP)/Rout = 3 mL/min.

In conclusion, the physiological mechanisms underlying the postural regulation of ICP remain unclear. An improved understanding of these mechanisms would help us to better evaluate shunt systems, in particular the usefulness of anti-siphon devices, and help to improve the management of patients with CSF disorders.

References

1. Janny P (1950) La pression intracrânienne chez l'homme. Thesis, Paris, pp 1–80
2. Lundberg N (1960) Continuous recording and control of ventricular fluid pressure in neurosurgical practice. Acta Psychiatr Scand Suppl 36(149):1–193
3. Chapman PH, Cosman ER, Arnold MA (1990) The relationship between ventricular fluid pressure and body position in normal subjects and subjects with shunts: a telemetric study. Neurosurgery 26(2):181–189
4. Magnaes B (1976) Body position and cerebrospinal fluid pressure. Part 1: clinical studies on the effect of rapid postural changes. J Neurosurg 44(6):687–697
5. Raabe A, Czosnyka M, Piper I, Seifert V (1999) Monitoring of intracranial compliance: correction for a change in body position. Acta Neurochir 141(1):31–36; discussion 35–36
6. Kenning JA, Toutant SM, Saunders RL (1981) Upright patient positioning in the management of intracranial hypertension. Surg Neurol 15(2):148–152
7. Antes S, Tschan CA, Heckelmann M, Breuskin D, Oertel J (2016) Telemetric intracranial pressure monitoring with the raumedic neurovent P-tel. World Neurosurg 91:133–148
8. Holmlund P, Eklund A, Koskinen L-OD, Johansson E, Sundström N, Malm J, Qvarlander S (2018) Venous collapse regulates intracranial pressure in upright body positions. Am J Phys Regul Integr Comp Phys 314(3):R377–R385
9. Petersen LG, Petersen JCG, Andresen M, Secher NH, Juhler M (2016) Postural influence on intracranial and cerebral perfusion pressure in ambulatory neurosurgical patients. Am J Phys Regul Integr Comp Phys 310(1):R100–R104
10. Qvarlander S, Sundström N, Malm J, Eklund A (2013) Postural effects on intracranial pressure: modeling and clinical evaluation. J Appl Physiol Bethesda Md 115(10):1474–1480

11. Czosnyka M, Pickard JD (2004) Monitoring and interpretation of intracranial pressure. J Neurol Neurosurg Psychiatry 75(6):813–821
12. Davson H, Welch K, Segal MB (1987) The physiology and pathophysiology of the cerebrospinal fluid. Churchill Livingstone, Edinburgh
13. Magnaes B (1976) Body position and cerebrospinal fluid pressure. Part 2: clinical studies on orthostatic pressure and the hydrostatic indifferent point. J Neurosurg 44(6):698–705
14. Hogan QH, Prost R, Kulier A, Taylor ML, Liu S, Mark L (1996) Magnetic resonance imaging of cerebrospinal fluid volume and the influence of body habitus and abdominal pressure. Anesthesiology 84(6):1341–1349
15. Tunturi AR (1978) Elasticity of the spinal cord, pia, and denticulate ligament in the dog. J Neurosurg 48(6):975–979
16. Usubiaga JE, Moya F, Usubiaga LE (1967) Effect of thoracic and abdominal pressure changes on the epidural space pressure. Br J Anaesth 39(8):612–618
17. Ejike JC, Kadry J, Bahjri K, Mathur M (2010) Semi-recumbent position and body mass percentiles: effects on intra-abdominal pressure measurements in critically ill children. Intensive Care Med 36(2):329–335
18. De Keulenaer BL, De Waele JJ, Powell B, Malbrain MLNG (2009) What is normal intra-abdominal pressure and how is it affected by positioning, body mass and positive end-expiratory pressure? Intensive Care Med 35(6):969–976
19. Hirasawa Y, Bashir WA, Smith FW, Magnusson ML, Pope MH, Takahashi K (2007) Postural changes of the dural sac in the lumbar spines of asymptomatic individuals using positional stand-up magnetic resonance imaging. Spine 32(4):E136–E140
20. Schmid MR, Stucki G, Duewell S, Wildermuth S, Romanowski B, Hodler J (1999) Changes in cross-sectional measurements of the spinal canal and intervertebral foramina as a function of body position: in vivo studies on an open-configuration MR system. AJR Am J Roentgenol 172(4):1095–1102
21. Lee RR, Abraham RA, Quinn CB (2001) Dynamic physiologic changes in lumbar CSF volume quantitatively measured by three-dimensional fast spin-echo MRI. Spine 26(10):1172–1178
22. Gehlen M, Kurtcuoglu V, Schmid Daners M (2017) Is posture-related craniospinal compliance shift caused by jugular vein collapse? A theoretical analysis. Fluids Barriers CNS 14(1):5
23. Alperin N, Hushek SG, Lee SH, Sivaramakrishnan A, Lichtor T (2005) MRI study of cerebral blood flow and CSF flow dynamics in an upright posture: the effect of posture on the intracranial compliance and pressure. Acta Neurochir Suppl 95:177–181
24. Alperin N, Lee SH, Sivaramakrishnan A, Hushek SG (2005) Quantifying the effect of posture on intracranial physiology in humans by MRI flow studies. J Magn Reson Imaging JMRI 22(5):591–596
25. Magnaes B (1978) Movement of cerebrospinal fluid within the craniospinal space when sitting up and lying down. Surg Neurol 10(1):45–49
26. Löfgren J, Zwetnow NN (1973) Cranial and spinal components of the cerebrospinal fluid pressure-volume curve. Acta Neurol Scand 49(5):575–585
27. Marmarou A, Shulman K, LaMorgese J (1975) Compartmental analysis of compliance and outflow resistance of the cerebrospinal fluid system. J Neurosurg 43(5):523–534
28. Bedford THB (1935) The effect of increased intracranial venous pressure on the pressure of the cerebrospinal fluid. Brain 58(4):427–447
29. Davson H (1966) Formation and drainage of the cerebrospinal fluid. Sci Basis Med Annu Rev 1:238–259
30. Cirovic S, Walsh C, Fraser WD, Gulino A (2003) The effect of posture and positive pressure breathing on the hemodynamics of the internal jugular vein. Aviat Space Environ Med 74(2):125–131
31. Holt JP (1941) The collaps factor in the measurement of venous pressure. Am J Phys 134:292–299
32. El-Shafei IL, el-Rifaii MA (1987) Ventriculojugular shunt against the direction of blood flow. I. Role of the internal jugular vein as an antisiphonage device. Childs Nerv Syst 3(5):282–284
33. Wåhlin A, Ambarki K, Birgander R, Alperin N, Malm J, Eklund A (2010) Assessment of craniospinal pressure-volume indices. AJNR Am J Neuroradiol 31(9):1645–1650
34. Klarica M, Rados M, Draganic P, Erceg G, Oreskovic D, Maraković J, Bulat M (2006) Effect of head position on cerebrospinal fluid pressure in cats: comparison with artificial model. Croat Med J 47(2):233–238
35. Poca MA, Sahuquillo J, Topczewski T, Lastra R, Font ML, Corral E (2006) Posture-induced changes in intracranial pressure: a comparative study in patients with and without a cerebrospinal fluid block at the craniovertebral junction. Neurosurgery 58(5):899–906; discussion 899–906
36. Holmlund P, Johansson E, Qvarlander S, Wåhlin A, Ambarki K, Koskinen L-OD, Malm J, Eklund A (2017) Human jugular vein collapse in the upright posture: implications for postural intracranial pressure regulation. Fluids Barriers CNS 14(1):17
37. Batson OV (1944) Anatomical problems concerned in the study of cerebral blood flow. Fed Proc 3:139–144
38. Gisolf J, van Lieshout JJ, van Heusden K, Pott F, Stok WJ, Karemaker JM (2004) Human cerebral venous outflow pathway depends on posture and central venous pressure. J Physiol 560(Pt 1):317–327
39. Valdueza JM, von Münster T, Hoffman O, Schreiber S, Einhäupl KM (2000) Postural dependency of the cerebral venous outflow. Lancet Lond Engl 355(9199):200–201
40. Iwabuchi T, Sobata E, Suzuki M, Suzuki S, Yamashita M (1983) Dural sinus pressure as related to neurosurgical positions. Neurosurgery 12(2):203–207

Differences in Cerebrospinal Fluid Dynamics in Posttraumatic Hydrocephalus Versus Atrophy, Including Effect of Decompression and Cranioplasty

Virginia Levrini, Afroditi D. Lalou, Zofia H. Czosnyka, Angelos G. Kolias, Laurent Gergelé, Matthew Garnett, Peter J. Hutchinson, and Marek Czosnyka

Introduction

Undiagnosed posttraumatic hydrocephalus (PTH) can delay and limit the extent of recovery in traumatic brain injury (TBI) patients [1, 2]. The clinical picture in these patients' presentation is difficult to tease out due to the long recovery courses and heterogeneity of injuries and brain insults. The predominant means to assess for PTH currently are imaging (CT/MRI) and high-volume lumbar punctures. However, imaging is poor at distinguishing between PTH and ex-vacuo ventriculomegaly in the context of atrophy and lumbar puncture opening pressures can be unreliable [3–7]. Although ICP monitoring can be a useful tool for CSF dynamics analysis, it is an invasive technique [4–8].

The use of volume infusion to help distinguish posttraumatic hydrocephalus was described by Marmarou et al. [2]. They used intracranial pressure (ICP) and resistance to CSF outflow (Rout) calculated using the bolus-injection method, alongside evidence of ventriculomegaly on imaging, to suggest shunting in patients with opening pressures greater than 15 mmHg or Rout greater than 6 mmHg*min/mL. In view of the possible limitations of the bolus-infusion method, that it may be measuring compartmental compliance opposed to that of the entire system and higher calculation of outflow conductance (Cout = 1/Rout), we aimed to investigate CSF dynamics in this cohort using constant-rate infusion tests [9, 10]. Additionally, to the best of our knowledge, infusion test parameters other than Rout in PTH and atrophy have not been described in detail. A case report by Czosnyka et al. described low-baseline AMP with abnormal reactivity to infusion and raised PVI index to likely signify an absence of vascular bed reactivity biologically [9]. We aimed to analyze various CSF dynamics parameters using constant-rate infusion studies in TBI patients with a comparison to idiopathic NPH (iNPH) and with attention to the effect of cranioplasty on CSF dynamics.

Material and Methods

Patient Selection

Our patient sample was obtained via searching for patients that had undergone TBI in our infusion study database at Cambridge University Hospital. All these patients had possible features of PTH and ventriculomegaly on imaging. We divided patients into two groups depending on CSF dynamics: group A, "likely PTH"; and group B, "likely atrophy". These were compared to a group of iNPH shunt-responsive patients (group C), who had undergone infusion studies between 2003 and 2018 [7]. These groups, based on CSF dynamics, were then compared to imaging. The data from some patients from group C has been previously reported in Lalou et al. [11].

Data Collection and Analysis

The infusion study database provided us with the following parameters: ICP baseline (ICPb), ICP at plateau (ICPp), resistance to outflow (Rout) and peak-to-peak amplitude of ICP (AMP). Patient notes (kept on the computer system EPIC and LADR) were searched to obtain the

V. Levrini (✉) · A. D. Lalou · Z. H. Czosnyka · A. G. Kolias · M. Garnett
P. J. Hutchinson · M. Czosnyka
Division of Neurosurgery, Department of Clinical Neuroscience, University of Cambridge, Addenbrooke's Hospital, Cambridge, UK

L. Gergelé
Division of Neurosurgery, Department of Clinical Neuroscience, University of Cambridge, Addenbrooke's Hospital, Cambridge, UK

Department of Intensive Care, Ramsay Générale de Santé, Hôpital Privé de la Loire, Saint Etienne, France

B. Depreitere et al. (eds.), *Intracranial Pressure and Neuromonitoring XVII*, Acta Neurochirurgica Supplement 131,
https://doi.org/10.1007/978-3-030-59436-7_66,

relevant patient demographics and clinical information. R software version 3.5.2. was used for statistical analysis, with comparison between groups being tested using non-parametric tests, with p-values <0.05 being considered significant.

Results

Groupings

In total, 50 TBI patients underwent 52 infusion tests. Table 1 shows the number of patients, demographics, and the range of time intervals between trauma and infusion study for patients in the three groups. As can be seen, the three groups showed heterogeneity in both age and TBI interval. Unfortunately, the date of TBI could not be retrieved in 11 cases. Severity of TBI, as measured by initial GCS, was "severe" in 35 cases, "mild" in 6, and in the remaining cases we could not retrieve this information.

All patients in group A had either never undergone decompressive craniectomy or had a cranioplasty in situ for over 1 month. Group B consisted of patients who had undergone decompressive craniotomy, had a cranioplasty inserted less than a month previously, or had an intact cranial vault with an atrophic CSF dynamics pattern. Rout and dAMP were significantly higher in Group A than B, but significantly lower than Group C [45 iNPH patients]. RAP baseline in Group A was 0.57 ± 0.16, increasing to 0.9 ± 0.07 during infusion, indicating depleted compensatory reserve, versus 0.11 ± 0.04 and 0.27 ± 0.11 in Group B, indicating ample compensatory reserve [1, 2, 10, 12]. Comparisons between these two groups are shown in Table 2 and Fig. 1.

Imaging

All patients had imaging in the form of either a CT or MRI scan, which was reported by a neuroradiologist. These reports differed from the CSF dynamics in several cases. Encephalomalacia or ex-vacuo ventriculomegaly was reported in 12 out of 36 patients in group A (the "likely PTH" group). In comparison, 9 subjects with a recent cranioplasty in groups B ("likely atrophy" group) had reports that described ventriculomegaly.

Effect of Cranioplasty

In all 6 patients who had undergone infusion testing both before and after cranioplasty, baseline and infusion parameters increased after the cranioplasty was inserted. Figure 2 shows the average increase in the various CSF dynamics parameters post-cranioplasty.

Table 2 Comparison of CSF dynamics in group A ('possible PTH'), group B ('possible atrophy') and group C (iNPH)

Mean	Group A (N = 36)	Group B (N = 16)	p-Value
ICPb (mmHg)	9.31 ± 4.12	5.84 ± 3.13	0.00557
Rout (mmHg/ml/min)	13.41 ± 5.19	4.2 ± 2.03	3.345×10^{-12}
AMPb (mmHg)	0.55 ± 0.39	0.21 ± 0.17	0.001272
dAMP (mmHg)	1.5 ± 1.12	0.21 ± 0.2	1.539×10^{-07}
RAPb	0.57 ± 0.18	0.11 ± 0.04	6.522×10^{-07}
RAPinf	0.9 ± 0.07	0.27 ± 0.11	2.749×10^{-07}

Table 1 Table showing the demographics and characteristics of groups A-C

	Group A ('possible PTH')	Group B ('possible atrophy')	Group C (iNPH)
No. Tests	36	16 (9 decompression ± recent cranioplasty; 7 no decompression/cranioplasty >1 month)	45
Sex	24 male, 12 female	14 male, 2 female	26 male, 19 female
Age (years)	53 ± 17	48 ± 16	66 ± 13
Study via	26 LP; 10 Ommaya	6 LP, 5 Ommaya, 1 EVD	28 LP, 17 Ommaya
TBI interval	10 days–33.5 years	3 months–5 years	N/A
Characteristics	All had normal or high Rout, AMP, dAMP and RAP	Rout, AMP, dAMP, and RAP appeared identical between the 9 decompressed/recent cranioplasty patients and the 7 possibly atrophic patients	Undergone CSF infusion tests prior to shunting and responded positively to VPS

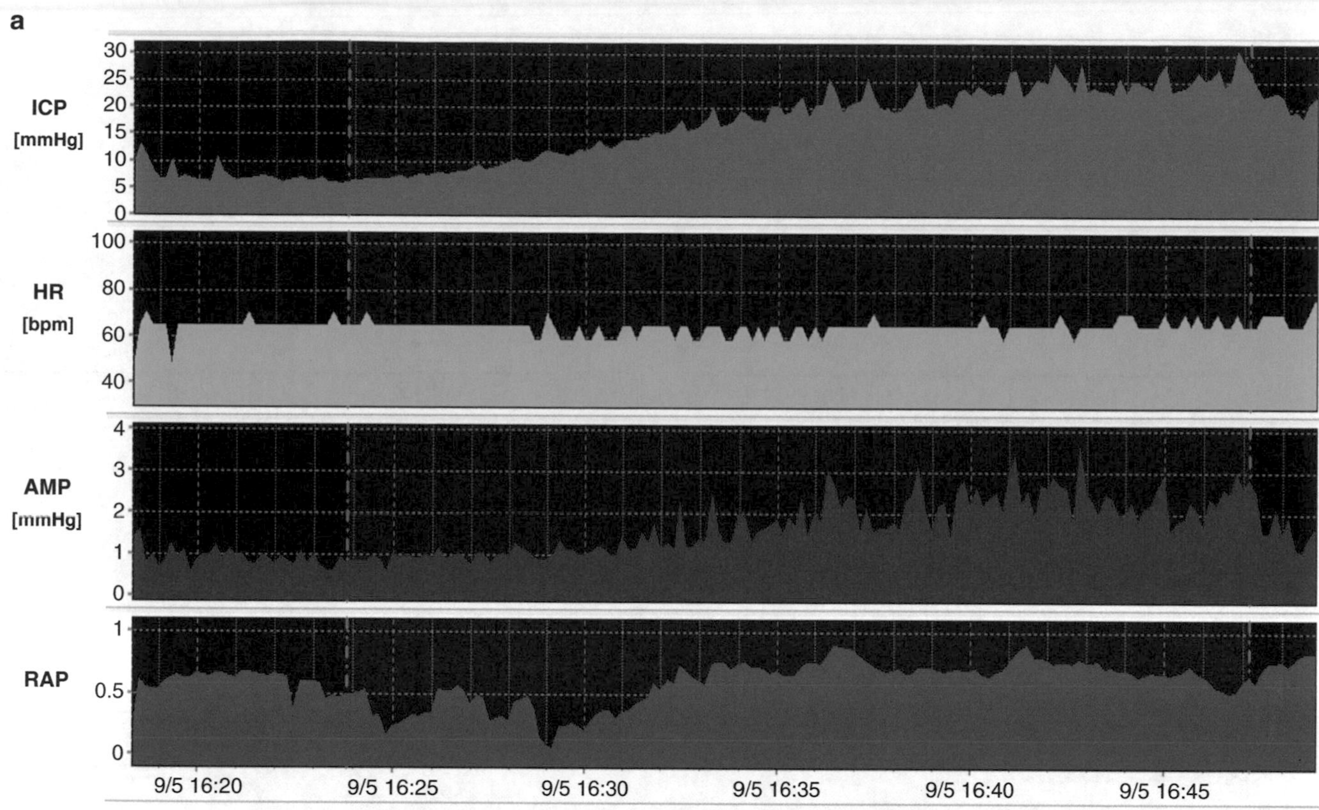

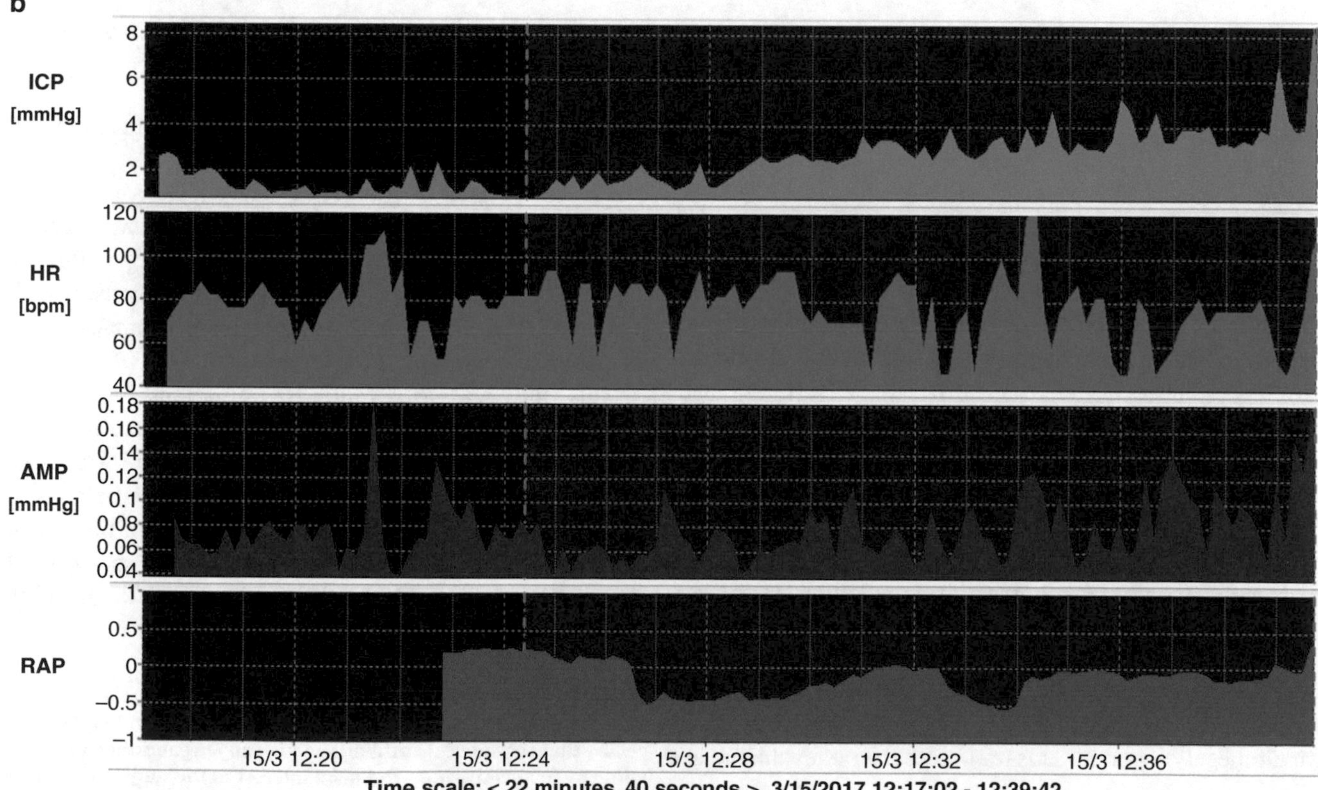

Fig. 1 Example of CSF dynamics in Post Traumatic Hydrocephalus versus atrophy. *Upper panel (possible PTH) Fig. 1a.*: ICP increasing briskly after start of infusion, with a Rout around 11–13 mmHg*min/mL. AMP at baseline ~1 mmHg, also reacting briskly to infusion until a plateau of 5.6 mmHg. RAP at baseline ~0.6, clearly increasing to almost 1 after infusion of only a few mLs, indicating exhaustion of compensatory reserve. *Lower panel (possible atrophy) Fig. 1b*: Picture of CSF dynamics identical to the decompressed patients: Low Rout (ICP increased from a baseline of 1.3–3.6 mmHg) with very low AMP at baseline (0.08), barely reacting to infusion (AMP plateau 0.09 mmHg). RAP at baseline low (<0.6), never reaching 0.6 despite infusion of >25 mLs

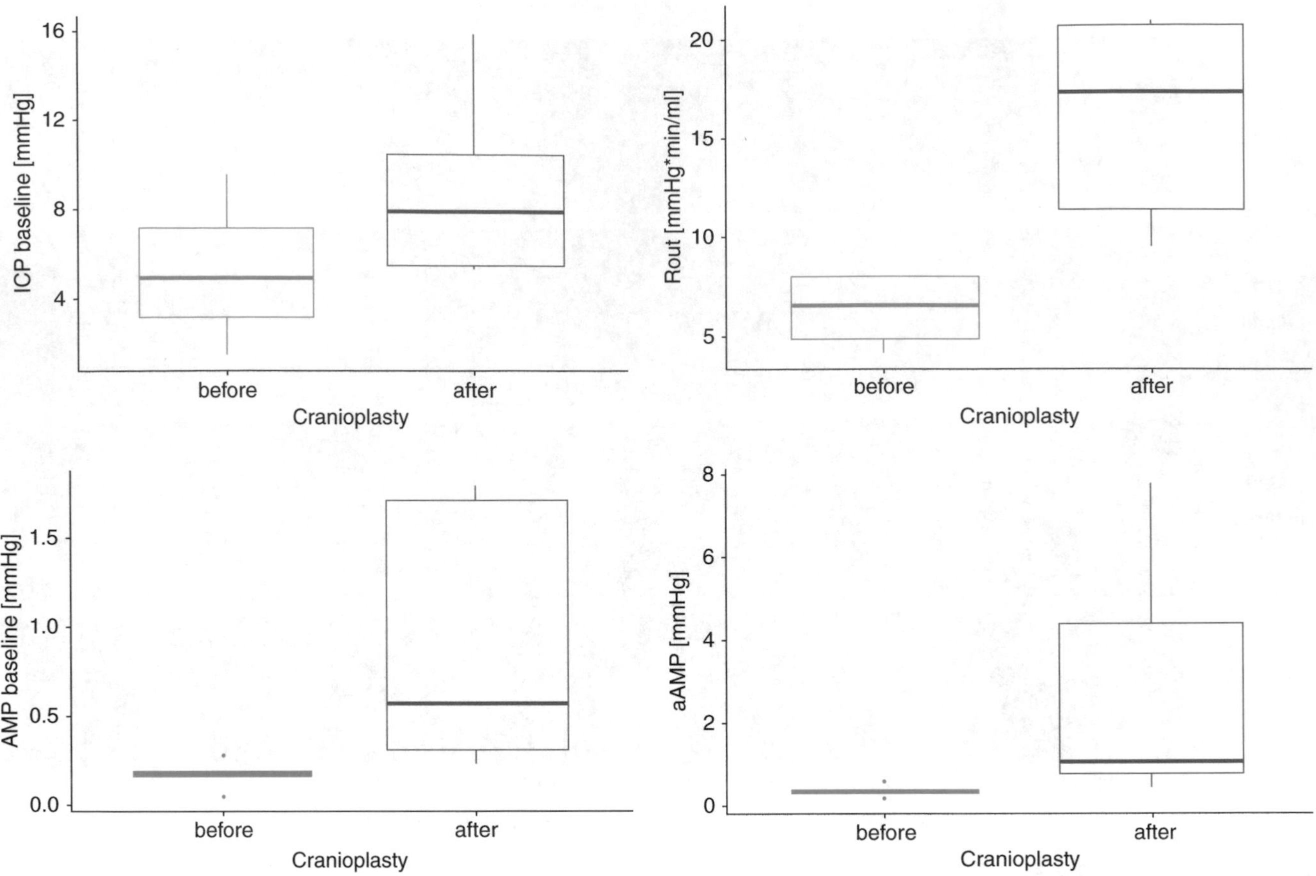

Fig. 2 Changes in CSF dynamic parameters after cranioplasty insertion in $N = 6$. All demonstrated parameters, including ICP, Rout, AMP baseline and dAMP increased

Discussion

Infusion studies can be a useful tool in the detection of PTH. Analysis of CSF dynamics in TBI patients allowed separation of subjects into two groups depending on Rout (using Rout <6 mmHg*min/ml as a threshold for atrophy) and other parameters. There was a statistically significant difference between the Rout, AMP, dAMP, RAPb, and RAPinf parameters in groups A and B. In particular, there was a salient difference between the dAMP values of group B compared to groups A and C. dAMP in group B was 0.22 ± 0.22 mmHg, compared to values of 1.5 mmHg and above in the other groups.

Notably, the grouping of patients into likely PTH or atrophic groups differed if done according to CSF dynamics compared to imaging. There were considerable proportions of patients in group A who had ex-vacuo ventriculomegaly/encephalomalacia reported, and in group B who had ventriculomegaly reported. This reinforces the notion that imaging is a poor tool in aiding diagnosis of PTH and atrophy in TBI patients.

The comparison of group A ("likely PTH") to group C (iNPH patients) found Rout and AMP to be significantly lower in group A. These lower values could possibly be explained by a coexistence of PTH due to deficits in CSF reabsorption in a brain with areas of encephalomalacia and an element of vascular bed dysfunction in TBI.

This study was not without its limitations. Our patient population was heterogenous, with varying time intervals between investigation and date of TBI, and unfortunately certain details were not retrievable from our databases. However, it does suggest that there is a role for the use of infusion studies in TBI patients who have suspected PTH and suspicion of PTH should not be based on imaging alone.

Conflict of Interest **MC has a partial financial interest in licensing ICM+ software (Cambridge Enterprise, UK). All other authors certify that they have no affiliations with any organisation or entity with any financial or non-financial interest in the subject matter or materials discussed in this manuscript.**

References

1. Manet R, Payen JF, Guerin R, Martinez O, Hautefeuille S, Francony G, Gergelé L (2017) Using external lumbar CSF drainage to treat communicating external hydrocephalus in adult patients after acute traumatic or non-traumatic brain injury. Acta Neurochir 159(10):2003–2009
2. Marmarou A, Abd-Elfattah Foda MA, Bandoh K, Yoshihara M, Yamamoto T, Tsuji O, Zasler N, Ward JD, Young HF (1996) Posttraumatic ventriculomegaly: hydrocephalus or atrophy? A new approach for diagnosis using CSF dynamics. J Neurosurg 85:1026–1035
3. Avery RA, Shah SS, Licht DJ, Seiden J et al (2010) Reference range for cerebrospinal fluid opening pressure in children. N Engl J Med 363:891–893
4. Cartwright C, Igbaseimokumo U (2015) Lumbar puncture opening pressure is not a reliable measure of intracranial pressure in children. J Child Neurol 30(2):170–173
5. Czosnyka M, Czosnyka ZH, Momjian S, Pickard JD (2004) Cerebrospinal fluid dynamics. Physiol Meas 25:R51–R76
6. Owler BK, Fong KCS, Czosnyka Z (2001) Importance of ICP monitoring in the investigation of CSF circulation disorders. Br J Neurosurg 15(5):439–440
7. Pickard J (2007) Lumbar infusion study: National Institute for Clinical Health Excellence guideline. 1–24
8. Kasprowicz M, Lalou DA, Czosnyka M, Garnett M, Czosnyka Z (2016) Intracranial pressure, its components and cerebrospinal fluid pressure–volume compensation. Acta Neurol Scand 134(3):168–180
9. Czosnyka M et al (2000) Post-traumatic hydrocephalus: influence of craniectomy on the CSF circulation. J Neurol Neurosurg Psychiatry 68(2):246–248
10. Czosnyka Z, Czosnyka M, Owler B, Momjian S, Kasprowicz M, Schmidt EA, Smielewski P, Pickard JD (2005) Clinical testing of CSF circulation in hydrocephalus. Acta Neurochir Suppl C 95:247–251
11. Lalou AD, Czosnyka M, Donnelly J, Pickard JD, Nabbanja E, Keong NC, Garnett M, Czosnyka ZH (2018) Cerebral autoregulation, cerebrospinal fluid outflow resistance, and outcome following cerebrospinal fluid diversion in normal pressure hydrocephalus. J Neurosurg 130:154–162
12. Kim DJ, Czosnyka Z, Keong N, Radolovich DK, Smielewski P, Sutcliffe MPF, Pickard JD, Czosnyka M (2009) Index of cerebrospinal compensatory reserve in hydrocephalus. Neurosurgery 64(3):494–501

Global Cerebral Autoregulation, Resistance to Cerebrospinal Fluid Outflow and Cerebrovascular Burden in Normal Pressure Hydrocephalus

Afroditi D. Lalou, Shadnaz Asgari, Matthew Garnett, Eva Nabbanja, Marek Czosnyka, and Zofia H. Czosnyka

Introduction

Despite criticism and alternative theories, CSF circulation is still one of the main pathophysiological hypotheses of normal pressure hydrocephalus (NPH). Studies related to the resistance to CSF outflow (Rout) and other components of the intracranial compartment are therefore essential until the complex puzzle of NPH is unravelled further. Moreover, shunting, with its hydrodynamic implications, remains the mainstay of management of hydrocephalus, via drainage and reduction of Rout [1, 2].

Whether other elements of the circulation or metabolism are disturbed, such as the regulatory mechanisms of CBF, cannot be concluded based on previous studies. An unknown state of cerebral hemodynamics, combined with a persistently unknown state of CSF dynamics, reveals a need for direction on rigorous research with detailed knowledge of these aspects and improved sample sizes.

Furthermore, in 2005, the NPH guidelines study group concluded that a single standard for the prognostic evaluation of idiopathic NPH (iNPH) was lacking. New guidelines are yet to be developed. Even the label of NPH remains therefore uncertain, the concept of NPH as a whole recently coming to question [3]. Among the burning questions in NPH are the behavior of Rout related to age and the etiology of NPH (idiopathic, secondary, and all causes under secondary), as well as its differentiation with cerebrovascular disease. These questions are extremely difficult to address, given the relative rarity of disease and the complexity of the ageing population.

A. D. Lalou (✉) · M. Garnett · E. Nabbanja · M. Czosnyka
Z. H. Czosnyka
Neurosurgery Unit, Department of Clinical Neurosciences, University of Cambridge, Cambridge, UK
e-mail: adl43@cam.ac.uk

S. Asgari
Biomedical Engineering Department, California State University, Long Beach, CA, USA

So far, Rout and possibly PRx and ABP have been the strongest predictors of outcome in NPH. None, however, is accurate enough as a single prognostication parameter. We have previously published a few studies of the relationship between global cerebral autoregulation and Rout, including mean arterial blood pressure [ABP] [4, 5]. Given the established relationship between NPH and disturbed cerebral blood flow (CBF) [6–8], and the quantitative interaction between Rout and PRx as a measure of global autoregulation, we aimed to model all parameters relevant to Rout and explore their combined effect on outcome prediction.

Material and Methods

Patients, Data Collection, and Processing

We used the data from a total of 88 patients (84 identical to those reported in Lalou et al. [5]). They were all NPH patients of various etiologies (predominantly iNPH) who had been selected for shunting after undergoing investigations at Cambridge University Hospital hydrocephalus clinic. Criteria for shunting included Rout, as well as responses to the spinal tap test and to extended lumbar drainage. Based on data recorded from their letters in the follow-up clinic, we classified them into CSF diversion responders and non-responders. The clinic follow-up letter depicts the final improvement presentation of the patient according to subjective reporting from the patients themselves and those closer to them, as well as objective findings from the clinical examination and gait assessment from physiotherapists [5, 9].

We had monitored ABP noninvasively using the Finometer® PRO in all patients during the entirety of the infusion test and were therefore able to calculate mean ABP, as well as PRx [10]. During infusion, a rise in ICP and a subsequent increase in the magnitude of slow waves of ICP [11] influences PRx calculation. However, as previously shown, detrending ICP

B. Depreitere et al. (eds.), *Intracranial Pressure and Neuromonitoring XVII*, Acta Neurochirurgica Supplement 131,
https://doi.org/10.1007/978-3-030-59436-7_67, © Springer Nature Switzerland AG 2021

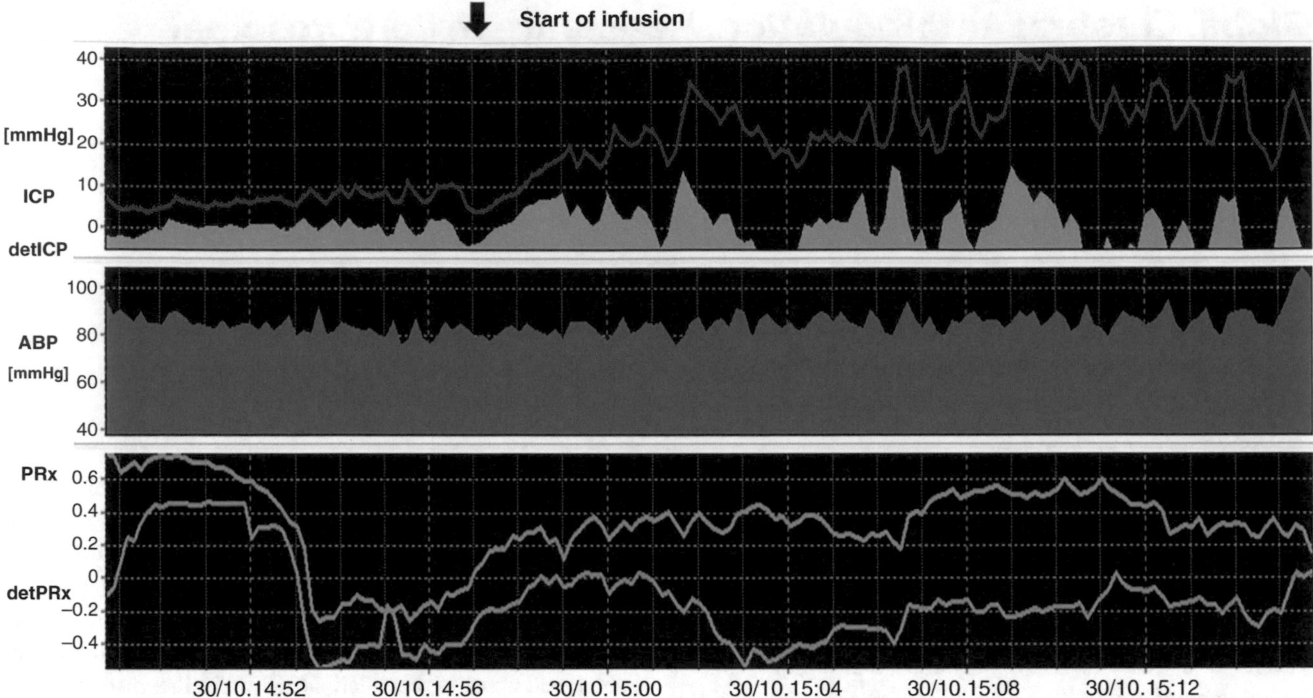

Fig. 1 ICP and PRx calculation during infusion, with detrending of the signals. Monitoring of ABP during infusion allows for PRx calculation over a 30–45-min window. ICP required detrending to avoid the influence of increasing ICP on PRx calculation. *ABP* arterial blood pressure, *detICP* detrended ICP, *detPRx* detrended PRx

during infusion will minimize that influence, and PRx can be calculated during the entire period of the test, on a total window of 30–45 min (baseline + infusion phase) [5].

ABP recording during infusion, ICP detrending and the result PRx detrending are shown in Fig. 1.

Statistical Analysis

We used the Fisher discrimination ratio (FDR) to revalidate the predictive power of individual parameters. Following that, we incorporated those stronger parameters in multilinear regression to model the known co-linearities and interactions between age, Rout, ABP, and PRx. All statistics were performed by ADL (author) and SA (co-author) using R version 3.6.0 and Matlab.

Results

Predictive Power of Individual Parameters

Sixty-nine patients had a favorable outcome after shunting, whereas 19 did not improve at all on follow-up.

ABP demonstrated better predictive power than Rout in the Fisher discriminant analysis. Using the multivariable logistic regression model created to test the predictive power of each value, we extracted that ABP was an independent predictor of outcome, with an odds ratio of 1.1, 95% confidence interval 1–1.2 and p-value = 0.01.

The plot of FDR values for all measured variables is shown in Fig. 2.

Predictive Power of Combined Variables

The strongest relationship was detected with the multilinear regression model combining the interaction between PRx, ABP, and Rout, and age correction was applied: Linear Model: Rout ~ PRx*ABP + age.

($N = 88$; $R = -0.56$; $p = 8.188 \times 10^{-0.5}$)

When testing this model as an outcome separator, the results showed strong relationship in the responders group ($R = -0.62$; $p = 8.986 \times 10^{-6}$, $N = 69$) and an absent correlation ($R = -0.15$; $p = 0.69$) in non-responders ($N = 19$).

The ROC curve and predictive values of the above linear model are shown in Fig. 3.

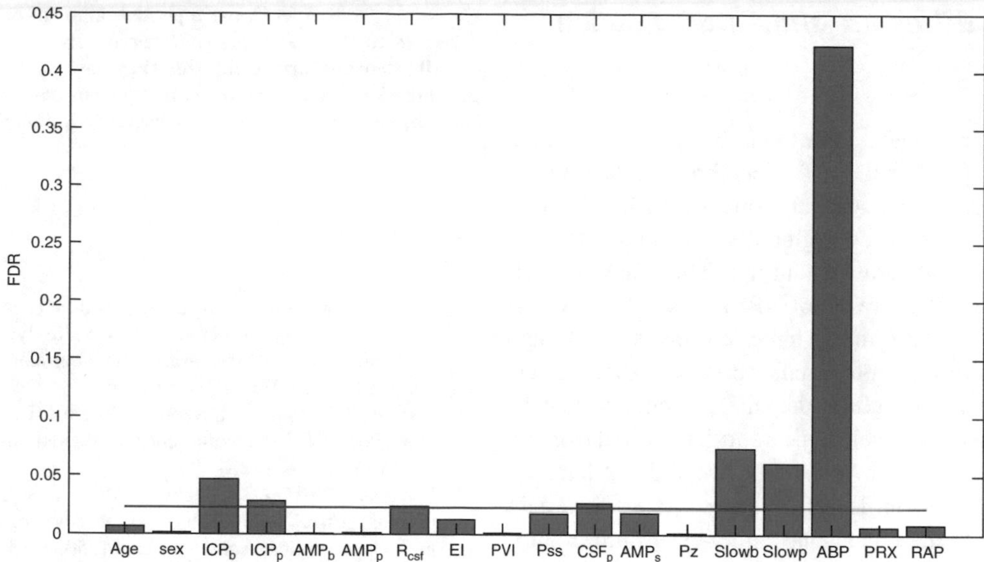

Fig. 2 Fisher discriminant analysis of measured parameters during infusion. The red line represents the predictive power of Rout. Some parameters, including ICP baseline and magnitude of slow waves, and ABP in particular, demonstrate higher predictive power than Rout. *ICPb* ICP baseline, *ICPp* ICP plateau, *AMPb* AMP baseline, *AMPp* AMP plateau, *Rcsf* Resistance to CSF outflow (Rout), *El* elasticity, *PVI* pressure-volume index, *Pss* sagittal sinus pressure, *CSFp* CSF production rate, *AMPs* slope of amplitude-pressure line, *Slowb* slow wave magnitude at baseline, *Slowp* slow wave magnitude at plateau, *ABP* arterial blood pressure, *RAP* correlation coefficient between ICP and AMP (compensatory reserve index)

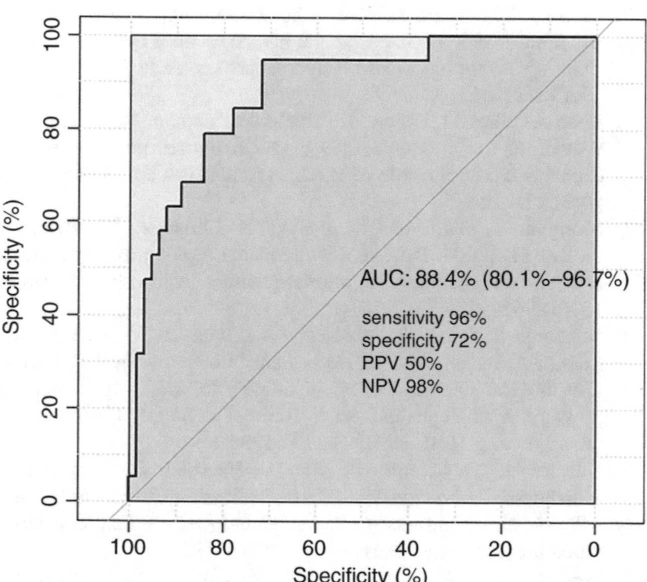

Fig. 3 ROC curve and predictive values for the linear interaction model between Rout, ABP, and PRx. For $N = 88$ patients (69 shunt responders and 19 non-responders), the interaction between Rout, ABP, and PRx in the form of decreasing Rout, in combination with high PRx and ABP could very accurately predict a poor outcome, with a high NPV of 98%

Discussion

We have provided a quantitative means of assessing the cerebrovascular profile of possible NPH patients and potentially more dementias with ventriculomegaly that clinically mimic NPH or could coexist with it.

To date, there is a vast pool of evidence validating a relationship between reduced regional CBF in the areas proximate to and in direct relationship with the ventricles [8, 12–15]. There is still a lot of work required to achieve the creation of a practical, bedside tool assessing CBF and autoregulation in such patients, if they are clinically useful at all as a diagnostic or predictive measure. We have shown in this paper a practical and low-cost method that could provide additional information to the cerebral hemodynamic state, as well as the CSF circulatory profile. It does not require any additional time of monitoring besides a standard infusion test and could be used to validate prospectively in randomized trials.

Influence of Hypertension and Autoregulation on Rout

While both age and PRx have been shown in multiple occasions to directly correlate with Rout [16, 17], ABP did not correlate with Rout despite being a stronger outcome predictor than Rout. At the same time, the inverse relationship between Rout and PRx could be driven by an influence of vascular disease and stronger disease burden on Rout, or an interaction derived from independent pathophysiologies [18]. Interestingly, the effect of age is possibly excluded because it is related with increased Rout and not related to PRx.

Arterial Blood Pressure and Autoregulation in NPH

The role of cerebrovascular disease has been suggested since early on in NPH [7]. It is likely that cerebrovascular disease, causing dysautoregulation and subsequently significant ischemia in several regions or even globally, can contribute to an unfavorable outcome after shunting. The question still remains whether this is a result of NPH, or is rather a contribution of uncontrolled primary hypertension related to age leading to coexisting cerebrovascular disease. From our current results, we can conclude that the presence of uncontrolled hypertension in itself appears to lead to unfavorable results after shunting. Unfortunately, we did not have an available objective identifier of cerebrovascular disease in those patients. On the other hand, globally disturbed autoregulation in itself was not associated with unfavorable outcome, unless it was combined with the effect of ABP. This finding appears intuitive, as a non-autoregulating brain would be exposed to such effects of increasing and decreasing ABP; it is of significance though, to be able to demonstrate that effect clinically, as a clear negative influence on outcome.

Clinical Applications

Prospective validation of the above results is required, ideally using both invasive and noninvasive ABP monitoring for optimal absolute values of ABP.

Ethical Approval and Consent to Participate

In line with the protocol in Cambridge University Hospitals NHS Foundation Trust, this retrospective study was conducted without separate approval from an ethics committee. All patients were investigated with infusion test within the neurosciences department, as a part of routine clinical assessment.

Consent for Publication

As per our ethics statement, this was a retrospective study, not requiring separate approval from an ethics committee. All data form part of an anonymized, retrospective cohort and are not identifiable.

Conflict of Interest **M.C. has a partial financial interest in licensing ICM+ software (Cambridge enterprise, UK).**

All other authors certify that they have no affiliations with any organization or entity with any financial or non-financial interest in the subject matter or materials discussed in this manuscript.

References

1. Czosnyka M, Czosnyka Z, Agarwal-harding KJ, Pickard JD (2012) Modeling of cerebrospinal fluid dynamics: Legacy of Professor Anthony Marmarou. Acta Neurochir 113:9–14. https://doi.org/10.1007/978-3-7091-0923-6
2. Petrella G, Czosnyka M, Keong N, Pickard JD, Czosnyka Z (2008) How does CSF dynamics change after shunting? Acta Neurol Scand 118(3):182–188
3. Espay AJ, Da Prat GA, Dwivedi AK et al (2017) Deconstructing normal pressure hydrocephalus: ventriculomegaly as early sign of neurodegeneration. Ann Neurol 82(4):503–513
4. Czosnyka ZH, Czosnyka M, Whitfield PC, Donovan T, Pickard JD, Milhorat TH, Selman WR, Gjerris F, Juhler M (2002) Cerebral autoregulation among patients with symptoms of hydrocephalus. Neurosurgery 50(3):526–533
5. Lalou AD, Czosnyka M, Donnelly J, Pickard JD, FMedSci NE, Keong NC, Garnett M, Czosnyka ZH (2018) Cerebral autoregulation, cerebrospinal fluid outflow resistance, and outcome following cerebrospinal fluid diversion in normal pressure hydrocephalus. J Neurosurg 130(1):154–162
6. Bakker SLM, Boon AJW, Wijnhoud AD, Dippel DWJ, Delwel EJ, Koudstaal PJ (2002) Cerebral hemodynamics before and after shunting in normal pressure hydrocephalus. Acta Neurol Scand 106(3):123–127
7. Boon AJ, Tans JT, Delwel EJ, Egeler-Peerdeman SM, Hanlo PW, Wurzer HA, Hermans J (1999) Dutch normal-pressure hydrocephalus study: the role of cerebrovascular disease. J Neurosurg 90(2):221–226
8. Momjian S, Owler BK, Czosnyka Z, Czosnyka M, Pena A, Pickard JD (2004) Pattern of white matter regional cerebral blood flow and autoregulation in normal pressure hydrocephalus. Brain 127(5):965–972
9. Nabbanja E, Czosnyka M, Keong NC, Garnett M, Pickard JD, Lalou DA, Czosnyka Z (2018) Is there a link between ICP-derived infusion test parameters and outcome after shunting in normal pressure hydrocephalus? Acta Neurochir Suppl 126:229–232. https://doi.org/10.1007/978-3-319-65798-1_46
10. Kasprowicz M, Schmidt E, Kim DJ, Haubrich C, Czosnyka Z, Smielewski P, Czosnyka M (2010) Evaluation of the cerebrovascular pressure reactivity index using non-invasive Finapres arterial blood pressure. Physiol Meas 31(9):1217–1228
11. Weerakkody RA, Czosnyka M, Zweifel C, Castellani G, Smielewski P, Keong N, Haubrich C, Pickard J, Czosnyka Z (2010) Slow vasogenic fluctuations of intracranial pressure and cerebral near infrared spectroscopy-an observational study. Acta Neurochir 152(10):1763–1769
12. Mori K, Maeda M, Asegawa S, Iwata J (2002) Quantitative local cerebral blood flow change after cerebrospinal fluid removal in patients with normal pressure hydrocephalus measured by a double injection method with N-isopropyl-p-[(123)I] iodoamphetamine. Acta Neurochir 144(3):255–262; discussion 262–3
13. Owler BK, Pickard JD (2001) Normal pressure hydrocephalus and cerebral blood flow: a review. Acta Neurol Scand 104:325–342
14. Tullberg M, Hellström P, Piechnik SK, Starmark JE, Wikkelsö C (2004) Impaired wakefulness is associated with reduced anterior

cingulate CBF in patients with normal pressure hydrocephalus. Acta Neurol Scand 110(5):322–330

15. Virhammar XJ, Laurell XK, Ahlgren XA, Larsson XE (2017) Arterial spin-labeling perfusion MR imaging demonstrates regional CBF decrease in idiopathic normal pressure hydrocephalus. Am J Neuroradiol 38:2081–2088
16. Czosnyka M, Czosnyka ZH, Whitfield PC, Donovan T, Pickard JD (2009) Age dependence of cerebrospinal pressure—volume compensation in patients with hydrocephalus. J Neurosurg 94(3):482–486
17. Stoquart-ElSankari S, Balédent O, Gondry-Jouet C, Makki M, Godefroy O, Meyer M-E (2007) Aging effects on cerebral blood and cerebrospinal fluid flows. J Cereb Blood Flow Metab 27(9):1563–1572
18. Czosnyka Z, Owler B, Keong N, Santarius T, Baledent O, Pickard JD, Czosnyka M (2011) Impact of duration of symptoms on CSF dynamics in idiopathic normal pressure hydrocephalus. Acta Neurol Scand 123(6):414–418

Comparison of Assessment for Shunting with Infusion Studies Versus Extended Lumbar Drainage in Suspected Normal Pressure Hydrocephalus

Virginia Levrini, Matthew Garnett, Eva Nabbanja, Marek Czosnyka, Zofia H. Czosnyka, and Afroditi D. Lalou

Introduction

Normal pressure hydrocephalus (NPH) is characterized by a clinical triad of gait disturbance, short-term memory deterioration, and urinary incontinence, with radiological evidence of ventriculomegaly. The treatment of choice is a shunt, after which patients should see an improvement in these symptoms. The tools available for the selection of patients with queried NPH for shunting are currently ICP monitoring, infusion studies, a CSF tap test, and extended lumbar drainage (ELD). These can be used alone or in combination.

CSF infusion studies and ELD have been shown to have a high positive predictive value, but low negative predictive value. Walchenbach et al. [1] found CSF tap test had a positive predictive value of 100% and negative predictive value of 32%. They found ELD to have a positive predictive value of 87% and negative predictive value of 36%. Table 1 shows the positive and negative predictive values of infusions tests found in different studies.

Although the coupling of CSF diversion test with specialist neurocognitive assessment and gait analysis has been shown to be a good predictor of shunt responsiveness, an element of subjectivity in these tests remains [3–5]. We aimed to investigate predicting improvement post-shunting by infusion tests versus ELD with emphasis on the dynamics of ELD responders.

V. Levrini (✉) · M. Garnett · E. Nabbanja · M. Czosnyka
Z. H. Czosnyka · A. D. Lalou
Division of Neurosurgery, Department of Clinical Neuroscience, University of Cambridge, Addenbrooke's Hospital, Cambridge, UK

Table 1 Table illustrating the positive and negative predictive values found for response to shunting in NPH with infusion tests in various studies

References	NPH	Aetiology	Rout	PPV	NPV
Borgesen et al. [15]	80	Mixed	≥12	96–100%	>95%
Borgesen et al. [19]	183	Mixed	≥12	NA	100%
Boon et al. [20]	101	iNPH	≥12 and ≥18	80 and 92%	34%
Kahlon et al. [21]	68	iNPH	≥14	80%	NA
Wikkelsø et al. [17]	115	iNPH	≥12 and ≥18	86 and 94%	18 and 18%
Nabbanja et al. [22]	310	Mixed	≥13 and ≥18	NA	NA

PPV positive predictive value, *NPV* negative predictive value. Reproduced with license from "cerebral autoregulation, resistance and outcome after CSF diversion" [2]

Material and Methods

We retrospectively recruited 83 patients from our NPH database at Cambridge University Hospital (CUH) who had undergone both a lumbar infusion study and ELD assessment between 2014 and 2018. All subjects had signed consent forms for their data to be used for research purposes. Constant-rate infusion studies were carried out via Ommaya reservoir in 5 cases and via lumbar puncture using an 18-gauge pink needle in 78 cases. ICM+ software is used routinely to record and process the data (University of Cambridge Enterprise Ltd). The constant-rate infusion study method used has been previously described in numerous publications ranging over 40 years [6–8].

ELD protocol involved placement of a lumbar catheter for a duration of 5 days, with 100 mL of CSF drained per

B. Depreitere et al. (eds.), *Intracranial Pressure and Neuromonitoring XVII*, Acta Neurochirurgica Supplement 131,
https://doi.org/10.1007/978-3-030-59436-7_68, © Springer Nature Switzerland AG 2021

day. Assessment of gait was done by physiotherapists with the Tinnetti tool and a 10-m timed walking test before drain placement and within 24 h after ELD removal. Subjective perception of symptom (gait, cognition, and urinary function) improvement or deterioration by the patient and mainly those closest to them (family and/or carers) was also asked at clinic follow-up. VL (author) collected the data from physiotherapy assessments from patient notes and documentation of improvement from electronic inpatient records and clinic letters. These were compared to CSF hydrodynamics. We used R software (version 3.5.2.) to perform all statistics.

We explored Rout thresholds >11 mmHg*min/mL and <11, as well as different thresholds based on shunt and ELD response. As initially described from studies in physiological individuals, the average normal Rout is around 7 mmHg*min/mL [9] and with a possible calculation error of ±3 mmHg|*min/mL [10], values >10 or below 4 would most likely be unphysiological, and values between 4 and 10 should be within the normal range.

Results

Of the 83 patients, 62 had Rout >11 mmHg/mL/min and 21 had Rout <11 mmHg/mL/min. In the Rout >11 group, 28 showed physiotherapy-documented improvement following ELD, 24 either did not respond or did worse following ELD, and assessments were unavailable for 10 patients. 28 of 62 (34% of total) patients were selected for shunting. Seven patients declined shunting and the remaining 21 patients were shunted and available for follow-up. Of these 21 patients, 19 showed improvement following shunting. Eight patients with Rout >20 mmHg/mL/min showed no response to ELD and were not shunted.

Figure 1 demonstrates the number of patients with resistances above or below 11 who were included, showed improvement following ELD, were shunted, and showed improvement following shunting.

In the Rout <11 group, all 5 patients who were shunted and showed improvement at follow-up had Rout >6 mmHg/mL/min. Two patients deteriorated significantly following ELD. Pre-ELD they were mobilizing independently or with the aid of a walking stick, but on discharge had to be transferred to a local hospital for rehabilitation because they could no longer mobilize.

Overall, 24/26 ELD responders also responded positively to shunting, which yields a 92% PPV for ELD.

ICP amplitude did not differ at baseline or plateau between ELD responders and non-responders (baseline: 0.95 ± 0.61 vs. 0.79 ± 0.64; p = 0.8161 plateau: 4.09 ± 1.64 vs. 3.69 ± 0.97; p = 0.9049). ICP baseline was 8.96 ± 3.81 vs. 10.53 ± 3.9; p = 0.1862, elasticity was 0.21 ± 0.1 vs. 0.25 ± 0.13; p = 0.6143 and compliance [1/(E*ICPbaseline)] did not differ between the two groups.

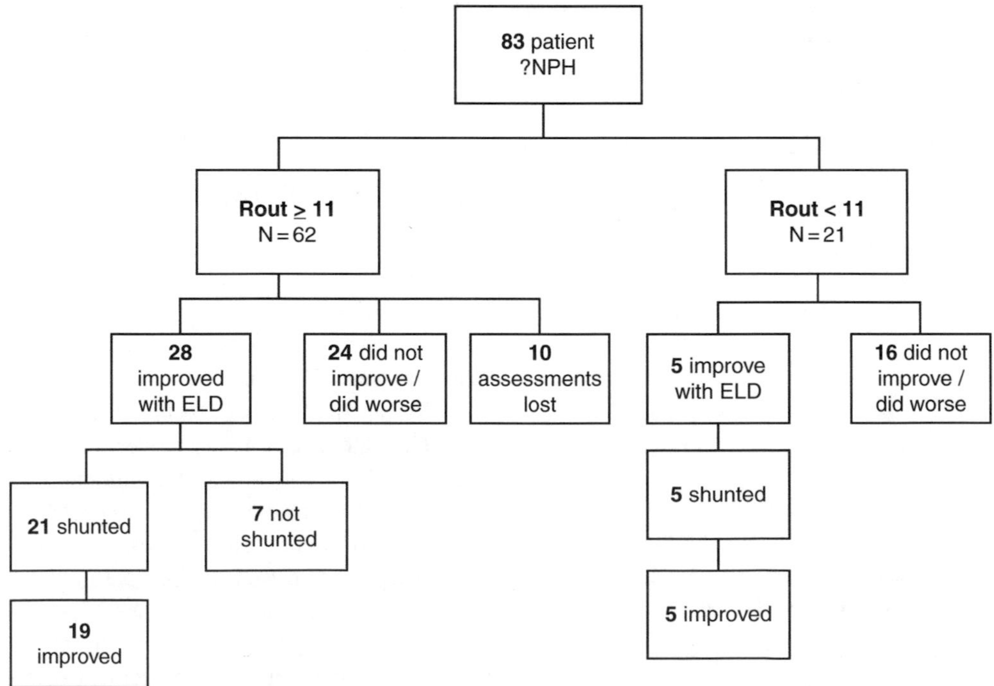

Fig. 1 Response to extended lumbar drainage and to shunting in the patient groups with resistance above and below 11 mmHg/mL/min. *NPH* normal pressure hydrocephalus, *ELD* extended lumbar drainage, *Rout* resistance to CSF outflow

Discussion

We have provided the first preliminary comparison between objective, CSF dynamics testing and ELD in NPH. Overall, there are marked differences between the two assessments, which would be of interest to investigate in the future.

Rout ≥11 and >20 Versus ELD Response

There was marked discrepancy between CSF hydrodynamics and ELD response, including 8 patients with Rout >20 mmHg/mL/min who showed no response to ELD. The reasons for this disparity could lie in part with our assessment of response following ELD. Some centers couple ELD with multiple tests from neuropsychologists, as well as physiotherapists, to assess and quantify any possible improvement in all areas of the NPH triad. At our center, the assessment is focused on improvement in gait, which has been shown to usually improve first and more prominently than cognition and urinary incontinence [11–13]. Additionally, the timing of assessment could play a role in the level of response we see to ELD. All our physiotherapy assessments were carried out within 24 h of removing the lumbar catheter. Response to CSF diversion is known to be variable [14–17]. An NPH subject is considered shunt-responsive if they show improvement within 3 months of the shunt being inserted. However, we measure the improvement of our ELD candidates just six days after the first day of diversion. Although the subjective family reports of patient improvement are just that, subjective, at least part of the 18 cases where physiotherapy and family disagreed could be due to the diverse timing of their respective observation periods. In view of this and of previously reported low negative predictive values of ELD, it could be argued that the eight patients with Rout >20 mmHg/mL/min who showed no ELD response could merit further consideration: Would their response to ELD change if the timing of their assessment did?

Rout <6 Versus ELD Response

There was a subgroup of patients that the two tests agreed on: patients with a Rout <6 mmHg/mL/min. All patients with Rout <6 mmHg/mL/min showed no improvement with ELD. As such, ELD assessment in this subgroup of patients is unadvisable.

CSF Dynamics in ELD Responders Vs. Non-responders

Besides Rout, no other CSF dynamic parameter on its own appears to correlate with ELD response. However, our current numbers are low and, in the future, it would be of interest to explore those parameters and to combine several parameters. Nonetheless, ELD re-confirms a high PPV, although infusion tests also have shown a very high PPV. Improving on NPV is a challenge that would be difficult to address in our current clinical setting, unless an appropriate trial is performed to assess and improve on the NPV of both ELD and infusion tests.

Clinical Significance

ELD investigations tend to be safe and a good approximation of shunt response [1, 18]. The addition of ELD in combination with infusion tests in investigating NPH could provide significant opportunities for understanding NPH further. This is due to the opportunity to clearly look into all "responders" versus "non-responders," whereas in the past surgery would be the only determinant of such response, without any insight into the non-shunted patients. By continuing to investigate patients in such a way, we will possibly be able to obtain new insights from infusion tests that were not available before. It is also for this reason that, if ELD were to be used, it would be required to be used in the best and most accurate way, as its PPV and especially NPV are still awaiting confirmation and should ideally be able to reflect response to shunt surgery as accurately as possible.

Conflict of Interest **M.C. has a partial financial interest in licensing ICM+ software (Cambridge enterprise, UK).**

All other authors certify that they have no affiliations with any organization or entity with any financial or non-financial interest in the subject matter or materials discussed in this manuscript.

References

1. Walchenbach R, Geiger E, Thomeer RTWM, Vanneste JAL (2002) The value of temporary external lumbar CSF drainage in predicting the outcome of shunting on normal pressure hydrocephalus. J Neurol Neurosurg Psychiatry 72(4):503–506
2. Lalou AD, Czosnyka M, Donnelly J, Pickard JD, Nabbanja E, Keong NC, Garnett M, Czosnyka ZH (2018) Cerebral autoregulation, cerebrospinal fluid outflow resistance, and outcome following cerebrospinal fluid diversion in normal pressure hydrocephalus. J Neurosurg 130(1):154–162

3. Allali G, Laidet M, Armand S, Assal F (2018) Brain comorbidities in normal pressure hydrocephalus. Eur J Neurol 25(3):542–548. https://doi.org/10.1111/ene.13543
4. Koivisto AM, Alafuzoff I, Savolainen S, Sutela A, Rummukainen J, Kurki M, Jääskeläinen JE, Soininen H, Rinne J, Leinonen V (2013) Poor cognitive outcome in shunt-responsive idiopathic normal pressure hydrocephalus. Neurosurgery 72(1):1–8; discussion 8. https://doi.org/10.1227/NEU.0b013e31827414b3
5. Peterson KA, Savulich G, Jackson D, Killikelly C, Pickard JD, Sahakian BJ (2016) The effect of shunt surgery on neuropsychological performance in normal pressure hydrocephalus: a systematic review and meta-analysis. J Neurol 263(8):1669–1677. https://doi.org/10.1007/s00415-016-8097-0
6. Czosnyka Z, Czosnyka M, Owler B, Momjian S, Kasprowicz M, Schmidt EA, Smielewski P, Pickard JD (2005) Clinical testing of CSF circulation in hydrocephalus. Acta Neurochir Suppl 95:247–251
7. Czosnyka M, Whitehouse H, Smielewski P, Simac S, Pickard JD (1996) Testing of cerebrospinal compensatory reserve in shunted and non-shunted patients: a guide to interpretation based on an observational study. J Neurol Neurosurg Psychiatry 60(5): 549–558
8. Katzman R, Hussey F (1970) A simple constant-infusion manometric test for measurement of CSF absorption. I Rationale and method. Neurology 20(6):534–544
9. Ekstedt J (1978) CSF hydrodynamic studies in man 2 Normal hydrodynamic variables related to CSF pressure and flow. J Neurol Psychiatry 41:345–353
10. Swallow DMA, Fellner N, Varsos GV, Czosnyka M, Smielewski P, Pickard JD, Czosnyka Z (2014) Repeatability of cerebrospinal fluid constant rate infusion study. Acta Neurol Scand 130(2):131–138
11. Liu A, Sankey EW, Jusué-Torres I, Patel MA, Elder BD, Goodwin CR, Hoffberger J, Lu J, Rigamonti D (2016) Clinical outcomes after ventriculoatrial shunting for idiopathic normal pressure hydrocephalus. Clin Neurol Neurosurg 143:34–38. https://doi.org/10.1016/j.clineuro.2016.02.013
12. Sankey EW, Jusué-Torres I, Elder BD, Goodwin CR, Batra S, Hoffberger J, Lu J, Blitz AM, Rigamonti D (2015) Functional gait outcomes for idiopathic normal pressure hydrocephalus after primary endoscopic third ventriculostomy. J Clin Neurosci 22:1303–1308. https://doi.org/10.1016/j.jocn.2015.02.019
13. Vakili S, Moran D, Hung A et al (2016) Timing of surgical treatment for idiopathic normal pressure hydrocephalus: association between treatment delay and reduced short-term benefit. Neurosurg Focus 41:E2. https://doi.org/10.3171/2016.6.FOCUS16146
14. Børgesen SE, Albeck MJ, Gjerris F, Czosnyka M, Laniewski P (1992) Computerized infusion test compared to steady pressure constant infusion test in measurement of resistance to CSF outflow. Acta Neurochir 119(1–4):12–16
15. Borgesen SE, Gjerris F (1982) The predictive value of conductance to outflow of CSF in normal pressure hydrocephalus. Brain 105:65–86
16. Keong NCH, Pena A, Price SJ, Czosnyka M, Czosnyka Z, Pickard JD (2016) Imaging normal pressure hydrocephalus: theories, techniques, and challenges. Neurosurg Focus 41(3):E11
17. Wikkelsø C, Hellström P, Klinge P et al (2013) The European iNPH Multicentre Study on the predictive values of resistance to CSF outflow and the CSF Tap Test in patients with idiopathic normal pressure hydrocephalus. J Neurol Neurosurg Psychiatry 84(5):562–568
18. Nakajima M, Miyajima M, Ogino I, Sugano H, Akiba C, Domon N, Karagiozov KL, Arai H (2015) Use of external lumbar cerebrospinal fluid drainage and lumboperitoneal shunts with strata NSC valves in idiopathic normal pressure hydrocephalus: a single-center experience. World Neurosurg 83(3):387–393. https://doi.org/10.1016/j.wneu.2014.08.004
19. Borgesen SE, Gjerris F, Schmidt J (1989) Measurement of resistance to CSF outflow by subarachnoid perfusion. AlfredBenzon Symposium 27: Outflow of cerebrospinal fluid. Gjerris F, Borgesen SE, Sorensen PS, eds. Copenhagen: Munksgaard 121–133
20. Boon AJW, Tans JT, Delwel EJ, Egeler-Peerdeman SM, Hanlo PW, Wurzer HAL et al (1997) Dutch normal-pressure hydrocephalus study: prediction of outcome after shunting by resistance to outflow of cerebrospinal fluid. J Neurosurg 87(5):687–93
21. Kahlon B, Sundbärg G, Rehncrona S (2002) Comparison between the lumbar infusion and CSF tap tests to predict outcome after shunt surgery in suspected normal pressure hydrocephalus. J Neurol Neurosurg Psychiatry 73(6):721–726
22. Nabbanja E, Czosnyka M, Keong NC, Garnett M, Pickard JD, Lalou DA et al (2018) Is there a link between ICP-derived infusion test parameters and outcome after shunting in normal pressure hydrocephalus? Vol. 126, Acta Neurochirurgica, Supplementum

The Role of Cerebrospinal Fluid Dynamics in Normal Pressure Hydrocephalus Diagnosis and Shunt Prognostication

Afroditi D. Lalou, Shadnaz Asgari, Marek Czosnyka, Eva Nabbanja, Matthew Garnett, and Zofia H. Czosnyka

Introduction

NPH is a heterogeneous disease characterized radiologically by enlarged ventricles and clinically by Hakim's triad: gait disturbance, urinary incontinence, and dementia. Since its first description in 1965 [1], the works of Marmarou [2, 3] and the development of the lumbar infusion test by Katzman [4] set the path for studying the CSF dynamics of the patients presenting with this clinical syndrome. Resistance to CSF outflow (Rout) has been investigated in several prospective studies and the European iNPH randomized trial [5]. Studies such as those from Borgensen et al. [6, 7] and the Dutch normal pressure hydrocephalus [8, 9] demonstrated that increased Rout (>12 mmHg*min/mL and >18 mmHg*min/mL, respectively) was characteristic of NPH and strongly predictive of outcome after shunting. Unfortunately, many centers—despite guidelines, clinical, and paraclinical tests—discovered that shunting response varied from 40–80%, with the latter being the most frequent in modern, specialized centers [2, 5, 8–16]. However, the newest iNPH trial [5] failed to show the high prognostic value of previously suggested Rout values for shunting.

Overall, there has been no objective overview of all CSF dynamic parameters and a lack of objective description of NPH with parameters outside Rout. From the data available in Cambridge, one of the main modern centers to utilize infusion tests in NPH, we have aimed to begin to understand the problems with Rout as well with other CSF dynamics assessed through the infusion test, on their own or combined. As such, we have attempted to assess the relationship of all infusion-derived parameters with shunt response and to identify sources of discrepancy between NPH diagnosis and shunt response-defined diagnosis using CSF dynamics.

Material and Methods

We analyzed the data of 369 NPH patients (154 females, 70 ± 11 years old) who were either shunted (332 patients) or had ETV (37 patients) with infusion tests and clinical follow-up at Addenbrooke's Hospital in Cambridge between 1998 and 2018. The 6-month patients' outcome was marked using a simple numerical scale: (1) long-term improvement (sustained improvement at 6 months); (2) temporary improvement (improvement at 3 months not sustained at 6 months); and (3) no improvement. For simplicity, in our analysis we combined the outcome scales 1 and 2 to indicate patients with improvement and compared them with those patients who showed no improvement. In addition to age and gender, the following ten baseline and infusion-derived variables were considered: ICP_b (baseline ICP), ICP_p (Plateau ICP), AMP_b (baseline amplitude), AMP_p (plateau amplitude), R_{out} (CSF resistance), El (Elasticity), PVI (pressure volume index), Pss (sagittal sinus pressure), CSF_p (CSF Production Rate), and AMP_s (Amplitude/pressure slope).

We conducted a correlation analysis among all variables. We also determined the patients' outcomes (improvement versus no improvement at 6 months) by applying a threshold on R_{out} and compared our results with those of existing literature (Bergensen 1982 [7], Boon 1997 [8], and Wikkelso 2013 [5]) in terms of sensitivity, specificity, positive predictive

A.D. Lalou and S. Asgari contributed equally to this work.

A. D. Lalou (✉) · M. Czosnyka · E. Nabbanja · M. Garnett
Z. H. Czosnyka
Division of Neurosurgery, Department of Clinical Neuroscience, University of Cambridge, Addenbrooke's Hospital, Cambridge, UK
e-mail: adl43@cam.ac.uk

S. Asgari
Biomedical Engineering Department, California State University, Long Beach, CA, USA

B. Depreitere et al. (eds.), *Intracranial Pressure and Neuromonitoring XVII*, Acta Neurochirurgica Supplement 131,
https://doi.org/10.1007/978-3-030-59436-7_69,

value (PPV), negative predictive value (NPV), overall accuracy, and likelihood ratio.

Finally, we employed Chi-Statistics (by applying non-parametric Kruskal Wallis test) as a measure of separability between improvement and no improvement outcomes to determine a subset of variables that achieved the highest accuracy in prediction of outcome (using a Bayesian classifier with fivefold cross validation and bootstrapping).

Results

292 out of 369 patients (79%) in our dataset had improvement after shunting. Figure 1 illustrates the results of the correlation analysis of all baseline and infusion-derived variables using a color bar where correlations with significant p-value (smaller than 0.05) are indicated with letters on the plot as follows:

- "W" indicates significant weak correlation (when correlation value <0.4)
- "M" indicates significant moderate correlation (when $0.4 \leq$ correlation value <0.7)
- "S" indicates significant strong correlation (when $0.7 \leq$ correlation value)

We observe that several variables have significant correlation with each other. For example, R_{out} has significant but weak correlation with age, ICP_b, AMP_b, and CSF_p. However, the correlation of R_{out} and ICP_p (AMP_p) is significant and strong (moderate).

Figure 2 presents the result of outcome prediction using a threshold value on R_{out} in our dataset and compares it with those of existing studies. While Bergensen 1982 results inconsistent with other studies, our results fall in between those of Boon 1997 and Wikkelso 2013.

Figure 3a shows the values of Chi-statistics obtained for different R_{out} thresholds. We observe that Rout threshold of 18 achieves the highest Chi-statistics. By adjusting the threshold based on age using ($9 + 0.08 \times$ age) formula [17] the Chi-Square increased from 8.6 (p-value = 0.003) to 9.7 (p-value = 0.002). Figure 3b demonstrates the correlation of R_{out} and shunt outcome for the subjects with R_{out} above the corresponding threshold. The threshold of 18 results in the highest absolute value of correlation.

Finally, we investigated the predictive power of CSF dynamic parameters by applying a Bayesian classifier with fivefold cross-validation and bootstrapping to a subset of variables in our dataset which showed significant Chi-Statistics values (more than 5). Using these variables (ICP_b, ICP_p, R_{out}, CSF_p, AMP_s), we achieved an overall accuracy of 0.70 ± 0.09 in prediction of the shunt outcome.

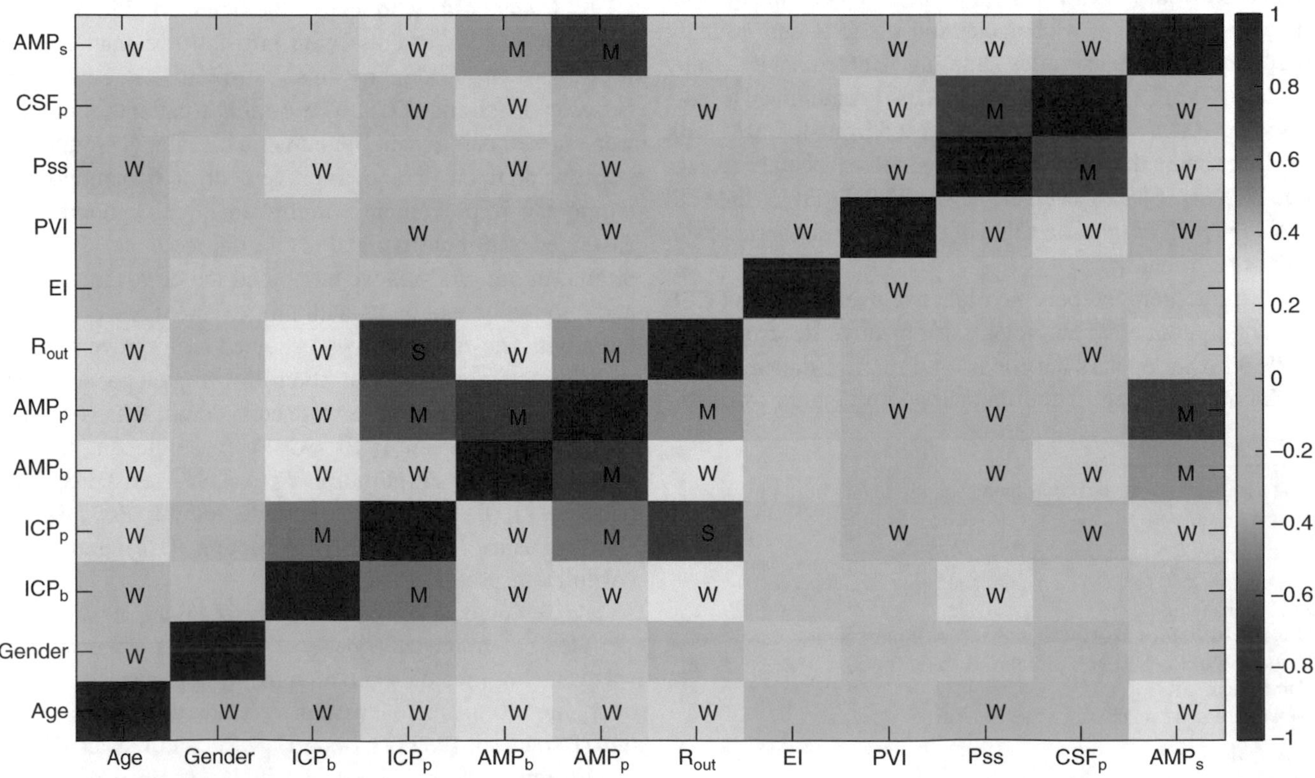

Fig. 1 Results of correlation analysis among all variables

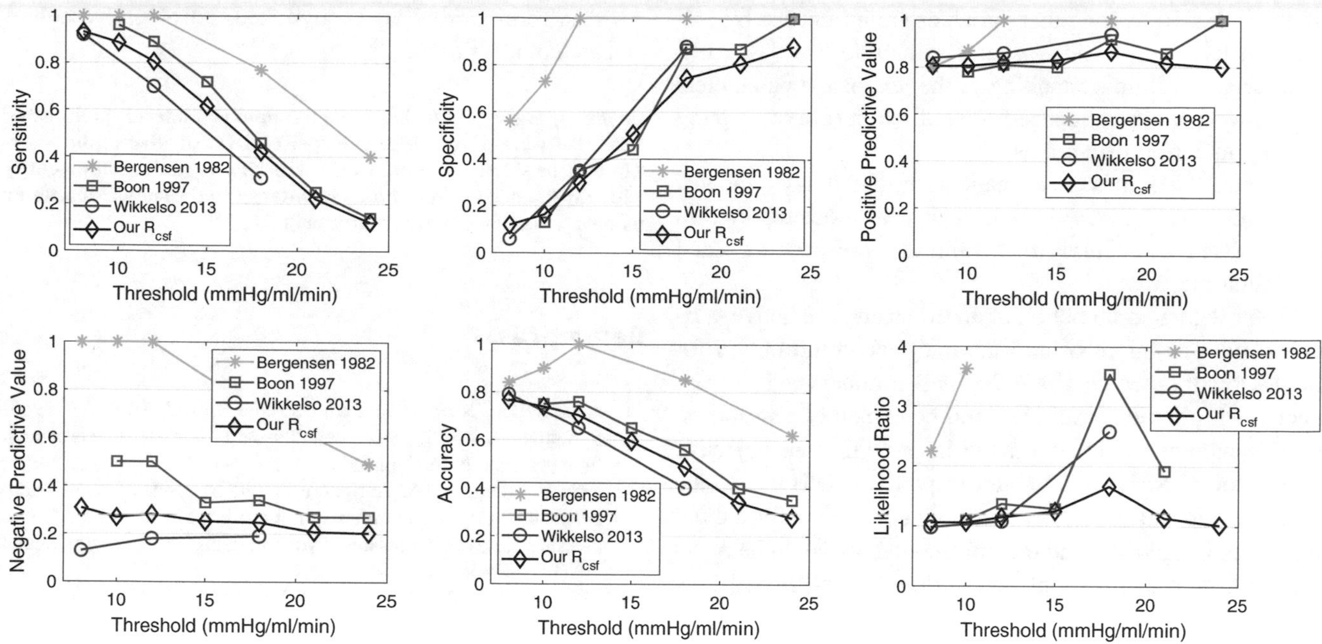

Fig. 2 Comparison of our dataset Shunt outcome prediction results using Rout with those of existing literature: (**a**) sensitivity, (**b**) specificity, (**c**) PPV, (**d**) NPV, (**e**) overall accuracy, (**f**) likelihood ratio

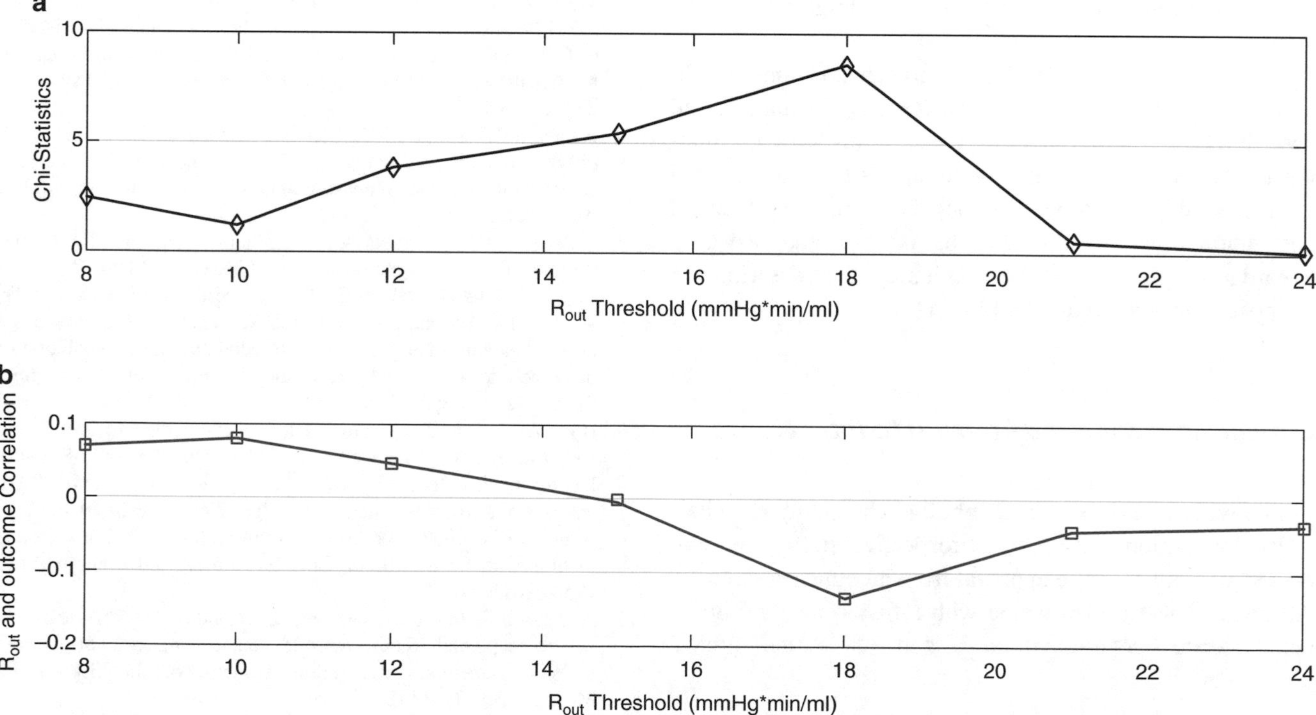

Fig. 3 Optimal threshold value on Rout for prediction of outcome: (**a**) Chi-Statistics versus the threshold value on R_{out}, (**b**) correlation of R_{out}, with improvement versus no improvement outcomes

Discussion

We have provided the detailed account of the predictive value of a combination of CSF pressure and dynamic variables in NPH using machine learning methodology. The traditional Rout thresholds of 13 and 18 mmHg*min/mL seem to remain similar in NPH, requiring individualization within the known range of 10–21 mmHg*min/mL [4]. CSF dynamics are not meant to provide generic outcome predictions, but to describe pathological processes of the CSF, as well as the cerebral vascular circulation. It is therefore not a surprise that Rout and other variables are influenced by factors such as age and vascular comorbidities [18, 19]. Similarly, a full understanding of the rest of the parameters and how they are influenced is required before attempting further outcome correlations.

Around 80% of shunted patients in our dataset showed improvement. This rate is consistent with those reported in [15] based on just the clinical presentation and ventriculomegaly.

Even with a combination of all the strong predictive variables, the maximum overall accuracy we could obtain for prediction of outcome was 70%. These numbers and discrepancies with clinical realities could be explained as follows: CSF dynamics might be limited in providing an objective descriptor of NPH and/or shunt-responsive NPH due to the way we currently diagnose, follow-up, and define shunt response. Considering all the information we could be missing on how much a shunt in situ drains in NPH and how occult NPH shunt malfunction/obstruction or inadequate drainage may be, shunt response should be carefully reconsidered and redefined. We might want to ask: Is NPH indeed such a complex entity and so much more than a CSF disorder that there could be no measured CSF circulation and pressure-volume compensation descriptor, or is shunt response-driven definition of NPH misleading and far from ideal?

Another issue might be that the objective testing of CSF dynamics should be followed by objective definition and post-shunting description of response. No response to shunting rarely receives rigorous follow-up, as there are limited tools available. Postoperative objective shunt assessment with shunt infusion tests could be an extra and easy step toward a completed assessment, as it provides a descriptor of the post-shunting circulation [20, 21].

Ethical Approval and Consent to Participate

In line with the protocol in Cambridge University Hospitals NHS Foundation Trust, this retrospective study was conducted without separate approval from an ethics committee. All patients were investigated with infusion test within the neurosciences department, as a part of routine clinical assessment.

Consent for Publication

As per our ethics statement, this was a retrospective study, not requiring separate approval from an ethics committee. All data form part of an anonymized, retrospective cohort and are not identifiable.

Conflict of Interest **M.C. has a partial financial interest in licensing ICM+ software (Cambridge enterprise, UK). All other authors certify that they have no affiliations with any organisation or entity with any financial or non-financial interest in the subject matter or materials discussed in this manuscript.**

References

1. Adams RD, Fisher CM, Hakim S, Ojeman RG, Sweet W (1965) Symptomatic occult hydrocephalus with "normal" cerebrospinal fluid pressure. N Engl J Med 273(3):117–126
2. Eide P, Fremming A, Sorteberg A (2003) Lack of relationship between resistance to cerebrospinal fluid outflow and intracranial pressure in normal pressure hydrocephalus. Acta Neurol Scand 108(14):381–388
3. Marmarou A, Maset AL, Ward JD, Chois S, Brooks D, Lutz HA, Moulton RJ, Muizelaar JP, De Salles A, Young H (1987) Contribution of CSF and vascular factors to elevation of ICP in severely head-injured patients. J Neurosurg 66(6):883–890
4. Swallow DMAA, Fellner N, Varsos GV, Czosnyka M, Smielewski P, Pickard JD, Czosnyka Z (2014) Repeatability of cerebrospinal fluid constant rate infusion study. Acta Neurol Scand 130(2):131–138
5. Wikkelsø C, Hellström P, Klinge P et al (2013) The European iNPH Multicentre Study on the predictive values of resistance to CSF outflow and the CSF Tap Test in patients with idiopathic normal pressure hydrocephalus. J Neurol Neurosurg Psychiatry 84(5):562–568
6. Børgesen SE, Albeck MJ, Gjerris F, Czosnyka M, Laniewski P (1992) Computerized infusion test compared to steady pressure constant infusion test in measurement of resistance to CSF outflow. Acta Neurochir 119(1–4):12–16
7. Czosnyka M, Czosnyka Z, Momjian S, Pickard JD (2004) Cerebrospinal fluid dynamics. Physiol Meas 25(5):R51–R76
8. Boon a J, Tans JT, Delwel EJ, Egeler-Peerdeman SM, Hanlo PW, Wurzer HA, Avezaat CJ, de Jong DA, Gooskens RH, Hermans J (1997) Dutch normal-pressure hydrocephalus study: prediction of outcome after shunting by resistance to outflow of cerebrospinal fluid. J Neurosurg 87(5):687–693
9. Boon AJW, Tans JTJ, Delwel EJ, Egeler-Peerdeman SM, Hanlo PW, Wurzer HAL, Hermans J (2000) The Dutch Normal-Pressure Hydrocephalus Study. How to select patients for shunting? An analysis of four diagnostic criteria. Surg Neurol 53(3):201–207
10. Andersson N (2007) Cerebrospinal fluid infusion methods. Online in: http://umu.diva-portal.org/smash/record.jsf?pid=diva2%3A140775&dswid=-9117
11. Andersson N, Malm J, Bäcklund T, Eklund A (2005) Assessment of cerebrospinal fluid outflow conductance using constant-pressure infusion—a method with real time estimation of reliability. Physiol Meas 26(6):1137–1148
12. Bech-Azeddine R, Gjerris F, Waldemar G, Czosnyka M, Juhler M (2005) Intraventricular or lumbar infusion test in adult communicating hydrocephalus? Practical consequences and clinical outcome of shunt operation. Acta Neurochir 147(10):1027–1036
13. Kahlon B, Sundbärg G, Rehncrona S (2002) Comparison between the lumbar infusion and CSF tap tests to predict outcome after shunt surgery in suspected normal pressure hydrocephalus. J Neurol Neurosurg Psychiatry 73(6):721–726

14. Kasprowicz M (2010) Evaluation of the cerebrovascular pressure reactivity index using non-invasive finapres arterial blood pressure. Physiol Meas 31(9):1217–1228. https://doi.org/10.1088/0967-3334/31/9/011
15. Meier U, Miethke C (2003) Predictors of outcome in patients with normal-pressure hydrocephalus. J Clin Neurosci 10(4):453–459
16. Vanneste J (1994) Editorial: Three decades of normal pressure hydrocephalus: are we wiser now? J Neurol Neurosurg Psychiatry 57:1021–1025
17. Nabbanja E, Czosnyka M, Keong NC, Garnett M, Pickard JD, Lalou DA, Czosnyka Z (2018) Is there a link between ICP-derived infusion test parameters and outcome after shunting in normal pressure hydrocephalus? Acta Neurochir Suppl 126:229–232. https://doi.org/10.1007/978-3-319-65798-1_46
18. Lavinio A, Schmidt EA, Haubrich C, Smielewski P, Pickard JD, Czosnyka M (2007) Noninvasive evaluation of dynamic cerebrovascular autoregulation using finapres plethysmograph and transcranial Doppler. Stroke 38(2):402–404
19. Lalou AD, Czosnyka M, Donnelly J, Pickard JD, Nabbanja E, Keong NC, Garnett M, Czosnyka ZH (2019) Cerebral autoregulation, cerebrospinal fluid outflow resistance, and outcome following cerebrospinal fluid diversion in normal pressure hydrocephalus. J Neurosurg 130(1):154–162
20. Petrella G, Czosnyka M, Keong N, Pickard JD, Czosnyka Z (2008) How does CSF dynamics change after shunting? Acta Neurol Scand 118(3):182–188
21. Petrella G, Czosnyka M, Smielewski P, Allin D, Guazzo EP, Pickard JD, Czosnyka ZH (2009) In vivo assessment of hydrocephalus shunt. Acta Neurol Scand 120(5):317–323

Part X

Spinal Cord Injury

Safety and Feasibility of Lumbar Cerebrospinal Fluid Pressure and Intraspinal Pressure Studies in Cervical Stenosis: A Case Series

Carl Moritz Zipser, José Miguel Spirig, José Aguirre, Anna-Sophie Hofer, Nikolai Pfender, Markus Hupp, Armin Curt, Mazda Farshad, and Martin Schubert

Introduction

Degenerative cervical myelopathy (DCM) is a common age-related, non-traumatic spinal cord disorder characterized by progressive neurological impairment, neuropathic pain, and bladder dysfunction [1–4]. In DCM, age- and stress-related spondylotic alteration is thought to inflict spinal compression due to ossification, ligament hypertrophy, disc herniation, and/or osteophyte formation with concurrently restricted segmental blood flow and loss of microvascular integrity contributing to pathogenesis [5–7]. Somatosensory evoked potentials (SSEPs), motor evoked potentials (MEPs) and contact-heat evoked potentials (CHEPs) are routinely performed before surgery to quantify the extent of spinal cord dysfunction and to estimate the degree of demyelination and axonal degeneration [8–10]. In patients with moderate or severe disability, current guidelines recommend surgical decompression [11, 12], with the goal of symptom remission and halting disease progression. However, the effects of decompression on spinal pressure and spinal hemodynamics, both of which might be relevant for peri- and postoperative function and recovery following spinal cord injury, are not known. The assessment of cerebrospinal fluid pressure (CSFP) has a long history in suspected spinal cord compression. It was first introduced for the diagnostic work-up of spine tumors, but almost vanished from the diagnostic repertoire with the introduction of CT and MRI scanning [13–16]. However, MRI is not a method that allows the assessment of pressure and is therefore less suited to distinguish the grade of functional deterioration as a consequence of structural compression. CSFP on the other side has not been investigated during operative decompression following DCM. In acute traumatic spinal cord injury (SCI), it was demonstrated that lumbar CSFP and CSF pulsation is decreased prior to, and restores following, decompression [17]. In addition, spinal cord perfusion pressure (SCPP) was calculated in acute SCI using CSFP [18], and intra-spinal pressure (ISP), i.e., pressure at the level of injury [19]. SCPP can be calculated from CSFP or ISP and the mean arterial pressure (MAP), and the optimum SCPP can be determined as the nadir of spinal autoregulation function (sPRx) over the SCPP [18, 20]. In other words: an ideal corridor of optimal SCPP was determined as a correlate of preserved spinal autoregulation. Spinal perfusion within this corridor was related to better outcome following acute SCI [20]. We hypothesize that CSFP or ISP and SCPP correlate with the functional impairment and degree of spinal compression as determined with structural MR-imaging. We additionally assume pressure release following successful decompression.

C. M. Zipser (✉) · N. Pfender · M. Hupp · A. Curt · M. Schubert
Department of Neurology and Neurophysiology, Balgrist University Hospital, Zurich, Switzerland

Balgrist University Hospital, University Spine Center, Zurich, Switzerland
e-mail: carlmoritz.zipser@balgrist.ch

J. M. Spirig · M. Farshad
Balgrist University Hospital, University Spine Center, Zurich, Switzerland

J. Aguirre
Department of Anesthesiology, Balgrist University Hospital, Zurich, Switzerland

A.-S. Hofer
Department of Neurosurgery, University Hospital Zurich, Zurich, Switzerland

Institute for Regenerative Medicine, University of Zurich, Zurich, Switzerland

Materials and Methods

Patients

Four patients with DCM were enrolled. Inclusion criteria were (1) presence of DCM, (2) age between 18 and 80 years, (3) written informed consent (IC), (4) any extent of functional

B. Depreitere et al. (eds.), *Intracranial Pressure and Neuromonitoring XVII*, Acta Neurochirurgica Supplement 131,
https://doi.org/10.1007/978-3-030-59436-7_70, © Springer Nature Switzerland AG 2021

or neurological impairment induced by spinal cord disorder due to DCM, (5) eligibility for surgical decompression, and (6) eligibility for spinal pressure monitoring. Exclusion criteria are (1) neurological impairment unrelated to spinal cord dysfunction, (2) contraindications to magnetic stimulation, e.g., epilepsy, (3) contraindications to MRI, e.g., cardiac pacemaker, (4) pregnancy, (5) previous cervical surgery in the past, and (6) psychiatric disorders that alter ability to give IC or potentially interfere with the measurements. The study protocol conformed to the latest revision of the Declaration of Helsinki and was approved by the local Ethics Committee of the University Hospital of Zurich (KEK-ZH-No.: PB_2016_00623).

Nurick score [21] was rated in every patient and fine motor skills were quantified with Graded Redefined Assessment of Strength, Sensibility and Prehension (GRASSP) [22] (Table 1). In one patient the ISP was measured peri- and postoperatively (level of stenosis C3-C6, subject 1), in two patients the CSFP was obtained peri- and postoperatively (level of stenosis C4–C5, subject 2; C4–C6, subject 3) and in another patient the CSFP was recorded at bedside prior to surgery (level of stenosis C3–C5, subject 4). This patient refused peri- and postoperative CSFP recording. Demographics are summarized in Table 1. During recording, we performed Queckenstedt's test (bilateral jugular vein compression), and Valsalva maneuver.

Technical Setup

To measure ISP, a subdural Codman® microsensor® was introduced and subsequently connected to a Codman DirectLink ICP box linked to a Philips X2-Pat.Interface + MX 700 Monitor. The arterial blood pressure (ABP) was recorded concomitantly from a radial artery catheter kept at the same horizontal level as the injured segment of the spinal cord. The measurements were performed continuously for 24 h after the intervention. ISP and ABP were analyzed offline using ICM+® software (University of Cambridge). To measure CSFP at the lumbar level, a lumbar catheter was inserted (Neuromedex® Lumbalkatheter 4.5F) and connected to the pressure monitors (Neuromedex® VentrEX), digitally converted and linked to the Philips Interface. Based on established procedures, calculations were performed as follows: The MAP was calculated from the systolic and diastolic ABP. ISP/CSFP and MAP were employed to continually calculate the SCPP (SCPP = MAP-ISP and SCPP = MAP-CSFP respectively). Spinal pressure reactivity (sPRx), a calculated measure of spinal cord vascular reactivity, is the correlation coefficient between mean ISP and MAP calculated over a 5-min period; spinal autoregulation of the vasculature is considered preserved/intact when sPRx is minimal, i.e., below or equal to 0 [20]. In all patients, preoperative neurophysiological exams were performed in order to specifically test for spinal and segmental spinothalamic conductance (i.e., somatosensory, motor, and contact heat evoked cortical potentials; SSEPs, MEPs, CHEPs, respectively).

Results

Clinical Characteristics and Neurophysiology

All patients suffered from cervical spinal canal stenosis as assessed by sagittal and transversal T2-weighted MRI (Fig. 1). Patients were between 55 and 74 years of age and all had sensory disturbance, neuropathic pain, neurogenic bladder disorder, and fine motor skill impairment at first presentation (clinical characteristics and demographics are summarized in Table 1). The GRASSP was abnormal in three patients, ranging from relatively mild impairment, left 61/100 pts/right 62/100 pts and left 64/100 pts/right 59/100 pts (subjects 1, 2), to more severe impairment, left 47/100 pts/right 51/100 pts (subject 3); GRASSP was not assessed in subject 4. The patients did not experience any adverse events associated with the lumbar catheter or subdural probe. Evoked potentials were performed to evaluate spinal cord integrity. Baseline tibial SEPs were abnormal in all patients and MEPs of the lower extremities were abnormal in three patients. CHEPs of the cervical dermatomes were abnormal in three subjects, but were not acquired in the patient tested at the bedside.

ISP Measurement

During subdural monitoring, ISP and MAP were reliably measured throughout the examination period of 24 h. Peak-to-peak amplitudes of pulse-wave-related pressure fluctuations were about 1–1.5 mmHg and peaks were consistently associated with systolic blood pressure peaks (Fig. 2a). The ISP curves were modulated by respiration intraoperatively and corresponded to the breathing frequency of the respirator. Valsalva maneuver increased baseline ISP by 10 mmHg and changed curve morphology (not depicted). With the patient in a flat and supine position, distinct peaks I-II-III as previously described were detected postoperatively [19] (Fig. 2b). A characteristic U-shaped curve of sPRx over SCPP was obtained over 10 h overnight, indicating optimum SCPP in this patient during this time at 72.5 mmHg (not depicted).

Table 1 Demographics and clinical characteristics

ID	Age[a]	Sex	Level of stenosis	Nurick Score	Pressure assessment	Surgical procedure	Sensory disturbance	Gait disorder	NBD	Pain	Impairment of fine motor skills (GRASSP)	tSEP/ LE-MEP pathologic	CHEPS pathologic
1	56	M	C3–C6	1	ISP IOM	Microsurgical decompression, laminectomy C4–6, laminotomy C3	X	X	X	X	X	X/X	X
2	55	M	C4–C5	1	CSFP IOM	Microsurgical decompression, ventral spondylodesis C4/5, C5/6	X		X	X	X	X/	X
3	61	F	C4–C6	2	CSFP IOM	Dorsal laminectomy C4-6	X	X	X	X	X	X/X	X
4	74	F	C3–C5	3	CSFP PRE	Microsurgical decompression laminotomy C3, laminectomy C4/C5	X	X	X	X	X	X/X	NP

X indicates presence of disorder

Abbreviations: *CHEPS* contact-heat evoked potentials (i.e. spinothalamic test), *CSFP* cerebrospinal fluid pressure, *IOM* intraoperative monitoring, *ISP* intraspinal pressure, *LE-MEP* lower extremity motor evoked potentials, *NBD* neurogenic bladder disorder, *NP* not performed, *PRE* pre-operative (i.e. bedside), *tSEP* tibial somatosensory evoked potentials

[a]In years

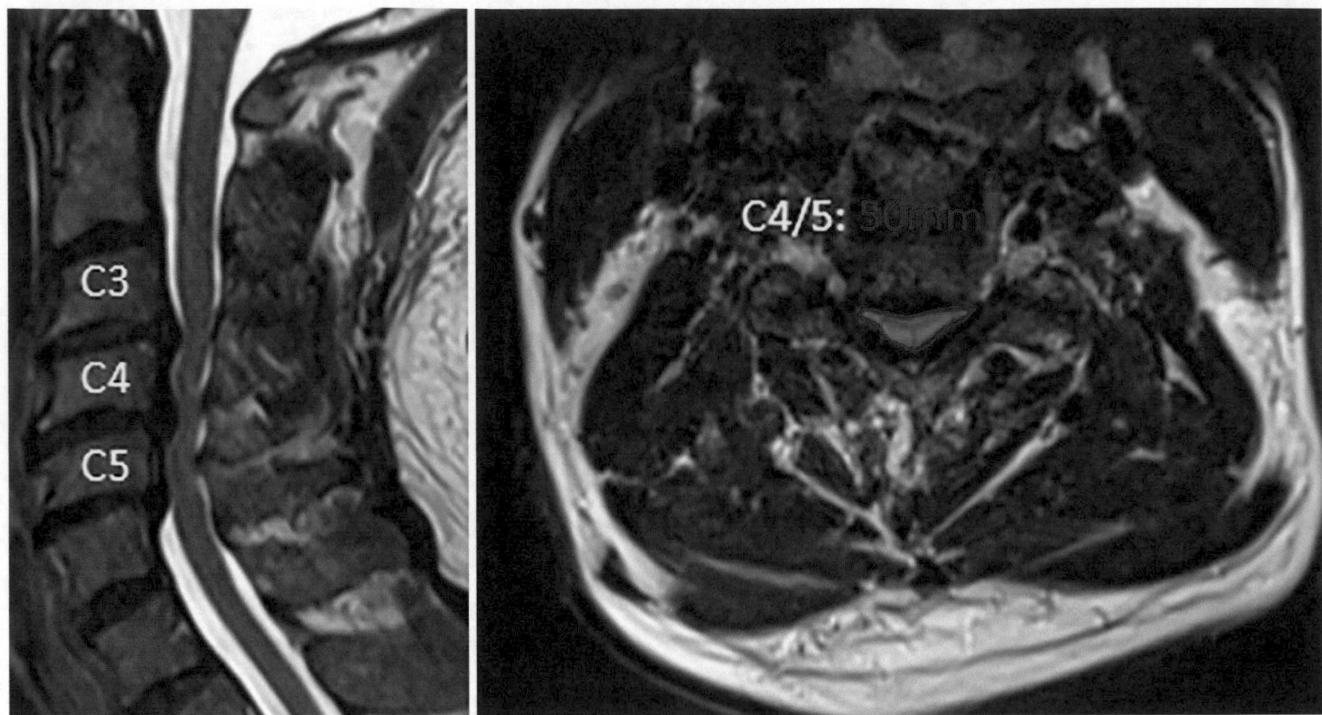

Fig. 1 Sagittal and transversal MRI of subject 1 revealing C3–C6 cervical stenosis

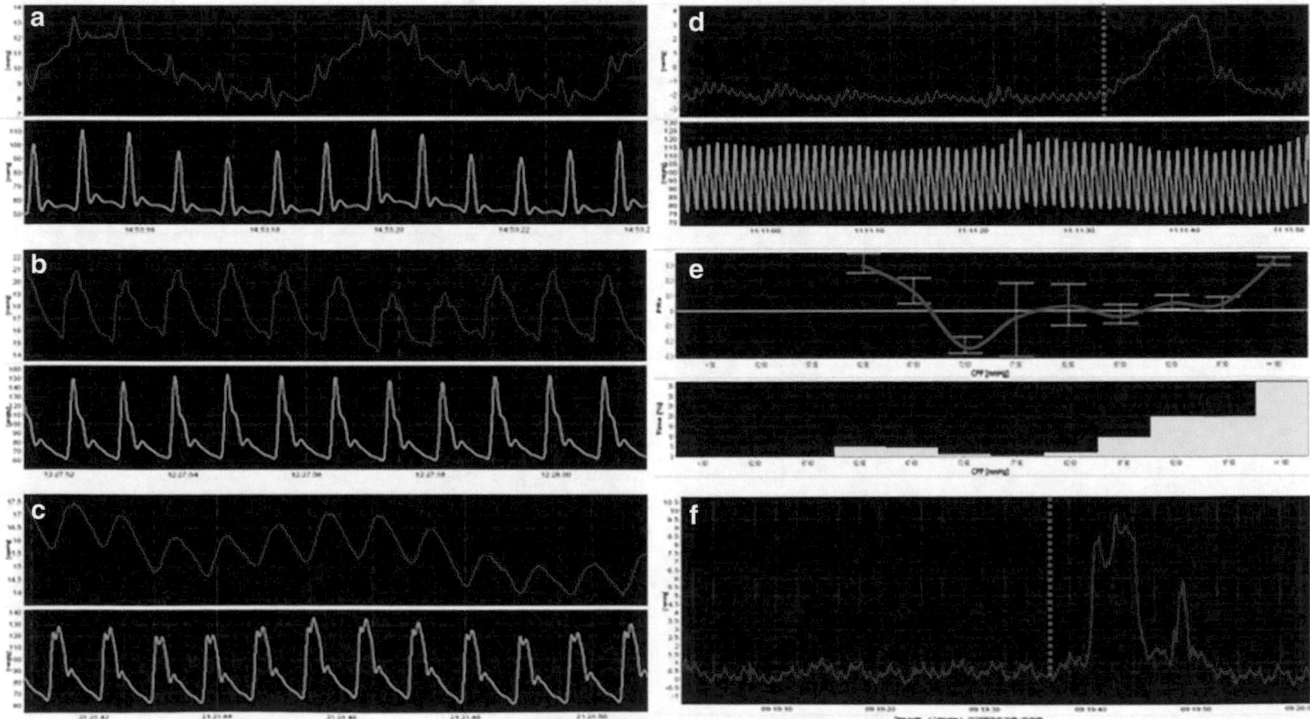

Fig. 2 (**a**–**f**) Red traces: ISP/CSFP; green traces: blood pressure. (**a**) Intraoperative ISP over 10 s, note respiratory modulation of ISP (subject 1). (**b**) Postoperative ISP over 10 s, note distinct peaks I–II–III (subject 1). (**c**) Postoperative CSFP over 10 s (subject 2). (**d**) Postoperative Queckenstedt's test (dotted blue line) increased about 4 mmHg (subject 3). (**e**) Optimum SCPP of 72.5 mmHg calculated over 6 h, estimated by the nadir of the sPRx (blue line); SCPP was >100 mmHg in 35% of the time indicating hyper-perfusion (yellow blocks (subject 3). (**f**) Bedside Valsalva maneuver (dotted blue line) prior to decompression (subject 4)

CSFP Measurements

In one patient with intraoperative CSFP measurement (patient 2), quality of intraoperative data was low due to artefacts, whereas the data quality was good in the other patient (patient 3). Postoperative data for both patients was free of artefacts (Fig. 2c, d). CSFP peaks were modulated by respiration and related to the systolic blood pressure peaks (Fig. 2c). Preoperative spine inclination and reclination did not change CSFP significantly (not depicted). Postoperative Valsalva maneuver peaked at about 57 mmHg in patient 2 (not depicted). Postoperative Queckenstedt's test was responsive in both patients undergoing CSFP recordings, indicating successful decompression (Fig. 2d). Pulse-wave related CSFP fluctuations showed peak-to-peak amplitudes that were between 0.5 and 1.5 mmHg. The optimum SCPP was about 75 mmHg when a characteristic U-shaped curve of sPRx over SCPP was obtained during 6–10 h in patients 2 and 3 (Fig. 2e); we detected a postoperative hyper-perfusion for most times in the first 24 h in patient 3. In patient 4, preoperative Queckenstedt's test was not responsive, i.e., during jugular vein compression baseline CSFP did not increase (not depicted). In this patient, pressure raised to a maximum of 10 mmHg during Valsalva maneuver (Fig. 2f), which was clearly below the values measured in the other patients after decompression.

Discussion

To the best of our knowledge this case series presents first data of ISP/CSFP and SCPP monitoring in DCM during decompressive surgery and after cervical decompression. Lumbar CSFP and subdural ISP measurements were safe and well tolerated over 24 h. Cervical spinal canal stenosis with myelopathy was confirmed by MRI and quantified with clinical and neurophysiological measures. The bedside CSFP analysis confirmed suspected cervical stenosis by non-responsive Queckenstedt's and Valsalva tests. Postoperative effects of decompression were determined with high CSFP rise during Valsalva maneuver and responsive Queckenstedt's test, which is consistent with prior studies [23]. Our results are also consistent with findings of abnormal CSF velocity and waveform in DCM derived from phase-contrast magnetic resonance imaging [24]. Both CSFP and ISP analysis allowed the estimation of the optimum perfusion pressure according to algorithms established in acute SCI. Values obtained from our patients ranged between 70 and 75 mmHg, which strongly resemble previous reports from traumatic SCI patients [18, 20]. Currently, evidence-based recommendations on blood pressure regimens in DCM do not exist; hence, as with spinal hemodynamics in acute SCI, more evidence is certainly needed [25–28].

With regard to Valsalva maneuver, we detected a CSFP increase of more than 40 mmHg in supine position with high temporal resolution. Previous investigators report pressure rise during Valsalva maneuver of more than 20 mmHg, and maximum of 35 mmHg, but suspected the average rise to exceed 20 mmHg when examined in larger cohorts [29]. Our findings support this notion. Much lower increases with a similarly steep slope were seen with Queckenstedt's test. These findings point out different mechanisms of how Valsalva and Queckenstedt's affect CSF dynamics. In our patients we could not determine whether pressure increase is only related to surgical decompression. Therefore, to identify surgery-related changes and to account for specific test effects on CSF dynamics, for systematic future evaluations we perform both *pre- and postoperative* Queckenstedt's test and Valsalva maneuver.

We conclude that CSFP/ISP and SCPP measurements are feasible, safe, and functionally promising approaches to individually monitor intradural pressure in DCM before, during, and after surgical decompression. Furthermore, results derived from this method may indicate changes in intrathecal pressure, thereby revealing postoperative complications such as critical edema and hemorrhage. Thus, countermeasures could be initiated at an early stage. Our findings encourage further research.

Conflict of Interest **The authors declare that they have no conflict of interest.**

References

1. Davies BM, McHugh M, Elgheriani A, Kolias AG, Tetreault L, Hutchinson PJ, Fehlings MG, Kotter MR (2017) The reporting of study and population characteristics in degenerative cervical myelopathy: a systematic review. PLoS One 12:e0172564. https://doi.org/10.1371/journal.pone.0172564
2. Davies BM, Mowforth OD, Smith EK, Kotter MR (2018) Degenerative cervical myelopathy. BMJ (Clin Res Ed) 360:k186. https://doi.org/10.1136/bmj.k186
3. Yamaguchi S, Mitsuhara T, Abiko M, Takeda M, Kurisu K (2018) Epidemiology and overview of the clinical spectrum of degenerative cervical myelopathy. Neurosurg Clin N Am 29:1–12. https://doi.org/10.1016/j.nec.2017.09.001
4. Fehlings MG, Tetreault LA, Wilson JR, Skelly AC (2013) Cervical spondylotic myelopathy: current state of the art and future directions. Spine 38:S1–S8. https://doi.org/10.1097/BRS.0b013e3182a7e9e0
5. Fehlings MG, Tetreault L, Hsieh PC, Traynelis V, Wang MY (2016) Introduction: degenerative cervical myelopathy: diagnostic, assessment, and management strategies, surgical complications, and outcome prediction. Neurosurg Focus 40:E1. https://doi.org/10.3171/2016.3.Focus16111

6. Akter F, Kotter M (2018) Pathobiology of degenerative cervical myelopathy. Neurosurg Clin N Am 29:13–19. https://doi.org/10.1016/j.nec.2017.09.015
7. Tetreault L, Goldstein CL, Arnold P, Harrop J, Hilibrand A, Nouri A, Fehlings MG (2015) Degenerative cervical myelopathy: a spectrum of related disorders affecting the aging spine. Neurosurgery 77(Suppl 4):S51–S67. https://doi.org/10.1227/neu.0000000000000951
8. Fujimoto K, Kanchiku T, Imajo Y, Suzuki H, Funaba M, Nishida N, Taguchi T (2017) Use of central motor conduction time and spinal cord evoked potentials in the electrophysiological assessment of compressive cervical myelopathy. Spine 42:895–902. https://doi.org/10.1097/brs.0000000000001939
9. Liu H, MacMillian EL, Jutzeler CR, Ljungberg E, MacKay AL, Kolind SH, Madler B, Li DKB, Dvorak MF, Curt A, Laule C, Kramer JLK (2017) Assessing structure and function of myelin in cervical spondylotic myelopathy: evidence of demyelination. Neurology 89:602–610. https://doi.org/10.1212/wnl.0000000000004197
10. Jutzeler CR, Ulrich A, Huber B, Rosner J, Kramer JLK, Curt A (2017) Improved diagnosis of cervical spondylotic myelopathy with contact heat evoked potentials. J Neurotrauma 34:2045–2053. https://doi.org/10.1089/neu.2016.4891
11. Fehlings MG, Tetreault LA, Kurpad S, Brodke DS, Wilson JR, Smith JS, Arnold PM, Brodt ED, Dettori JR (2017) Change in functional impairment, disability, and quality of life following operative treatment for degenerative cervical myelopathy: a systematic review and meta-analysis. Global Spine J 7:53s–69s. https://doi.org/10.1177/2192568217710137
12. Fehlings MG, Tetreault LA, Riew KD, Middleton JW, Aarabi B, Arnold PM, Brodke DS, Burns AS, Carette S, Chen R, Chiba K, Dettori JR, Furlan JC, Harrop JS, Holly LT, Kalsi-Ryan S, Kotter M, Kwon BK, Martin AR, Milligan J, Nakashima H, Nagoshi N, Rhee J, Singh A, Skelly AC, Sodhi S, Wilson JR, Yee A, Wang JC (2017) A clinical practice guideline for the management of patients with degenerative cervical myelopathy: recommendations for patients with mild, moderate, and severe disease and nonmyelopathic patients with evidence of cord compression. Global Spine J 7:70s–83s. https://doi.org/10.1177/2192568217701914
13. Magnaes B, Hauge T (1980) Surgery for myelopathy in cervical spondylosis: safety measures and preoperative factors related to outcome. Spine 5:211–214. https://doi.org/10.1097/00007632-198005000-00002
14. Pearce JM (2006) Queckenstedt's manoeuvre. J Neurol Neurosurg Psychiatry 77:728. https://doi.org/10.1136/jnnp.2005.083618
15. Tachibana S, Iida H, Yada K (1992) Significance of positive Queckenstedt test in patients with syringomyelia associated with Arnold-Chiari malformations. J Neurosurg 76:67–71. https://doi.org/10.3171/jns.1992.76.1.0067
16. Williams B (1976) Cerebrospinal fluid pressure changes in response to coughing. Brain J Neurol 99:331–346. https://doi.org/10.1093/brain/99.2.331
17. Kwon BK, Curt A, Belanger LM, Bernardo A, Chan D, Markez JA, Gorelik S, Slobogean GP, Umedaly H, Giffin M, Nikolakis MA, Street J, Boyd MC, Paquette S, Fisher CG, Dvorak MF (2009) Intrathecal pressure monitoring and cerebrospinal fluid drainage in acute spinal cord injury: a prospective randomized trial. J Neurosurg Spine 10:181–193. https://doi.org/10.3171/2008.10.Spine08217
18. Squair JW, Belanger LM, Tsang A, Ritchie L, Mac-Thiong JM, Parent S, Christie S, Bailey C, Dhall S, Street J, Ailon T, Paquette S, Dea N, Fisher CG, Dvorak MF, West CR, Kwon BK (2017) Spinal cord perfusion pressure predicts neurologic recovery in acute spinal cord injury. Neurology 89:1660–1667. https://doi.org/10.1212/wnl.0000000000004519
19. Werndle MC, Saadoun S, Phang I, Czosnyka M, Varsos GV, Czosnyka ZH, Smielewski P, Jamous A, Bell BA, Zoumprouli A, Papadopoulos MC (2014) Monitoring of spinal cord perfusion pressure in acute spinal cord injury: initial findings of the injured spinal cord pressure evaluation study*. Crit Care Med 42:646–655. https://doi.org/10.1097/ccm.0000000000000028
20. Chen S, Smielewski P, Czosnyka M, Papadopoulos MC, Saadoun S (2017) Continuous monitoring and visualization of optimum spinal cord perfusion pressure in patients with acute cord injury. J Neurotrauma 34:2941–2949. https://doi.org/10.1089/neu.2017.4982
21. Nurick S (1972) The pathogenesis of the spinal cord disorder associated with cervical spondylosis. Brain J Neurol 95:87–100. https://doi.org/10.1093/brain/95.1.87
22. Kalsi-Ryan S, Beaton D, Curt A, Duff S, Popovic MR, Rudhe C, Fehlings MG, Verrier MC (2012) The graded redefined assessment of strength sensibility and prehension: reliability and validity. J Neurotrauma 29:905–914. https://doi.org/10.1089/neu.2010.1504
23. Kaplan L, Kennedy F (1950) The effect of head posture on the manometrics of the cerebrospinal fluid in cervical lesions: a new diagnostic test. Brain J Neurol 73:337–345. https://doi.org/10.1093/brain/73.3.337
24. Bae YJ, Lee JW, Lee E, Yeom JS, Kim KJ, Kang HS (2017) Cervical compressive myelopathy: flow analysis of cerebrospinal fluid using phase-contrast magnetic resonance imaging. Eur Spine J 26:40–48. https://doi.org/10.1007/s00586-016-4874-9
25. Gallagher MJ, Hogg FRA, Zoumprouli A, Papadopoulos MC, Saadoun S (2019) Spinal cord blood flow in patients with acute spinal cord injuries. J Neurotrauma 36:919–929. https://doi.org/10.1089/neu.2018.5961
26. Menacho ST, Floyd C (2019) Current practices and goals for mean arterial pressure and spinal cord perfusion pressure in acute traumatic spinal cord injury: defining the gaps in knowledge. J Spinal Cord Med 16:1–7. https://doi.org/10.1080/10790268.2019.1660840
27. Rashnavadi T, Macnab A, Cheung A, Shadgan A, Kwon BK, Shadgan B (2019) Monitoring spinal cord hemodynamics and tissue oxygenation: a review of the literature with special focus on the near-infrared spectroscopy technique. Spinal Cord 57:617–625. https://doi.org/10.1038/s41393-019-0304-2
28. Squair JW, Belanger LM, Tsang A, Ritchie L, Mac-Thiong JM, Parent S, Christie S, Bailey C, Dhall S, Charest-Morin R, Street J, Ailon T, Paquette S, Dea N, Fisher CG, Dvorak MF, West CR, Kwon BK (2019) Empirical targets for acute hemodynamic management of individuals with spinal cord injury. Neurology 93:e1205–e1211. https://doi.org/10.1212/wnl.0000000000008125
29. Neville L, Egan RA (2005) Frequency and amplitude of elevation of cerebrospinal fluid resting pressure by the Valsalva maneuver. Can J Ophthalmol 40:775–777. https://doi.org/10.1016/s0008-4182(05)80100-0

Correction to: Comparison of Two Algorithms Analysing the Intracranial Pressure Curve in Terms of the Accuracy of Their Start-Point Detection and Resistance to Artefacts

Anna-Li Schönenberg-Tu, Benjamin Pätzold, Adam Lichota, Christa Raak, Ghaith Al Assali, Friedrich Edelhäuser, Dirk Cysarz, Martin Marsch, and Wolfram Scharbrodt

Correction to: B. Depreitere et al. (eds.), Intracranial Pressure and Neuromonitoring XVII, Acta Neurochirurgica Supplement 131 https://doi.org/10.1007/978-3-030-59436-7

The original version of Chapter 46 was revised.

We have now correctly added Dr. Wolfram Scharbrodt as an author for this chapter.

The updated online version of this chapter can be found at https://doi.org/10.1007/978-3-030-59436-7_46

B. Depreitere et al. (eds.), *Intracranial Pressure and Neuromonitoring XVII*, Acta Neurochirurgica Supplement 131,
https://doi.org/10.1007/978-3-030-59436-7_71,

Correction to: Why Hydrocephalus Patients Suffer When the Weather Changes: A New Hypothesis

Andreas Spiegelberg, Lennart Stieglitz, and Vartan Kurtcuoglu

Correction to: Chapter 59 in: B. Depreitere et al. (eds.), Intracranial Pressure and Neuromonitoring XVII, Acta Neurochirurgica Supplement 131, https://doi.org/10.1007/978-3-030-59436-7_59

The original version of Chapter 59 was revised.

The double quote in Equation (1) has been replaced with capital delta (Δ).

$$\Delta \text{paCO}_2 = 0.033 \bullet \Delta p_{\text{at}}. \quad (1)$$

The updated version of the chapter can be found at https://doi.org/10.1007/978-3-030-59436-7_59

B. Depreitere et al. (eds.), *Intracranial Pressure and Neuromonitoring XVII*, Acta Neurochirurgica Supplement 131,
https://doi.org/10.1007/978-3-030-59436-7_72,

Printed in the United States
by Baker & Taylor Publisher Services